P9-DXM-961

The Sanford Guides are updated annually and published by:

ANTIMICROBIAL THERAPY, INC.
P.O. Box 276, 11771 Lee Highway,
Sperryville, VA 22740-0276 USA
Tel 540-987-9480 Fax 540-987-9486
Email: info@sanfordguide.com   www.sanfordguide.com

Acknowledgements
Thanks to Ushuaia Solutions, SA, Argentina; Alcom Printing, Harleysville, PA and Fox Bindery, Quakertown, PA for design and production of this edition of the Sanford Guide.

Note to Readers
Since 1969, the Sanford Guide has been independently prepared and published. Decisions regarding the content of the Sanford Guide are solely those of the editors and the publisher. We welcome questions, comments and feedback concerning the Sanford Guide. All of your feedback is reviewed and taken into account in updating the content of the of the Sanford Guide.

Every effort is made to ensure the accuracy of the content of this guide. However, current full prescribing information available in the package insert for each drug should be consulted before prescribing any product. The editors and publisher are not responsible for errors or omissions or for any consequences from application of the information in this book and make no warranty, express or implied, with respect to the currency, accuracy, or completeness of the contents of this publication. Application of this information in a particular situation remains the professional responsibility of the practitioner.

**For the most current information, subscribe to webedition.sanfordguide.com
or Sanford Guide mobile device applications**

**Check our website for content-related notices:
http://www.sanfordguide.com**

Printed in the United States of America
ISBN 978-1-930808-84-3
Pocket Edition (English)

QUICK PAGE GUIDE TO THE SANFORD GUIDE

SANFORD GUIDE ®

The Sanford Guide
To Antimicrobial Therapy
2015

45th Edition

THE SANFORD GUIDE TO ANTIMICROBIAL THERAPY 2015
45TH EDITION

Editors

David N. Gilbert, M.D.
Chief of Infectious Diseases
Providence Portland Medical Center, Oregon
Professor of Medicine, Oregon Health
Sciences University

Henry F. Chambers, M.D.
Professor of Medicine
Director, Clinical Research Services
UCSF Clinical and Translational Sciences Institute
University of California at San Francisco

George M. Eliopoulos, M.D.
Chief, James L. Tullis Firm,
Beth Israel Deaconess Hospital,
Professor of Medicine,
Harvard Medical School,
Boston, Massachusetts

Michael S. Saag, M.D.
Director, UAB Center for AIDS Research,
Professor of Medicine and Director,
Division of Infectious Diseases,
University of Alabama, Birmingham

Contributing Editors

Douglas Black, Pharm. D.
Associate Professor
of Pharmacy,
University of Washington,
Seattle

Brian S. Schwartz, M.D.
Associate Professor
of Medicine
University of California
at San Francisco

David O. Freedman, M.D.
Director, Travelers Health Clinic,
Professor of Medicine,
University of Alabama,
Birmingham

Andrew T. Pavia, M.D.
George & Esther Gross Presidential Professor
Chief, Division of Pediatric Infectious Diseases
University of Utah, Salt Lake City

Managing Editor

Jeb C. Sanford

Memoriam

Jay P. Sanford, M.D.
1928-1996

Merle A. Sande, M.D.
1935-2007

Robert C. Moellering, Jr., M.D.
1936-2014

Publisher

Antimicrobial Therapy, Inc.

—TABLE OF CONTENTS—

2

ABBREVIATIONS

3TC = lamivudine
AB,% = percent absorbed
ABC = abacavir
ABCD = amphotericin B colloidal dispersion
ABLC = ampho B lipid complex
ADF = after dialysis
ADV = adefovir
AG = aminoglycoside
AIDS = Acquired Immune Deficiency Syndrome
AM-CL = amoxicillin-clavulanate
AM-CL-ER = amoxicillin-clavulanate extended release
AMK = amikacin
Amox = amoxicillin
Amp = ampicillin
Ampho B = amphotericin B
AM-SB = ampicillin-sulbactam
AP = atovaquone proguanil
AP Pen = antipseudomonal penicillins
APAG = antipseudomonal aminoglycoside
ARDS = acute respiratory distress syndrome
ARF = acute rheumatic fever
ASA = aspirin
ATS = American Thoracic Society
ATV = atazanavir
AUC = area under the curve
Azithro = azithromycin
bid = 2x/per day
BL/BLI = beta-lactam/beta-lactamase inhibitor
BSA = body surface area
BW = body weight
C&S = culture & sensitivity
CARB = carbapenems
CAPD = continuous ambulatory peritoneal dialysis
CDC = Centers for Disease Control
Cefpodox = cefpodoxime proxetil
Ceftaz = ceftazidime
Ceph = cephalosporin
CFB = ceftobiprole
CFP = cefepime
Chloro = chloramphenicol
CIP = ciprofloxacin; **CIP-ER** = CIP extended release
Clarithro = clarithromycin; **ER** = extended release
Clav = clavulanate
Clinda = clindamycin
CLO = clofazimine
CMV = cytomegalovirus
CO = chloroquine phosphate
Cobi = cobicistat
CrCl = creatinine clearance
CrCln = CrCl normalized for BSA
CRRT = continuous renal replacement therapy
CSD = cat-scratch disease

CSF = cerebrospinal fluid
CXR = chest x-ray
d4T = stavudine
Dapto = daptomycin
DBPCT = double-blind placebo-controlled trial
dc = discontinue
ddC = zalcitabine
ddI = didanosine
DIC = disseminated intravascular coagulation
div = divided
DLV = delavirdine
Dori = doripenem
DOT = directly observed therapy
Doxy = doxycycline
DR = delayed release
DRSP = drug-resistant S. pneumoniae
DS = double strength
EBV = Epstein-Barr virus
EES = erythromycin ethyl succinate
EFZ = efavirenz
EMB = ethambutol
ENT = entecavir
ER = extended release
ERTA = ertapenem
Erythro = erythromycin
ESBLs = extended-spectrum β-lactamases
ESR = erythrocyte sedimentation rate
ESRD = endstage renal disease
Flu = fluconazole
Flucyt = flucytosine
FOS-APV = fosamprenavir
FQ = fluoroquinolone
FTC = emtricitabine
G = generic
GAS = Group A Strep
Gati = gatifloxacin
GC = gonorrhea
Gemi = gemifloxacin
Gent = gentamicin
GNB = gram-negative bacilli
Griseo = griseofulvin
HEMO = hemodialysis
HHV = human herpesvirus
HIV = human immunodeficiency virus
HLR = high-level resistance
H₂O = history of
HSCT = hematopoietic stem cell transplant
HSV = herpes simplex virus
IA = injectable agent/anti-inflammatory drugs
IDV = indinavir
IFN = interferon

IM = intramuscular
IMP = imipenem-cilastatin
INH = isoniazid
Inv = investigational
IP = intraperitoneal
IT = intrathecal
Itra = itraconazole
IV = intravenous
IVDU = intravenous drug user
IVIG = intravenous immune globulin
Keto = ketoconazole
kg = kilogram
LAB = liposomal ampho B
LCM = lymphocytic choriomeningitis virus
LCR = ligase chain reaction
Levo = levofloxacin
LP/R = lopinavir/ritonavir
mcg (or μg) = microgram
MDR = multi-drug resistant
MER = meropenem
Metro = metronidazole
Mino = minocycline
mL = milliliter
Moxi = moxifloxacin
MQ = mefloquine
MSSA/MRSA = methicillin-sensitive/resistant S. aureus
MTB = Mycobacterium tuberculosis
NB = name brand
NF = nitrofurantoin
NAI = not FDA-approved (indication or dose)
NFR = nelfinavir
NNRTI = non-nucleoside reverse transcriptase inhibitor
NRTI = nucleoside reverse transcriptase inhibitor
NSAIDs = non-steroidal
NUS = not available in the U.S.
NVP = nevirapine
O Ceph 1, 2, 3 = oral cephalosporins
Oflox = ofloxacin
P Ceph 1, 2, 3, 4 = parenteral cephalosporins
P Ceph 3 AP = parenteral cephalosporins with antipseudomonal activity
PCR = polymerase chain reaction
PEP = post-exposure prophylaxis
PI = protease inhibitor
PIP = piperacillin
PIP-TZ = piperacillin-tazobactam
po = oral dosing
PO = primaquine
PRCT = Prospective randomized controlled trials
PTLD = post-transplant lymphoproliferative disease
Pts = patients
Pyri = pyrimethamine
PZA = pyrazinamide

ABBREVIATIONS (2)

qid = 4x per day
QS = quinine sulfate
Quinu-dalfo = Q-D = quinupristin-dalfopristin
q[x]h = every [x] hours, e.g., q8h = every 8 hrs
R = resistant
RFB = rifabutin
Rick = Rickettsia
RIF = rifampin
RSV = respiratory syncytial virus
RTI = respiratory tract infection
RTV = ritonavir
rx = treatment
SA = Staph. aureus sc = subcutaneous
SD = serum drug level after single dose
Sens = sensitive (susceptible)

SM = streptomycin
SQV = saquinavir
SS = steady state serum level
STD = sexually transmitted disease
subcut = subcutaneous
Sulb = sulbactam
Sx = symptom(s)
Tazo = tazobactam
TBc = tuberculosis
TC-CL = ticarcillin-clavulanate
TDF = tenofovir
TEE = transesophageal echocardiography
Teico = teicoplanin
Telith = telithromycin
Tetra = tetracycline
Ticar = ticarcillin

tid = 3x per day
TMP-SMX = trimethoprim-sulfamethoxazole
TNF = tumor necrosis factor
Tobra = tobramycin
TPV = tipranavir
TST = tuberculin skin test
UTI = urinary tract infection
Vanco = vancomycin
VISA = vancomycin intermediately resistant S. aureus
VL = viral load
Vori = voriconazole
VZV = varicella-zoster virus
ZDV = zidovudine

ABBREVIATIONS OF JOURNAL TITLES

AAC: Antimicrobial Agents & Chemotherapy
Adv PID: Advances in Pediatric Infectious Diseases
AHJ: American Heart Journal
AIDS Res Hum Retrovir: AIDS Research & Human Retroviruses
AJG: American Journal of Gastroenterology
AJM: American Journal of Medicine
AJRCCM: American Journal of Respiratory Critical Care Medicine
AJTMH: American Journal of Tropical Medicine & Hygiene
Aliment Pharmacol Ther: Alimentary Pharmacology & Therapeutics
Am J Hlth Pharm: American Journal of Health-System Pharmacy
Amer J Transpl: American Journal of Transplantation
AnEM: Annals of Emergency Medicine
AnIM: Annals of Internal Medicine
Ann Pharmacother: Annals of Pharmacotherapy
AnSurg: Annals of Surgery
Antivir Ther: Antiviral Therapy
ArDerm: Archives of Dermatology
ArIM: Archives of Internal Medicine
ARRD: American Review of Respiratory Disease
BMJ: British Medical Journal
BMT: Bone Marrow Transplantation
Brit J Derm: British Journal of Dermatology
Can JID: Canadian Journal of Infectious Diseases
Canad Med J: Canadian Medical Journal
CCM: Critical Care Medicine
CCTID: Current Clinical Topics in Infectious Disease
CDSR: Cochrane Database of Systematic Reviews
CID: Clinical Infectious Diseases
Clin Micro Inf: Clinical Microbiology and Infection
CMN: Clinical Microbiology Newsletter
Clin Micro Rev: Clinical Microbiology Reviews
CMAJ: Canadian Medical Association Journal
COID: Current Opinion in Infectious Disease
Curr Med Res Opin: Current Medical Research and Opinion

Derm Ther: Dermatologic Therapy
Dermatol Clin: Dermatologic Clinics
Dig Dis Sci: Digestive Diseases and Sciences
DMID: Diagnostic Microbiology and Infectious Disease
EID: Emerging Infectious Diseases
EJCMID: European Journal of Clin. Micro. & Infectious Diseases
Eur J Neurol: European Journal of Neurology
Exp Mol Path: Experimental & Molecular Pathology
Exp Rev Anti Infect Ther: Expert Review of Anti-Infective Therapy
Gastro: Gastroenterology
Hpt: Hepatology
ICHE: Infection Control and Hospital Epidemiology
IDC No. Amer: Infectious Disease Clinics of North America
IDCP: Infectious Diseases in Clinical Practice
IJAA: International Journal of Antimicrobial Agents
Inf Med: Infections in Medicine
J AIDS & HR: Journal of AIDS and Human Retrovirology
J Clin Immunol: Journal of Allergy and Clinical Immunology
J Am Ger Soc: Journal of the American Geriatrics Society
J Chemother: Journal of Chemotherapy
J Clin Micro: Journal of Clinical Microbiology
J Clin Virol: Journal of Clinical Virology
J Derm Treat: Journal of Dermatological Treatment
J Hpt: Journal of Hepatology
J Inf: Journal of Infection
J Infect Micro: Journal of Medical Microbiology
J Med Immunol Inf: Journal of Microbiology,
    Immunology, & Infection
J Ped: Journal of Pediatrics
J Viral Hep: Journal of Viral Hepatitis
JAC: Journal of Antimicrobial Chemotherapy
JACC: Journal of American College of Cardiology
JAIDS: JAIDS Journal of Acquired Immune Deficiency Syndromes
JAMA: Journal of the American Medical Association

JAVMA: Journal of the Veterinary Medicine Association
JCI: Journal of Clinical Investigation
JCM: Journal of Clinical Microbiology
JIC: Journal of Infection and Chemotherapy
JID: Journal of Infectious Diseases
JNS: Journal of Neurosurgery
JTMH: Journal of Tropical Medicine and Hygiene
Lnc: Lancet
LnID: Lancet Infectious Disease
Mayo Clin Proc: Mayo Clinic Proceedings
Med Lett: Medical Letter
Med Mycol: Medical Mycology
MMWR: Morbidity & Mortality Weekly Report
NEJM: New England Journal of Medicine
Neph Dial Transpl: Nephrology Dialysis Transplantation
OFID: Open Forum Infectious Diseases
Ped Ann: Pediatric Annals
Peds: Pediatrics
Pharmacother: Pharmacotherapy
PIDJ: Pediatric Infectious Disease Journal
QJM: Quarterly Journal of Medicine
Scand Resp Inf: Scandinavian Journal of Infectious Diseases
Sem Resp Inf: Seminars in Respiratory Infections
SGO: Surgery Gynecology and Obstetrics
SMJ: Southern Medical Journal
Surg Neurol: Surgical Neurology
Transpl Inf Dis: Transplant Infectious Diseases
Transpl: Transplantation
TRSM: Transactions of the Royal Society of Medicine

TABLE 1 – CLINICAL APPROACH TO INITIAL CHOICE OF ANTIMICROBIAL THERAPY*

Treatment based on presumed site or type of infection. In selected instances, treatment and prophylaxis are based on identification of pathogens.
Regimens should be reevaluated based on pathogen isolated, antimicrobial susceptibility determination, and individual host characteristics. *(Abbreviations on page 2)*

ANATOMIC SITE/DIAGNOSIS/ MODIFYING CIRCUMSTANCES	ETIOLOGIES* (usual)	SUGGESTED REGIMENS*		ADJUNCT DIAGNOSTIC OR THERAPEUTIC MEASURES AND COMMENTS
		PRIMARY	ALTERNATIVE†	
ABDOMEN: See Peritoneum, page 47; Gallbladder, page 17; and Pelvic Inflammatory Disease, page 26				
BONE: Osteomyelitis. Microbiologic diagnosis is essential. If blood culture negative, need culture of bone. Culture of sinus tract drainage not predictive of bone culture. Review: *Ln 364:369, 2004.*				
Hematogenous Osteomyelitis				
Empiric therapy—Collect bone and blood cultures before empiric therapy For comprehensive review of antimicrobial penetration into bone, see *Clinical Pharmacokinetics 48:89, 2009.*				
Newborn (<4 mos.)	S. aureus, Gm-neg. bacilli, Group B strep, Kingella kingae in children	MRSA possible: **Vanco** ± (**Ceftaz or CFP**)	MRSA unlikely: (**Nafcillin or oxacillin**) + (**Ceftaz or CFP**)	Severe allergy or toxicity: (**Linezolid**^AMA 10 mg/kg IV/po q8h + **aztreonam**).
Children (>4 mos.) — Adult: Osteo of extremity (*NEJM 370:352, 2014*)	S. aureus, Group A strep, Gm-neg. bacilli rare, Kingella kingae in children	MRSA possible: **Vanco** 40 mg/kg/day q6h	MRSA unlikely: (**Nafcillin or oxacillin**) 150 mg/kg/day div q6h (max 12 gm).	Severe allergy or toxicity. **Clinda** or **TMP-SMX** or **linezolid**^AMA. Adults: **ceftaz** 2 gm IV q8h. **CFP** 2 gm IV q12h. *See Table 10B for adverse reactions to drugs.*
		Add **Ceftaz** or **CFP** if Gm-neg. bacilli on Gram stain **Adult doses below.**		
Adult (>21 yrs) **Vertebral osteo ± epidural abscess**: other sites **Blood & bone cultures essential**	S. aureus most common but variety other organisms. In Turkey: Brucella & M.TBc common	MRSA possible: **Vanco** 15-20 mg/kg IV q8-12h for trough of 15-20 μg/mL + (**Ceftriaxone** 2 gm q24h OR **CFP** 2 gm q8h OR **Levo** 750 mg q24h)	MRSA unlikely: **Nafcillin** OR **oxacillin** 2 gm IV q4h + (**Ceftriaxone** 2 gm q24h OR **CFP** 2 gm q8h OR **Levo** 750 mg q24h)	**Dx: MRI early to look for epidural abscess.** For comprehensive review of vertebral osteomyelitis see *NEJM 362:11, 2010.* Whenever possible empirical therapy should be administered after cultures are obtained.
Specific therapy—Culture and in vitro susceptibility results known				
	MSSA	**Nafcillin** or **oxacillin** 2 gm IV q4h or **cefazolin** 2 gm IV q8h	**Vanco** 15-20 mg/kg IV q8-12h for trough of 15-20 μg/mL ± **RIF** 300-450 mg po/IV bid	**Vanco** 15-30 mg/kg IV q8-12h for trough of 15-20 mg/mL OR **Dapto** 6 mg/kg q24h IV ± **RIF** 300-450 mg q24h + Other options if susceptible in vitro and allergy/toxicity issues (see *NEJM 362:11, 2010*):
	MRSA—See Table 6, page 79; IDSA Guidelines CID 52:e18-55, 2011; CID 52:285-92, 2011	**CIP** 400 mg IV q12h OR **CIP** 750 mg PO bid	**Vanco** 15-20 mg/kg IV q8-12h for trough of 15-20 μg/mL ± **RIF** 300-450 mg bid.	**Linezolid** 600 mg q12h IV/po ± **RIF** 300 mg po/IV bid OR **Dapto** 6 mg/kg 2q 24h IV ± **RIF** 300-450 mg po/IV bid	1) **TMP-SMX** 8-10 mg/kg po/IV div q8h + **RIF** 300-450 mg bid: limited data, particularly for MRSA (see *AAC 53:2672, 2009*); 2) **CIP** 750 mg po bid or **Levo** 750 mg po/IV q24h) + **RIF** 300 mg po bid]; 3) Linezolid assoc. with optic & peripheral neuropathy with long-term use; 4) **Fusidic acid**^NUS 500 mg IV q8h + **RIF** 300 mg po bid *(CID 42:394, 2006)*. **Ceftriaxone** 2 gm IV q24h *(CID 54:585, 2012)*; 5) Daptomycin 6 mg/kg IV q24h (some recommend 8-10 mg/kg dose)
Hemoglobinopathy: Sickle cell/thalassemia	Salmonella; other Gm-neg. bacilli		**Levo** 750 mg IV/PO q24h	Thalassemia: transfusion and iron chelation risk factors. Because of decreasing levels of susceptibility to fluoroquinolones among Salmonella spp. and growing resistance among other gram-negative bacilli, would add a second agent (e.g., third-generation cephalosporin) until susceptibility test results available.

* **DOSAGES SUGGESTED** are for adults (unless otherwise indicated) with clinically severe (often life-threatening) infections. Dosages also assume normal renal function, and not severe hepatic dysfunction.

† **ALTERNATIVE THERAPY INCLUDES** these considerations: allergy, pharmacology/pharmacodynamics, compliance, costs, local resistance profiles.

TABLE 1 (2)

ANATOMIC SITE/DIAGNOSIS/ MODIFYING CIRCUMSTANCES	ETIOLOGIES (usual)	SUGGESTED REGIMENS*		ADJUNCT DIAGNOSTIC OR THERAPEUTIC MEASURES AND COMMENTS
		PRIMARY	ALTERNATIVE¹	
BONE *(continued)*				
Contiguous Osteomyelitis Without Vascular Insufficiency				
Empiric therapy: Get cultures!				
Foot bone osteo due to nail through tennis shoe	P. aeruginosa	**CIP** 750 mg po bid or **Levo** 750 mg po q24h	**Ceftaz** 2 gm IV q8h or **CFP** 2 gm IV q8h	See *Skin—Nail puncture, page 56.* Need debridement to remove foreign body.
Long bone, post-internal fixation of fracture	S. aureus, Gm-neg. bacilli, P. aeruginosa	**Vanco** 15-20 mg/kg q8-12h IV q8-12h for trough of 15-20 μg/mL + (**ceftaz** or **CFP**). See **Comment**	**Linezolid** 600 mg IV/po bid[NAI] + (**ceftaz** or **CFP**). See **Comment**	Often necessary to remove hardware after union to achieve eradication. May need revascularization. **Regimens listed are empiric.** Adjust after culture data available. If susceptible Gm-neg. bacillus, **CIP** 750 mg po bid or **Levo** 750 mg po q24h. For other S. aureus options: See *Hem. Osteo. Specific Therapy, page 4.*
Osteonecrosis of the jaw	Probably rare adverse reaction to bisphosphonates	Infection may be secondary to bone necrosis and loss of overlying mucosa. Treatment: minimal surgical debridement, chlorhexidine rinses, antibiotics (e.g. PIP-TZ). Evaluate for concomitant actinomycosis, for which specific long-term antibiotic treatment would be warranted (CID 49:1729, 2009).		
Prosthetic joint	See *prosthetic joint, page 33*			
Spinal implant infection	S. aureus, coag-neg staphylococci, gram-neg bacilli	Onset within 30 days: culture, treat for 3 mos (CID 55:1481, 2012).	Onset after 30 days remove implant, culture & treat	See CID 55:1481, 2012
Sternum, post-op	S. aureus, S. epidermidis, occasionally gram-negative bacilli	**Vanco** 15-20 mg/kg q8-12h IV for trough of 15-20 μg/mL	**Linezolid** 600 mg po/IV[NAI] bid	Sternal debridement for cultures & removal of necrotic bone. For S. aureus options: Hem. Osteo. Specific Therapy, page 4. If setting or gram stain suggests possibility of gram-negative bacilli, add appropriate coverage based on local antimicrobial susceptibility profiles (e.g., cefepime, pip-tazo).
Contiguous Osteomyelitis With Vascular Insufficiency.				
Most pts are **diabetics** with peripheral neuropathy & infected skin ulcers (see *Diabetic foot, page 16*)	Polymicrobic (Gm+ cocci (to include MRSA) (aerobic & anaerobic) and Gm-neg. bacilli (aerobic & anaerobic)	Debride overlying ulcer & submit bone for histology & culture. Select antibiotic based on culture results & treat for 6 weeks. **No empiric therapy unless acutely ill.** If acutely ill, see suggestions, Diabetic foot, page 16. Revascularize if possible.		**Diagnosis of osteo:** Culture bone biopsy (gold standard). Poor concordance of culture results between swab of ulcer and bone – need concordance of culture & bone (CID 42:57–62, 2006). Sampling by needle puncture inferior to bone biopsy (CID 48:888, 2009). Osteo more likely if ulcer >2 cm², positive probe to bone, ESR >70 & abnormal plain x-ray (JAMA 299:806, 2008). **Treatment:** (1) Revascularize if possible; (2) Culture bone; (3) Specific antimicrobial(s). Reviews: (1) CID 47:528, 2006; (3) Plast Reconstr Surg 117: (7 Suppl) 212S, 2006.
Chronic Osteomyelitis: Specific therapy By definition, implies presence of dead bone. **Need valid cultures**	S. aureus, Enterobacteriaceae, P. aeruginosa	**Empiric rx not indicated.** Base systemic rx on results of chronic osteo, rx as acute hematogenous osteo. Surgical debridement important.	Base acute exacerbation of chronic sensitivity testing.	**Important adjuncts:** removal of orthopedic hardware, surgical debridement, revascularization, muscle flaps, distraction osteogenesis (Ilizarov) techniques. Antibiotic-impregnated cement & hyperbaric oxygen adjunctive. **NOTE: RIF + (vanco or β-lactam)** effective in animal model and in a clinical trial of S. aureus chronic osteo. The contribution of rifampin-containing regimens in this setting is not clear, however (AAC 53:2672, 2009).

Abbreviations on page 2.   *NOTE: All dosage recommendations are for adults (unless otherwise indicated) and assume normal renal function. § Alternatives consider allergy, PK, compliance, local resistance, cost

TABLE 1 (3)

ANATOMIC SITE/DIAGNOSIS/ MODIFYING CIRCUMSTANCES	ETIOLOGIES (usual)	SUGGESTED REGIMENS*		ADJUNCT DIAGNOSTIC OR THERAPEUTIC MEASURES AND COMMENTS
		PRIMARY	ALTERNATIVE§	
BREAST: Mastitis—Obtain culture: need to know if MRSA present. Review with definitions: Review of breast infections: BMJ 342:d396, 2011.				
Postpartum mastitis (Recent Cochrane Review: Cochrane Database Syst Rev 2013 Feb 28;2:CD005458; see also CID 54:71, 2012)				
Mastitis without abscess	S. aureus; less often S. pyogenes (Gp A or B), E. coli, bacteroides species, maybe Corynebacterium sp. & selected coagulase-neg. staphylococci (e.g., S. lugdunensis)	**NO MRSA:** **Outpatient: Dicloxacillin** 500 mg qid **or cephalexin** 500 mg qid. **Inpatient: Nafcillin/oxacillin** 2 gm IV q4-6h	**MRSA Possible:** **Outpatient: TMP-SMX-DS** tabs 1-2 po bid or, if susceptible, **clinda** 300 mg po tid **Inpatient: Vanco** 1 gm IV q12h; if over 100 Kg, 1.5 gm IV q12h.	If no abscess & controllable pain. ↑ freq of nursing may hasten response.
Mastitis with abscess				For painful abscess I&D is standard; needle aspiration reported successful. Resume breast feeding from affected breast as soon as pain allows. (Breastfeed Med 9:239, 2014)
Non-puerperal mastitis with abscess	S. aureus; less often peptostreptococcus, & selected coagulase-neg. staphylococci	See regimens for Postpartum mastitis, page 6.		Smoking and diabetes may be risk factors (BMJ 342:d396, 2011). **If subareolar & odoriferous,** most likely anaerobes; need to **add metro** 500 mg IV po/bid. If not subareolar, staph. Need pretreatment aerobic/anaerobic cultures. Surgical drainage for abscess. **I&D standard.** Corynebacterium sp. assoc. with chronic granulomatous mastitis (CID 35:1434, 2002; CID 59:410, 2014).
Breast implant infection	Acute: S. aureus, S. pyogenes. TSS reported. Chronic: Look for rapidly growing Mycobacteria	Acute **Vanco** 15-20 mg/kg IV q8-12h.	Chronic: Await culture results. See Table 12A for mycobacteria treatment.	Lancet Infect Dis 5:94, 462, 2005. Coag-negative staph also common (Aesthetic Plastic Surg 31:325, 2007).
CENTRAL NERVOUS SYSTEM				
Brain abscess				
Primary or contiguous source In 51 pts, 30 positive by standard culture; using molecular diagnostics, 80 bacterial taxa & many polymicrobic (CID 54:202, 2012). Review: NEJM 371:447, 2014. Mild infection: NEJM 371:150, 2014.	Streptococci (60-70%), bacteroides (20-40%), Enterobacteriaceae 25-33%), S. aureus (10-15%), S. anginosus grp. Rare: Nocardia (below). Listeria. See S. aureus Comment	[P Ceph 3 {(cefotaxime 2 gm IV q4h or ceftriaxone 2 gm IV q12h)} + (metro 7.5 mg/kg q6h or 15 mg/kg IV q12h)] Duration of rx unclear; treat until response by neuroimaging (CT/MRI)	For MSSA: **(Nafcillin** or **oxacillin** 2 gm IV q4h + **(ceftriaxone** or **cefotaxime)** For MRSA: **Vanco** 15-20 mg/kg (V q 8-12h for trough of 15-20 mcg/mL) + **(ceftriaxone** or **cefotaxime)**	If CT scan suggests cerebritis or abscesses <2.5 cm and pt neurologically stable and conscious, start antibiotics and observe. Otherwise, surgical drainage necessary. If blood cultures or other clinical data do not yeld a likely etiologic agent, aspirate even small abscesses for diagnosis if this can be done safely. Experience with Pen G (HD) + metro without ceftriaxone or nafcillin/oxacillin has been good. We use ceftriaxone because of frequency of isolation of Enterobacteriaceae. **S. aureus rare without positive blood culture.** **If S. aureus, use vanco until susceptibility known.** Strep. anginosus group (Strep. milleri) may be microaerophilic or anaerobic, group has propensity to produce abscesses. Ceph/metro does not cover listeria. Empirical coverage, de-escalated based on culture results. **Aspiration of abscess usually necessary for dx & rx. If P. aeruginosa suspected, substitute (Cefepime or Ceftazidime) for (Ceftriaxone or Cefotaxime).**
Post-surgical, post-traumatic. Review: NEJM 371:447, 2014.	S. aureus. Enterobacteriaceae	See Table 13A, page 148		
HIV-1 infected (AIDS)	Toxoplasma gondii			

TABLE 1 (4)

ANATOMIC SITE/DIAGNOSIS/ MODIFYING CIRCUMSTANCES	ETIOLOGIES (usual)	SUGGESTED REGIMENS*		ADJUNCT DIAGNOSTIC OR THERAPEUTIC MEASURES AND COMMENTS
		PRIMARY	ALTERNATIVE§	
CENTRAL NERVOUS SYSTEM/Brain abscess *(continued)*				
Nocardia: Haematogenous abscess	N. farcinia, N. asteroides & N. brasiliensis See AAC 58:795, 2014 for other species.	**TMP-SMX:** 15 mg/kg/day of TMP, & 75 mg/kg/day of SMX, IV/po div in 2-4 doses + **Imipenem** 500 mg IV. If multiorgan involvement some add **amikacin** 7.5 mg/kg q12h. After 3-6 wks of IV therapy, switch to po therapy. Immunocompetent pts: **TMP-SMX, minocycline** or **AM-CL** x 3+ months. Immunocompromised pts: Treat with 2 drugs x 1 yr.	**Linezolid** 600 mg IV or po q12h + meropenem 2 gm q8h	Measure peak sulfonamide levels: target 100-150 mcg/mL, 2 hrs post dose. **Linezolid** 600 mg po bid reported effective. For in vitro susceptibility testing: Wallace (+1) 903-877-7680 or U.S. CDC (+1) 404-639-3158. In vitro resistance to TMP-SMX may be increasing (*Clin Infect Dis* 51:1445, 2010), but whether this is associated with worse outcomes is not known; TMP-SMX remains a drug of choice for CNS nocardia infection. If sulfonamide resistant or sulfa-allergic, **amikacin** plus one of: **IMP, MER, ceftriaxone** or **cefotaxime**. N. farcinia is resistant to third-generation cephalosporins, which should not be used for treatment of infection caused by this organism.
Subdural empyema: In adult 60-90% is extension of sinusitis or otitis media. Rx same as primary brain abscess. Surgical emergency: must drain. Review in *LnID* 7:62, 2007.				
Encephalitis/encephalopathy IDSA Guideline: *CID* 47:303, 2008; Int'l diagnosis consensus: *CID* 57:1114, 2013. (For Herpes see *Table 14A, page 161* and for rabies, *Table 20B, page 216*)	H. simplex (42%), VZV (15%), M. TB (15%), Listeria (10%) (*CID* 49:1838, 2009). Other: arbovirus, West Nile, rabies, Lyme, Parvo B19, Cat-scratch, Mycoplasma, EBV and others.	Start IV **acyclovir** while awaiting results of CSF PCR for H. simplex. For amebic encephalitis see *Table 13A*. Start **Doxy** if setting suggests R. rickettsii, Anaplasma, Ehrlichia or Mycoplasma.		Review of all etiologies: *LnID* 10:835, 2010. **Anti-NMDAR** (N-Methyl-D-Aspartate Receptor) encephalitis (*Ann Neurol* 75:317, 2014), autoimmune encephalitis, more common than individual viral etiologies as a cause of encephalitis in the California Encephalitis Project cohort (*CID* 54:899, 2012.) Clinical review: *Chest* 145:1143, 2014.
Meningitis, "Aseptic": Pleocytosis of up to 100s of cells, CSF glucose normal, neg. culture for bacteria (see *Table 14A, page 158*) Ref: *CID* 47:783, 2008	Enteroviruses, HSV-2, LCM, HIV, other viruses, drugs (NSAIDs, metronidazole, carbamazepine, lamotrigine TMP-SMX, IVIG, azathioprine, detuximab, infliximab]), rarely leptospirosis	For all but leptospirosis, IV fluids and analgesics. D/C drugs that may be etiologic. For lepto (**doxy** 100 mg IV/po q12h) **Acyclovir** 5-10 mg/kg IV q8h sometimes given for HSV-2 meningitis (Note: distinct from HSV encephalitis where early rx is mandatory).	For all but leptospirosis, IV fluids and analgesics. D/C drugs that may be etiologic. For lepto (**Pen G** 5 million units IV q6h) or (**AMP** 0.5–1 gm IV q6h) Repeat LP if suspect partially-treated bacterial meningitis.	If available, PCR of CSF for enterovirus. HSV-2 unusual without concomitant genital herpes (Mollaret's syndrome). For lepto, positive epidemiologic history and concomitant hepatitis, conjunctivitis, dermatitis, nephritis. For list of implicated drugs: *Int Med* 25:331, 2006.

Abbreviations on page 2.   *NOTE: All dosage recommendations are for adults (unless otherwise indicated) and assume normal renal function. § Alternatives consider allergy, PK, compliance, local resistance, cost

TABLE 1 (5)

ANATOMIC SITE/DIAGNOSIS/ MODIFYING CIRCUMSTANCES	ETIOLOGIES (usual)	SUGGESTED REGIMENS*		ADJUNCT DIAGNOSTIC OR THERAPEUTIC MEASURES AND COMMENTS
		PRIMARY	ALTERNATIVE†	
Meningitis, Bacterial, Acute: Goal is empiric therapy, then CSF exam within 30 min. If focal neurologic deficit, give empiric therapy, then head CT, then LP. (NEJM 354:44, 2006; LnID 10:32, 2010) **NOTE:** In children, treatment caused CSF cultures to turn neg. in 2 hrs with meningococci & partial response with pneumococci in 4 hrs (Peds 108:1169, 2001. For distribution of pathogens by age group, see NEJM 364:2016, 2011.				
Empiric Therapy—CSF Gram stain is negative—Immunocompetent				
Age: Preterm to <1 mo LnID 10:32, 2010	Group B strep 49%, E. coli 18%, listeria 7%, misc. Gm-neg. 10%, misc. Gm-pos. 10%	AMP 100 mg/kg IV q6h + cefotaxime 50 mg/kg IV q6h	AMP 100 mg/kg IV q6h + gentamicin 2.5 mg/kg IV q8h	Regimens active vs. Group B strep, most coliforms, & listeria. If premature infant with long nursery stay: staph, aureus, enterococci, and resistant coliforms potential pathogens. **Optional empiric regimens except for listeria: nafcillin + (cefazidime or cefotaxime). If high risk of MRSA,** use vanco + cefotaxime. Alter regimen after culture/sensitivity data available.
		Intraventricular treatment not recommended. Repeat CSF exam/culture 24–36 hr after start of therapy		
Age: 1 mo–50 yrs Hearing loss is most common neurologic sequelae (LnID 10:32, 2010)	S. pneumo, meningococci, H. influenzae now uncommon, listeria unlikely if young adult & immunocompetent (add ampicillin if suspect listeria: 2 gm IV q4h)	Adult dosage: [(Cefotaxime 2 gm IV q4-6h OR ceftriaxone 2 gm IV q12h)] + (dexamethasone) + vanco. **Dexamethasone:** 0.15 mg/kg IV q6h x 2-4 days. **Give with, or just before, 1st dose of antibiotic to block TNF production** (see Comment). See footnote¹ for Vanco Adult dosage and⁴ for ped. dosage	[MER 2 gm IV q8h] (Peds: 40 mg/kg IV q8h)] + IV dexamethasone + vanco **Dexamethasone:** 0.15 mg/kg IV q6h x 2-4 days. Give with, or just before, 1st dose of antibiotic to block TNF production (see Comment).	Value of **dexamethasone** shown in children with H. influenzae and adults with S. pneumoniae in some studies (NEJM 357:2431 & 2441, 2007; LnID 4:139, 2004). In the Netherlands, adoption of dexamethasone treatment in adult pneumococcal meningitis led to reduced mortality and hearing loss compared with historical control group (Neurology 75:1533, 2010). For patients with severe **β-lactam allergy**, see below (Empiric Therapy)—positive gram stain and Specific Therapy) for alternative therapies
Age: >50 yrs or alcoholism or other debilitating assoc diseases or impaired cellular immunity	S. pneumo, listeria, Gm-neg. bacilli. Note absence of meningococcus.	AMP 2 gm IV q4h) + (ceftriaxone 2 gm IV q12h or cefotaxime 2 gm IV q4-6h) + vanco + IV dexamethasone. **For Vanco dose,** see footnote¹. **Dexamethasone dose:** 0.15 mg/kg IV q6h x 2-4 days; 1st dose before, or concomitant with, 1st dose of antibiotic.	MER 2 gm IV q8h + vanco + IV dexamethasone. *For severe pen. Allergy: **Dexamethasone dose:** 0.15 mg/kg IV q6h x 2-4 days; 1st dose before, or	For patients with severe β-lactam allergy, see below (Empiric Therapy-positive gram stain and Specific Therapy) for alternative therapies that can be substituted to cover likely pathogens.
Post-neurosurgery Ventriculostomy/lumbar catheter; ventriculoperitoneal (atrial) shunt) or Penetrating trauma w/o basilar skull fracture	S. epidermidis, S. aureus, P. acnes. Fastidious, variable and aerobic gram-neg bacilli, including: P. aeruginosa & A. baumannii (may be multi-drug resistant)	Vanco (to achieve trough level of 15-20 μg/mL) + (Cefepime or Ceftaz 2 gm IV q8h)	Vanco (to achieve trough level of 15-20 μg/mL) + [MER 2 gm IV q8h]	• Remove infected shunt and place external ventricular catheter for drainage or pressure control. • Intraventricular therapy used if the shunt cannot be removed or cultures fail to clear with systemic therapy. Logic for intraventricular therapy: achieve 10-20 ratio of CSF concentration to MIC of infecting bacteria. Use only preservative-free drug. Clamp/close catheter for 1 hr after dose. For potential toxicities see CMR 23:858, 2010. • **Systemically ill patient:** systemic therapy + pathogen-directed intraventricular therapy once culture results are available • **Not systemically ill,** indolent Gram-positive: can D/C systemic vancomycin and treat with daily intraventricular therapy
		• If severe Pen/Ceph allergy, for possible gram-neg, substitute either: Aztreonam 2 gm IV q6-8h or CIP 400 mg IV q8-12h. **If IV therapy inadequate, may need intraventricular therapy:** Intraventricular daily doses (CID 39:1267, 2004; CMR 23:858, 2010): **Adult:** Vanco 10-20 mg; **Peds:** Vanco 5-20 mg (or 5 mg q12h). **Polymyxin B** 5 mg. **Peds: Gent** 1-2 mg; **Adult:** Gent 4-8 mg; **Tobra** 5-20 mg; **Gent** 4-8 mg (or 5 mg q12h). **Polymyxin B** 2 mg. **Alternative approach:** 1) systemically ill patient: systemic therapy + pathogen-directed intraventricular therapy once culture results are available; 2) not systemically ill, indolent Gram-positive: can D/C systemic vancomycin and treat with daily intraventricular therapy		• **Shunt reimplantation:** 1) If coagulase-negative staphylococci, diphtheroids, or P. acnes may immediately reimplant new shunt after CSF cultures are negative, no further systemic therapy needed. 2) For Staph. aureus and Gram-negative bacilli, may internalize shunt after 3 serial CSF cultures are negative and then treat with systemic therapy for an additional week. Ref: N Engl J Med 362:146, 2010.
		Amikacin 30 mg; **Colistin** 10 mg (or		
Trauma with basilar skull fracture	S. pneumoniae, H. influenzae, S. pyogenes	Vanco (to achieve trough level of 15-20 μg/mL) q6h x 2-4 d (1st dose with or before 1st antibiotic dose)) + (Ceftriaxone 2 gm IV q12h or Cefotax 2 gm IV q6h + (Dexamethasone 0.15 mg/kg IV		

¹ **Vanco adult dose:** 15-20 mg/kg IV q8-12h to achieve trough level of 15-20 μg/mL.
² **Dosage of drugs used to treat children ≥1 mo of age: Cefotaxime** 50 mg/kg per day IV q6h; **ceftriaxone** 50 mg/kg IV q6h to achieve trough level of 15-20 μg/mL; **vanco** 15 mg/kg IV q6h to achieve trough level of 15-20 μg/mL. § Alternatives consider allergy; PK compliance, local resistance, cost

Abbreviations on page 2.

*NOTE: All dosage recommendations are for adults (unless otherwise indicated) and assume normal renal function.

TABLE 1 (6)

ANATOMIC SITE/DIAGNOSIS/ MODIFYING CIRCUMSTANCES	ETIOLOGIES (usual)	SUGGESTED REGIMENS* PRIMARY	ALTERNATIVE§	ADJUNCT DIAGNOSTIC OR THERAPEUTIC MEASURES AND COMMENTS
CENTRAL NERVOUS SYSTEM/Meningitis, Bacterial, Acute (continued)				
Empiric Therapy—Positive CSF Gram stain				
Gram-positive diplococci	S. pneumoniae	(**ceftriaxone** 2 gm IV q12h or **cefotaxime** 2 gm IV q4-6h) + **vanco** 15-20 mg/kg IV q8-12h (to achieve 15-20 mcg/mL trough) + timed **dexamethasone** 0.15 mg/kg IV q6h x2-4 days.		Alternatives: **MER** 2 gm IV q8h or **Moxi** 400 mg IV q24h. Dexamethasone does not block penetration of vanco into CSF (CID 44:250, 2007).
Gram-negative diplococci	N. meningitidis	(**Cefotaxime** 2 gm IV q4-6h or **ceftriaxone** 2 gm IV q12h)		Alternatives: **Pen G** 4 mill. units IV q4h or **AMP** 2 gm IV q4h or **Moxi** 400 mg IV q24h or **chloro** 1 gm IV q6h
Gram-positive bacilli or coccobacilli	Listeria monocytogenes	**AMP** 2 gm IV q4h ± **gentamicin** 2 mg/kg IV loading dose then 1.7 mg/kg q8h		If pen-allergic, use **TMP-SMX** 5 mg/kg q6-8h
Gram-negative bacilli	H. influenzae, coliforms, or P. aeruginosa	(**Ceftazidime** or **cefepime** 2 gm IV q8h) ± **gentamicin** 2 mg/kg IV 1st dose then 1.7 mg/kg IV q8h (See Comment)		Alternatives: **CIP** 400 mg IV q8-12h; **MER** 2 gm IV q8h; **Aztreonam** 2 gm IV q6-8h. Consider adding intravenous **Gentamicin** to the **β-lactam** or **CIP** if gram-stain and clinical setting suggest P. aeruginosa or resistant coliforms.
Specific Therapy—Positive culture of CSF with in vitro susceptibility results available. Interest in monitoring/reducing intracranial pressure: CID 38:384, 2004				
H. influenzae	β-lactamase positive	**Ceftriaxone** 2 gm IV q12h (adult), 50 mg/kg IV q12h (peds)		Pen. allergic: **Chloro** 12.5 mg/kg IV q6h (max. 4 gm/day.); **CIP** 400 mg IV q8-12h; **Aztreonam** 2 gm q6-8h.
Listeria monocytogenes (CID 43:1233, 2006)		**AMP** 2 gm IV q4h ± **gentamicin** 2 mg/kg IV loading dose, then 1.7 mg/kg IV q8h		Pen. allergic: **TMP-SMX** 20 mg/kg per day div. q6-12h. Alternative: **MER** 2 gm IV q8h. Success reported with **linezolid** + **RIF** (CID 40:907, 2005) after AMP rx for brain abscess with meningitis.
N. meningitidis	Pen G 0.1-1 mcg per mL	**Pen G** 4 million units IV q4h or **AMP** 2 gm IV q4h		Rare isolates chloro-resistant. FQ-resistant isolates encountered. Alternatives: **Ceftriaxone** 2 gm IV q12h; **chloro** 1 gm IV q6h
S. pneumoniae **NOTES:** 1. Assumes dexamethasone just prior to 1st dose & x 4 days 2. If MIC ≥1, repeat CSF exam after 24-48h. 3. Treat for 10-14 days	Pen G MIC <0.1 mcg/mL	**Pen G** 4 million units IV q4h or **AMP** 2 gm IV q4h		
	0.1-1 mcg/mL	**Ceftriaxone** 2 gm IV q12h or **cefotaxime** 2 gm IV q4-6h		Alternatives: **Cefepime** 2 gm IV q8h or **MER** 2 gm IV q8h
	≥2 mcg/mL	**Vanco** 15-20 mg/kg IV q8-12h (15-20 mg/kg trough target) + (**ceftriaxone** or **cefotaxime** as above)		Alternatives: **Moxi** 400 mg IV q24h
	Ceftriaxone MIC ≥1 mcg/mL	**Vanco** 15-20 mg/kg IV q8-12h (15-20 µg/mL trough target) + (**ceftriaxone** or **cefotaxime** as above)		Alternatives: **Moxi** 400 mg IV q24h; If MIC to ceftriaxone >2 mcg/mL, add **RIF** 600 mg po/IV 1x/day to **vanco** + (**ceftriaxone** or **cefotaxime**).
E. coli, other coliforms, or P. aeruginosa	Consultation advised— need susceptibility results	(**Ceftazidime** or **cefepime** 2 gm IV q8h) ± **gentamicin**		Alternatives: **CIP** 400 mg IV q8-12h; **MER** 2 gm IV q8h. For intraventricular therapy: drug dosing, see Meningitis, Post-neurosurgery, page 8.
Prophylaxis for H. influenzae and N. meningitidis				
Haemophilus influenzae type B Household and/or day care contact: residing with index case for 24 hrs in a day. Day care contact or same day care facility as index case for 5-7 days before onset		**Children: RIF** 20 mg/kg po (not to exceed 600 mg) q24h x 4 doses. **Adults (non-pregnant): RIF** 600 mg q24h x 4 days		Household: If there is one unvaccinated contact age ≤4 yrs in the household, give RIF to all household contacts except pregnant women. Child Care Facilities: With 1 case, if attended by unvaccinated children ≤2 yrs, consider prophylaxis if all contacts >2 yrs: no prophylaxis. If ≥2 cases in 60 days & unvaccinated children attend, prophylaxis recommended for children & personnel (Am Acad Ped Red Book 2006, page 313).

Abbreviations on page 2.   *NOTE: All dosage recommendations are for adults (unless otherwise indicated) and assume normal renal function. § Alternatives consider allergy, PK, compliance, local resistance, cost

TABLE 1 (7)

ANATOMIC SITE/DIAGNOSIS/ MODIFYING CIRCUMSTANCES	ETIOLOGIES (usual)	SUGGESTED REGIMENS*		ADJUNCT DIAGNOSTIC OR THERAPEUTIC MEASURES AND COMMENTS
		PRIMARY	ALTERNATIVE§	
CENTRAL NERVOUS SYSTEM/Meningitis, Bacterial, Acute/Prophylaxis for H. influenzae and N. meningitidis (continued)				
Prophylaxis for Neisseria meningitidis exposure (close contact) **NOTE:** CDC reports **CIP-resistant group B meningococcus** from selected counties in N. Dakota & Minnesota. **Avoid CIP.** Use **ceftriaxone** or **RIF**, or single 500 mg dose of **azithro** (MMWR 57:173, 2008).		**Ceftriaxone** 250 mg IM x 1 dose (child <15 yrs 125 mg IM x 1) **OR RIF** 600 mg po q12h x 4 doses. (Children ≥1 mo 10 mg/kg po q12h x 4 doses, <1 mo 5 mg/kg q12h x 4 doses) **OR** if not CIP-resistant, **CIP** 500 mg po x 1 dose (adult)		**Spread by respiratory droplets**, not aerosols, hence close contact req. ↑ risk if close contact for at least 4 hrs during wk before illness onset (e.g., housemates, day care contacts, cellmates) or exposure to pt's nasopharyngeal secretions (e.g., kissing, mouth-to-mouth resuscitation, intubation, nasotracheal suctioning).
Meningitis, chronic Defined as symptoms + CSF pleocytosis for ≥4 wks	MTB cryptococcosis, other fungal, neoplastic, Lyme, syphilis, Whipple's disease	Treatment depends on etiology. No urgent need for empiric therapy, but when TB suspected treatment should be expeditious.		Long list of possibilities: bacteria, parasites, fungi, viruses, neoplasms, vasculitis, and other miscellaneous etiologies—see *Neuro Clin* 28:1061, 2010. See *NEJM* 370:2408, 2014 for diagnosis of neuroleptospirosis by next generation sequencing technologies.
Meningitis, eosinophilic *LnID* 8:621, 2008	Angiostrongyliasis, gnathostomiasis, Baylisascaris	Corticosteroids	Not sure antihelmintic therapy works	1/3 lack peripheral eosinophilia. Need serology to confirm diagnosis. Steroid ref.: *LnID* 8:621, 2008. Automated CSF count may not correctly identify eosinophils (*CID* 48: 322, 2009).
Meningitis, HIV-1 infected (AIDS) See *Table 11*, SANFORD GUIDE TO HIV/AIDS THERAPY	As in adults, >50 yrs: also consider cryptococcci, M. tuberculosis, syphilis, HIV aseptic meningitis, Listeria monocytogenes	If etiology not identified: treat as adult >50 yrs + obtain CSF/serum cryptococcal antigen (see Comments)	For crypto rx, see *Table 11A*, page 119	C. neoformans most common etiology in AIDS patients. H. influenzae, pneumococci, listeria, TBc, syphilis, viral, histoplasma & coccidioides also need to be considered. Obtain blood cultures.
EAR				
External otitis				
Chronic	Usually 2° to seborrhea	Eardrops: [(**polymyxin B** + **neomycin** + **hydrocortisone**) + **selenium sulfide shampoo**]		Control seborrhea with dandruff shampoo containing selenium sulfide (Selsun) + (ketoconazole shampoo) + (medium potency steroid solution, triamcinolone 0.1%)
Fungal	Candida species	**Fluconazole** 200 mg po x 1 dose & then 100 mg po x 3-5 days.		
"Necrotizing (malignant) otitis externa" Risk groups: Diabetes mellitus, AIDS, chemotherapy.	Pseudomonas aeruginosa in >95% (*Otol & Neurology* 34:620, 2013)	**CIP** 400 mg IV q8h, 750 mg po q8-12h for only early disease	**PIP-TZ** 3.375 gm q4h or extended infusion dose (3.375 gm over 4h q8h) + **Tobra**	Very high ESRs are typical. Debridement usually required. R/O osteomyelitis: CT or MRI scan. If bone involved, treat for 6-8 wks. Other alternatives if P. aeruginosa is susceptible: **IMP** 0.5 gm q6h or **MER** 1 gm IV q8h or **CFP** 2 gm IV q12h or **Ceftaz** 2 gm IV q8h.
"Swimmer's ear"; occlusive devices (earphones); contact dermatitis, psoriasis *Pediatr Rev* 28:77, 2007; Cochrane Database Sys Rev 2010, CD004740	Acute infection usually 2° S. aureus (11%); other: Pseudomonas (11%), Anaerobes (2%), S. epidermidis (46%), candida (8%)	Mild: eardrops: **acetic acid** + **propylene glycol** + **HC** (**Vosol HC**) 5 gtts 3-4x/day until resolved. Moderate, severe: Eardrops **CIP** + **HC** (**Cipro HC Otic**) 3 gtts bid x 7 days. Alternative: Finavofloxacin 0.3% otic suspension 4 gtts q12h x 7d. (for P. aeruginosa and S. aureus).		Rx includes gentle cleaning. Recurrences prevented (or decreased) by drying with alcohol drops (1/3 white vinegar, 2/3 rubbing alcohol) after swimming, then antibiotic drops or 2% acetic acid solution. Ointments should not be used in ear. Do not use neomycin or other aminoglycoside drops if tympanic membrane punctured.

Abbreviations on page 2.   *NOTE: All dosage recommendations are for adults (unless otherwise indicated) and assume normal renal function. PK, compliance, local resistance, cost

*NOTE: All dosage recommendations are for adults (unless otherwise indicated) and assume normal renal function. § Alternatives consider allergy, PK, compliance, local resistance, cost

TABLE 1 (8)

ANATOMIC SITE/DIAGNOSIS/ MODIFYING CIRCUMSTANCES	ETIOLOGIES (usual)	SUGGESTED REGIMENS*		ADJUNCT DIAGNOSTIC OR THERAPEUTIC MEASURES AND COMMENTS
		PRIMARY	ALTERNATIVE†	
EAR (continued)				
Otitis media—infants, children, adults (Cochrane review: Cochrane Database Syst Rev. Jan 31;1:CD000219, 2013); American Academy of Pediatrics Guidelines: Pediatrics 131:e964, 2013)				
Acute Two PRDB trials indicate efficacy of antibiotic rx if age < 36 mos & definite AOM (NEJM 364:105, 116 & 168, 2011)				
Initial empiric therapy of acute otitis media (AOM) NOTE: **Treat children <2 yrs old.** If > 2 yrs old, afebrile, no ear pain, neg./questionable exam—consider analgesic treatment and antimicrobials. Favorable results in mostly afebrile pts with waiting 48hrs before deciding on antibiotic use (JAMA 296:1235, 1290, 2006)	Overall detection in middle ear fluid: No pathogen 4% Virus 70% Bact. + virus 66% Bacteria 92% Bacterial pathogens from middle ear: S. pneumo 49%, H. influenzae 29%, M. catarrhalis 28%. Ref.: CID 43:1417 & 1423, 2006. Children 6 mos-3 yrs. 2 episodes AOM/yrs & 63% are virus positive (CID 46:815 & 824, 2008).	If NO antibiotics in prior month: Amox HD[3]	**If allergic to β-lactam drugs?** If history unclear or rash, effective oral ceph OK; avoid ceph if IgE-mediated allergy, e.g., anaphylaxis. High failure rate with azithro, clarithro, erythro if etiology is S. pneumoniae, H. influenzae. Clindamycin has some limited efficacy against S. pneumo and H. influenza. **Up to 50% S. pneumo resistant to macrolides.** **Spontaneous resolution occurred in:** 90% pts infected with M. catarrhalis, 50% with H. influenzae, 10% with S. pneumoniae; overall 80% resolve within 2–14 days (Ln 363:465, 2004).	
		If NO antibiotics in prior month: Amox HD[3] or AM-CL extra-strength[4] or cefdinir or cefpodoxime or cefprozil or cefuroxime axetil For dosage, see footnote[4] **All doses see pediatric**	**Received antibiotics in prior month:** Amox HD[3] or AM-CL extra-strength[4] or cefdinir or cefpodoxime or cefprozil or cefuroxime axetil For dosage, see footnote[4] **All doses see pediatric**	Risk of drug-resistant S. pneumo if age < 2 yrs, antibiotics last 3 mos, &/or daycare attendance. Selection of drug based on (1) effectiveness against β-lactamase producing H. influenzae & M. catarrhalis & (2) effectiveness against vs. **resistant S. pneumo.** inc. DRSP. **Cefaclor, loracarbef, & ceftibuten less active vs. resistant S. pneumo.** than other agents listed. No benefit of antibiotics in treatment of otitis media with effusion (Cochrane Database Syst Rev. Sep 12;9:CD009163, 2012). For persistent otitis media, hydrocortisone/bacitracin/colistin eardrops[NUS] 5 drops tid x 7 d more effective than no AM-CL (NEJM:370:723, 2014). Benefit for AOM.	
Duration of rx: <2 yrs old x 10 days; >2 yrs old x 5-7 days. Appropriate duration unclear. 5 days may be inadequate for severe disease (NEJM 347:1169, 2002) **For adult dosages, see Sinusitis, page 50, and Table 10A**					
Treatment for clinical failure after 3 days	Drug-resistant S. pneumoniae main concern	**NO antibiotics in month prior to last 3 days:** AM-CL high dose or cefdinir or cefpodoxime or cefprozil or cefuroxime axetil x 3 days	**Antibiotics in month prior to last 3 days:** (IM ceftriaxone) or cefdinir (clindamycin) and/or tympanocentesis] See clindamycin Comments	Clindamycin not active vs. H. influenzae or M. catarrhalis. S. pneumo resistant to macrolides are usually also resistant to clindamycin. Definition of failure: no change in ear pain, fever, bulging TM or otorrhea after 3 days of therapy. Tympanocentesis will allow culture. **Newer FQs active vs. drug-resistant S. pneumo (DRSP), but not approved for use in children (PIDJ 23:390, 2004). Vanco is active vs. DRSP.**
			For dosage, see footnote[4] **All doses see pediatric** Duration of rx as above	
After >48hrs of nasotracheal intubation	Pseudomonas sp. klebsiella, enterobacter	**Ceftazidime** or **CFP** or **IMP** or **MER** or (**PIP-TZ**) or **TC-CL** or **CIP.** (For dosages, see Ear, Necrotizing (malignant) otitis externa, page 10)		With nasotracheal intubation >48 hrs, about ½ pts will have otitis media with effusion.

Abbreviations on page 2.   *NOTE: All dosage recommendations are for adults (unless otherwise indicated) and assume normal renal function.

---

[3] **Amoxicillin UD or HD** = amoxicillin usual dose or high dose. **AM-CL HD** = amoxicillin-clavulanate high dose. **Dosages in footnote[4].** Data supporting amoxicillin HD: PIDJ 22:405, 2003

[4] **Drugs & peds dosage** (all drugs usually specified) **for acute otitis media: Amoxicillin UD** = 40 mg/kg per day div q12h or q8h; **AM-CL HD** = 90 mg/kg per day div q12h. **Amoxicillin HD** = 90 mg/kg per day div q12h or q8h. **Cefuroxime axetil** 30 mg/kg per day div q12h. **Ceftriaxone** 50 mg/kg per day IM x 3 days. **Clindamycin** 20-30 mg/kg per day div q8h. Extra-strength AM-CL oral suspension (Augmentin ES-600) available with 600 mg AM & 42.9 mg CL/5 mL—dose. 90/6.4 mg/kg per day div bid. **Cefprozil** 15 mg/kg q12h. DRSP but no activity vs H. influenzae). Other drugs suitable for drug (e.g., **penicillin**) - **sensitive S. pneumo: TMP-SMX** 4 mg/kg of TMP q12h. **Erythro-sulfisoxazole** 50 mg/kg per day of erythro div q6-8h. **Clarithro** 15 mg/kg per day div q12h; **azithro** 10 mg/kg per day x 1 & then 5 mg/kg per day x 2-5. Other FDA-approved regimens: 10 mg/kg q24h x 3 days & 30 mg/kg x 1 **Cefdinir** 7 mg/kg q12h or q8h; **torcarbef** 15 mg/kg per day q8h; **cefpodoxime proxetil** 10 mg/kg per day as single dose; **cefaclor** 40 mg/kg per day div q8h. † Alternatives consider allergy; PK, compliance, local resistance, cost

TABLE 1 (9)

ANATOMIC SITE/DIAGNOSIS/ MODIFYING CIRCUMSTANCES	ETIOLOGIES* (usual)	SUGGESTED REGIMENS* PRIMARY	SUGGESTED REGIMENS* ALTERNATIVE†	ADJUNCT DIAGNOSTIC OR THERAPEUTIC MEASURES AND COMMENTS
EAR, Otitis Media (continued)				
Prophylaxis: acute otitis media *J Laryngol Otol 126:874, 2012*	Pneumococci, H. influenzae, M. catarrhalis, Staph. aureus, Group A strep (see Comment)	**Sulfisoxazole** 50 mg/kg po at bedtime or **amoxicillin** 20 mg/kg po q24h	**Use of antibiotics to prevent otitis media is a major contributor to emergence of antibiotic-resistant S. pneumo!** Pneumococcal protein conjugate vaccine decreases freq AOM due to vaccine serotypes. Adenoidectomy at time of tympanostomy tubes ↓ need for future hospitalization for AOM (NEJM 344:1188, 2001).	
Mastoiditis. Complication of acute or chronic otitis media. If chronic, look for cholesteatoma (Keratoma)				
Acute		Obtain cultures, then empiric therapy.		• Diagnosis: CT or MRI
Generally too ill for outpatient therapy. Complication ref: *Otolaryngol Clin No Amer 39:1237, 2006*	1st episode: S. pneumoniae H. influenzae M. catarrhalis	1st episode: **Ceftriaxone** 2 gm IV once daily OR **Levofloxacin** 750 mg IV once daily		• Look for complication: osteomyelitis, suppurative lateral sinus thrombophlebitis, purulent
	If secondary to chronic otitis media: S. aureus P. aeruginosa S. pneumoniae	Acute exacerbation of chronic otitis media: Surgical debridement of auditory canal, then [**Vancomycin** (dose to achieve trough of 15–20 mcg/mL) + **Pip-Tazo** 3.375 gm IV q6h] OR [**Vancomycin** (dose as above) + **Ciprofloxacin** 400 mg IV q8h]		meningitis, brain abscess. ENT consultation for possible mastoidectomy S. aureus (J Otolaryng Head Neck Surg 38:483, 2009)
Chronic				
Generally not ill enough for parenteral antibiotics	As per 1st episode and: S. aureus P. aeruginosa Anaerobes Fungi	Culture ear drainage. May need surgical debridement. Topical Fluoroquinolone ear drops.		• Diagnosis: CT or MRI
EYE				
Eyelid: Little reported experience with CA-MRSA (See Cochrane Database Syst Rev 5:CD005556, 2012)				
Blepharitis	Etiol. unclear. Factors include Staph. aureus & Staph. epidermidis, seborrhea, rosacea, & dry eye	Lid margin care with baby shampoo & warm compresses q24h. Artificial tears if assoc. dry eye (see Comment)		Usually topical ointments of no benefit. If associated rosacea, add doxy 100 mg po bid for 2 wks and then q24h.
Hordeolum (Stye)				
External (eyelash follicle)	Staph. aureus	Hot packs only. Will drain spontaneously		Infection of superficial sebaceous gland.
Internal (Meibomian glands): Can be acute, subacute or chronic.	Staph. aureus, MSSA Staph. aureus, MRSA-CA Staph. aureus, MRSA-HA	Oral **dicloxacillin** + hot packs TMP-SMX-DS, tabs ii po bid **Linezolid** 600 mg po bid possible therapy if multi-drug resistant.		Also called acute meibomianitis. Rarely drain spontaneously. I&D and culture. Role of fluoroquinolone eye drops is unclear. MRSA often resistant to lower conc.; may be susceptible to higher concentration of FQ in ophthalmologic solutions of gati, levo or moxi.
Conjunctiva: Review: JAMA 310:1721, 2013				
Conjunctivitis of the newborn (**ophthalmia neonatorum**): by day of onset post-delivery—all dose pediatric				
Onset 1st day	Chemical due to silver nitrate prophylaxis	None		Usual prophylaxis is erythro ointment; hence, silver nitrate irritation rare.
Onset 2–4 days	N. gonorrhoeae	**Ceftriaxone** 25–50 mg/kg IV x 1 dose (see Comment), not to exceed 125 mg		Treat mother and her sexual partners. Hyperpurulent. Topical rx inadequate. **Treat neonate for concomitant Chlamydia trachomatis.**
Onset 3–10 days	Chlamydia trachomatis	Erytho base or ethylsuccinate syrup 12.5 mg/kg po q6h x 14 days. No topical rx needed.		Diagnosis by antigen detection. Alternative: **Azithro suspension** 20 mg/kg po q24h x 3 days. Treat mother & sexual partner

Abbreviations on page 2.   *NOTE: All dosage recommendations are for adults (unless otherwise indicated) and assume normal renal function. § Alternatives consider allergy, PK, compliance, local resistance, cost

TABLE 1 (10)

ANATOMIC SITE/DIAGNOSIS/ MODIFYING CIRCUMSTANCES	ETIOLOGIES (usual)	SUGGESTED REGIMENS* PRIMARY	ALTERNATIVE†	ADJUNCT DIAGNOSTIC OR THERAPEUTIC MEASURES AND COMMENTS
EYE/Conjunctiva (continued)				
Onset 2–16 days	Herpes simplex types 1, 2	Topical anti-viral rx under direction of ophthalmologist.		Also give Acyclovir 60 mg/kg/day IV div 3 doses (Red Book online, accessed Jan 2011).
Ophthalmia neonatorum prophylaxis		**erythro** 0.5% ointment x 1 or **tetra** 1% ointmentAUS x 1 application		
Pink eye (viral conjunctivitis) Usually unilateral	Adenovirus (types 8 & 7 in children, 8, 11 & 19 in adults)	No treatment. If symptomatic, artificial tears may help.		Highly contagious. Onset of ocular pain and photophobia in an adult suggests associated keratitis—rare.
Inclusion conjunctivitis (adult) Usually unilateral & concomitant genital infection	Chlamydia trachomatis	**Azithro** 1 g once	**Doxy** 100 mg po bid x 7 days	Oculogenital disease. Diagnosis NAAT. Urine NAAT for both GC & chlamydia. Treat sexual partner. May need to repeat dose of azithro.
Trachoma—a chronic bacterial keratoconjunctivitis linked to poverty	Chlamydia trachomatis	**Azithro** 20 mg/kg po single dose—78% effective in children; Adults: 1 gm po.	**Doxy** 100 mg po bid x minimum of 21 days or **tetracycline** 250 mg po qid x 14 days.	Starts in childhood and can persist for years with subsequent damage to cornea. Topical therapy of marginal benefit. Avoid doxy/tetracycline in young children. Mass treatment works (NEJM 358:1777 & 1870, 2008; JAMA 299:778, 2008).
Suppurative conjunctivitis: Children and Adults (Eyedrops speed resolution of symptoms: Cochrane Database Syst Rev. Sep 12;9:CD001211, 2012)				
JAMA 310:1721, 2013	Staph. aureus, S. pneumoniae, H. influenzae, Viridans Strep., Moraxella sp.	FQ ophthalmic solns: **CIP** (generic), others expensive [Besi, Gati, Levo, Moxi] All 1–2 gtts q2h while awake 1st 2 days, then q4–8h up to 7 days.	**Polymyxin** solution 1–2 gtts q3–6 h x 7–10 days.	**FQs** best spectrum for empiric therapy. High concentrations ↑ likelihood of activity vs. S. aureus—even MRSA. **TMP** spectrum may include MRSA. Polymyxin S spectrum only Gm-neg. bacilli but no ophthal. prep of only **TMP**. Most S. pneumo resistant to **gent** & tobra.
Gonococcal (peds/adults)	N. gonorrhoeae	**Ceftriaxone** 25–50 mg/kg IV/IM (not to exceed 125 mg) as one dose in children. 1 gm IM/IV as one dose in adults		
Cornea (keratitis): Usually serious and often sight-threatening. Prompt ophthalmologic consultation essential for diagnosis, antimicrobial and adjunctive therapy! Herpes simplex most common etiology in developed countries; bacterial and fungal infections more common in underdeveloped countries.				
Viral				
H. simplex	H. simplex, types 1 & 2	**Trifluridine** ophthalmic soln, one drop q2h up to 9 drops/day until re-epithelialized, then one drop q4h up to 5x/day for total not to exceed 21 days.	**Ganciclovir** 0.15% ophthalmic gel. Indicated for acute herpetic keratitis. One drop 5 times per day while awake until corneal ulcer heals; then, one drop three times per day for 7 days. **Vidarabine** ointment— useful in children Use 5x/day for up to 21 days (currently listed as discontinued in U.S.).	Approx 30% recurrence rate within one year; consider prophylaxis with acyclovir 400 mg bid for 12 months to prevent recurrences (Arch Ophthal 130:108, 2012)
Varicella-zoster ophthalmicus	Varicella-zoster virus	**Famciclovir** 500 mg bid or **valacyclovir** 1 gm po tid x 10 days	**Acyclovir** 800 mg po 5x/day x 10 days	Clinical diagnosis most common: dendritic figures with fluorescein staining in patient with varicella-zoster of ophthalmic branch of trigeminal nerve.

*NOTE: All dosage recommendations are for adults (unless otherwise indicated) and assume normal renal function. § Alternatives consider allergy, PK, compliance, local resistance, cost

Abbreviations on page 2.

TABLE 1 (11)

ANATOMIC SITE/DIAGNOSIS/ MODIFYING CIRCUMSTANCES	ETIOLOGIES (usual)	SUGGESTED REGIMENS* PRIMARY	SUGGESTED REGIMENS* ALTERNATIVE†	ADJUNCT DIAGNOSTIC OR THERAPEUTIC MEASURES AND COMMENTS
EYE/Cornea (keratitis) (continued)				
Bacterial Acute: No comorbidity	S. aureus, S. pneumo., S. pyogenes, Haemophilus sp.	**All treatment listed for bacterial, fungal, protozoan is topical unless otherwise indicated** **Moxi:** ophthalmic 0.5%: 1 drop q1h for the first 48h then taper according to response	**Gatt:** ophthalmic 0.3%: 1 drop q1h for the first 48h then taper according to response	Regimens vary; some start rx by appling drops q5 min for 5 doses; some apply drops q15-30 min for or several hours; some extend interval to q2h during sleep. In a clinical trial, drops were applied q1h for 43-72h, then q2h through day 6, then q2h during waking hours on days 7-9, then q6h until healing (Cornea 29:751, 2010). **Note:** despite high concentrations, may fail vs. MRSA. Prior use of fluoroquinolones associated with increased MICs (JAMA Ophthalmol. 131:310, 2013); high MICs associated with poorer outcome (Clin Infect Dis 54:1381, 2012). **Cornea abrasions:** treated with Tobra, Gent, or CIP gtts qid for 3-5 days; referral to ophthalmologist recommended cornea infiltrate or ulcer, visual loss, lack of improvement or worsening symptoms (Am Fam Physician. 87:114, 2013).
Contact lens users	P. aeruginosa	**CiP** 0.3% ophthalmic solution or **LEVO** 0.5% ophthalmic solution 1-2 gtts hourly x24-72h; taper based on response.	**Gent** or **Tobra** 0.3% ophthalmic solution 1-2 gtts hourly x24h then taper based on clinical response.	Specific therapy guided by results of alginate swab culture.
Dry cornea, diabetes, immunosuppression	Staph. aureus, S. epidermidis, S. pneumoniae, S. pyogenes, Enterobacteriaceae, listeria	**CiP** 0.3% ophthalmic solution 1-2 gtts hourly x24-72 hrs, taper based on clinical response.	**Vanco** (50 mg/mL) + **Ceftaz** (50 mg/mL) hourly for 24-72h, taper depending upon response. See Comment.	
Fungal	Aspergillus, fusarium, candida and others.	**Natamycin** (5%): 1 drop, every 1-2 h for several days; then q3-4h for several days; can reduce frequency depending upon response.	**Amphotericin B** (0.15%): 1 drop every 1-2 hours for several days; can reduce frequency depending upon response.	Obtain specimens for fungal wet mount and cultures. Numerous other treatment options (1% topical Itra or 1% oral Itra 100 mg bid for 3 wks, topical voriconazole 1% hourly for 2 wks, topical miconazole 1% 5x a day, topical silver sulphadiazine 0.5-1.0% 5x a day) appear to have similar efficacy (Cochrane Database Syst Rev 2:004241, 2012).
Mycobacteria: Post-refractive eye surgery	Mycobacterium chelonae	**Gati** or **Moxi** eye drops: 1 gtt qid, probably in conjunction with other active antimicrobials		Used in conjunction with other topical and/or systemic anti-mycobacterial agents (J Cataract Refract Surg 33:1978, 2007; Ophthalmology 113:950, 2006).
Protozoan Soft contact lens users. Ref: CID 35:434, 2002.	Acanthamoeba, sp.	Optimal regimen uncertain. Suggested regimen: **[Chlorhexidine** 0.02% or Polyhexamethylene biguanide 0.02%] + (Propamidine isethionate 0.1% or Hexamidine 0.1%) drops. Apply one drop every hour for 48h, then one drop every hour only while awake for 72h, then one drop every two hours while awake for 3-4 weeks, then reducing frequency based on response (Ref: Am J Ophthalmol 148:487, 2009; Curr Op Infect Dis 23:590, 2010).		Uncommon. Trauma and soft contact lenses are risk factors. To obtain suggested drops: Leiter's Park Ave Pharmacy (800-292-6773; www.leiterx.com). Cleaning solution outbreak: MMWR 56: 532, 2007.

Abbreviations on page 2.

*NOTE: All dosage recommendations are for adults (unless otherwise indicated) and assume normal renal function. § Alternatives consider allergy, PK, compliance, local resistance, cost

TABLE 1 (12)

ANATOMIC SITE/DIAGNOSIS/ MODIFYING CIRCUMSTANCES	ETIOLOGIES (usual)	SUGGESTED REGIMENS*		ADJUNCT DIAGNOSTIC OR THERAPEUTIC MEASURES AND COMMENTS
		PRIMARY	**ALTERNATIVE¹**	
EYE/Cornea (keratitis) *(continued)*				
Lacrimal apparatus				
Canaliculitis	Actinomyces most common. Rarely, Arachnia, fusobacterium, nocardia, candida	Remove granules & irrigate with **pen G** (100,000 mcg/mL). **Child: AM-CL or cefprozil or cefuroxime.**	If fungi, irrigate with **nystatin** approx. 5 mcg/mL; 1 gtt tid	Digital pressure produces exudate at punctum; Gram stain confirms diagnosis. Hot packs to punctal area qid. M. chelonae reported after use of intracanalicular plugs (*Ophth Plast Reconstr Surg 24: 241, 2008*).
Dacryocystitis (lacrimal sac)	S. pneumo, S. aureus, H. influenzae, S. pyogenes, P. aeruginosa	Often consequence of obstruction of lacrimal duct. Empiric systemic antimicrobial therapy based on Gram stain of aspirate—see Comment.		Need ophthalmologic consultation. Surgery may be required. Can be acute or chronic. Culture to detect MRSA.
Endophthalmitis: Endogenous (secondary to bacteremia or fungemia, post-operative) and exogenous (post-injection, post-operative) types				
Bacterial: Haziness of vitreous key to diagnosis. Needle aspirate of both vitreous and aqueous humor for culture prior to therapy. Intravitreal administration of antimicrobials essential.				
Postocular surgery (cataracts) Early, acute onset (incidence 0.05%)	S. epidermidis 60%, Staph. aureus, streptococci & enterococci each 5–10%, Gm-neg. bacilli 6%	**Immediate ophthal. consult.** If only light perception or worse, immediate vitrectomy + intravitreal vanco 1 mg & intravitreal ceftazidime		2.25 mg. No clear data on intravitreal steroid. May need to repeat intravitreal antibiotics in 2–3 days. Can usually leave lens in. Adjunctive systemic antibiotics (e.g., Vancomycin, Ceftazidime, Moxifloxacin or Gatifloxacin¹⁰ᴺ) not of proven value, but recommended in endogenous infection.
Low grade, chronic	Propionibacterium acnes, S. epidermidis, S. aureus (rare)	Intraocular **vanco**. Usually requires vitrectomy, lens removal.		
Post filtering blebs for glaucoma	Strep. species (viridans & others), H. influenzae	Intravitreal agent (e.g., **Vanco** 1 mg + **Ceftaz** 2.25 mg) and a topical agent. Consider a systemic agent such as **Amp-Sulb** or **Cefuroxime** or **Ceftaz** (add **Vanco** if MRSA is suspected).		
Post-penetrating trauma	Bacillus sp. S. epiderm.	Intravitreal agent as above + systemic **clinda** or **vanco**. Use topical antibiotics post-surgery (tobra & cefazolin drops).		
None, suspect hematogenous	S. pneumoniae, Staph. aureus, Grp B Strep, K. pneumo	(**cefotaxime** 2 gm IV q4h or **ceftriaxone** 2 gm IV q24h) + **vanco** 30–60 mg/kg/day in 2-3 div doses to achieve target trough serum concentration of (15-20 mcg/mL) pending cultures. Intravitreal antibiotics as with early post-operative.		
IV heroin abuse	Bacillus cereus, Candida sp.	Intravitreal agent + systemic agent based on etiology and antimicrobial susceptibility.		
Mycotic (fungal): Broad-spectrum antibiotics, often corticosteroids, indwelling venous catheters	Candida sp., Aspergillus sp.	Intravitreal **ampho B** 0.005–0.01 mg in 0.1 mL. Also see Table 11A, page 117 for concomitant systemic therapy. See Comment		Patients with Candida spp. chorioretinitis usually respond to systemically administered antifungals (*Clin Infect Dis 53:262, 2011*). Intravitreal amphotericin and/or vitrectomy may be necessary for those with vitritis or endophthalmitis (*Br J Ophthalmol 92:466, 2008; Pharmacotherapy 27:1711, 2007*).
Retinitis				
Acute retinal necrosis	Varicella zoster, Herpes simplex	IV **acyclovir** 10–12 mg/kg IV q8h x 5–7 days, then 800 mg po 5x/day x 6 wks		Strong association of VZ virus with atypical necrotizing herpetic retinopathy.
HIV+ (AIDS) CD4 usually <100/mm³	Cytomegalovirus	See Table 14A, page 160		Occurs in 5–10% of AIDS patients

Abbreviations on page 2.   *NOTE: All dosage recommendations are for adults (unless otherwise indicated) and assume normal renal function. § Alternatives consider allergy, PK, compliance, local resistance, cost

TABLE 1 (13)

ANATOMIC SITE/DIAGNOSIS/ MODIFYING CIRCUMSTANCES	ETIOLOGIES* (usual)	SUGGESTED REGIMENS*		ADJUNCT DIAGNOSTIC OR THERAPEUTIC MEASURES AND COMMENTS
		PRIMARY	ALTERNATIVE†	
EYE/Retinitis *(continued)*				
Progressive outer retinal necrosis	VZV, H. simplex, CMV (rare)	**Acyclovir** 10-12 mg/kg IV q8h for 1-2 weeks, then **valacyclovir** 800 mg po tid, or **famciclovir** 500 mg po tid, or **acyclovir** 800 mg po tid. Ophthalmology consultation imperative: approaches have also included intra-vitreal injection of anti-virals (foscarnet, ganciclovir implant). In rare cases due to CMV use **ganciclovir/valganciclovir** (see CMV retinitis, Table 14A).		Most patients are highly immunocompromised (HIV with low CD4 or transplantation). In contrast to Acute Retinal Necrosis, lack of intraocular inflammation or arteritis. May be able to stop oral antivirals when CD4 recovers with ART (Ocul Immunol Inflammation 15:425, 2007).
Orbital cellulitis *(see page 54 for erysipelas, facial)*	S. pneumoniae, H. influenzae, M. catarrhalis, S. aureus, anaerobes, group A strep, occ. Gm-neg. bacilli post-trauma	**Vancomycin** 15-20 mg/kg IV q8-12h (target **vancomycin** trough serum concentrations of 15-20 µg/mL) + ((**Ceftriaxone** 2 gm IV q24h + **Metronidazole** 1 gm IV q12h) OR **Piperacillin-Tazobactam** 4.5 gm IV q8h)	**If** penicillin/ceph allergy: **Vanco** + **levo** 750 mg IV once daily + **metro** IV. Problem is frequent inability to make microbiologic diagnosis. Image orbit (CT or MRI). Risk of cavernous sinus thrombosis. If vanco intolerant, another option for s. aureus is dapto 6 mg/kg IV q24h.	
FOOT				
"Diabetic foot"—Two thirds of patients have triad of neuropathy, deformity and pressure-induced trauma. IDSA Guidelines CID 54:e132, 2012.				
Ulcer without inflammation	Colonizing skin flora	No antibacterial therapy.		**General:** 1. Glucose control, eliminate pressure on ulcer 2. **Assess for peripheral vascular disease** 3. Caution in patients with diabetes, as many have risk factors for hyperkalemia (e.g., advanced age, reduced renal function, concomitant medications) (Arch Intern Med 170:1045, 2010).
Mild infection	S. aureus (assume MRSA), S. agalactiae (Gp B), S. pyogenes predominate	**Oral therapy.** Diclox or cephalexin or AM-CL (not MRSA) Doxy or TMP-SMX-DS (MRSA, strep) CLINDA (covers MSSA, MRSA, strep)		**Principles of empiric antibacterial therapy:** 1. Obtain culture. Cover for MRSA in moderate, severe infections pending culture data, local epidemiology. 2. Severe limb and/or life-threatening infections require initial parenteral therapy with predictable activity vs. Gm-positive cocci including MRSA, coliforms & other aerobic Gm-neg. rods, & anaerobic Gm-neg. bacilli. 3. **NOTE:** The regimens listed are suggestions consistent with above principles. Other alternatives exist & may be appropriate for individual patients.
Moderate infection. **Osteomyelitis** See Comment.	As above, plus coliforms possible	**Oral:** As above **Parenteral therapy:** (based on prevailing susceptibilities: (**AM-SB** or **TC-CL** or **PIP-TZ** or **ERTA** or other carbapenem) plus (**vanco** until MRSA ruled out as below) until MRSA excluded)	Dosages in footnotes[5]	Is there an associated osteomyelitis? Risk increased if ulcer area >2 cm², positive probe to bone. ESR > 70 and abnormal plain x-ray. Negative MRI reduces likelihood of osteomyelitis (JAMA 299:806, 2008). MRI is best imaging modality (CID 47:519 & 528, 2008).
Extensive local inflammation plus systemic toxicity.	As above, plus anaerobic bacteria. Role of enterococci unclear.	**Parenteral therapy:** (**Vanco** plus (β-lactam/β-lactamase inhibitor)) or (**vanco** plus **Dori** or **IMP** or **MER**)). Other alternatives: 1. **Dapto** or **linezolid** for vanco 2. **CIP** or **Levo** or **Moxi** or **aztreonam** plus **metronidazole** for β-lactam/β-lactamase inhibitor	Dosages in footnotes[6,7]	
		Assess for arterial insufficiency!		

[5] **TMP-SMX-DS** 1-2 tabs po bid, **minocycline** 100 mg po bid, **Pen VK** 500 mg po qid, (O **Ceph** 2, 3: **cefprozil** 500 mg po bid, **cefuroxime axetil** 500 mg po q12h, **cefdinir** 300 mg po q12h or 600 mg po q24h, **cefpodoxime** 200 mg po q12h), **CIP** 750 mg po bid, **Levo** 750 mg po qd, **Diclox** 500 mg po q24h, **Cephalexin** 500 mg po q6h, **AM-CL** 875/125 mg bid, **Doxy** 100 mg bid, **CLINDA** 300-450 mg tid

[6] **AM-CL-ER** 2000/125 mg po q12h, **TMP-SMX-DS** 1-2 tabs po bid, **CIP** 750 mg po bid, **Levo** 750 mg po q24h, **Moxi** 400 mg po q24h, **linezolid** 600 mg po bid.

[7] **Vanco** 1 gm IV q12h, (**parenteral β-lactam/β-lactamase inhibitors: AM-SB** 3 gm IV q6h, **PIP-TZ** 3.375 gm IV q6h or 4.5 gm IV q8h or 4 hr infusion of 3.375 gm q8h; **TC-CL** 3.1 gm IV q6h); **carbapenems: Doripenem** 500 mg IV q8h (1 hr infusion) q8h, **ERTA** 1 gm IV q24h, **IMP** 1 gm IV q6h, **MER** 1 gm IV q8h, **daptomycin** 6 mg per kg IV q24h, **linezolid** 600 mg IV q12h, **aztreonam** 2 gm IV q8h, **CIP** 400 mg IV q12h, **Levo** 750 mg IV q24h, **metro** 1 gm IV loading dose & then 0.5 gm IV q6h or 1 gm IV q12h.

*NOTE: All dosage recommendations are for adults (unless otherwise indicated) and assume normal renal function. § Alternatives consider allergy, PK, compliance, local resistance, cost

TABLE 1 (14)

ANATOMIC SITE/DIAGNOSIS/ MODIFYING CIRCUMSTANCES	ETIOLOGIES (usual)	SUGGESTED REGIMENS*		ADJUNCT DIAGNOSTIC OR THERAPEUTIC MEASURES AND COMMENTS
		PRIMARY	ALTERNATIVE†	
FOOT (continued)				
Onychomycosis: See Table 11, page 121, fungal infections				
Puncture wound: Nail/Toothpick	P. aeruginosa (Nail), S. aureus, Strept (Toothpick)	Cleanse. Tetanus booster. Observe.		See page 4. 1–2% evolve to osteomyelitis.
GALLBLADDER				
Cholecystitis, cholangitis, biliary sepsis, or common duct obstruction (partial): 2° to tumor, stones, stricture). Cholecystitis Ref: NEJM 358:2804, 2008.	Enterobacteriaceae 68%, enterococci 14%, bacteroides 10%, Clostridium sp. 7%, rarely candida	**(PIP-TZ or AM-SB or TC-CL)** If life-threatening: **IMP** or **MER or Dori** Dosages in footnote* on page 16. * Add vanco for empiric activity vs. enterococci	**(P Ceph 3* + metro)** or **(Aztreonam* + metro)** or **(CIP* + metro) or Moxi**	In severely ill pts, antibiotic therapy complements adequate biliary drainage. 15-30% pts will require decompression: surgical, percutaneous or ERCP-placed stent. Gallbladder bile is culture pos in 40-60% (J Infect 51:128, 2005). No benefit to continuation of antibiotics after surgery in pts with acute calculous cholecystitis (JAMA 312:145, 2014).
GASTROINTESTINAL				
Gastroenteritis—Empiric Therapy (laboratory studies not performed or culture, microscopy, toxin results NOT AVAILABLE)				
Premature infant with necrotizing enterocolitis	Associated with intestinal flora	Treatment should cover broad range of intestinal bacteria using drugs appropriate to age and local susceptibility patterns, rationale as in diverticulitis/peritonitis, page 22.		Pneumatosis intestinalis, if present on x-ray confirms diagnosis. Bacteremia-peritonitis in 30-50%. If Staph. epidermidis isolated, add vanco (IV). For review and general management, see NEJM 364:255, 2011.
Mild diarrhea (≤3 unformed stools/day, minimal associated symptomatology).	Bacterial (see Severe, below), viral (norovirus), parasitic. Viral usually causes mild to moderate disease. For traveler's diarrhea, see page 20	Fluids only + lactose-free diet, avoid caffeine		**Rehydration: For po fluid replacement**, see Cholera, page 19. **Antimotility** (Do not use if fever, bloody stools, or suspicion of HUS): Loperamide (Imodium) 4 mg po, then 2 mg after each loose stool to max. of 16 mg per day. Bismuth subsalicylate (Pepto-Bismol) 2 tablets (262 mg) po qid.
Moderate diarrhea (≥4 unformed stools/day &/or systemic symptoms)		Antimotility agents (see Comments) + fluids		**Hemolytic uremic syndrome (HUS):** Risk in **children** infected with E. coli 0157:H7 is 6-9%. Early treatment with TMP-SMX or FQs ↑ risk of HUS.
Severe diarrhea (≥6 unformed stools/day, &/or temp ≥101°F, tenesmus, blood, or fecal leukocytes)	Shigella, salmonella, C. jejuni, Shiga toxin + E. coli, toxin-positive C. difficile, Klebsiella oxytoca, E. histolytica. For typhoid fever, see page 61	**FQ (CIP** 500 mg po q12h or **Levo** 500 mg q24h) times 3-5 days	**TMP-SMX-DS** po bid times 3-5 days. Campylobacter resistance to TMP-SMX common in tropics.	**Norovirus:** Etiology of over 90% of non-bacterial diarrhea (± nausea/vomiting). Lasts 12-60 hrs. Hydrate. No effective antiviral. **Other potential etiologies:** Cryptosporidia—no treatment in immuno-competent host. Cyclospora—usually chronic diarrhea, responds to TMP-SMX (see Table 13A).
NOTE: Severe or febrile bloody diarrhea should ↑ suspicion of Shiga-toxin E. coli 0157:H7 and others (MMWR 58 (RR-12):1, 2009).		If recent antibiotic therapy (C. difficile toxin colitis possible): **Metro** 500 mg po tid times 10-14 days	**Vanco** 125 mg po qid times 10-14 days	Klebsiella oxytoca identified as cause of antibiotic-associated hemorrhagic colitis (cytotoxin positive): NEJM 355:2418, 2006.

Abbreviations on page 2.   *NOTE: All dosage recommendations are for adults (unless otherwise indicated) and assume normal renal function. § Alternatives consider allergy, PK, compliance, local resistance, cost

TABLE 1 (15)

ANATOMIC SITE/DIAGNOSIS/ MODIFYING CIRCUMSTANCES	ETIOLOGIES (usual)	SUGGESTED REGIMENS*		ADJUNCT DIAGNOSTIC OR THERAPEUTIC MEASURES AND COMMENTS
		PRIMARY	ALTERNATIVE§	
GASTROINTESTINAL *(continued)*				
Gastroenteritis—Specific Therapy (results of culture, microscopy, toxin assay AVAILABLE) *(Ref.: NEJM 370:1532, 2014)*				
If culture negative, probably **Norovirus** (Norwalk) other virus *(EID 17:1381, 2011)* — see **NOTE:** WBC > 15,000 suggestive of C. difficile in hospitalized patient. Norovirus, page 166	**Aeromonas/Plesiomonas**	CIP 750 mg po bid x3 days.	TMP-SMX DS tab 1 po bid X 3 days	Although no absolute proof, increasing evidence for Plesiomonas as cause of diarrheal illness *(NEJM 361:1560, 2009)*.
	Amebiasis (Entamoeba histolytica, Cyclospora, Cryptosporidia and Giardia), see *Table 13A*			
	Campylobacter jejuni History of fever in 53-83%. Self-limited diarrhea in normal host.	Azithro 500 mg po q24h x 3 days.	Erytho stearate 500 mg po qid x 5 days or CIP 500 mg po bid (CIP resistance increasing).	**Post-Campylobacter Guillain-Barré;** assoc. 15% of cases *(Lin 366:1653, 2005)*. Assoc. with small bowel lymphoproliferative disease; may respond to antimicrobials *(NEJM 350:239, 2004)*. **Reactive arthritis** another potential sequelae. See *Traveler's diarrhea, page 20*.
	Campylobacter fetus Diarrhea uncommon. More systemic disease in debilitated hosts	Gentamicin (*See Table 10D*)	AMP 100 mg/kg/day IV div q6h or IMP 500 mg IV q6h	Draw blood cultures: in bacteremic pts, 33% of C. fetus resistant to FQs *(CID 47:790, 2008)*. Meropenem inhibits C. fetus at low concentrations in vitro. Clinical review: *CID 56:1579, 2014*.
Differential diagnosis of toxin-producing diarrhea: • C. difficile • Klebsiella oxytoca • S. aureus • Shiga toxin producing E. coli (STEC) • Enterotoxigenic B. fragilis *(CID 47:797, 2008)* More on C. difficile: *Treatment review:* *CID 51:1306, 2010. SHEA/IDSA treatment guidelines: ICHE 31:431, 2010. ESCMID guidelines: Clin Microbiol Infect 15:1067, 2009; AnIM 155:839, 2011.*	**C. difficile** toxin positive antibiotic-associated colitis. po meds okay, WBC <15,000; no increase in serum creatinine.	Metro 500 mg po tid or 250 mg po tid x 10-14 days	**Probiotics** (lactobacillus or saccharomyces) inconsistent results *(AnIM 157:878, 2012; Lancet 382:1249, 2013).* **Vanco** 125 mg po qid x 10-14 days	**D/C antibiotic if possible; avoid antimotility agents, hydration, enteric isolation.** Recent review suggests antimotility agents can be used cautiously in certain pts with mild disease who are receiving rx *(CID 48: 598, 2009)*. **Relapse in 10-20%.**
	Post-treatment relapse			
	po meds okay. Sicker. WBC >15,000; ≥50% increase in baseline creatinine	Vanco 125 mg po qid x 10-14 days. Use IV vanco po. See Table 10A page 100.	Fidaxomicin 200 mg po bid x 10 days	Vanco superior to metro in sicker pts. Relapse in 10-20%. Fidaxomicin had lower rate of recurrence than Vanco for diarrhea with non-NAP1 strains *(N Engl J Med 364:422, 2011).*
	Post-treatment relapse	**1st relapse** Metro 500 mg po tid x 10 days	Teicoplanin^NUS 400 mg po bid x 10 days	**Vanco taper** (all doses 125 mg po): week 1- bid, week 2 - q24h; week 3 - qod, then every 3rd day for 5 doses *(NEJM 359: 1932, 2008)*. Another option: After initial vanco, **rifaximin**^NUS 400-800 mg po daily divided bid or tid x 2 wks.
		2nd relapse Metro 125 mg po qid x 14 days, then immediately start taper *(See Comments)*		**Fecal transplant** more efficacious than vancomycin (15/16 [93%] versus 7/26 [27%]) in curing recurrent C. difficile infection *(New Engl J Med 368:407, 2013).*
	Post-op ileus; severe disease with toxic megacolon *(NEJM 359:1932, 2008)*	Metro 500 mg IV q6h + vanco 500 mg IV q6h via nasogastric tube or naso-small bowel tube) + retrograde via catheter in cecum. See Comments.		For vanco instillation into bowel, add 500 mg vanco to 1 liter of saline and perfuse at 1-3 mL/min to maximum of 2 gm in 24 hrs *(CID 690, 2002)*. **Note: IV vanco not effective.** Indications for colectomy, see *ICHE 31:431, 2010.* Reported successful use of tigecycline^NUS IV to treat severe C. diff refractory to standard rx *(CID 48:1732, 2009).*
				No data on efficacy of Fidaxomicin in severe life-threatening disease.
	Enterohemorrhagic E. coli (EHEC). Some produce Shiga toxin (**STEC**) and cause **hemolytic uremic syndrome (HUS).** Strains: 0157:H7, 0104:H4 and others. Classically bloody diarrhea and afebrile	**Hydration:** avoid antiperistaltic drugs. 25% increased risk of HUS in children given TMP-SMX. Role of antibiotics in age 10-18 given TMP-SMX, beta lactam, metronidazole and azithromycin in STEC-HUS *(CID 55:33, 2012)*. In uncontrolled study, antibiotic treatment of STEC outbreak, shorter excretion of STEC, fewer seizures, lower mortality *(BMJ 345:e565, 2012)*. If on empiric antibiotics, then D/C STEC, reasonable to discontinue antibiotics. Avoid antibiotics in age < 10 yrs with bloody diarrhea. When antibiotics used, azithromycin may be the safest choice *(JAMA 307:1046, 2012).*		• HUS more common in children 1 & 2 in age < 10 yrs; 6-9% overall. • Diagnosis: EIA for Shiga toxins 1 & 2 in stool *(MMWR 58:849-12, 2009).* • Treatment: In vitro and in vivo data, that exposure of STEC to TMP-SMX, beta lactam, or CIP causes burst of Shiga toxin production as bacteria die *(JID 181:664, 2000).* • HUS bad disease: 10% mortality, 50% some degree of permanent renal damage *(CID 38:1298, 2004).*
(Continued on next page)				

Abbreviations on page 2.   *NOTE: All dosage recommendations are for adults (unless otherwise indicated) and assume normal renal function. PK: compliance, local resistance, cost*

§ *Alternatives consider allergy, PK, compliance, local resistance, cost*

TABLE 1 (16)

ANATOMIC SITE/DIAGNOSIS/ MODIFYING CIRCUMSTANCES	ETIOLOGIES (usual)	SUGGESTED REGIMENS* PRIMARY	SUGGESTED REGIMENS* ALTERNATIVE§	ADJUNCT DIAGNOSTIC OR THERAPEUTIC MEASURES AND COMMENTS
GASTROINTESTINAL/Gastroenteritis—Specific Therapy (continued)				
(Continued from previous page)				
	Klebsiella oxytoca— antibiotic-associated diarrhea	Responds to stopping antibiotic		Suggested that stopping NSAIDs helps. Ref.: NEJM 355:2418, 2006.
	Listeria monocytogenes	Usually self-limited. Value of oral antibiotics (e.g., ampicillin or TMP-SMX) unknown, but their use might be reasonable in populations at risk for serious listeria infections. Those with bacteremia/meningitis require parenteral therapy; see pages 9 & 60.		Recognized as a cause of food-associated febrile gastroenteritis. Not detected in standard stool cultures. Populations at † risk of severe systemic disease: pregnant women, neonates, the elderly, and immunocompromised hosts (MMWR 57:1097, 2008).
	Salmonella, non-typhi— For typhoid (enteric) fever, see page 61. Fever in 71–91%, history of bloody stools in 34%	If pt asymptomatic or illness mild, antimicrobial therapy not indicated. **Treat** if age <1 yr or >50 yrs, if immunocompromised, if vascular grafts or prosthetic joints, bacteremic, hemoglobinopathy, or hospitalized with fever and/or severe diarrhea (see typhoid fever, page 61). **CIP 500 mg bid) or (Levo 500 mg q24h) x 7-10 days (14 days if immunocompromised).**	**Azithro 500 mg once daily x 7 days (14 days if immunocompromised).**	†resistance to TMP-SMX and chloro. Ceftriaxone, cefotaxime usually active if IV therapy required (see footnote 11, page 25, for dosage). CLSI has established new interpretive breakpoints for susceptibility to CIP: susceptible strains, MIC < 0.06 μg/mL (Clin Infect Dis 55:1107, 2012). **Primary treatment of enteritis is fluid and electrolyte replacement.**
	Shigella Fever in 58%, history of bloody stools 51%	**CIP 750 mg po bid x 3 days**	**Azithro 500 mg once daily x 3 days**	Recent expert review recommended adult CIP dose of 750 mg po once daily for 3 days (NEJM 361:1560, 2009). Infection due to S. flexneri resistant to CIP, ceftriaxone and cefotaxime has been reported (MMWR 59:1619, 2010). CIP superior to ceftriaxone in children (JJ/D 3:537, 2003).
		Peds doses: Azithro 10 mg/kg/day once daily x 3 days. For severe disease, ceftriaxone 50–75 mg/kg per day x 2–5 days. CIP suspension 10 mg/kg bid x 5 days.		**Immunocompromised children & adults: Treat for 7-10 days.** Azithro superior to cefixime in trial in children (LnID 9:37, 2009).
	Spirochetosis (Brachyspira pilosicoli)	Benefit of treatment unclear. Susceptible to **metro, ceftriaxone** and **Moxi**.		Anaerobic intestinal spirochete that colonizes colon of domestic & wild animals plus humans. Called enigmatic disease due to uncertain status (Digest Dis & Sci 58:202, 2013).
	Vibrio cholerae Treatment decreases volume losses & duration of excretion	**Primary therapy is rehydration.** Select antibiotics based on susceptibility of locally prevailing isolates. Options include: **Doxycycline** 300 mg po single dose **OR Azithromycin** 1 gm po single dose **OR Tetracycline** 500 mg po qid x 3 days **OR Erythromycin** 500 mg po qid x 3 days.	**For pregnant women: Azithromycin** 1 gm po single dose **OR Erythromycin** 500 mg po qid x 3 days **For children: Azithromycin** 20 mg/kg po as single dose; for other age-specific alternatives, see CDC website http://www.cdc.gov/haiticholera/haiti.htm	**Antimicrobial therapy shortens duration of illness, but rehydration is paramount.** When IV hydration is needed, use Ringer's lactate. Switch to PO repletion with Oral Rehydration Salts (ORS) as soon as able to take oral fluids. ORS are commercially available for reconstitution in potable water. If not available, WHO suggests a substitute can be made by dissolving ½ teaspoon salt and 6 level teaspoons of sugar per liter of potable water (http://www.who.int/cholera/technical/en/). CDC recommendations for other aspects of management developed for Haiti outbreak can be found at http://www.cdc.gov/haiticholera/hcp_gongtohaiti.htm. Isolates from this outbreak demonstrate reduced susceptibility to ciprofloxacin and resistance to sulfisoxazole, nalidixic acid and furazolidone.

§ Alternatives consider allergy, PK, compliance, local resistance, cost

*NOTE: All dosage recommendations are for adults (unless otherwise indicated) and assume normal renal function.

TABLE 1 (17)

ANATOMIC SITE/DIAGNOSIS/ MODIFYING CIRCUMSTANCES	ETIOLOGIES* (usual)	SUGGESTED REGIMENS*		ADJUNCT DIAGNOSTIC OR THERAPEUTIC MEASURES AND COMMENTS
		PRIMARY	ALTERNATIVE†	
GASTROINTESTINAL/Gastroenteritis—Specific Therapy *(continued)*				
	Vibrio parahaemolyticus	Antimicrobial rx does not shorten course. Hydration.		Shellfish exposure common. Treat severe disease: **FQ, doxy, P Ceph 3**.
	Vibrio vulnificus	Usual presentation is skin lesions & bacteremia; life-threatening; treat early: **ceftaz + doxy**—see page 54; *Levo or CIP + ceftaz or cefotaxime. Ref: Epidemiol Infect. 142:878, 2014.*		
	Yersinia enterocolitica Fever in 68%, bloody stools in 26%	No treatment unless severe. If severe, combine **doxy** 100 mg IV bid + (**tobra** or **gent** 5 mg/kg per day once q24h). **TMP-SMX** or **FQs** are alternatives.		Mesenteric adenitis pain can mimic acute appendicitis. Lab diagnosis difficult: requires "cold enrichment" and/or yersinia selective agar. Desferrioxamine therapy increases severity; discontinue if pt on it. Iron overload states predispose to yersinia.
Gastroenteritis—Specific Risk Groups—Empiric Therapy				
Anoreceptive intercourse	Herpes viruses, gonococci, chlamydia, syphilis. *See Genital Tract, page 22*			
Proctitis (distal 15 cm only)				
Colitis	Shigella, salmonella, campylobacter, E. histolytica *(see Table 13A)*			*See Specific GI pathogens, Gastroenteritis, above.*
HIV-1 infected (AIDS): >10 days diarrhea	G. lamblia			
	Acid fast: Cryptosporidium parvum, Cyclospora cayetanensis			See Table 13A
	Other: Isospora belli, microsporidia (Enterocytozoon bieneusi, Septata intestinalis)			
Neutropenic enterocolitis or "typhlitis" *(CID 56:711, 2013)*	Mucosal invasion by Clostridium septicum. Occasionally caused by C. sordellii or P. aeruginosa	Appropriate agents include PIP-TZ, IMP, MER, DORI plus bowel rest.		Tender right lower quadrant may be clue, but may be diffuse or absent in immunocompromised. Need surgical consult. Surgical resection controversial but may be necessary. **NOTE:** Resistance of clostridia to clindamycin reported. PIP-TZ, IMP, MER, DORI should cover most pathogens.
Traveler's diarrhea. self-medication. Patient often afebrile	**Acute:** 60% due to diarrheagenic E. coli; shigella, salmonella, campylobacter, C. difficile, amebiasis *(see Table 13A).* **If chronic:** cyclospora, cryptosporidia, giardia, isospora	**CIP** 750 mg po bid for 1-3 days **OR Levo** 500 mg po q24h for 1-3 days **OR Oflox** 300 mg po bid for 3 days **OR Rifaximin** 200 mg po tid for 3 days **OR Azithro** 1000 mg po once or 500 mg po q24h for 3 days OR Ceftriaxone 10 mg/kg/day as a single dose for 3 days. Avoid FQs. **For pediatrics:** Azithro 10 mg/kg/day as a single dose for 3 days or Ceftriaxone 50 mg/kg/day as single dose for 3 days. Avoid FQs. **For pregnancy:** Use Azithro. Avoid FQs.		**Antimotility agent:** For non-pregnant adults with no fever or blood in stool, add loperamide 4 mg po x 1, then 2 mg po after each loose stool to a maximum of 16 mg per day. **Comments:** Rifaximin approved only for ages 12 and older. Works only for diarrhea due to non-invasive E. coli; do not use if fever or bloody stool. **References:** NEJM 361:1560, 2009; BMJ 337: a1746, 2008; http://wwwnc.cdc.gov/travel/yellowbook/2012/chapter-2-the-pre-travel-consultation/travelers-diarrhea.htm.
Prevention of Traveler's diarrhea	Not routinely indicated. Current recommendation is to take **FQ + Imodium** with 1° loose stool.			

Abbreviations on page 2.   *NOTE: All dosage recommendations are for adults (unless otherwise indicated) and assume normal renal function. †Alternatives consider allergy; PK, compliance, local resistance, cost

TABLE 1 (18)

ANATOMIC SITE/DIAGNOSIS/ MODIFYING CIRCUMSTANCES	ETIOLOGIES (usual)	SUGGESTED REGIMENS*		ADJUNCT DIAGNOSTIC OR THERAPEUTIC MEASURES AND COMMENTS
		PRIMARY	ALTERNATIVE[†]	
GASTROINTESTINAL (continued)				
Gastrointestinal Infections by Anatomic Site: Esophagus to Rectum				
Esophagitis	Candida albicans, HSV, CMV	See SANFORD GUIDE TO HIV/AIDS THERAPY and Table 11A.		
Duodenal/Gastric ulcer; gastric cancer, MALT lymphomas (not 2°NSAIDs) Ref: Gut 61:646, 2012; Med Lett 9:55, 2012.	**Helicobacter pylori** See Comment Prevalence of pre-treatment resistance increasing	**Sequential therapy:** **Rabeprazole** 20 mg + **amox** 1 gm) bid x 5 days, then: (**rabeprazole** 20 mg + **clarithro** 500 mg + **tinidazole** 500 mg) bid for another 5 days. See footnote[a]. Can modify by substituting Levo for Clarithro (JAMA 309:578, 2013; Ln 381:205, 2013).	**Quadruple therapy (10-14 days):** Bismuth (see footnote[b]), bismuth subsalicylate 2 tabs qid + tetracycline 500 mg qid + **metro** 500 mg bid + **omeprazole** 20 mg bid.	**Comment:** In many locations, 20% failure rates with previously recommended **triple** regimens (**PPI + Amox + Clarithro**) are not acceptable. With 10 days of quadruple therapy (**omeprazole** 20 mg po twice daily) + (3 capsules po four times per day, each containing **Bismuth subcitrate potassium** 140 mg + **Metro** 125 mg + **Tetracycline** 125 mg)), eradication rates were 93% in a per protocol population and 80% in an intention-to-treat population, both significantly better than with 7-day triple therapy regimen (PPI + Amox + Clarithro) (Lancet 377:905, 2011). Exercise caution regarding potential interactions with other drugs. contraindications in pregnancy and warnings for other special populations. **Dx: Stool antigen**—Monoclonal EIA >90% sens. & 92% specific. Other tests: if endoscoped, rapid urease &/or histology &/or culture; urea breath test, but some office-based tests underperform. Testing ref: BMJ 344:44, 2012. **Test of cure:** Repeat stool antigen and/or urea breath test >8 wks post-treatment. **Treatment outcome:** Failure rate of triple therapy 20%.
		100% compliance/94% eradication rate reported: (**Pantoprazole** 40 mg + **Clarithro** 500 mg + **Amox** 1000 mg + **Metro** 500 mg) po bid x 7 d (AAC 58:5936, 2014).		In vitro susceptibility testing and collected clinical experience (JAC 69:219, 2014). In vitro resistance to TMP-SMX plus frequent clinical failures & relapses. Frequent in vitro resistance to carbapenems. Complete in vitro resistance to Ceftriaxone.
Small intestine: Whipple's disease (NEJM 356:55, 2007; LnID 8:179, 2008) Treatment: (AAC 69:219, 2014. See Infective endocarditis, culture-negative, page 30.	Tropheryma whipplei	(**Doxycycline** 100 mg po bid + **Hydroxychloroquine** 200 mg po(t id) x 1 year; then **Doxycycline** 100 mg po bid for life Immune reconstitution inflammatory response (IRIS) reactions occur. Thalidomide therapy may be better than steroids for IRIS reaction (J Infect 60:79, 2010)		

[*] Can substitute other proton pump inhibitors for omeprazole or rabeprazole–all bid: **esomeprazole** 20 mg (FDA-approved), **lanzoprazole** 30 mg (FDA-approved), **pantoprazole** 40 mg (not FDA-approved for this indication).

[a] **Bismuth preparations:** (1) In U.S., **bismuth subsalicylate (Pepto-Bismol)** 262 mg/tabs; adult dose for helicobacter is 2 tabs (524 mg). qid. (2) Outside U.S., colloidal bismuth subcitrate (De-Nol) 120 mg chewable tablets; dose is 1 tablet qid. In the U.S. bismuth subcitrate is available in combination cap only (Pylera: each cap contains bismuth subcitrate 140 mg + Metro 125 mg + Tetracycline 125 mg), given as 3 caps po 4x daily for 10 days **together with** a twice daily PPI.

[b] *NOTE: All dosage recommendations are for adults (unless otherwise indicated) and assume normal renal function. PK, compliance, local resistance, cost*

Abbreviations on page 2. *NOTE: All dosage recommendations are for adults (unless otherwise indicated) and assume normal renal function. § Alternatives consider allergy; PK, compliance, local resistance, cost*

TABLE 1 (19)

ANATOMIC SITE/DIAGNOSIS/ MODIFYING CIRCUMSTANCES	ETIOLOGIES (usual)	SUGGESTED REGIMENS* PRIMARY	SUGGESTED REGIMENS* ALTERNATIVE¹	ADJUNCT DIAGNOSTIC OR THERAPEUTIC MEASURES AND COMMENTS

GASTROINTESTINAL/Gastrointestinal Infections by Anatomic Site: Esophagus to Rectum *(continued)*

Diverticulitis, perirectal abscess. Peritonitis Also see *Peritonitis, page 47*	Enterobacteriaceae, occasionally P. aeruginosa, Bacteroides sp., enterococci	**Outpatient rx—mild diverticulitis, drained perirectal abscess:** [**TMP-SMX-DS** bid **or** (**CIP** 750 mg bid **or Levo** 750 mg q24h)] + **metro** 500 mg q6h. All po x 7–10 days. **Mild-moderate disease—Inpatient—Parenteral Rx:** (e.g., focal periappendiceal peritonitis, periverticular abscess, endomyometritis) **PIP-TZ** 3.375 gm IV q6h **or** 4.5 gm IV q8h **or TC-CL** 3.1 gm IV q6h **or ERTA** 1 gm IV q24h **or MOXI** 400 mg IV q24h. **Severe life-threatening disease, ICU patient:** **IMP** 500 mg IV q6h **or MER** 1 gm IV q8h **or Dori** 500 mg q8h (1-hr infusion). **Severe penicillin/cephalosporin allergy: aztreonam** 2 gm IV q6h (to q8h) [**metro** (500 mg q6h) or (1 gm IV q12h) **OR** [(**CIP** 400 mg IV q12h or (**Levo** 750 mg IV q24h) + **metro**].	[**AM-CL-ER** 1000/62.5 mg 2 tabs po bid x 7–10 days **OR Moxi** 400 mg po q24h x 7–10 days] [(**CIP** 400 mg IV q12h) or **Levo** 750 mg IV q24h)] + (**metro** 500 mg IV q6h or 1 gm IV q12h) **OR Moxi** 400 mg IV q24h. **AMP + metro + CIP** 400 mg IV q12h **or Levo** 750 mg IV q24h) **OR** [**AMP** 2 gm IV q6h + **metro** 500 mg + **aminoglycoside¹⁰** (see *Table 10D, page 110*)]	Must "cover" both Gm-neg, aerobic & Gm-neg, anaerobic bacteria. **Drugs active only vs. anaerobic Gm-neg. bacilli:** clinda, metro. **Drugs active only vs. aerobic Gm-neg. bacilli:** APAG, P. Ceph 2/3/4 (see *Table 10A, page 96*), aztreonam, APAG, CIP. **Drugs active vs. both aerobic/anaerobic Gm-neg. bacteria:** cefoxitin cefotetan, TC-CL, PIP-TZ, AM-SB, ERTA, Dori, IMP, MER, Moxi, & tigecycline. **Increasing resistance of B. fragilis group**
					Moxi	Cefoxitin	Cefotetan		Clindamycin	42–80	34–45	19–35	% Resistant:	42–80	34–45	48–60	19–35
				Ref: Anaerobe 17:147, 2011; AAC 56:1247, 2012; Surg Infect 10:111, 2009. **Resistance (B. fragilis):** Metro, PIP-TZ rare. Resistance to FQ increased in enteric bacteria, particularly if any FQ used recently. **Ertapenem** poorly active vs. P. aeruginosa/Acinetobacter sp. **Concomitant surgical treatment important,** esp. with moderate-severe disease. **Role of enterococci remains debatable.** Probably pathogenic in infections of biliary tract. Probably need drugs active vs. enterococci in pts with valvular heart disease. **Tigecycline: Black Box Warning:** All cause mortality higher in pts treated with tigecycline (2.5%) than comparators (1.8%) in meta-analysis of clinical trials. Cause of mortality risk difference of 0.6% (95% CI 0.1, 1.2) not established. Tigecycline should be reserved for use in situations when alternative treatments are not suitable *(FDA MedWatch Sep 27, 2013)*

GENITAL TRACT: Mixture of empiric & specific treatment. Divided by sex of the patient. For sexual assault (rape), see *Table 15A, page 192 & MMWR 59 (RR-12), 2010.* **See Guidelines for Dx of Sexually Transmitted Diseases,** *MMWR 59 (RR-12), 2010 www.cdc.gov/std/treatment.*

Both Women & Men:				
Chancroid	H. ducreyi	**Ceftriaxone** 250 mg IM single dose **OR azithro** 1 gm po single dose	**CIP** 500 mg bid po x 3 days **OR erythro base** 500 mg qid po x 7 days.	In HIV+ pts, failures reported with single dose azithro *(CID 21:409, 1995).* Evaluate after 7 days, ulcer should objectively improve. Symptoms improve in 7 days. All patients treated for chancroid should be tested for HIV and syphilis. All sex partners of pts with chancroid should be examined and treated if they have evidence of disease or have had sex with index pt within the last 10 days.

---

¹⁰ **Aminoglycoside = antipseudomonal aminoglycoside, e.g., amikacin, gentamicin, tobramycin**

Abbreviations on page 2.   *NOTE: All dosage recommendations are for adults (unless otherwise indicated) and assume normal renal function. § Alternatives consider allergy, PK, compliance, local resistance, cost*

TABLE 1 (20)

ANATOMIC SITE/DIAGNOSIS/ MODIFYING CIRCUMSTANCES	ETIOLOGIES (usual)	SUGGESTED REGIMENS*		ADJUNCT DIAGNOSTIC OR THERAPEUTIC MEASURES AND COMMENTS
		PRIMARY	ALTERNATIVE[1]	
GENITAL TRACT/Both Women & Men (continued)				
Chlamydia, et al, non-gono-coccal or post-gonococcal urethritis, cervicitis NOTE: **Assume concomitant** Chlamydia conjunctivitis, see page 12.	Chlamydia 50%, Mycoplasma genitalium (30%). Other known etiologies (10–15%): trichomonas, herpes simplex virus, see JID 206:357, 2012.	**(Doxy** 100 mg bid po x 7 days) **or azithro** 1 gm po as single dose). Evaluate & treat sex partner. **In pregnancy: Azithromycin** 1 gm po single dose **OR amox** 500 mg po tid x 7 days.	**Erythro base** 500 mg po x 7 days) **or** (**Ofloxacin** 300 mg po bid x7 days) or **Levo** 500 mg po q24h x 7 days. **In pregnancy: Erythro base** 500 mg po qid for 7 days **Doxy & FQs contraindicated**	**Diagnosis:** NAAT for C. trachomatis & N. gonorrhoeae on urine or cervix or urethral specimens (AnIM 142:914, 2005). Test all urethritis/cervicitis pts for HIV & syphilis. **For proctitis:** prefer **doxy** x 7d (Sex Trans Dis H, 2014). Evaluate & treat sex partners. Azithromycin 1 gm was superior to doxycycline for chlamydia & N. genitalium male urethritis (CID 48:1649, 2009), but may select resistance leading to ↑ failure of multi-dose azithromycin retreatment regimens (CID 48:1655, 2009).
Recurrent/persistent urethritis	C. trachomatis (43%), M. genitalium (30%), T. vaginalis (13%) (CID 52:163, 2011).	**Metro** 2 gm po X 1 dose + Azithro 1 gm po X 1 dose	**Tinidazole** 2 gm po X 1 + **Azithromycin** 1 gm po X 1	High failure rate of M. genitalium (CID 56:934, 2013). Can try **Moxi** 400 mg po once daily x 10 days if Azithro failure (PLoS One 3:e3618, 2008). New FQ resistance in Japan (JAC 69:2376, 2014).
Gonorrhea (MMWR 59 (RR-12): 49, 2010). FQs no longer recommended for treatment of gonococcal infections (MMWR 59 (RR-12):49, 2010). **Cephalosporin resistance:** JAMA 309:163 & 185, 2013.				
Conjunctivitis (adult)	N. gonorrhoeae	**Ceftriaxone** 1 gm IM x1 dose		Consider one-time saline lavage of eye.
Disseminated gonococcal infection (DGI, dermatitis-arthritis syndrome)	N. gonorrhoeae	**Ceftriaxone** 1 gm IV q24h— see Comment	**Cefotaxime** 1 gm IV q8h IV) or (**Ceftizoxime** 1 gm IV q8h IV) —see Comment. FQs may be effective if susceptible organism.	Continue IM or IV regimen for 24hr after symptoms ↓, Owing to high-level resistance to oral cephalosporins and fluoroquinolones in the community, "Step-down" therapy should be avoided unless susceptibilities are known and demonstrate full activity of cephalosporin or fluoroquinolone R/O meningitis/ endocarditis. **Treat presumptively for concomitant C. trachomatis.** Ref. JID 157:1281, 1988.
Endocarditis Dx: NAAT	N. gonorrhoeae	**Ceftriaxone** 1–2 gm IV q24h x 4 wks	Due to resistance concerns, **do not use FQs**	Pharyngeal GC more difficult to eradicate. Some suggest test of cure culture after 1 wk. **Spectinomycin[NUS], cefixime, cefpodoxime & cefuroxime not effective**
Pharyngitis	N. gonorrhoeae	**Ceftriaxone** 250 mg IM x1 PLUS (**Azithro** 1 gm po x 1) or **doxy** 100 mg po bid x 7 days]		Screen for syphilis.
Urethritis, cervicitis, proctitis (uncomplicated) For prostatitis, see page 27. **Diagnosis:** Nucleic acid amplification test (NAAT) on vaginal swab, urine or urethra. Resistance in MSM (MMWR 62:103, 2013; AnIM 158:321, 2013).	N. gonorrhoeae (50% of pts with urethritis, cervicitis have concomitant C. trachomatis—**treat for both unless NAAT indicates single pathogen)** greatest in MSM	[(**Ceftriaxone** 250 mg IM x1) + (**doxy** 100 mg po bid x 7 days)]. Add **Azithro** or **Doxy** even if chlamydia ruled out. **Alternative: Azithro** 2 gm po x 1. Severe PenI/Ceph allergy: (**Gem** 240 mg IM + **Azithro** 2 gm po) x 1 dose OR (**Gemi** 320 mg + **Azithro** 2 gm) po x 1 dose (CID 59:1083, 2014)(nausea in >20%)	**Other alternatives for GC (Test of Cure recommended one week after Rx for ALL of these regimens listed below):** • **Cefixime** 400 mg po x1 OR **Cefpodoxime** 400 mg po x 1 (Note: not effective for pharyngeal disease); oral cephalosporin use is no longer recommended due to emergence of resistance. MMWR 61:590, 2012. • Other single-dose cephalosporins: ceftizoxime 500 mg IM, cefotaxime 500 mg IM, cefoxitin 2 gm IM + probenecid 1 gm po. • **Azithro** 1 gm x 1 effective for chlamydia but need 2 gm for GC; not recommended for GC due to GI side-effects, expense & rapid emergence of resistance
Granuloma inguinale (Donovanosis)	Klebsiella (formerly Calymmatobacterium) granulomatis	**Doxy** 100 mg po bid x 3–4 wks	**TMP-SMX** one DS tablet po x 3 wks **OR** Erythro 500 mg po qid x 3 wks **OR** CIP 750 mg po bid x 3 wks **OR** Azithro 1 gm p.o q.wk x 3 wks	Clinical response usually seen in 1 wk. **Rx until all lesions healed**, may take 4 wks. Treatment failures & recurrence seen with doxy & TMP-SMX. Report of efficacy with FQ and chloro. Ref.: CID 25:24, 1997. Relapse can occur 6-18 months after apparently effective Rx. ↑ improvement with evidence in first few days; some experts add gentamicin 1 mg/kg IV q8h.

Abbreviations on page 2.   *NOTE: All dosage recommendations are for adults (unless otherwise indicated) and assume normal renal function.   § Alternatives consider allergy, PK, compliance, local resistance, cost

TABLE 1 (21)

ANATOMIC SITE/DIAGNOSIS/ MODIFYING CIRCUMSTANCES	ETIOLOGIES (usual)	SUGGESTED REGIMENS* PRIMARY	ALTERNATIVE§	ADJUNCT DIAGNOSTIC OR THERAPEUTIC MEASURES AND COMMENTS
GENITAL TRACT/Both Women & Men (continued)				
Herpes simplex virus	See Table 14A, page 161			
Human papilloma virus (HPV)	See Table 14A, page 166			
Lymphogranuloma venereum	Chlamydia trachomatis, serovars: L1, L2, L3	**Doxy** 100 mg po bid x 21 days	**Erythro** 0.5 gm po qid x 21 days or **Azithro** 1 gm po qwk X 3 weeks (clinical data lacking)	Dx based on serology; biopsy contraindicated because sinus tracts develop. Nucleic acid ampli tests for C. trachomatis will be positive. In MSM, presents as fever, rectal ulcer, anal discharge (CID 39:996, 2004; Dis Colon Rectum 52:507, 2009).
Phthirus pubis (**pubic lice, "crabs"**) & scabies	Phthirus pubis & Sarcoptes scabiei	See Table 13A, page 153		
Syphilis Diagnosis: JAMA 312:1922, 2014; treatment: JAMA 312:1905, 2014 **Early**: primary, secondary, or latent (<1 yr). Screen with treponema-specific antibody or RPR/VDRL, see JCM 50:2 & 148, 2012; CID 58:1116, 2014. NOTE: Test all pts with syphilis for HIV; test all HIV patients for latent syphilis.	T. pallidum	**Benzathine pen G (Bicillin L-A)** 2.4 million units IM x 1 or **Azithro** 2 gm po x 1 dose (See Comment)	**Doxy** 100 mg po bid x 14 days) or **tetracycline** 500 mg po qid x 14 days) or **ceftriaxone** 1 gm IM/IV q24h x 10-14 days). Follow-up mandatory.	If early or congenital syphilis, **quantitative VDRL at 0, 3, 6, 12 & 24 mos** after rx. If 1° or 2° syphilis, VDRL should ↓ 2 tubes at 6 mos, 3 tubes 12 mos, & 4 tubes 24 mos. Update on congenital syphilis (MMWR 59:413, 2010). Early latent: 2 tubes ↓ at 12 mos. With 1°, 50% will be RPR seronegative at 12 mos, 24% neg. FTA/ABS at 2-3 yrs. (AnIM 114:1005, 1991). If fail to fall, consider CSF; if CSF (+), treat as neurosyphilis; if CSF is negative, retreat with benzathine Pen G 2.4 mu IM weekly x 3 wks. If no other options: **Azithro** 2 gm po x 1 dose (equivalent to **benzathine Pen G** 2.4 mu x 1 dose in early syphilis (J Infect Dis 201:1729, 2010). **Azithro-resistant syphilis** documented in California, Ireland, & elsewhere (CID 44:S130, 2007; AAC 54:583, 2010).
More than 1 yr's duration (Early: of later secondary duration, cardiovascular, late benign gumma)	For penicillin desensitization method, see Table 7, page 80 and MMWR 59 (RR-12); 26, 2010. NOTE: Test all pts with syphilis for HIV; test all HIV patients for latent syphilis.	**Benzathine pen G (Bicillin L-A)** 2.4 million units IM q week X 3 = 7.2 million units total	**Doxy** 100 mg po bid x 28 days) or **tetracycline** 500 mg po qid x 28 days; **Ceftriaxone** 2 gm IM daily for 10-14 days MAY be an alternative. (No clinical data, consult an ID specialist)	NOTE: Use of benzathine procaine penicillin is inappropriate! No published data on efficacy of alternatives. **Indications for LP (CDC): neurologic symptoms, treatment failure, any eye or ear involvement, other evidence of active syphilis (aortitis, gumma, iritis).**
Neurosyphilis—Very difficult to treat. Includes ocular (retrobulbar neuritis) syphilis. **Alt need CSF exam.** CID 44:S130, 2007.		**Pen G** 18-24 million units per day either as continuous infusion or as 3-4 million units IV q4h x 10-14 days.	(**Procaine pen G** 2.4 million units IM q24h + **probenecid** 0.5 gm po qid) both x 10-14 days—See Comment	**Ceftriaxone** 2 gm (IV or IM) q24h x 14 days. 23% failure rate reported (AJM 93:481, 1992). For penicillin allergy: either desensitize to penicillin or obtain infectious diseases consultation. **Serologic criteria for response to rx: 4-fold or greater ↓ in VDRL titer over 6-12 mos.** (CID 28 (Suppl. 1):S21, 1999).
HIV infection (AIDS) CID 44:S130, 2007.	Treatment same as HIV uninfected with closer follow-up. Treat early neurosyphilis regardless of CD4 count. MMWR 56:625, 2007.			See Syphilis discussion in MMWR 59 (RR-12), 2010. Treat for neurosyphilis if CSF VDRL negative but >20 CSF WBCs (STD 39:291, 2012).
Pregnancy and syphilis	Same as for non-pregnant, some recommend 2nd dose benzathine pen G 1 wk after initial dose esp. in 3rd trimester or with 2° syphilis		Skin test for penicillin allergy. Desensitize if necessary. Parenteral pen G is only therapy with documented efficacy	Monthly quantitative VDRL or equivalent. If 4-fold ↑, re-treat. Doxy, tetracycline contraindicated. Erythro not recommended because of high risk of failure to cure fetus.

Abbreviations on page 2.

*NOTE: All dosage recommendations are for adults (unless otherwise indicated) and assume normal renal function. § Alternatives consider allergy, PK, compliance, local resistance, cost

TABLE 1 (22)

ANATOMIC SITE/DIAGNOSIS/ MODIFYING CIRCUMSTANCES	ETIOLOGIES (usual)	SUGGESTED REGIMENS* PRIMARY	SUGGESTED REGIMENS* ALTERNATIVE[1]	ADJUNCT DIAGNOSTIC OR THERAPEUTIC MEASURES AND COMMENTS
GENITAL TRACT/Both Women & Men (continued)				
Congenital syphilis: (Update on Congenital Syphilis: MMWR 59 (RR-12): 36, 2010)	T. pallidum	**Aqueous crystalline pen G** 50,000 units/kg per dose IV q12h x 7 days, then q8h for 10 days total.	**Procaine pen G** 50,000 units/kg IM q24h for 10 days	Another alternative: Ceftriaxone ≤30 days old, 75 mg/kg IV/IM q24h (use with caution in infants with jaundice); or > 30 days old 100 mg/kg IV/IM q24h. Treat 10-14 days. If symptomatic, ophthalmologic exam indicated. If more than 1 day of rx missed, restart entire course. **Need serologic follow-up!**
Warts, anogenital	See Table 14A, page 166			
Women:				
Amnionitis, septic abortion	Bacteroides, esp. Prevotella bivius; Group B, A strepto-cocci; Enterobacteriaceae; C. trachomatis	[(Cefoxitin or TC-CL or Dori[NAI] or IMP or MER or AM-SB or ERTA or PIP-TZ) + doxy] OR [Clinda + (aminoglycoside or ceftriaxone)] **Note:** in US and Europe, 1/3 of Grp B Strep resistant to clindamycin.		D&C of uterus. In septic abortion, Clostridium perfringens may cause fulminant intravascular hemolysis. In postpartum patients with enigmatic fever and/or pulmonary emboli, consider septic pelvic vein thrombophlebitis (see Vascular, septic pelvic vein thrombophlebitis, page 67). After discharge: doxy or clinda for C. trachomatis.
				Criteria for diagnosis: 1) (muco) purulent endocervical exudate and/or 2) sustained endocervical bleeding after passage of cotton swab. >10 WBC/hpf of vaginal fluid is suggestive. Intracellular gram-neg diplococci are specific but insensitive. If in doubt, send swab or urine for culture, EIA or nucleic acid amplification test and treat for both.
Cervicitis, mucopurulent Treatment based on results of nucleic acid amplification test	N. gonorrhoeae Chlamydia trachomatis	Treat for Gonorrhea, page 23 Treat for non-gonococcal urethritis, page 23		
Endomyometritis/septic pelvic phlebitis				
Early postpartum (1st 48 hrs) (usually after C-section)	Bacteroides, esp. Prevotella bivius; Group B, A strepto-cocci; Enterobacteriaceae; C. trachomatis	[(Cefoxitin or TC-CL or ERTA or IMP or MER or AM-SB or PIP-TZ) + doxy] OR [Clinda + (aminoglycoside, see footnote[1]]		See Comments under Amnionitis, septic abortion, above
Late postpartum (48 hrs to 6 wks) (usually after vaginal delivery)	Chlamydia trachomatis, M. hominis	**Doxy** 100 mg IV or po q12h times 14 days		Tetracyclines not recommended in nursing mothers; discontinue nursing. M. hominis sensitive to tetra, clinda, not erythro.
Fitzhugh-Curtis syndrome	C. trachomatis, N. gonorrhoeae	Treat as for pelvic inflammatory disease immediately below.		Perihepatitis (violin-string adhesions). Sudden onset of RUQ pain. Associated with salpingitis. Transaminases elevated in < 30% of cases.
Pelvic actinomycosis; usually tubo-ovarian abscess	A. israelii most common	**AMP** 50 mg/kg/day IV div 3-4 doses x 4-6 wks, then **Pen VK** 2-4 gm/day po x 3-6 mos.	**Doxy** or **ceftriaxone** or **clinda.**	Complication of intrauterine device (IUD). Remove IUD. Can use Pen G 10-20 million units/day x 4-6 wks.

---

[1] **P Ceph 2 (cefotetan** 2 gm IV q6-8h; **cefotetan** 2 gm IV q12h; **cefuroxime** 2 gm IV q8h); **TC-CL** 3.1 gm IV q4-6h; **AM-SB** 3 gm IV q6h; **PIP-TZ** 3.375 gm q6h or for nosocomial pneumonia: 4.5 gm IV q6h or 4-hr infusion of 3.375 gm q8h; **doxy** 100 mg IV/po q12h; **clinda** 450-900 mg IV q8h; **aminoglycoside (gentamicin,** see Table 10D, page 110); **P Ceph 3 (cefotaxime** 2 gm IV q8h; **ceftriaxone** 2 gm IV q24h); **ertapenem** 500 mg IV q8h (1-hr infusion); **ertapenem** 1 gm IV q24h; **IMP** 0.5 gm IV q6h; **MER** 1 gm IV q8h; **azithro** 500 mg IV q24h; **linezolid** 600 mg IV/po q12h; **vanco** 1 gm IV q12h 2 gm IV q24h); **doripenem** 500 mg IV q8h (1-hr infusion); **azithro** 600 mg IV q24h and assume normal renal function. § Alternatives consider allergy, PK compliance, local resistance, cost

Abbreviations on page 2. *NOTE: All dosage recommendations are for adults (unless otherwise indicated) and assume normal renal function. § Alternatives consider allergy, PK compliance, local resistance, cost

TABLE 1 (23)

ANATOMIC SITE/DIAGNOSIS/ MODIFYING CIRCUMSTANCES	ETIOLOGIES (usual)	SUGGESTED REGIMENS* PRIMARY	ALTERNATIVE†	ADJUNCT DIAGNOSTIC OR THERAPEUTIC MEASURES AND COMMENTS
GENITAL TRACT/Women (continued)				
Pelvic Inflammatory Disease (PID), salpingitis, tubo-ovarian abscess Outpatient rx; limit to pts with temp <38°C, WBC <11,000 per mm³, minimal evidence of peritonitis, active bowel sounds & able to tolerate oral nourishment CID 44:953 & 961, 2007; MMWR 59 (RR-12):63, 2010 & www.cdc.gov/std/treatment	N. gonorrhoeae, chlamydia, bacteroides, Enterobacteriaceae, streptococci, especially S. agalactiae. Less commonly: G. vaginalis, Haemophilus influenzae, cytomegalovirus (CMV), M. genitalium, U. urealyticum	**Outpatient rx:** [(**ceftriaxone** 250 mg IM x 1) or (**cefoxitin** 2 gm IM with **probenecid** 1 gm po both as single dose) plus (**doxy** 100 mg po bid x 14 days)], **OR** **cefoxitin** 2 gm IM with **probenecid** 1 gm po both as single dose) plus (**doxy** 100 mg po bid x 14 days)	**Inpatient regimens:** [(**Cefotetan** 2 gm IV q12h or **cefoxitin** 2 gm IV q6h) + **doxy** 100 mg IV/po q12h] (**Clinda** 900 mg IV q8h) + **gentamicin** 2 mg/kg loading dose, then 1.5 mg/kg q8h or 4.5 mg/kg once per day), then **doxy** 100 mg po bid x 14 days	Another alternative parenteral regimen: **AM-SB** 3 gm IV q6h + **doxy** 100 mg IV/po q12h Remember: Evaluate and treat sex partner. FQs not recommended due to increasing resistance (MMWR 59 (RR-12), 2010 & www.cdc.gov/std/treatment). Suggest initial inpatient evaluation/therapy for pts with tubo-ovarian abscess. For inpatient regimens, continue treatment until satisfactory response for ≥24-hr before switching to outpatient regimen. Improved routine testing for chlamydia and N. gonorrhea among outpatients resulted in reduced hospitalization and ectopic pregnancy rates (J Adolescent Health 51:80, 2012)
Vaginitis—MMWR 59 (RR-12):63, 2010				
Candidiasis Pruritus, thick cheesy discharge, pH 4.5 See Table 11A, page 117	Candida albicans 80–90%. C. glabrata, C. tropicalis may be particularly—they are less susceptible to azoles	**Oral azoles: Fluconazole** 150 mg po x 1; **itraconazole** 200 mg po x 1 day or 200 mg po x 1 day. For milder cases, topical therapy with one of the over the counter preparations usually is successful (e.g., clotrimazole, butoconazole, miconazole, or tioconazole) as creams or vaginal suppositories.	**Intravaginal azoles:** variety of strengths—from 1 dose to 14 days... vaginal suppositories (all azoles): butoconazole, clotrim, micon, tiocon, tercon (doses: Table 11A)	Nystatin vag. tabs tabs 14 days less effective. Other rx for azole-resistant strains: gentian violet, boric acid. For recurrent candidiasis (4 or more episodes per yr), 6 mos. suppression with **fluconazole** 150 mg po q week or **itraconazole** 100 mg po q24h or **clotrimazole** vag. suppositories 500 mg q week.
Trichomoniasis Copious frothy discharge, pH >4.5 Treat sexual partners—see Comment	Trichomonas vaginalis **Dx:** NAAT & PCR available; wet mount is less sensitive, but can try	**Metro** 2 gm as single dose or 500 mg po bid x 7 days OR **Tinidazole** 2 gm single dose. **Pregnancy:** See Comment	**For rx failure:** Re-treat with **metro** 500 mg po bid x 7 days. If 2nd "failure": **metro** 2 gm po x 3-5 days. If still failing, use **Tinidazole** 2 gm po q24h x 5 days.	**Treat male sexual partners (2 gm metronidazole as single dose).** Nearly 20% men with NGU are infected with trichomonas (JID 188:465, 2003). For alternative option in refractory cases, see CID 33:1341, 2001. **Pregnancy:** No data indicating metro teratogenic or mutagenic. For discussion of treating trichomonas, including issues in pregnancy, see MMWR 59 (RR-12), 2010.
Bacterial vaginosis (BV) Malodorous vaginal discharge, pH >4.5	Etiology uncertain: associated with Gardnerella vaginalis, mobiluncus, Mycoplasma hominis, Prevotella sp., Atopobium vaginae et al.	**Metro** 0.5 gm po bid x 7 days or **metro vaginal gel** 1% (1 applicator intravaginally) 1X/day x 5 days OR **Tinidazole** (2 gm po once daily x 2 days or 1 gm po once daily x 5 days) OR **clinda vaginal cream** 5 gm intravaginally at bedtime x 7 days	**Clinda** 0.3 gm po bid x 7 days or **clinda ovules** 100 mg vaginally at bedtime x 3 days.	Reported 50% 1 cure rate if abstain from sex or use condoms: CID 44:213 & 220, 2007. Treatment of male sex partner **not** indicated unless balanitis present. Metro extended release tabs 750 mg po q24h x 7 days available: no published data. **Pregnancy:** Oral metro or oral **clinda** 7-day regimens (see Canadian OB GYN practice guidelines in J ObstetGynCan 30:702, 2008). If recurrent BV, can try adding **boric acid** to suppressive regimen: Metro 0.5 gm po bid x 7 days, then vaginal boric acid gelatin capsule 600 mg hs x 21 days, followed by Metro vaginal gel 2x/week x 16 weeks (Sex Trans Dis 36:732, 2009).

¹² 1 applicator contains 5 gm of gel with 37.5 mg metronidazole

Abbreviations on page 2.   *NOTE: All dosage recommendations are for adults (unless otherwise indicated) and assume normal renal function. § Alternatives consider allergy; PK, compliance, local resistance, cost

TABLE 1 (24)

ANATOMIC SITE/DIAGNOSIS/ MODIFYING CIRCUMSTANCES	ETIOLOGIES (usual)	SUGGESTED REGIMENS*		ADJUNCT DIAGNOSTIC OR THERAPEUTIC MEASURES AND COMMENTS
		PRIMARY	ALTERNATIVE§	
GENITAL TRACT (continued)				
Men: **Balanitis**	Candida 40%, Group B strep, gardnerella	**Metro** 2 gm po as a single dose OR **Fluc** 150 mg po x1 OR **tinra** 200 mg po bid x 1 day.		Occurs in 1/4 of male sex partners of women infected with candida. Exclude circinate balanitis (Reiter's syndrome); (non-infectious) responds to hydrocortisone cream.
Epididymo-orchitis				
Age <35 years	N. gonorrhoeae, Chlamydia trachomatis	(**Ceftriaxone** 250 mg IM x 1 + **doxy** 100 mg po bid x 10 days) + bed rest, scrotal elevation, analgesics.		Enterobacteriaceae occasionally encountered. Test all pts age < 35 yrs for HIV and syphilis.
Age >35 years or homosexual men (insertive partners in anal intercourse)	Enterobacteriaceae (coliforms)	**Levo** 500-750 mg IV/po once daily) OR (**cipro** 500 mg po bid) or (400 mg IV twice daily) for 10-14 days. **AM-SB, P Ceph 3, TC-CL, PIP-TZ** (Dosage: see footnote page 25) Also: bed rest, scrotal elevation, analgesics		Midstream pyuria and scrotal pain and edema. NOTE: Do urine NAAT (nucleic acid amplification test) to ensure absence of N. gonorrhoeae with concomitant risk of FQ-resistant gonorrhoeae or of chlamydia if using agents without reliable activity. Other causes include: mumps, brucella, TB, intravesicular BCG, B. pseudomallei, coccidioides, Behçet's.
Non-gonococcal urethritis	See Chlamydia et al, Non-gonococcal urethritis, Table 1(26), page 23			
Prostatitis—Review. CID 50:1641, 2010.				
Acute	N. gonorrhoeae, C. trachomatis	(**ceftriaxone** 250 mg IM x 1 OR **cefixime** 400 mg po x 1) then **doxy** 100 mg bid x 10 days.		FQs no longer recommended for gonococcal infections. Test for HIV. In AIDS pts, prostate may be focus of Cryptococcus neoformans.
Uncomplicated (with risk of STD; age < 35yrs)	Enterobacteriaceae (coliforms)	**FQ** (dosage: see Epididymo-orchitis >35 yrs, above) or **TMP-SMX** 1 DS tablet (160 mg TMP) po bid x 10-14 days (minimum). Some authorities recommend 4 weeks of therapy.		Treat as acute urinary infection, 14 days (not single dose regimen). Some recommend 3-4 wks therapy. If uncertain, do NAAT for C. trachomatis and N. gonorrhoeae. If resistant enterobacteriaceae, use ERTA 1 gm IV qd. If resistant pseudomonas, use IMP or MER (500 mg IV q6, or q8 respectively).
Uncomplicated with low risk of STD				
Chronic bacterial	Enterobacteriaceae 80%, enterococci 15%, P. aeruginosa	**FQ** (**CIP** 500 mg po bid x 4-6 wks. **Levo** 750 mg po q24h x 4 wks.		**With treatment failures** consider infected prostatic calculi. FDA approved dose of levo is 500 mg; editors prefer higher dose.
Chronic prostatitis/chronic pain syndrome	The most common prostatitis syndrome. Etiology is unknown.	**α-adrenergic blocking agents are controversial** (AnIM 133:367, 2000).		Pt has sx of prostatitis but negative cultures and no cells in prostatic secretions. Rev. JAC 46:157, 2000. In randomized double-blind study, CIP and an alpha-blocker of no benefit (AnIM 141:581 & 639, 2004).
HAND (Bites: See Skin)				
Paronychia				
Nail biting, manicuring	Staph. aureus (maybe MRSA)	Incision & drainage; culture	**TMP-SMX-DS** 1-2 tabs po bid while waiting for culture result.	See Table 6 for alternatives. Occasionally—candida, gram-negative rods.
Contact with saliva— dentists, anesthesiologists, wrestlers	Herpes simplex (Whitlow)	**Acyclovir** 400 mg tid po x 10 days	**Famciclovir** or **valacyclovir** See Comment	Gram stain and routine culture negative. Famciclovir/valacyclovir for primary genital herpes; see Table 14A, page 161.
Dishwasher (prolonged water immersion)	Candida sp.	**Clotrimazole** (topical)		Avoid immersion of hands in water as much as possible.

Abbreviations on page 2.   *NOTE: All dosage recommendations are for adults (unless otherwise indicated) and assume normal renal function. PK: compliance, local resistance, cost
§ Alternatives consider allergy, PK, compliance, local resistance, cost

TABLE 1 (25)

ANATOMIC SITE/DIAGNOSIS/ MODIFYING CIRCUMSTANCES	ETIOLOGIES (usual)	SUGGESTED REGIMENS* PRIMARY	ALTERNATIVE[1]	ADJUNCT DIAGNOSTIC OR THERAPEUTIC MEASURES AND COMMENTS
HEART				
Infective endocarditis—Native valve—empiric rx awaiting cultures—No IV illicit drug use Valvular or congenital heart disease but no modifying circumstances See Table 15C, page 197 for prophylaxis	**NOTE: Diagnostic criteria** include evidence of continuous bacteraemia (multiple positive blood cultures), new murmur (worsening of old murmur) of valvular insufficiency, definite emboli, and echocardiographic (transthoracic or transesophageal) evidence of valvular vegetations. Refs: *Circulation* 111:3167, 2005; *Eur Heart J* 30:2369, 2009. For antimicrobial prophylaxis, see Table 15C, page 197.			
	Viridans strep 30–40%, "other" strep 15–25%, enterococci 5–18%, staphylococci 20–35% (including coag-neg staphylococci–CID 46:232, 2008).	[(**Pen G** 20 million units IV q24h, continuous or div. q4h) or (**AMP** 12 gm IV q24h, continuous or div. q4h) + **gentamicin** 1 mg/kg IV q4h] + **gentamicin** 1 mg/kg IM or IV q4h (see Comment)	Vanco 30–60 mg/kg/d in 2-3 divided doses to achieve trough of 15-20 mcg/mL+ **gentamicin** 1 mg/kg IM or IV q4h **OR dapto** 6 mg/kg IV q24h	If patient not acutely ill and not in heart failure, wait for blood culture results. If initial 3 blood cultures neg. after 24–48 hrs, obtain 2–3 more blood cultures before empiric therapy started. **Nafcillin/oxacillin + gentamicin** may not cover enterococci, hence addition of penicillin G pending cultures. When blood cultures +, modify regimen to specific therapy for organism. **Gentamicin** used for synergy; peak levels need not exceed 4 mcg per mL. **Surgery indications:** See *NEJM* 368:1425, 2013. Role of surgery in pts with left-sided endocarditis & large vegetation (*NEJM* 366:2466, 2012). No difference in 15 yr survival between bioprosthetic and mechanical valve (*JAMA* 312:1323, 2014).
Infective endocarditis—Native valve—IV illicit drug use ± evidence rt-sided endocarditis — empiric therapy	S. aureus (MSSA & MRSA). All others rare	**Vanco** 15-20 mg/kg q8-12h to achieve target trough concentrations of 15-20 mcg/mL recommended for serious infections.	**Dapto** 6 mg/kg IV q24h Approved for right-sided endocarditis.	Target **gent levels:** peak 3 mcg/mL, trough <1 mcg/mL. If very obese pt, recommend consultation for dosage adjustment. Infuse vanco over ≥1 hr to avoid "red man" syndrome. **S. bovis suggests occult bowel pathology (new name: S. gallolyticus).** Since relapse rate may be greater in pts ill for >3 mos. prior to start of rx, the penicillin-gentamicin synergism theoretically may be advantageous in this group.
Infective endocarditis—Native valve—culture positive				
Viridans strep, S. bovis (S. gallolyticus) with penicillin G MIC ≤0.12 mcg/mL	Viridans strep, S. bovis (S. gallolyticus subsp. gallolyticus)	[**Pen G** 12–18 million units/day IV divided q4h x **2 wks**) PLUS (**gentamicin** IV 1 mg/kg q8h IV x **2 wks**)] **OR Pen G** 12–18 million units/day IV, divided - q4h x 4 wks	[(**Ceftriaxone** 2 gm IV q24h + **gentamicin** 1 mg per kg IV q8h **x 2 wks**). If allergy: pen G or ceftriax, use **vanco** 15 mg/kg IV q12h to 2 gm/day max unless serum levels measured **x 4 wks**	Can use cefazolin for pen G in pt with allergy that is not IgE-mediated (e.g., anaphylaxis). Alternatively, can use vanco. (See Comment above for gent and vanco). **NOTE: If necessary to remove infected valve culture neg., 2 weeks antibiotic treatment post-op sufficient** (CID 41:187, 2005).
Viridans strep, S. bovis, S. gallolyticus with penicillin G MIC >0.12 to ≤0.5 mcg/mL **NOTE:** Inf. Dis. consultation suggested	Viridans strep, S. bovis, nutritionally variant streptococci, (e.g. S. abiotrophia.) tolerant strep[13]	[(**Pen G** 18 million units/day IV divided q4h) x **4 wks** PLUS Gent 1 mg/kg IV q8h **x 2 wks** **NOTE: Low dose of Gent**	[(**Vanco** 15 mg/kg IV q12h to max of 2 gm/day unless serum levels measured **x 4 wks**	**4 wks of rx if symptoms <3 mos.; 6 wks of rx if symptoms >3 mos.** Vanco for non-allergic pts; do not use cephalosporins. Do not give gent once-q24h for enterococcal endocarditis. Target gent levels: peak 3 mcg/mL, trough <1 mcg/mL. Vanco target serum levels: peak 20–50 mcg/mL, trough 5–12 mcg/mL.
For viridans strep or S. bovis with pen G MIC >0.5 and enterococci susceptible to AMP/pen G, vanco, gentamicin (synergy positive) **NOTE:** Inf. Dis. consultation suggested	"Susceptible" enterococci, viridans strep, S. bovis, nutritionally variant streptococci (new names e.g. Abiotrophia sp. & Granulicatella sp.)	[(**Pen G** 18-30 million units/day IV divided q4h x **4-6 wks**) PLUS (**gentamicin** 1 mg/kg q8h IV x **4-6 wks**)] **OR** [**AMP** 12 gm/day IV divided q4h x **4-6 wks** + **gent** as above	**Vanco** 15 mg/kg IV q12h to max of 2 gm/day unless serum levels measured **PLUS gentamicin** 1 mg/kg IV x **4-6 wks** **NOTE: Low dose of Gent**	**NOTE:** Because of ↑ frequency of resistance (see below), all enterococci causing endocarditis should be tested in vitro for susceptibility to penicillin, gentamicin and vancomycin plus β lactamase production

[13] Tolerant streptococci = MBC 32-fold greater than MIC

Abbreviations on page 2. *NOTE: All dosage recommendations are for adults (unless otherwise indicated) and assume normal renal function. § Alternatives consider allergy; PK, compliance, local resistance, cost

TABLE 1 (26)

ANATOMIC SITE/DIAGNOSIS/ MODIFYING CIRCUMSTANCES	ETIOLOGIES (usual)	SUGGESTED REGIMENS* PRIMARY	SUGGESTED REGIMENS* ALTERNATIVE†	ADJUNCT DIAGNOSTIC OR THERAPEUTIC MEASURES AND COMMENTS
HEART/infective endocarditis—Native valve—culture positive *(continued)*				
Enterococci: MIC streptomycin >2000 mcg/mL; MIC gentamicin >500–2000 mcg/mL; no resistance to penicillin	Enterococci, high-level aminoglycoside resistance	**E. faecalis:** Pen G or AMP IV as above **x 8–12 wks** (approx. 50% cure) success in single case: **AMP + Dapto** (AAC 56:6064, 2012; Eur J Clin Micro Inf Dis 30:807, 2011).	**E. faecalis: Ceftriaxone** 2 gm IV q12h, **AMP** 2 gm IV q4h) x 7-8 wks (CID 56:1261, 2013)	10–25% E. faecalis and 45–60% E. faecium resistant to high gent levels. May have to consider surgical removal of infected valve. Theory of efficacy of combination of Amp + Ceftriaxone: sequential blocking of PBPs 4&5 (Amp) and 2&3 (ceftriaxone).
Enterococci: pen G MIC >16 mcg/mL; no gentamicin resistance	Enterococci, intrinsic pen G/AMP resistance (E. faecium or E. faecalis)	(**Vanco** 15 mg/kg IV q12h (check levels if >2 gm) **+ Gent** 1 mg/kg q8h x 6 wks (see Comment) Vanco alternative: **AM-SB** 3 gm IV q6h.		Desired vanco serum levels: trough 5–12 mcg/mL. **Gentamicin** used for synergy; peak levels need not exceed 4 mcg/mL.
Enterococci: Pen/AMP resistant + high-level gent/strep resistant + vanco resistant; usually VRE	Enterococci, vanco-resistant, usually E. faecium	**E. faecium: Linezolid** 600 mg IV/po q12h x 8 wks or **Quinu-dalfo** 7.5 mg/kg IV (central line) q8h x min 8 wks	**E. faecalis:** (IMP 500 mg IV q6h + **AMP** 2 gm IV q12h + **Ceftriaxone** 2 gm IV q12h + **AMP** 2 gm IV q4h) x min 8 wks (CID 56:1261, 2013)	**Synercid** not active vs. E. faecalis. Linezolid bacteriostatic; failures have occurred. Dapto bactericidal in vitro but sparse clinical data (CID 41:1134, 2005). Cure of single E. faecalis pt: AMP + Dapto (AAC 56:6064, 2012; Eur J Clin Micro Infect Dis 30:807, 2011). Teicoplanin active vs. subset of vanco-resist enterococci, but NUS.
Consultation suggested				
Staphylococcal endocarditis Aortic &/or mitral valve infection—MSSA Surgery indications: see Comment page 28.	Staph. aureus, methicillin-sensitive	**Nafcillin** (oxacillin) 2 gm IV q4h **x 4–6 wks**	(**Cefazolin** 2 gm IV q8h) OR **Vanco** 30-60 mg/kg/d in 2-3 divided doses to achieve trough of 15-20 mcg/mL **x 4–6 wks**	If IgE-mediated penicillin allergy, 10% cross-reactivity to cephalosporins (AnIM 141:16, 2004). **Cefazolin** and **Nafcillin** probably similar in efficacy and Cefazolin better tolerated (AAC 55:5122, 2011)
Aortic and/or mitral valve infection—MRSA	Staph. aureus, methicillin-resistant	**Vanco** 30-60 mg/kg per day in 2-3 divided doses to achieve target trough concentrations of 15-20 mcg/mL recommended for serious infections.	**Dapto** 8-10 mg/kg IV q24h (NOT FDA approved for this indication or dose)	In clinical trial (NEJM 355:653, 2006): high failure rate with both vanco and daptomycin in small numbers of pts. For other alternatives, see Table 6, pg 79. Daptomycin references: JAC 68:936 & 2921, 2013. Case reports of success with Telavancin (JAC 65:1315, 2010; JAC 54:5369, 2010; JAC (Jun 9) 2011) and ceftaroline (JAC 67:1267, 2012; J Infect Chemo online 7/14/12).
Tricuspid valve infection (usually IVDUs): MSSA	Staph. aureus, methicillin-sensitive	**Nafcillin** (oxacillin) 2 gm IV q4h **PLUS gentamicin** 1 mg/kg IV q8h x 2 wks. **NOTE: low dose of gent**	**If penicillin allergy: Vanco** 30-60 mg/kg IV q24h (divided if concomitant left-sided endocarditis) **x 4 wks OR Dapto** 6 mg/kg IV q24h x 4 wks	**2-week regimen not long enough** if metastatic infection (e.g., osteo) or left-sided endocarditis. **Dapto** is used treat for at least 4 weeks. **Dapto** resistance can occur de novo, or during vanco, or after/during dapto therapy. Cefazolin 2 gm q8h also an option. Fewer adverse events and discontinuations vs nafcillin (Clin Infect Dis 59:369, 2014).

*NOTE: All dosage recommendations are for adults (unless otherwise indicated) and assume normal renal function. §Alternatives consider allergy; PK, compliance, local resistance, cost

Abbreviations on page 2.

TABLE 1 (27)

ANATOMIC SITE/DIAGNOSIS/ MODIFYING CIRCUMSTANCES	ETIOLOGIES (usual)	SUGGESTED REGIMENS* PRIMARY	SUGGESTED REGIMENS* ALTERNATIVE¹	ADJUNCT DIAGNOSTIC OR THERAPEUTIC MEASURES AND COMMENTS
HEART/Infective endocarditis—Native valve—culture positive *(continued)*				
Tricuspid valve, methicillin-resistant	**Staph. aureus, methicillin-resistant**	Vanco 15-20 mg/kg q8-12h to achieve target trough concentrations of 15-20 mg/mL; recommended for serious infections **x 4-6 wks**	**Dapto** 6 mg/kg IV q24h x 4-6 wks equiv to **vanco** for rt-sided endocarditis; both vanco & dapto did poorly if lt-sided endocarditis (*NEJM* 355: 653, 2006) (See Comments & table 6, page 79)	**Linezolid:** Limited experience (see *JAC* 58:273, 2006) in patients with few treatment options; 64% cure rate; clear failure in 21%, thrombocytopenia in 31%. **Dapto** dose of 8-12 mg/kg may help in selected cases, but not FDA-approved.
Slow-growing fastidious Gm-neg. bacilli–any valve	**HACEK group** (see Comments).	**Ceftriaxone** 2 gm IV q24h x 4 wks **OR** **CIP** 400 mg IV q12h or 500 mg po bid x 4 wks (Bartonella resistant – see below).	**AM-SB** 3 gm IV q6h x 4 wks or **CIP** (400 mg po bid) x 4 wks	**HACEK** (acronym for **H**aemophilus parainfluenzae, **H. (aphrophilus) aggregatibacter, Actinobacillus, Cardiobacterium, Eikenella, Kingella**). Penicillinase-positive HACEK organisms should be susceptible to AM-SB + ceftriaxone. Ref: *Circulation* 111:e394, 2005.
	Bartonella species–any valve	B. henselae, B. quintana	(**Doxy** 100 mg IV/po bid + **RIF** 300 mg IV/po q12h) x 8-8 wks	**Dx:** Immunofluorescent antibody titer ≥1:800; blood cultures only occ. positive, or PCR of tissue from surgery. **Surgery:** Over ½ pts require valve surgery; relation to cure unclear. B. quintana transmitted by body lice among homeless.
Infective endocarditis—"culture negative" Fever, valvular disease, and ECHO vegetations ± emboli and neg. cultures		Etiology in 348 cases studied by serology, culture, histopath. Leading etiologic diagnoses: C. burnetii 48%, Bartonella sp. 28%, and rarely (Abiotrophia elegans (nutritionally variant strep), Mycoplasma hominis, Legionella pneumophila, Tropheryma whipplei—together 1%), & rest without etiology identified (most on antibiotic). (See *CID* 51:131, 2010 for approach to work-up. Chronic Q fever: *JCM* 52:1637, 2014.		**Dx:** Immunofluorescent antibody titer ≥1:800; blood cultures only occ. positive, or PCR of tissue from surgery. **Surgery:** Over ½ pts require valve surgery; relation to cure unclear. B. quintana transmitted by body lice among homeless.
Infective endocarditis—Prosthetic valve—empiric therapy (cultures pending)				
Early (<2 mos post-op)	S. epidermidis, S. aureus. Rarely, Enterobacteriaceae, diphtheroids, fungi	**Vanco** 15-20 mg/kg IV q8-12h + **gentamicin** 1 mg/kg IV q8h + **RIF** 600 mg po q24h		Early surgical consultation advised especially if etiology is S. aureus, evidence of heart failure, presence of diabetes and/or renal failure, or concern for valve ring abscess (*JAMA* 297:1354, 2007; *CID* 44:364, 2007).
Late (>2 mos post-op)	S. epidermidis, viridans strep, enterococci, S. aureus			
Infective endocarditis—Prosthetic valve—positive blood cultures Treat for 6 weeks, even if suspect Viridans Strep. **Surgical consultation advised:** Indications for surgery: severe heart failure, S. aureus infection, prosthetic dehiscence, resistant organism, emboli due to large vegetation (*JACC* 48:e1, 2006). See also, *Eur. J Clin Micro Infect Dis* 38:528, 2010.	Staph. epidermidis	(**Vanco** 15 mg /kg IV q12h + **RIF** 300 mg po q8h) x 6 wks + **gentamicin** 1 mg/kg IV q8h **x 14 days.**		If S. epidermidis is susceptible to nafcillin/oxacillin (or oxacillin) (not common), then substitute nafcillin (or oxacillin) for vanco.
	Staph. aureus	Methicillin sensitive: (**Nafcillin** 2 gm IV q4h + **RIF** 300 mg po q8h) **times 6 wks + gentamicin** 1 mg per kg IV q8h **times 14 days.** Methicillin-resistant: (**Vanco** 15-20 mg/kg IV q8-12h to achieve a target trough of 15-20 mg/mL) + **RIF** 300 mg po q8h) **times 6 wks** + **gentamicin** 1 mg/kg IV q8h **times 14 days.**		Treat for 6 weeks. To substitute CIP for aminoglycoside, but no clinical data.
	Viridans strep, enterococci	See infective endocarditis, native valve, culture positive, page 28.		
	Enterobacteriaceae or P. aeruginosa	**Aminoglycoside** (tobra IV [for P. aeruginosa]) + (**AP Pen** or **P Ceph 3 AP** or **P Ceph 4**)		In theory, could substitute CIP for aminoglycoside, but no clinical data.
	Candida, aspergillus	*Table 11, page 174*		High mortality. Valve replacement plus antifungal therapy standard therapy but some success with antifungal therapy alone.

*NOTE: All dosage recommendations are for adults (unless otherwise indicated) and assume normal renal function. § Alternatives consider allergy; PK, compliance, local resistance, cost

TABLE 1 (28)

ANATOMIC SITE/DIAGNOSIS/ MODIFYING CIRCUMSTANCES	ETIOLOGIES (usual)	SUGGESTED REGIMENS*		ADJUNCT DIAGNOSTIC OR THERAPEUTIC MEASURES AND COMMENTS
		PRIMARY	ALTERNATIVE§	
HEART *(continued)*				
Infective endocarditis—Q fever *IJID 10:527, 2010; NEJM 356:715, 2007.*	Coxiella burnetii	**Doxy** 100 mg po bid + **hydroxychloroquine** 600 mg/day for at least 18 mos *(Mayo Clin Proc 83:574, 2008). Pregnancy: Need long term* TMP-SMX *(see CID 45:548, 2007).*		**Dx:** Phase I IgG titer >800 plus clinical evidence of endocarditis. Treatment duration: 18 mos for native valve, 24 mos for prosthetic valve. Monitor serologically for 5 yrs.
Pacemaker/defibrillator infections	S. aureus (40%), S. epidermidis (40%), Gram-negative bacilli (5%), fungi (5%)	**Device removal + vanco** 15-20 mg/kg IV q8-12h+ **RIF** 300 mg po bid	**Device removal + dapto** 6 mg per kg IV q24h[14] ± **RIF** *(no data)* 300 mg po bid	**Duration of rx after device removal:** For "pocket" or subcutaneous infection, 10-14 days; if lead-assoc. endocarditis, 4-6 wks depending on organism. Device removal and absence of valvular vegetation assoc. with significantly higher survival at 1 yr *(JAMA 307:1727, 2012).*
Pericarditis, purulent— empiric therapy. *Ref: Medicine 88: 52, 2009.*	Staph. aureus, Strep. pneumoniae, Group A strep, Enterobacteriaceae	**Vanco + CIP** *(Dosage, see footnote[14])*	**Vanco + CFP** *(see footnote[14])*	Drainage required if signs of tamponade. Forced to use empiric vanco due to high prevalence of MRSA.
Rheumatic fever with carditis *Ref: Ln 366:155, 2005*	Post-infectious sequelae of Group A strep infection (usually pharyngitis)	ASA, and usually prednisone 2 mg/kg po q24h for symptomatic treatment of fever, arthritis, arthralgia. May not influence carditis.		Clinical features: Carditis, polyarthritis, chorea, subcutaneous nodules, erythema marginatum. *Prophylaxis: see page 61*
Ventricular assist device-related *CID 57:1438, 2013*	S. aureus, S. epidermidis, aerobic gm-neg bacilli, Candida sp.	After culture of blood, wounds, drive line, device pocket and maybe pump: **Vanco** 15-20 mg/kg IV q8-12h + **(Cip** 400 mg IV q12h or **levo** 750 mg IV q24h) + **fluconazole** 800 mg IV q24h		Can substitute **daptomycin** 10 mg/kg/d[14] for **vanco, cefepime** 2 gm IV q12h for FQ, and **vori, caspo, micafungin or anidulafungin)** for **fluconazole.** Modify regimen based on results of culture and susceptibility tests. Higher than FDA-approved Dapto dose because of potential emergence of resistance.
JOINT—*Also see Lyme Disease, page 58*				
Reactive arthritis **Reiter's syndrome** *(See Comment for definition)* *Occurs wks after infection with C. trachomatis, Campylobacter jejuni, Yersinia enterocolitica, Shigella/Salmonella sp.*		Only treatment is non-steroidal anti-inflammatory drugs		Definition: Urethritis, conjunctivitis, arthritis, and sometimes uveitis and rash. Arthritis: asymmetrical oligoarthritis of ankles, knees, feet, sacroiliitis. Rash: palms and soles—keratoderma blennorrhagica; circinate balanitis of glans penis. HLA-B27 positive predisposes to Reiter's.
Poststreptococcal reactive arthritis *(See Rheumatic fever, above)*	Immune reaction after strep pharyngitis. (1) arthritis onset in <10 days, (2) lasts months, (3) unresponsive to ASA	Treat strep pharyngitis and then NSAIDs *(prednisone needed in some pts)*		A reactive arthritis after a β-hemolytic strep infection in absence of sufficient Jones criteria for acute rheumatic fever. *Ref.: Mayo Clin Proc 75:144, 2000.*

[14] **Aminoglycosides** *(see Table 10D, page 110);* **IMP** 0.5 gm IV q6h, **MER** 1 gm IV q8h, **natcillin** or **oxacillin** 2 gm IV q4h, **TC-CL** 3.1 gm IV q6h, **PIP-TZ** 3.375 gm IV q6h or 4.5 gm IV q8h, **AM-SB** 3 gm IV q6h, **P Ceph 1** (cephalothin 2 gm IV q4h or cefazolin 2 gm IV q8h), **CIP** 750 mg po bid or 400 mg IV bid, **vanco** 1 gm IV q12h, **RIF** 600 mg po q24h, **aztreonam** 2 gm IV q24h, **CFP** 2 gm IV q12h

Abbreviations on page 2.   *NOTE: All dosage recommendations are for adults (unless otherwise indicated) and assume normal renal function. § Alternatives consider allergy, PK, compliance, local resistance, cost*

TABLE 1 (29)

ANATOMIC SITE/DIAGNOSIS/ MODIFYING CIRCUMSTANCES	ETIOLOGIES (usual)	SUGGESTED REGIMENS*		ADJUNCT DIAGNOSTIC OR THERAPEUTIC MEASURES AND COMMENTS
		PRIMARY	ALTERNATIVE§	
JOINT (continued)				
Septic arthritis: Treatment requires both adequate drainage of purulent joint fluid and appropriate antimicrobial therapy. **There is no need to inject antimicrobials into joints.** Empiric therapy after collection of blood and joint fluid for culture; review Gram stain of joint fluid.				
Infants <3 mos (neonate)	Staph. aureus, Enterobacteriaceae, Group B strep	**If MRSA not a concern: (Nafcillin** or **oxacillin**) + **P Ceph 3**	**If MRSA a concern: Vanco + P Ceph 3**	Blood cultures frequently positive. Adjacent bone involved in 2/3 pts. Group B strep and gonococci most common community-acquired etiologies.
Children (3 mos–14 yrs)	S. aureus 27%, S. pyogenes & S. pneumo 14%, H. influ 3%, Gm-neg. bacilli 6%, other (GC, N. mening.) 14%, unk 36%	**Vanco + (Cefotaxime, ceftizoxime or ceftriaxone)** until culture results available Steroids—see Comment		Marked ↓ in H. influenzae since use of conjugate vaccine. **NOTE:** Septic arthritis due to salmonella has no association with sickle cell disease, unlike salmonella osteomyelitis. 10 days of therapy as effective as a 30-day treatment course if there is a good clinical response and CRP levels normalize quickly *(CID 48:1201, 2009)*.
Adults (review Gram stain): See page 58 for Lyme Disease and page 58 for gonococcal arthritis				
Acute monoarticular At risk for sexually-transmitted disease	N. gonorrhoeae (see page 23), S. aureus, streptococci, rarely aerobic Gm-neg. bacilli	**Gram stain negative: Ceftriaxone** 1 gm IV q24h or **cefotaxime** 1 gm IV q8h or **ceftizoxime** 1 gm IV q8h	**If Gram stain shows Gm + cocci in clusters: vanco** 15-20 mg/kg IV q8-12h	For treatment comments, see *Disseminated GC, page 23*
Not at risk for sexually-transmitted disease	S. aureus, streptococci, Gm-neg. bacilli	**All empiric choices guided by Gram stain** **Vanco + P Ceph 3** | **Vanco + (CIP** or **Levo)** *For treatment duration, see Table 3, page 71* *For dosage, see footnote page 34*		Differential includes gout and chondrocalcinosis (pseudogout). **Look for crystals in joint fluid.** **NOTE:** *See Table 6 for MRSA treatment.*
Chronic monoarticular	Brucella, nocardia, myco-bacteria, fungi	See *Table 2 & Table 12*		
Polyarticular, usually acute	Gonococci, B. burgdorferi; acute rheumatic fever; viruses, e.g., hepatitis B, rubella vaccine, parvo B19	Gram stain usually negative for GC. If sexually active, culture urethra, cervix, anal canal, throat, blood, joint fluid, and then: **ceftriaxone** 1 gm IV q24h		If GC, usually associated petechiae and/or pustular skin lesions and tenosynovitis. Consider Lyme disease if exposure areas known to harbor infected ticks. *See page 58.* Expanded differential includes gout, pseudogout, reactive arthritis (HLA-B27 pos.).
Septic arthritis, post intra-articular injection	MSSE/MRSE 40%, MSSA/ MRSA 20%, P. aeruginosa, Propionibacteria, AFB	**NO empiric therapy.** Arthroscopy for culture/sensitivity, crystals, washout		Treat based on culture results x 14 days (assumes no foreign body present).

*NOTE: All dosage recommendations are for adults (unless otherwise indicated) and assume normal renal function.

Abbreviations on page 2.

*NOTE: All dosage recommendations are for adults (unless otherwise indicated) and assume normal renal function. § Alternatives consider allergy, PK, compliance, local resistance, cost

TABLE 1 (30)

ANATOMIC SITE/DIAGNOSIS/ MODIFYING CIRCUMSTANCES	ETIOLOGIES (usual)	SUGGESTED REGIMENS* PRIMARY	ALTERNATIVE§	ADJUNCT DIAGNOSTIC OR THERAPEUTIC MEASURES AND COMMENTS
JOINT (continued)				
Infected prosthetic joint (PJI) • Suspect infection if sinus tract w/ wound drainage, acutely painful prosthesis; chronically painful prosthesis, or high ESR/CRP assoc. w/painful prosthesis. Treat based on culture and sensitivity results. • **Empiric therapy is NOT recommended.** Treat based on culture and sensitivity results. • **3 surgical options:** 1) 1 stage exchange (debridement and prosthesis retention if < 3 wks or implantation < 30 days); 2) 1 stage, direct exchange; 3) 2 stage: debridement, removal, reimplantation • **IDSA Guidelines:** *CID 56:61, 2013.* • Data do not allow assessment of value of adding antibacterial cement to temporary joint spacers (*CID 55:474, 2012*). • Evidence of systemic absorption of Tobra from antibiotic-impregnated cement spacers (*CID 58:1783, 2014*).	MSSA/MSSE	**Debridement/Retention:** [(**Nafcillin** 2 gm IV q4h or **Oxacillin** 2 gm IV q4h IV) + **Rifampin** 300 mg po bid] OR **Cefazolin** 2 gm IV q8h + **Rifampin** 300 mg po bid] OR **Levofloxacin** 750 mg po q24h) + **Rifampin** 300 mg po bid] for 3-6 months (shorter duration for total hip arthroplasty) **2-stage exchange:** regimen as above for 4-6 wks	**Daptomycin** 6-8 mg/kg IV q24h OR **Linezolid** 600 mg po/IV bid ± **Rifampin** 300 mg po bid	**Confirm isolate susceptibility to fluoroquinolone and rifampin:** for fluoroquinolone-resistant isolate consider using other active highly bioavailable agent, e.g., TMP-SMX, Doxy, Doxycycline, Amoxicillin-Clavulanate, Clindamycin, or Linezolid. Enterococcal infection: addition of aminoglycoside optional.
	MRSA/MRSE	**Debridement/Retention: Vancomycin** 15-20 mg/kg IV q8-12h + **Rifampin** 300 mg po bid OR **Levofloxacin** 750 mg po q24h OR **Ciprofloxacin** 750 mg po bid OR **Levofloxacin** 750 mg po q24h) + **Rifampin** 300 mg po bid] for 3-6 months (shorter duration for total hip arthroplasty) **1-stage exchange:** IV/PO regimen as above for 3 mos **2-stage exchange:** regimen as above for 4-6 wks	**Daptomycin** 6-8 mg/kg IV q24h OR **Linezolid** 600 mg po/IV bid ± **Rifampin** 300 mg po bid	• *P. aeruginosa* infection: consider adding aminoglycoside if isolate is susceptible, (but if this improves outcome unclear.) • Prosthesis retention most important risk factor for treatment failure. (*Clin Microbiol Infect 16:1789, 2010*). (Linezolid 600 mg + Rifampin 300 mg) may be effective as salvage therapy if device removal not possible (*Antimicrob Agents Chemother 55:4308, 2011*). • If prosthesis is retained, consider long-term suppressive therapy, particularly for staphylococcal infections; depending on in vitro susceptibility options include TMP-SMX, Doxycycline, Minocycline, Amoxicillin, Ciprofloxacin, Cephalexin. • Culture yield may be increased by sonication of prosthesis (*N Engl J Med 357:654, 2007*). • Other treatment consideration: Rifampin is bactericidal vs. biofilm-producing bacteria. Never use Rifampin alone due to rapid development of resistance. Rifampin 300 mg po/IV bid + Fusidic acid* 500 mg po qid is another option (*JAC 65:1008, 2010*). If MRSA **Daptomycin** Watch for toxicity (Linezolid) if used for more than 2 weeks of therapy.
	Streptococci (Grps A, B, C, D,viridans, other)	**Debridement/Retention: Penicillin G** 20 million units IV continuous infusion q24h or in 6 divided doses OR **Ceftriaxone** 2 gm IV q24h x 4-6 weeks **1 or 2 stage exchange:** regimen as above for 4-6 weeks	**Vancomycin** 15 mg/kg IV q12h	
	Enterococci	**Debridement/Retention: Pen-susceptible: Ampicillin** 12 gm IV OR **Penicillin G** 20 million units IV continuous infusion q24h or in 6 divided doses x 4-6 weeks **Pen-resistant: Vancomycin** 15 mg/kg IV q12h x 4-6 weeks **1 or 2 stage exchange:** regimen as above for 4-6 wks	**Daptomycin** 6-8 mg/kg IV q24h OR **Linezolid** 600 mg po/IV bid	
	Propionibacterium acnes	**Debridement/Retention: Penicillin G** 20 million units IV continuous infusion or in 6 divided doses OR **Ceftriaxone** 2 gm IV q24h OR 2 gm IV q24h x 4-6 weeks **1 or 2 stage exchange:** regimen as above for 4-6 weeks	**Vancomycin** 15 mg/kg IV q12h OR **Clindamycin** 300-450 mg po/IV qid	
	Gm-neg enteric bacilli	**Debridement/Retention: Cefepime** 2 gm IV q24h OR other beta-lactam or **Ceftriaxone** 2 gm IV q24h OR **Cefepime** 2 gm IV q12h, based on susceptibility x 4-6 weeks **1 or 2 stage exchange:** regimen as above for 4-6 weeks	**Ciprofloxacin** 750 mg po bid or 400 mg IV q8h	
	P. aeruginosa	**Debridement/Retention: Cefepime** 2 gm IV q8h OR **Meropenem** 1 gm IV q8h + **Tobramycin** 5.1 mg/kg once daily x 4-6 wks **1 or 2 stage exchange:** regimen as above for 4-6 weeks	**Ciprofloxacin** 750 mg po bid or 400 mg IV q8h	
Rheumatoid arthritis	**TNF inhibitors** (adalimumab, certolizumab, etanercept, golimumab, infliximab), and other anti-inflammatory biologics (tofacitinib, rituximab, tocilizumab, abatacept) ↑ risk of TBc, fungal infection, legionella, listeria, and malignancies. See *J Infect Dis/J.org, 59:1, 2013* for full listing.			Empiric MRSA coverage recommended if risk factors are present and in high prevalence areas. Immunosuppression, not duration of therapy, is a risk factor for recurrence; 7 days of therapy.
Septic bursitis: **Olecranon bursitis; prepatellar bursitis**	Staph. aureus >80%, M. tuberculosis (rare). M. marinum (rare)	(**Nafcillin** 2 gm IV q4h or **Cefazolin** 2 gm IV q8h if **MSSA**)	(**Vanco** 15-20 mg/kg IV q12h or **linezolid** 600 mg bid) if **MRSA**	patients undergoing one-stage bursectomy (*JAC 65:1008, 2010*). If MSSA **Dicloxacillin** 500 mg po qid as oral step-down. If MRSA **Daptomycin** 6 mg/kg IV q24h.

Other doses, see footnote page 34

TABLE 1 (31)

ANATOMIC SITE/DIAGNOSIS/ MODIFYING CIRCUMSTANCES	ETIOLOGIES (usual)	SUGGESTED REGIMENS*		ADJUNCT DIAGNOSTIC OR THERAPEUTIC MEASURES AND COMMENTS
		PRIMARY	ALTERNATIVE†	
KIDNEY, BLADDER AND PROSTATE				
Acute uncomplicated urinary tract infection (cystitis-urethritis) in females: *NEJM 366:1028, 2012; CID 57:719, 2013; JAMA 312:1677, 2014.*				
NOTE: Resistance of *E. coli* to TMP-SMX approx. 15–20% & correlates with microbiological/clinical failure. **Recent reports of *E. coli* resistant to FQs.**	Enterobacteriaceae (E. coli), Staph. saprophyticus, Enterococci and/or Strep. Enterococcus in midstream urine often result in *NEJM 369:1883 & 1959, 2013*).	**<20% of Local *E. coli* resistant to TMP-SMX & no allergy: TMP-SMX-DS** x 3 days; if sulfa allergy: **nitrofurantoin** 100 mg po bid x 5 days OR **fosfomycin** 3 gm po x one dose. All plus **Pyridium**	**>20% Local *E. coli* resistant to TMP-SMX & sulfa allergy:** then 3 days of **CIP** 250 mg bid, **CIP-ER** 500 mg q24h, **Levo** 250 mg q24h, **Moxi** 400 mg q24h OR **Fruitifloxacin(NUS)** 600 mg q24h **OR Nitrofurantoin** 100 mg po bid x 7 days **Pyridium**	7-day course recommended **in pregnancy** [discontinue or do not use sulfonamides (TMP-SMX) near term (2 weeks before EDC) because of potential 1 in kernicterus]. If failure on 3-day course, culture and x 2 weeks. **Fosfomycin** 3 gm po times 1 less effective vs. *E. coli* than multi-dose TMP-SMX or FQ. Fosfo active vs. *E. faecalis*; poor activity vs. other coliforms. **Moxifloxacin:** Not approved for UTIs. Moxi equivalent to comparator drugs in unpublished clinical trials (on file with Bayer). Therapy of **ESBL producing *E. coli* and *Klebsiella* spp.** problematic because of multiple drug resistances: ESBL producers susceptible to fosfomycin, ertapenem, and combo of amox-clav + cefdinir in vitro (AAC 53:1278, 2009). Amox-Clav or an oral cephalosporin are options, but generally less efficacious. **Phenazopyridine (Pyridium)**—non-prescription— may relieve dysuria: 200 mg tid po times 2 days. Hemolysis if G6PD deficient.
Risk factors for STD. Dipstick: positive leukocyte esterase or hemoglobin, neg. Gram stain **Recurrent** (3 or more episodes/ year) in young women	C. trachomatis	**Azithro** 1 gm po single dose	**Doxy** 100 mg po bid 7 days	Pelvic exam for vaginitis & herpes simplex, urine LCR/PCR for GC and C. trachomatis.
	Any of the above bacteria	Eradicate infection, then **TMP-SMX** 1 single-strength tab po q24h long term		A cost-effective alternative to continuous prophylaxis is self-administered single dose rx (TMP-SMX DS, 2 tabs, 320/1600 mg) at symptom onset. Another alternative: 1 DS tablet TMP-SMX post-coitus.
Child: ≤5 yrs old & grade 3–4 reflux	Coliforms	**TMP-SMX** 8-12 mg/kg/day (based on TMP comp) div q12h drug ages 1-17 yrs.		**CIP** approved as alternative
Recurrent UTI in postmenopausal women	E. coli & other Enterobacteriaceae, enterococci, S. saprophyticus	Treat as for uncomplicated UTI. Evaluate for potentially correctable urologic factors—see Comment. **Nitrofurantoin** more effective than vaginal cream in decreasing frequency; but Editors worry about pulmonary fibrosis with long-term NF rx.		Definition: ≥3 culture + symptomatic UTIs in 1 year or 2 UTIs in 6 months. Urologic factors: (1) cystocele, (2) incontinence, (3) ↑ residual urine volume (250 mL).
Acute uncomplicated pyelonephritis (usually women 18–40 yrs. temperature >102°F, frequent costovertebral tenderness). **for obstructive uropathy or other complicating pathology.**				[NOTE: Culture of urine and blood indicated prior to therapy.] **If male, look**
Moderately ill (outpatient) **NOTE:** May need one IV dose due to nausea.	Enterobacteriaceae (most likely E. coli), enterococci (Gm stain of uncentrifuged urine may allow identification of Gm-neg. bacilli vs. Gm+ cocci)	**FQ** po times 5-7 days; **CIP** 500 mg bid or **CIP-ER** 1000 mg q24h, **Levo** 750 mg q24h, **Oflox** 400 mg q24h, possibly **Moxi** q24h—see comment.	**AM-CL, O Ceph. or TMP-SMX-DS po.** Treat for 14 days. Dosage in footnotes[15] FQs: **CIP** 500 mg IV q12h; **levo** 750 mg IV q24h; **metro** 500 mg q6h or 15 mg/kg q12h.	7 day course of **Cipro** 500 mg bid as effective as 14 day course in women (*Lancet 380:484, 2012*) **PIP-TZ** 3.375 gm IV q6h; **PIP** 3 gm IV q4-6h; **PIP** 3 gm IV q6h for pseudomonas **aztreonam** 2 gm IV q8h; Carbapenems: **DORI** 500 mg IV q8h (1 hr infusion); **ERTA** 1 gm IV q24h; **IMP** 0.5 gm IV q12h (max 4 gm/day); **MER** 1 gm IV q8h for severe infection); **cefotetin** 2 gm IV q8h; **Gati** 400 mg IV q24h; **levo** 750 mg IV q24h; **gentamicin**—see Table 10D, page 110; **linezolid** 600 mg IV/po q12h; **metro** 500 mg po q6h or 15 mg/kg q12h. Beta-lactams less effective than FQ or TMP-SMX. Fruitifloxacin 600 mg q24h an option where available.

[15] **AM-CL** 875/125 mg q12h or 500/125 mg po q12h or 2000 /125 mg po bid; Antipseudomonal penicillins; **AM-SB** 3 gm IV q6h; **PIP** 3 gm IV q4-6h; **PIP** 3 gm IV q6h for pneumonia); **TC-CL** 3.1 gm IV q6h; Antipseudomonal cephalosporins: **ceftaz** 2 gm IV q8h; **CFP** 2 gm IV q12h; Ceftolozane-tazobactam 1.5 gm IV q8h **aztreonam** 2 gm IV q8h; Carbapenems: **DORI** 500 mg IV q8h (1 hr infusion); **ERTA** 1 gm IV q24h; **IMP** 0.5 gm IV q12h (max 4 gm/day); **MER** 1 gm IV q8h for severe infection); **cefotetin** 2 gm IV q8h; Parenteral cephalosporins: **cefotaxime** 2 gm IV q8h; **cefotetin** 2 gm IV q8h; Oral cephalosporins—see *Table 10A page 99*; FQs: **CIP** 500 mg IV q12h; **levo** 750 mg IV q24h; **ceftriaxone** 1-2 gm IV q24h; **dicloxacillin** 500 mg po q6h; **Gati** 400 mg IV q24h; **levo** 750 mg IV q24h; **gentamicin**—see *Table 10D, page 110;* **linezolid** 600 mg IV/po q12h; **metro** 500 mg po q6h or 15 mg/kg q12h; **nafcillin/oxacillin** 2 gm IV q4h; **TMP-SMX** 2 mg/kg (TMP component) IV q6h; **vanco** 1 gm IV q12h (if over 100 kg, 1.5 gm IV q12h).

Abbreviations on page 2.

*NOTE: All dosage recommendations are for adults (unless otherwise indicated) and assume normal renal function. § Alternatives consider allergy, PK, compliance, local resistance, cost

TABLE 1 (32)

ANATOMIC SITE/DIAGNOSIS/ MODIFYING CIRCUMSTANCES	ETIOLOGIES (usual)	SUGGESTED REGIMENS*		ADJUNCT DIAGNOSTIC OR THERAPEUTIC MEASURES AND COMMENTS
		PRIMARY	ALTERNATIVE†	
KIDNEY, BLADDER AND PROSTATE/Acute uncomplicated pyelonephritis				
Acute pyelonephritis— Hospitalized	E. coli most common, enterococci 2nd in frequency	FQ (IV) or (AMP + gentami- cin) or ceftriaxone or PIP- TZ. Treat for 14 days.	TC-CL or PIP-TZ or ERTA or DORI. Treat for 14 days.	Treat IV until pt afebrile 24–48 hrs., then complete 2-wks course with oral drugs (as Moderately ill, above). DORI approved for 10 day treatment. If pt hypotensive, prompt imaging (Ultrasound or CT) is recommended to ensure absence of obstructive uropathy. NOTE: Cephalosporins & ertapenem not active vs. enterococci.
		Dosages in footnote[15] on page 34. Do not use cephalosporins for suspect or proven enterococcal infection		
Complicated UTI/catheters Obstruction, reflux, azotemia, transplant, **Foley catheter-related, R/O obstruction:** multi-drug resistant gram-neg bacilli. For IDSA Guidelines: CID 50:625, 2010.	Enterobacteriaceae, P. aeruginosa, enterococci, rarely S. aureus	(AMP + gent) or PIP-TZ or TC-CL or DORI or IMP or MER for up to 2-3 wks	(IV FQ CIP Gati, Levo) or (Ceftaz or CFP for 2-3 wks) or Ceftolozane- tazobactam x 7 days	Not all listed drugs predictably active vs. enterococci or P. aeruginosa. CIP approved in children (1-17 yrs) as alternative. Not 1st choice secondary to increased incidence joint adverse effects. Peds dose: 6-10 mg/kg (400 mg max) IV q8h or 10-20 mg/kg (750 mg max) po q12h.
		Switch to po FQ or TMP-SMX when possible For dosages, see footnote[15] on page 34.		Treat for 7 days for catheter-associated UTI if prompt resolution of symptoms and 10-14 days if delayed response; a 3-day course of therapy may be consider for women < 65 years of age (CID 50:625, 2010)
Asymptomatic bacteriuria. IDSA Guidelines: CID 40:643, 2005; U.S. Preventive Services Task Force AnIM 149:43, 2008.				
Preschool children	Aerobic Gm-neg. bacilli & Staph. hemolyticus	Base regimen on C&S, not empirical		Diagnosis requires ≥10⁴ CFU per mL urine of same bacterial species in 2 specimen's obtained 3-7 days apart.
Pregnancy		Screen 1st trimester. If positive: 3-7 days with **amox**, **nitrofurantoin**, **O ceph, TMP-SMX**, or **TMP** alone		Screen monthly for recurrence. Some authorities treat continuously until delivery (stop TMP-SMX 2 wks before EDC); ↑ resistance of E. coli to TMP-SMX.
Before and after invasive uro- logic intervention, e.g., Foley catheter	Aerobic Gm-neg. bacilli	Obtain urine culture and then x 3 days with TMP-SMX DS, bid. For prevention of UTI: Consider removal after 72 hrs (CID 46:243 & 251, 2008).		Clinical benefit of antimicrobial-coated Foley catheters is uncertain (AnIM 144:116, 2006; CID 60:625, 2010).
Neurogenic bladder – see "spinal cord injury" below		No therapy in asymptomatic patient; intermittent catheterization if possible.		Ref.: AJM 113(1A):67S, 2002.— Bacteriuria in spinal cord injured patient.
Asymptomatic, advanced age, male or female Ref. JAMA 312:1687, 2014		If no symptoms, no therapy indicated unless in conjunction with surgery to correct obstructive uropathy; measure residual urine vol. in females, prostate exam/PSA in males. No screening recommended in men and non-pregnant women (CID 55:771, 2012).		
Malacoplakia	E. coli	Bethanechol chloride • (CIP or TMP-SMX)		Chronic pyelo with abnormal inflammatory response.
Perinephric abscess Associated with staphylococcal bacteremia	Staph. aureus	If MSSA, **Nafcillin/ oxacillin**; If **MRSA: Vanco** 15- 20 mg/kg q8-12h **OR dapto** 6 mg/kg IV q24h		Drainage, surgical or image-guided aspiration
		or ceftriaxone (Dosage, see footnote page 34.)		
Associated with pyelonephritis	Enterobacteriaceae	See pyelonephritis, complicated UTI, above		Drainage, surgical or image-guided aspiration
Post Renal Transplant Obstructive Uropathy (CID 46:825, 2008)	Corynebacterium urealyticum	**Vanco** or **Teicoplanin**[NUS]		Organism can synthesize struvite stones. Requires 48-72 hr incubation to detect in culture
Prostatitis		See prostatitis, page 27		
Spinal cord injury pts with UTI	E. coli, Klebsiella sp., entero- cocci	**CIP** 250 mg po bid x 14 days		If fever, suspect assoc. pyelonephritis. Microbiologic cure greater after 14 vs. 3 days of CIP (CID 39:658 & 665, 2004); for asymptomatic bacteriuria see AJM 113(1A):67S, 2002.

Abbreviations on page 2.   *NOTE: All dosage recommendations are for adults (unless otherwise indicated) and assume normal renal function. § Alternatives consider allergy, PK, compliance, local resistance, cost

TABLE 1 (33)

ANATOMIC SITE/DIAGNOSIS/ MODIFYING CIRCUMSTANCES	ETIOLOGIES (usual)	SUGGESTED REGIMENS*		ADJUNCT DIAGNOSTIC OR THERAPEUTIC MEASURES AND COMMENTS
		PRIMARY	ALTERNATIVE†	
LIVER (for spontaneous bacterial peritonitis, see page 47)				
Cholangitis		See Gallbladder, page 17		
Cirrhosis & variceal bleeding	Esophageal flora	(**Norfloxacin** 400 mg po bid or **CIP** 400 mg IV q12h) x max. of 7 days	**Ceftriaxone** 1 gm IV once daily for max. of 7 days	Short term prophylactic antibiotics in cirrhotics with G-I hemorr, with or without ascites, decreases rate of bacterial infection &, ↑ survival (*Hepatology 46:922, 2007*).
Hepatic abscess Klebsiella liver abscess ref.: *Ln ID 12:881, 2012*	Enterobacteriaceae (esp. Klebsiella sp.), bacteroides, enterococci, Entamoeba histolytica, Yersinia enterocolitica (rare), Fusobacterium necrophorum (*Lemierre's*). For echinococcus, see Table 13, page 152. For cat-scratch disease (CSD), see pages 45 & 57	**Metro** + [(**ceftriaxone** or **cefotixin** **TC-CL** or **PIP-TZ** or **AM-SB** or **CIP** or **levo** (Dosage, see footnote[15] on page 34)	**Metro** (for amoeba) + either **IMP** **MER** or **Dori** (Dosage, see footnote[15] on page 34)	**Serological tests for amebiasis should be done on all patients**; if neg, surgical drainage of percutaneous aspiration. In pyogenic abscess, ½ have identifiable GI source or underlying biliary tract disease. If amoeba serology positive, treat with **metro** alone without surgery. Empiric **metro** included for both E. histolytica & bacteroides. **Hemochromatosis** associated with Yersinia enterocolitica liver abscess; regimens listed are effective for yersinia. Klebsiella pneumonia genotype K1 associated ocular & CNS Klebsiella infections.
Hepatic encephalopathy	Urease-producing gut bacteria	**Rifaximin** 550 mg po bid (take with lactulose)		Refs: *NEJM 362:1071, 2010; Med Lett 52:87, 2010.*
Leptospirosis	Leptospirosis, see page 60	See page 57		
Peliosis hepatis in AIDS pts	Bartonella henselae and B. quintana			
Post-transplant infected "biloma"	Enterococci (incl. VRE), candida, Gm-neg bacilli (P. aeruginosa 8%), anaerobes 5%	**Linezolid** 600 mg IV bid + **CIP** 400 mg IV q24h + **fluconazole** 400 mg IV q24h	**Dapto** 6 mg/kg per day + **Levo** 750 mg IV q24h + **fluconazole** 400 mg IV q24h	Suspect if fever & abdominal pain post-transplant. Exclude hepatic artery thrombosis. Presence of candida and/or VRE bad prognosticators.
Viral hepatitis	Hepatitis A, B, C, D, E, G	See Table 14F and Table 14G		
LUNG/Bronchi				
Bronchiolitis/wheezy bronchitis (expiratory wheezing)				
Infants/children (≤ age 5) See RSV, Table 14A page 167 Ref: *Ln 368:312, 2006*	< Age 2: Adenovirus; age 2–5: Respiratory syncytial virus, parainfluenza 3 virus, human metapneumovirus **Respiratory syncytial virus** 50%, parainfluenza 25%, human metapneumovirus	Antibiotics not useful; mainstay of therapy is oxygen. Ribavirin for severe disease: 6 gm vial (20 mg/mL) in sterile H₂O by SPAG-2 generator over 18–20 hrs daily times 3–5 days.	Antibiotics indicated only with associated sinusitis or heavy growth on throat culture for S. pneumo, Group A strep, H. influenzae or no improvement in 1 week. Otherwise rx is symptomatic.	RSV most important. Rapid diagnosis with antigen detection methods. For prevention (a humanized mouse monoclonal antibody), **palivizumab**. See Table 14A, page 167. RSV immune globulin is no longer available. Guidance from the American Academy of Pediatrics recommends use of Palivizumab only in newborn infants born at 29 weeks gestation (or earlier) and in special populations (e.g., those infants with significant heart disease). (*Pediatrics 2014;134:415–420*)
Bronchitis				
Infants/children (≤ age 5)	Usually viral. M. pneumoniae 5%, C. pneumoniae 5%. See Persistent cough	**Antibiotics not indicated.** Antitussive ± inhaled bronchodilators. Throat swab PCR available for Dx of mycoplasma or chlamydia.		
Adolescents and adults with acute tracheobronchitis (**Acute bronchitis**) Ref.: *JAMA 312:2678, 2014*	Usually viral. M. pneumoniae 5%, C. pneumoniae 5%. See Persistent cough (**Pertussis**)	**Antitussive ± bronchodilators.**	Purulent sputum alone not an indication for antibiotic therapy. Expect cough to last 2 weeks. If fever/rigors, get chest x-ray. **If mycoplasma documented, prefer doxy over macrolides due to increasing macrolide resistance (***JAC 68:506, 2013***).**	

*NOTE: All dosage recommendations are for adults (unless otherwise indicated) and assume normal renal function. § Alternatives consider allergy, PK, compliance, local resistance, cost

Abbreviations on page 2.

TABLE 1 (34)

ANATOMIC SITE/DIAGNOSIS/ MODIFYING CIRCUMSTANCES	ETIOLOGIES (usual)	SUGGESTED REGIMENS*		ADJUNCT DIAGNOSTIC OR THERAPEUTIC MEASURES AND COMMENTS
		PRIMARY	ALTERNATIVE¹	
LUNG/Bronchi/Bronchitis (continued)				
Persistent cough (>14 days), afebrile during community outbreak: Pertussis (whooping cough) 10–20% adults with cough >14 days have pertussis (Review: Chest 146:205, 2014)	Bordetella pertussis & occ. Bordetella parapertussis. Also consider asthma, gastroesophageal reflux, post-nasal drip, mycoplasma and also chlamydia.	**Peds doses:** Azithro OR clarithro OR erythro esto- late OR erythro base¹⁶ OR TMP-SMX (doses in footnote¹⁶)	**Adult doses:** Azithro 500 mg po x 1 dose, then 250 mg po q24h x 4 days OR erythro estolate 500 mg po qid times 14 days OR TMP-SMX-DS 1 tab po bid times 14 days OR clarithro 500 mg po bid or 1 gm ER (see JAMA times 1 day)	**3 stages of illness:** catarrhal (1–2 wks), paroxysmal coughing (2–4 wks), and convalescence (1–2 wks). Treatment may abort or eliminate pertussis in catarrhal stage, but does not shorten paroxysmal stage. **Diagnosis:** PCR on nasopharyngeal secretions or ↑ pertussis-toxin antibody. **Rx aimed at eradication of NP carriage.** In non-outbreak setting, likelihood of pertussis increased if ↑ post-tussive emesis or inspiratory whoop present (JAMA 304:890, 2010).
Pertussis: Prophylaxis of household contacts	Drugs and doses as per treatment immediately above.		Vaccination of newborn contacts.	Recommended by Am. Acad. Ped. (Red Book 2006 for all household & close contacts; community-wide prophylaxis not recommended).
Acute bacterial exacerbation of chronic bronchitis (ABECB), adults (almost always smokers with COPD) Ref: NEJM 359:2355, 2008.	Viruses 20–50%, C. pneumoniae 5%, H. pneumoniae <1%, role of S. pneumo, H. influenza & M. catarrhalis controversial. Tobacco use, air pollution contribute.	**Severe ABECB** = ↑ dyspnea, ↑ sputum viscosity/purulence. **Role of antimicrobial therapy is debated even for severe disease, but recent study of >80,000 patients shows value of antimicrobial therapy in patients hospitalized with severe disease (JAMA 303(20):2035, 2010). For mild or moderate disease, no antimicrobial treatment or maybe amox. doxy. TMP-SMX, or O Ceph. For severe disease, AM-CL, azithro/clarithro, or O Ceph or FQs with enhanced activity vs. drug-resistant S. pneumo (Gemi, Levo, Moxi or Pruliflox).** *Drugs & doses in footnote.	&/or low O₂ sat; (2) inhaled anticholinergic bronchodilator; (3) oral corticosteroid for just 5 days (JAMA 309:2223, 2013). (4) D/C tobacco use; Duration varies with drug: range 3–10 days. Limit Gemi to 5 days to decrease risk of rash. Azithro 250 mg daily x 1 yr modestly reduced frequency of acute exacerbations in pts with milder disease (JAMA 365:689, 2011).*	Options: (1) O₂ if pO₂ low or O₂ sat low, 1 sputum volume. For severe ABECB (1) consider chest x-ray, esp. if febrile **Complications: Influenza pneumonia, secondary bacterial pneumonia** Community MRSA and MSSA, S. pneumoniae, H. influenzae.
Fever, cough, myalgia during influenza season (See NEJM 360:2605, 2009 regarding novel H1N1 (Influenza A)	Influenza A & B	*See* Influenza, Table 14A, page 165.		
Bronchiectasis. Thorax 65(suppl1):i1, 2010; Am J Respir Crit Care 183:186:647, 2013.	H. influ, P. aeruginosa, and rarely S. pneumo.	Gemi, levo, or moxi x 7–10 days. *Dosage in footnote¹⁶.*		Many potential etiologies: obstruction, ↑ immune globulins, cystic fibrosis, dyskinetic cilia, tobacco, prior severe or recurrent necrotizing bronchitis; e.g. pertussis.
Acute exacerbation				**Caveats:** higher rates of macrolide resistance in oropharyngeal flora; potential for ↑ risk of a) cardiovascular deaths from macrolide-induced QTc prolongation, b) liver toxicity, or c) hearing loss (see JAMA 309:1295, 2013).
Prevention of exacerbation	Not applicable	Two randomized trials of **Erythro** 250 mg bid (JAMA 309:1260, 2013) or **Azithro** 250 mg qd (JAMA 309:1251, 2013) x 1 year showed significant reduction in the frequency of acute exacerbations, better preservation of lung function, and better quality of life versus placebo in adults with non-cystic fibrosis bronchiectasis.		**Pre-treatment screening:** baseline liver function tests, electrocardiogram; assess hearing; sputum culture to exclude mycobacterial disease.
Specific organisms	Aspergillus (see Table 11) MAI (Table 12) and P. aeruginosa (Table 5A)			

¹⁶ **ADULT DOSAGE: AM-CL** 875/125 mg po bid or 500/125 mg po q8h or 2000/125 mg po bid; **azithro** 500 mg po x 1 dose, then 250 mg q24h x 4 days or 500 mg po q24h x 3 days; *Oral cephalosporins:* **cefaclor** 500 mg po q8h or 500 mg extended release q12h; **cefdinir** 300 mg po q12h or 600 mg po q24h; **cefditoren** 200 mg po q12h; **cefixime** 400 mg po q24h; **cefpodoxime proxetil** 200 mg po q12h; **cefprozil** 500 mg po q12h; **ceftibuten** 400 mg po q24h; **cefuroxime axetil** 250 or 500 mg po q12h; **loracarbef** 400 mg po q12h; **clarithro** extended release 1000 mg po q24h; **erythro base** 40 mg/kg/day po div q6h; **erythro estolate** 40 mg/kg/day po div qid; FQs: **CIP** 750 mg po q24h; **gemi** 320 mg po q24h; **levo** 500 mg po q24h; **moxi** 400 mg po q24h (where available) **TMP-SMX** 1 DS tab po bid.

PEDS DOSAGE: azithro 10 mg/kg/day po on day 1, then 5 mg/kg po q24h x 4 days; **clarithro** 7.5 mg/kg po q12h; **erythro base** 40 mg/kg/day div q6h; **erythro estolate** 40 mg/kg/day div q8-12h; **TMP-SMX** (>6 mos. of age) 8 mg/kg/day (TMP component) po bid.

Abbreviations on page 2. *NOTE: All dosage recommendations are for adults (unless otherwise indicated) and assume normal renal function. § Alternatives consider allergy, PK, compliance, local resistance, cost*

Abbreviations on page 2.

TABLE 1 (35)

ANATOMIC SITE/DIAGNOSIS/ MODIFYING CIRCUMSTANCES	ETIOLOGIES (usual)	SUGGESTED REGIMENS* PRIMARY	SUGGESTED REGIMENS* ALTERNATIVE†	ADJUNCT DIAGNOSTIC OR THERAPEUTIC MEASURES AND COMMENTS
LUNG/Bronchi (continued)				
Pneumonia: CONSIDER TUBERCULOSIS IN ALL PATIENTS; ISOLATE ALL SUSPECT PATIENTS				
Neonatal: Birth to 1 month	**Viruses:** CMV, rubella, H. simplex **Bacteria:** Group B strep, listeria, coliforms, S. aureus, P. aeruginosa **Other:** Chlamydia trachomatis, syphilis	**AMP + gentamicin ± cefotaxime.** Add **vanco** if MRSA a concern. For chlamydia therapy, **erythro** 12.5 mg per kg po or IV qid times 14 days.		Blood cultures indicated. Consider C. trachomatis if afebrile pneumonia, staccato cough; IgM >1:8; therapy with erythro or sulfisoxazole. If MRSA documented, **vanco**, **TMP-SMX**, & **linezolid** alternatives. **Linezolid** dosage from birth to age 11 yrs is **10 mg per kg q8h.**
Age 1–3 months				
Pneumonitis syndrome, afebrile	Usually C. trachomatis, RSV, parainfluenza virus 3, human metapneumovirus, Bordetella, S. pneumoniae, S. aureus (rare)	**Outpatient: po erythro** 12.5 mg/kg q6h x 14 days or po **azithro** 10 mg/kg x dose, then 5 mg/kg x 4 days.	**Inpatient: If afebrile erythro** 10 mg/kg IV q6h or **azithro** 2.5 mg/kg IV q12h (see Comment). **If febrile** add **cefotaxime** 200 mg/kg per day div q8h	Pneumonitis syndrome: Cough, tachypnea, dyspnea, diffuse infiltrates, afebrile. Usually requires hospital care. Reports of hypertrophic pyloric stenosis after erythro under age 6 wks; not sure about azithro; bid azithro dosing theoretically might ↓ risk of hypertrophic pyloric stenosis. If lobar pneumonia, give AMP 200–300 mg per kg per day for S. pneumoniae. No empiric coverage for S. aureus, as it is rare etiology.
			For RSV, see Bronchiolitis, page 36	
Infants and Children, age > 3 months to 18 yrs (IDSA Treatment Guidelines: CID 53:617, 2011)				
Outpatient	RSV, human metapneumovirus, rhinovirus, influenza virus, adenovirus, parainfluenza virus, Mycoplasma, H. influenzae, S. pneumoniae, S. aureus (rare)	**Amox** 90 mg/kg in 2 divided doses x 5 days	**Azithro** 10 mg/kg x 1 dose(max 500 mg), then 5 mg/kg (max 250 mg) x 4 days OR **Amox-Clav** 90 mg/kg (Amox) in 2 divided doses x 5 days	Antimicrobial therapy not routinely required for preschool-aged children with CAP as most infections are viral etiologies.
Inpatient	As above	Fully immunized: **AMP** 50 mg/kg IV q6h Not fully immunized: **Cefotaxime** 150 mg/kg IV divided q8h	Fully immunized: **Cefotaxime** 150 mg/kg IV divided q8h	If atypical infection suspected, add **Azithro** 10 mg/kg x 1 dose (max 500 mg), then 5 mg/kg (max: 250 mg) x 4 days. If community MRSA suspected, add **Vanco** 15-20 mg/kg q8-12h OR **Clinda** 40 mg/kg/day divided q6-8h. Duration of therapy: 10-14 days. Depending on clinical response, may switch to oral agents as early as 2-3 days.

*NOTE: All dosage recommendations are for adults (unless otherwise indicated) and assume normal renal function. § Alternatives consider allergy; PK, compliance, local resistance, cost

TABLE 1 (36)

ANATOMIC SITE/DIAGNOSIS/MODIFYING CIRCUMSTANCES	ETIOLOGIES (usual)	SUGGESTED REGIMENS*		ADJUNCT DIAGNOSTIC OR THERAPEUTIC MEASURES AND COMMENTS
		PRIMARY	ALTERNATIVE[1]	

LUNG/Bronchi/Pneumonia (continued)

Adults (over age 18) — IDSA/ATS Guideline for CAP in adults: *CID 44 (Suppl 2); S27-S72, 2007; NEJM 370:543, 2014;*				**Azithro/clarithro:** Pro: appropriate spectrum of activity; q24h dosing; better tolerated than erythro.
NEJM 371:1619, 2014.	Varies with clinical setting.	**No co-morbidity;**	**Co-morbidity present: Respiratory FQ** (see	Con: Overall S. pneumo resistance in vitro 20–30%, higher if pen G resist. Slightly higher risk of cardiovascular events found in retrospective studies (BMJ 346:f1235, 2013); consider alternative regimen in setting of cardiovascular disease.
Community-acquired, not hospitalized	Atypicals—M. pneumoniae, et al (S. pneumo, viral	**azithro** 0.5 gm po times 1, then 0.25 gm per day **OR**	footnote[19])	
	No co-morbidity:	**clarithro** 500 mg po bid **or**		
Prognosis prediction: CURB-65	**Co-morbidity:**	**azithro-ER** 2 gm po times 1	(*azithro* or *clarithro*) +	
(*Thorax 58:377, 2003*)	Alcoholism: S. pneumo, anaerobes, coliforms	**OR**	higher dose **amox** or high dose	**Amoxicillin:**
	Bronchiectasis: see Cystic	**clarithro** 1 gm po q24h	**AM-CL OR**	Pro: Active 90–95% vs S. pneumo at 3–4 gm per day.
U: confusion = 1 pt	fibrosis, page 44	**OR if prior antibiotic within**	*(azithro* or *clarithro*) +	Con: No activity vs atypicals or β-lactamase positive organisms.
R: BUN >19 mg/dl = 1 pt	COPD: H. influenzae,	**3 months: (azithro or**	**AM-CL cefdinir, cefpodox**	
B: RR >30 /min = 1 pt	M. catarrhalis, S. pneumo	**clarithro) + (amox** 1 gm po	**ime, cefprozil)[1]**	**AM-CL:**
B: BP < 90 syst. = 1 pt	IVDU: Hematogenous	**tid or high dose AM-CL OR**		Pro: Spectrum of activity includes β-lactamase positive organisms.
Age ≥65 = 1 pt	S. pneumo	**Respiratory FQ**	*Doses in footnote[19]*	Con: Diarrhea—see footnote.
				Cephalosporins—po: Cefditoren, cefpodoxime, cefprozil, cefuroxime
If score = 1, ok for outpatient therapy; if >1,	Post-CVA aspiration: Oral flora, incl. S. pneumo	**Duration of rx:** S. pneumo—Not bacteremic: until afebrile 3 days—		& others—see footnote[19] Pro: Active 75–85% S. pneumo & H. influenzae. Cefuroxime least active & higher mortality rate when S. pneumo resistant.
hospitalize. The higher the score, the higher the mortality.	Post-influenza: S. pneumo, S. aureus	Bacteremic: 10–14 days reasonable		Con: Inactive vs. atypical pathogens.
	H1-influenza:	C. pneumoniae—Uncertain. Some reports suggest		**Doxycycline:**
Lab diagnosis of invasive pneumococcal disease:	S. pneumo, and S. aureus	clarithro (*J Med Micro 52:265, 2003*) Legionella—10–21 days		Pro: Active vs S. pneumo 18–20%, H. influenzae, atypicals, & bioterrorism agents (anthrax, plague, tularemia). Resistance of S. pneumo 18–20%. Some clinical data.
CID 57:e22, 2013. Antibiotic therapy decreases % pos. S. pneumo sputum cultures within 6 hrs (*CID 58:1782, 2014*).		Necrotizing pneumonia 2° to coliforms, S. aureus, anaerobes: ≥2 weeks		**FQs—Respiratory:** Gemi, Moxi, Levo & gemi S. pneumo. **NOTE: dose of Levo is 750 mg q24h.** Gemi only available po.
		Cautions: 1. **Local macrolide resistance to S. pneumoniae**		Con: Geographic pockets of resistance with clinical failure. Important drug-drug interactions (see *Table 22A, page 218*). Reversible rash in young females, given Gemi for >7 days.
Community-acquired, hospitalized—NOT in the ICU. Empiric therapy	Etiology by co-morbidity & risk factors as above.	**>25%, use alternative empiric therapy.** 2. **Esp. during influenza season, look for S. aureus.**		
	Culture sputum & blood.			**Ceftriaxone/cefotaxime:** Pro: Drugs of choice for pen-sens. S. pneumo, active H. influenzae,
Treat for minimum of 5 days, afebrile 48–72 hrs, with stable BP, adequate oral intake, and room air O₂ saturation of >90% (*CID 20:177, 2007*).	S. pneumo, urine antigen helpful (50–75% sens, 90% specif); Legionella urine antigen indicated. In general, the sicker the pt, the more valuable culture data. Look for S. aureus especially concomitant influenza and IVDU.	**Ceftriaxone** 1 gm IV q24h **or** **+ azithro** 500 mg IV q24h **OR** **Ertapenem** 1 gm IV q24h **plus** *azithro* 500 mg IV q24h	**Respiratory FQ** **Levo** 750 mg IV q24h **or** **Moxi** 400 mg IV q24h **Gatt** 400 mg IV q24h (gati no longer marketed in US due to serious hyperglycemic reactions)	M. catarrhalis, & MSSA. Con: Not active vs atypicals or pneumonia due to bioterrorism pathogens. **Ceftaroline:** (FDA approved at a dose of 600 mg q12h IV for 5-7 days for hospitalized patients with CAP). Pro: Clinical response rates at day 4 and clinical cure rates at days 8-15 post-treatment were similar for ceftaroline and ceftriaxone (*see ceftaroline package insert*). Con: More expensive; no data for MRSA yet.
		Administration of antibiotic within 6h associated with improved survival in pneumonia and severe sepsis (*Eur Respir J 39:156, 2012*); 1st dose in ER, first dose in ER [If diagnosis of pneumonia vague, cautionary: 1st dose in ER for admitting diagnosis of "uncertain" - (*Chest 130:16, 2006*).			

---

[17] Atypical pathogens: Chlamydophila pneumoniae, C. psittaci, Legionella sp., M. pneumoniae, C. burnetii (Q fever), (Ref: *LnID 3:709, 2003*)

[18] Respiratory FQs with enhanced activity vs. S. pneumo with high-level resistance to penicillin: **Gati**[lus] 400 mg IV/po q24h (no longer marketed in US due to hypo- and hyperglycemic reactions). **Gemi** 320 mg po q24h, **Levo** 750 mg IV/po q24h. Ketolide: **Moxi** 400 mg IV/po q24h (physicians warned about rare instances of hepatotoxicity).

[19] **O Ceph** dosage: **Cefdinir** 300 mg po q12h; **cefditoren pivoxil** 200 mg, 2 tabs po q12h; **cefpodoxime proxetil** 200 mg po q12h, **cefprozil** 500 mg po q12h, **high dose amox** 1 gm po tid; **high dose AM-CL**—use **AM-CL-ER** 1000/62.5 mg, 2 tabs po bid.

NOTE: All dosage recommendations are for adults (unless otherwise indicated) and assume normal renal function. § Alternatives consider allergy, PK, compliance, local resistance, cost

Abbreviations on page 2.   *NOTE: All dosage recommendations are for adults (unless otherwise indicated) and assume normal renal function. § Alternatives consider allergy, PK, compliance, local resistance, cost*

TABLE 1 (37)

ANATOMIC SITE/DIAGNOSIS/ MODIFYING CIRCUMSTANCES	ETIOLOGIES (usual)	SUGGESTED REGIMENS*		ADJUNCT DIAGNOSTIC OR THERAPEUTIC MEASURES AND COMMENTS
		PRIMARY	ALTERNATIVE†	
LUNG/Bronchi/Pneumonia/Adults (over age 18) *(continued)*				
Community-acquired, hospitalized—IN ICU, Empiric therapy 4 clinical settings: • **Severe COPD** • **Post-Influenza** • **Suspect gm-neg bacilli** • **Risk of Pen G-resistant S. pneumo**	**Severe COPD** (8-38%): S. pneumoniae (8-38%), H. influenzae, Moraxella sp. If admitted to ICU: S. pneumo (15-23%), S. aureus (1.2-8.7%), Legionella (0.6-5%), H. flu. Chest 133:610, 2008; Thorax 66:340, 2011; CID 50:202, 2010; Int J Antimicrob Agts 31:107, 2008. **Severe COPD pt with pneumonia:** S. pneumoniae, H. influenzae, Moraxella sp. Legionella sp. Rarely S. aureus. **Post-Influenza:** Most common S. pneumoniae, S. aureus.	(**Levo** 750 mg IV q24h or **Moxi** 400 mg IV q24h) (see Comment) **Gati** not available in US due to hypo- and hyperglycemic reactions	[**Ceftriaxone** 1 gm IV q24h + **azithro** 500 mg IV q24h) or **ERTA** 1 gm IV q24h + **azithro** 500 mg IV q24h *(see Comment)*	Improved outcome with β-lactam/macrolide combo vs. β-lactam alone (patients treated with fluoroquinolones were excluded) in hospitalized CAP of moderate severity, but not low-severity (Thorax 68:493, 2013). **Ertapenem** could substitute for ceftriaxone if need azithro for atypical pathogens. Do not use if suspect P. aeruginosa. **Legionella:** Not all Legionella species detected by urine antigen; if suspicious do PCR on airway secretions. (CID 57:1275, 2013). In patients with normal sinus rhythm and not receiving beta-blockers, relative bradycardia suggests Legionella, psittacosis, Q-fever, or typhoid fever.
		Pro-calcitonin: Several clinical trials and meta-analyses indicate that normal procalcitonin levels can be used to guide duration of antibiotic therapy. Safe to discontinue antibiotics when procalcitonin level has decreased to 0.1-0.2 mcg/mL. (CID 55:651, 2012; JAMA 309:717, 2013).		
Post-Influenza resistant influenzae? S. aureus, S. pneumoniae	Culture sputum, blood and maybe pleural fluid. Look for respiratory viruses. Urine antigen for both Legionella and S. pneumoniae. Sputum PCR for Legionella.	**Vanco** 15 mg/kg q8-12h + (**Levo** 750 mg IV q24h or **moxi** 400 mg IV q24h)	**Linezolid** 600 mg IV bid (**levo** or **moxi**)	**Nasal swab for MRSA PCR helpful; neg predictive value of 96.2%; if PCR neg, can de-escalate empiric vanco** (Arch Path Lab Med 137:1367, 2013). Nasal swab for S. aureus post-influenza (see Table 10D, page 110). FQ dose for P. aeruginosa. Staph gram stain or PCR may help. S. aureus post-influenza ref EID 12:894, 2006 Empiric therapy vs. MRSA decreases risk of mortality. (CCM 34:2069, 2006). **Risk factors:** alcoholism (Klebsiella pneumoniae), underlying chronic bronchiectasis (e.g. cystic fibrosis), chronic tracheostomy and/or mechanical ventilation, febrile neutropenia and pulmonary infiltrates, septic shock, underlying malignancy, or organ failure. **P. aeruginosa:**
Suspect aerobic gm-neg bacilli (see Comment). Hypoxic and/or hypotensive? S. pneumo & GNB		**Anti-pseudomonal beta-lactam²⁰‡** + (**respiratory FQ** or [**aztreonam + aminoglycoside**] + **azithro** if no P. aeruginosa	If severe IgE-mediated beta-lactam allergy: **aztreonam + FQ** or (**aztreonam + aminoglycoside + azithro**). advantage only one agent active vs. S. aureus; disadvantage: only one agent active vs. GNB	If need higher doses of **CIP** (400 mg IV q8h) and/or **PIP-TZ** 3.375 gm IV q4h.
		Empiric **Vanco** + **PIP-TZ.** advantage is activity vs. S. aureus; disadvantage: only one agent active vs. GNB		
Risk of Pen G-resistant S. pneumoniae: 2° antibiotic use in last 3 months.		**High dose IV amp** (or **Pen G**) + **azithro** + **respiratory FQ**	**Beta-lactam allergy: vanco** + **respiratory FQ**	If Pen G MIC≤4 mg/mL, vanco. Very rare event.
Health care-associated pneumonia (HCAP) Ref. CID 46 (Suppl 4):S296, 2008.	HCAP designates large diverse population of pts with many co-morbidities who reside in nursing homes, other long-term care facilities, require home IV therapy or are on dialysis (do NOT use to treat pneumonia). Pneumonia in these pts frequently resembles hospital-acquired pneumonia (below). Higher frequency of resistant bacteria than pts with CAP: MRSA (11.5%). MDR enterobacteriaceae (7.8%); P. aeruginosa (6.9%) (CID 57:1373, 2013).			

20 *Antipseudomonal beta-lactams:* **Aztreonam** 2 gm IV q6h; **piperacillin** 3 gm IV q6h; **piperacillin/tazobactam** 3.375 gm IV q4h or 4.5 gm IV q6h or 4-hr infusion of 3.375 gm q8h(high dose for Pseudomonas); **cefepime** 2 gm IV q12h; **ceftazidime** 2 gm IV q8h; **doripenem** 0.5 gm IV q8h (do NOT use to treat pneumonia); **imipenem/cilastatin** 500 mg IV q6h; **meropenem** 1 gm IV q8h; **gentamicin or tobramycin** 1 gm IV q8h (see *Table 10D, page 110*). FQ dose for P. aeruginosa: **CIP** 400 mg IV q8h or **levo** 750 mg IV q24h; **Respiratory FQs: levofloxacin** 750 mg IV q24h or **moxifloxacin** 400 mg IV q24h; **high-dose ampicillin** 2 gm IV q6h; **vanco** 15-20 mg/kg IV q8h (based on actual body wt) IV q8-12h (to achieve target trough concentration of 15-20 µg/mL).

Abbreviations on page 2.   *NOTE: All dosage recommendations are for adults (unless otherwise indicated) and assume normal renal function. § Alternatives consider allergy; PK, compliance, local resistance, cost

TABLE 1 (38)

ANATOMIC SITE/DIAGNOSIS/ MODIFYING CIRCUMSTANCES	ETIOLOGIES (usual)	SUGGESTED REGIMENS*		ADJUNCT DIAGNOSTIC OR THERAPEUTIC MEASURES AND COMMENTS
		PRIMARY	ALTERNATIVE[1]	
LUNG/Bronchi/Pneumonia/Adults (over age 18) (continued)				
Hospital-acquired—usually with mechanical ventilation (VAP) (empiric therapy) Proposed diagnostic approach: *CID 57:1742, 2013.*	Highly variable depending on culture results: S. pneumo, S. aureus, Legionella, coliforms, P. aeruginosa, Stenotrophomonas, Acinetobacter sp. (susceptibility to IMP/MER may be discordant (*CID 41:758, 2005*), anaerobes are possible. In some locales, GNB that have extended-spectrum beta-lactamase (ESBL) and/or carbapenemases *Diagnosis; see Comment*	**IMP** 0.5 gm IV q6h or **MER** 1 gm IV q8h) plus, if suspect legionella or suspect **respiratory FQ** (**Levo** or **Moxi**) for MRSA	If suspect P. aeruginosa, empirically select 2 drugs to increase likelihood that at least one will be active, e.g.: **IMP** or **CFP** or **PIP-TZ**[21] + (**CIP** or **tobra**) Ref: *CCM 35:1888, 2007*	**Dx of ventilator-associated pneumonia:** Fever & lung infiltrates often **not** pneumonia. Quantitative cultures helpful: bronchoalveolar lavage (>10⁴ per mL pos.) or protect. spec. brush (>10³ per mL pos.) Ref.: *AJRCCM 165:867, 2002; AnIM 132:621, 2000.* **Microbial etiology:** No empiric regimen covers all possibilities. Regimens listed above majority vs. S. pneumo, legionella, & most coliforms. Regimens **not active** vs. MRSA, Stenotrophomonas & others; *see below. Specific therapy when culture results known.* **Ventilator-associated pneumonia.—Prevention:** Keep head of bed elevated 30° or more. Remove N-G, endotracheal tubes as soon as possible. If available, continuous subglottic suctioning. Chlorhexidine oral care. Silver coated endotracheal tubes reported to reduce incidence of VAP. (*JAMA 300:805 & 842, 2008*). **Doripenem:** do not use q8h for VAP. Dori failed vs. IMP in prospective randomized double blind phase 3 trial.
		Dosages: See *Comment* on page 40. Duration of therapy, see *footnote[23]* Nasal swab PCR for MRSA helpful. If PCR neg., can dc empiric **vanco** (*CID 58:859, 2014*).		
Hospital- or community-acquired, neutropenic pt (<500 neutrophils per mm³)	Any of organisms listed under community- & hospital-acquired + fungi (aspergillus) + *See Table 11.*	See Hospital-acquired; *immediately above.* Vanco not included in initial therapy unless high suspicion of infected IV access or drug-resistant S. pneumo. Ampho not used unless still febrile after 3 days or high clinical likelihood. See *Comment*		
Pneumonia —Selected specific therapy after culture results (sputum, blood, pleural fluid, etc.) available. *Also See Table 2, page 68*				
Acinetobacter baumannii (*See also Table 10A*) Ref: *NEJM 358:1271, 2008*	Patients with VAP	Use **IMP** or **MER** if susceptible	If IMP resistant: **colistin** + (**IMP** or **MER**). Colistin Dose: *Table 10A, page 104*	Subbactam portion of AM-SB often active; Meropenem or Clinda for meningitis. 1. Meropenem preferred over Clinda for meningitis. 2. Pen G 4 million units IV (adults) or 67,000 units/kg (children, max 4 million units per dose) IV q4h can be substituted for Meropenem for pen-susceptible strain.
Actinomycosis	A. Israelii and rarely others	**AMP** 50 mg/kg/day IV div in 3-4 doses x 4-6 wks, then **Pen VK** 2-4 gm/day po x 3-6 wks	**Doxy** or **ceftriaxone** or **clinda**	Can use **Pen G** instead of AMP: 10-20 million units/day IV x 4-6 wks.
Anthrax **Inhalation** (applies to oro-pharyngeal & gastrointestinal forms): **Treatment** (Cutaneous: *See page 51*) Ref: *www.bt.cdc.gov; CDC panel recommendations for adults. Emerg Infect Dis 20(2) doi: 10.3201/eid2002.130687. American Academy of Pediatrics recommendations for children: Pediatrics 133:e1411, 2014.*	Bacillus anthracis **To report possible bioterrorism event:** 770-488-7100	**Adults (including pregnancy):** **CIP** 400 mg IV q12h or **Levo** 750 mg IV q24h or **Clindamycin** 900 mg IV q8h (see comments) + **raxibacumab** 40 mg/kg IV over 2 hrs). Switch to po after 2 wks if stable: **CIP** 500 mg q12h or Doxy 100 mg q12h to complete 60-day regimen	**Children:** **CIP** 10 mg/kg IV q8h (max 400 mg per dose) + **Linezolid** 10 mg/kg q8h (age <12 yr) or q12h (age ≥12 yr) + **Meropenem** 40 mg/kg IV q8h (max 2 gm per dose) (see comments) + **raxibacumab** 40-80 mg/kg IV over 2 hrs. Switch to po after 2 wks if stable: **CIP** 15 mg/kg q12h (<45 kg) or 500 mg q12h (>45 kg) or Doxy q12h to complete 60-day regimen dosage	3. For children <3 years: Linezolid preferred over Clinda. 4. Levo and Moxi are alternatives to CIP 5. For complete recommendations see *Emerg Infect Dis 20(2), doi: 10.3201/eid2002.130687 (adults) and Pediatrics 133:e1411, 2014 (children).*
Actinomycosis				

---

[21] **PIP-TZ** for P. aeruginosa pneumonia: 3.375 gm IV over 4 hrs & repeat q8h (*CID 44:357, 2007*) plus **tobra**.

Abbreviations on page 2.   *NOTE: All dosage recommendations are for adults (unless otherwise indicated) and assume normal renal function.*   PK, compliance, local resistance, cost

NOTE: All dosage recommendations are for adults (unless otherwise indicated) and assume normal renal function. §*Alternatives consider allergy, PK, compliance, local resistance, cost*

TABLE 1 (39)

ANATOMIC SITE/DIAGNOSIS/ MODIFYING CIRCUMSTANCES	ETIOLOGIES (usual)	SUGGESTED REGIMENS*		ADJUNCT DIAGNOSTIC OR THERAPEUTIC MEASURES AND COMMENTS
		PRIMARY	ALTERNATIVE§	
LUNG/Bronchi/Pneumonia/ Selected specific therapy after culture results (sputum, blood, pleural fluid, etc.) available. *(continued)*				
Anthrax, prophylaxis: See: *Emerg Infect Dis 2012;* doi: 10.3201/eid1802.111184. 60-3205 of **antimicrobial prophylaxis + 3-dose series of Biothrax Anthrax Vaccine Adsorbed.** Info: www.bt.cdc.gov		**Adults (including pregnancy):** CIP 500 mg po q12h or Doxy 100 mg po q12h x 60 days + 3-dose series of Biothrax Anthrax Vaccine Adsorbed	**Children: CIP** or **Doxy** (see Comment) CIP 10-15 mg per kg IV q12h x 60 days + 3-dose series of Biothrax Anthrax Vaccine Adsorbed (not FDA approved, to be made available on investigational basis)	1. Consider alternatives to Doxy for pregnant adult. 2. Alternatives should include Clinda, Levo, Moxi, and for pen-susceptible strains Amox or Pen VK.
Burkholderia (Pseudomonas) pseudomallei (etiology of melioidosis) Can cause primary or secondary skin infection See *NEJM 367:1035, 2012.*	Gram-negative	**Initial parenteral rx:** Ceftazidime 30-50 mg per kg IV q8h or IMP or MER 20 mg per kg IV q8h. Rx minimum 10 days & improving, then po therapy → see *Alternative* column	**Post-parenteral po rx: Adults** (see Comment for children): TMP-SMX 5 mg/kg (TMP component) bid + Doxy 2 mg/kg bid x 3 mos.	**Children ≤8 yrs old & pregnancy:** For oral regimen, use **AM-CL-ER** 1000/62.5, 2 tabs po bid times 20 wks. Even with compliance, relapse rate is 10%. Max. daily ceftazidime dose: 6 gm.
Haemophilus influenzae		**AMP IV, amox po, TMP-SMX, azithro/clarithro, doxy.** AM-CL, O Ceph 2/3, P Ceph 3, FQ Dosage: *Table 10A*		Tigecycline: No clinical data but active in vitro (*AAC 50:1555, 2006*) 25-35% strains β-lactamase positive. ↑ resistance to both TMP-SMX and doxy. See *Table 10A, page 96 for dosages.* High % of commensal H. hemolyticus misidentified as H. influenza (*JID 195:61, 2007*).
β-lactamase negative				
β-lactamase positive				
Klebsiella sp.—ESBL pos. & other coliforms[22] β-lactamase positive	β-lactamase positive	IMP or MER. If resistant, **Colistin + (IMP or MER)**		ESBL inactivates all cephalosporins, β-lactam/β-lactamase inhibitor drug activ'not predictable; co-resistance to FQs often aminoglycosides.
Legionella species Relative bradycardia common feature		**Azithro** 500 mg IV or **Levo** 750 mg IV or **Moxi** 400 mg IV See *Table 10A, pages 101 & 103 for dosages.* Treat for 7-14 days (*CID 39:1734, 2004*)		Legionella website: www.legionella.org. Two studies support superiority of **Levo** over macrolides (*CID 40:794 & 800, 2005*), *although not FDA-approved.* Meta-analysis favors a FQ (*CID 59:2354, 2014*).
Moraxella catarrhalis	93% β-lactamase positive	**AM-CL, O Ceph 2/3, P Ceph 2/3, macrolide[23], FQ, TMP-SMX. Doxy** another option. See *Table 10A, page 96 for dosages.*		
Nocardia pneumonia Expert Help: Wallace Lab (+1) 903-877-7680; CDC (+1) 404-639-3158 Ref: *Medicine 88:250, 2009.*	N. asteroides, N. brasiliensis	**TMP-SMX** 15 mg/kg/day IV/po in 2-4 divided doses + **Imipenem** 500 mg IV q6h for first 3-4 wks then po **TMP-SMX** 10 mg/kg/day in 2-4 divided doses x3-6 mos.	**IMP 500 mg IV q6h +** amikacin 7.5 mg/kg IV q12h x 3-4 wks & then po **TMP-SMX**	**Duration:** 3 mos. if immunocompetent; 6 mos. if immunocompromised. **Measure peak sulfonamide levels:** Target is 100-150 mcg/mL 2 hrs post po dose. **Linezolid** active in vitro (*Ann Pharmacother 41:1694, 2007*). In vitro resistance to TMP-SMX may be increasing (*Clin Infect Dis 51:1445, 2010*), but whether this is associated with worse outcomes is not known.
Pseudomonas aeruginosa Combination rx controversial: superior in animal model benefit in subset clinical trials (*AAC 57:1270, 2013; CID 57:208, 2013*).	Often ventilator-associated	**PIP-TZ** 3.375 gm IV q4h or prefer 4-hr infusion of 3.375 gm q8h) + **tobra** 5 mg/kg/day IV q24h (see *Table 10D, page 110*). Could substitute (**IMP MER**) for **PIP-TZ** if pt. strain is susceptible.		Options: **CFP** 2 gm IV q8h; **CIP** 400 mg IV q8h + **PIP-TZ**; **IMP** 500 mg IV q6h + **CIP** 400 mg IV q8h; if multi-drug resistant, **Colistin** IV + (**IMP or MER**) + **Colistin** by inhalation 80 mg bid (controversial, *CID 52:1278, 2011*). Also available for inhalation rx: **tobra** and **aztreonam**.

---

[22] Dogma on duration of therapy not possible with so many variables; i.e. certainty of diagnosis, infecting organism, severity of infection and number/severity of co-morbidities. Agree with efforts to de-escalate & shorten course. Treat at least 7-8 days. Need clinical evidence of response: fever resolution, improved oxygenation, failing WBC. Refs: *AJRCCM 171:388, 2005; CID 43:S75, 2005; COID 19:185, 2006.*

[23] **Macrolide** = azithromycin, clarithromycin and erythromycin.

Abbreviations on page 2.

*NOTE: All dosage recommendations are for adults (unless otherwise indicated) and assume normal renal function. § Alternatives consider allergy, PK, compliance, local resistance, cost

*Abbreviations on page 2.

*NOTE: All dosage recommendations are for adults (unless otherwise indicated) and assume normal renal function. § Alternatives consider allergy, PK, compliance, local resistance, cost

TABLE 1 (40)

ANATOMIC SITE/DIAGNOSIS/ MODIFYING CIRCUMSTANCES/	ETIOLOGIES (usual)	SUGGESTED REGIMENS*		ADJUNCT DIAGNOSTIC OR THERAPEUTIC MEASURES AND COMMENTS
		PRIMARY	ALTERNATIVE§	
LUNG/Bronchi/Pneumonia/ Selected specific therapy after culture results (sputum, blood, pleural fluid, etc.) available. *(continued)*				
Q Fever Acute atypical pneumonia. See *MMWR* 62 (3):1, 2013.	Coxiella burnetii	**Doxy** 100 mg po bid x 14 days	No valvular heart disease: **Doxy** 100 mg po bid + **hydroxychloroquine** 200 mg tid x 12 months (CID 57:836, 2013) Valvular heart disease:	In pregnancy: **TMP-SMX DS** 1 tab po bid throughout pregnancy.
Staphylococcus aureus Duration of treatment: 2-3 wks if just pneumonia; 4-6 wks if concomitant endocarditis and/or osteomyelitis. IDSA Guidelines, CID 52 (Feb 1):1, 2011.	Nafcillin/oxacillin susceptible	**Nafcillin/oxacillin** 2 gm IV q4h	**Vanco** 30-60 mg/kg/d IV in 2-3 divided doses or **linezolid** 600 mg IV q12h	Adjust dose of vancomycin to achieve target trough concentrations of 15-20 mcg/mL. Some authorities recommend a 25-30 mg/kg loading dose (actual body weight) in severely ill patients (CID 49:325, 2009).
	MRSA	**Vanco** 15-20 mg/kg IV q8-12h IV in 2-3 divided doses **or Linezolid** 600 mg IV/po q12h	**Dapto** not an option; pneumonia developed during dapto rx (CID 49:1286, 2009). **Ceftaroline** 600 mg IV q8h.	Prospective trial for MRSA pneumonia: cure rate with Linezolid (58%), Vanco (47%), p = 0.042; no difference in mortality with Linezolid **Televancin** 10 mg/kg IV x 60 min q24h another option. Perhaps lower efficacy if CrCl < 50mL/min (AAC 58:2030, 2014).
Stenotrophomonas maltophilia		**TMP-SMX** up to 20 mg/kg/day div q6h	**TC-CL** 3.1 gm IV q4h or **FQ**³ (AAC 58:176, 2014).	Potential synergy: **TMP-SMX** + **TC-CL** (JAC 62:889, 2008). Tigecycline may be another option (J Chemother 24:150, 2012).
Streptococcus pneumoniae	Penicillin-susceptible	**AMP** 2 gm IV q6h, **amox** 1 gm po tid, **pen G** IV²⁴ **doxy** IV (JAC 69:1441, 2014). See Table 10A, page 96 for other dosages.	**O Ceph 2, P Ceph 3** (resistance rare); high-dose IV **AMP. vanco** IV—see Table 5A, page 78	May add **Azithro** 500 mg IV/po qd until afebrile. (min. of 5 days) and/or until serum procalcitonin normal.
	Penicillin-resistant, high level	**FQs** with enhanced activity: **Gemi, Levo, Moxi**; **P Ceph 3** if all options not possible (e.g., allergy): high-dose IV **AMP, vanco** IV—see Table 10A. Treat until afebrile, 3-5 days (min. of 5 days). In CAP trial, **Ceftaroline** 600 mg IV q12h superior to Ceftriaxone (CID 51:1641, 2010).	**linezolid** active: 600 mg IV q12h. Dosages: See Table 10A. Treat until afebrile,	
Tularemia Inhalational tularemia Treatment Ref.: JAMA 285:2763, 2001 & www.bt.cdc.gov	Francisella tularemia	**(Streptomycin** 15 mg per kg IV bid) or **gentamicin** 5 mg per kg IV qd) times 10 days	**Doxy** 100 mg IV or po bid times 14-21 days or **CiP** 400 mg IV (or 750 mg po) bid times 14-21 days	Pregnancy: As for non-pregnant adults.
Postexposure prophylaxis		**Doxy** 100 mg po bid times 14 days	**CiP** 500 mg po bid times 14 days	Pregnancy: As for non-pregnant adults Pregnancy: **Tobramycin** should work.
Viral (interstitial) pneumonia suspected See Influenza, Table 14A, page 165. Ref.: Chest 133:1221, 2008.	Consider: **Influenza** adenovirus, coronavirus (SARS), hantavirus, metapneumovirus, parainfluenza virus, respiratory syncytial virus	**Oseltamivir** 75 mg po bid for 5 days or **zanamivir** two 5 mg inhalations twice a day for 5 days	**Doxy** 200 mg IV times 1, then 100 mg IV bid	No known efficacious drugs for adenovirus, coronavirus (SARS), hantavirus, metapneumovirus, parainfluenza or RSV. Need travel (SARS) & exposure (Hanta), history, RSV and human metapneumovirus as serious as influenza in the elderly (NEJM 352:1749 & 1810, 2005; CID 44:1152 & 1759, 2007).
Yersinia pestis (Plague) CID 49:736, 2009	Y. pestis. If aerosolized, suspect bioterror.	**Gentamicin** 5 mg/kg IV q24h	**Doxy** 200 mg IV q12h also an option. **Chloramphenicol**	**Cipro** 500 mg po bid or 400 mg IV q12h also an option. **Chloramphenicol** also effective but potentially toxic.

²⁴ **IV Pen G dosage:** no meningitis, 2 million units IV q4h. If concomitant meningitis, 4 million units IV q4h.

*NOTE: All dosage recommendations are for adults (unless otherwise indicated) and assume normal renal function. § Alternatives consider allergy, PK, compliance, local resistance, cost

Abbreviations on page 2.

TABLE 1 (41)

ANATOMIC SITE/DIAGNOSIS/ MODIFYING CIRCUMSTANCES	ETIOLOGIES (usual)	SUGGESTED REGIMENS*		ADJUNCT DIAGNOSTIC OR THERAPEUTIC MEASURES AND COMMENTS
		PRIMARY	ALTERNATIVE‡	
LUNG—Other Specific Infections				
Aspiration pneumonia/anaerobic lung infection/lung abscess	Transthoracic culture in 90 pts—% of total isolates: anaerobes 34%, Gm-pos. cocci 26%, S. milleri 16%, Klebsiella pneumoniae 25%, nocardia 3%	**Clindamycin** 300-450 mg po tid **OR Ampicillin-sulbactam** 3 g IV q6h OR **Carbapenem** (e.g., ertapenem 1 g IV q24h)	**Ceftriaxone** 1 gm IV q24h plus **metro** 500 mg IV q6h or 1 gm IV q12h	Typically anaerobic infection of the lung: aspiration pneumonitis, necrotizing pneumonia, lung abscess and empyema (REF: Anaerobe 18:235, 2012) other treatment options: PIP-TZ 3.325 g IV q6h (for mixed infections with resistant Gram-negative aerobes) or Moxi 400 mg IV/po q24h (CID 47:1764, 2005).
Chronic pneumonia with fever, night sweats and weight loss	M. tuberculosis, coccidiodomycosis, histoplasmosis	See Table 11, Table 12 for risk associated with TNF inhibitors, see CID 41(Suppl 3):S187, 2005		HIV+, foreign-born, alcoholism, contact with TB, travel into developing countries
Cystic fibrosis **Acute exacerbation of pulmonary symptoms** BMC Medicine 9:32, 2011	S. aureus or H. influenzae early in disease, P. aeruginosa later in disease Nontuberculous mycobacteria emerging as an important pathogen (Semin Respir Crit Care Med 34:124, 2013)	**For P. aeruginosa:** (Pods doses) **Tobra** 3.3 mg/kg q8h or 12 mg/kg IV q24h. Combine tobra with **PIP** or **ticarcillin** 100 mg/kg q6h) **or ceftaz** 50 mg/kg IV q8h to max of 6 gm per day; if resistant to above, **CIP/Levo** used if P. aeruginosa susceptible. See footnote¹ & Comment	**For S. aureus: (1) MSSA-oxacillin/nafcillin** 2 gm IV q4h; **(2) MRSA—vanco** 15-20 mg/kg (actual wt) IV q8-12h (to achieve target trough concentration of 15-20 μg/mL.	Cystic Fibrosis Foundation Guidelines: 1. Combination therapy for P. aeruginosa infection. 2. Once-daily dosing for aminoglycosides. 3. Need more data on continuous infusion beta-lactam therapy. 4. Routine use of steroid not recommended Inhalation options (P. aeruginosa suppression): 1) Nebulized tobra 300 mg bid x 28 days, no rx for 28 days, repeat; 2) inhaled tobra powder-hand held: 4-28 mg cap bid x 28 days, no rx for 28 days, repeat; Nebulized aztreonam (Cayston): 75 mg bid after pre-dose bronchodilator. Ref: Med Lett 56:51, 2014.
	Burkholderia (Pseudomonas) cepacia	**TMP-SMX** 5 mg per kg (TMP) IV q6h	**Chloro** 15-20 mg per kg IV/po q6h	B. cepacia has become a major pathogen. Patients develop progressive respiratory failure, 62% mortality at 1 yr. **Fail to respond to aminoglycosides**, piperacillin, & ceftazidime. Patients with B. cepacia should be isolated from other CF patients.
Empyema. IDSA Treatment Guidelines for Children, CID 53:617, 2011; exudative pleural effusion criteria (JAMA 311:2422, 2014).				For other alternatives, see Table 2
Neonatal	Staph. aureus	See Pneumonia, neonatal, page 38		
Infants/children (1 month–5 yrs)	Staph. aureus, Strep. pneumoniae, H. influenzae	See Pneumonia, age 1 month–5 years, page 36		Drainage indicated.
Child >5 yrs to ADULT—Diagnostic thoracentesis; chest tube for empyemas For dosage, see Table 10B or footnote page 25	Strep. pneumoniae, Strep. pyogenes, Staph. aureus; Group A strep	**Cefotaxime** or **ceftriaxone**† (Dosage, see footnote¹ page 25)	**Vanco**	Drainage indicated.
	Staph. aureus; Check for MRSA	**Nafcillin** or **oxacillin** if MSSA	**Vanco** or **linezolid** if MRSA	Usually complication of S. aureus pneumonia &/or bacteremia.
	Staph. aureus; H. influenzae	**Ceftriaxone**	**TMP-SMX** if MRSA	Pleomorphic Gm-neg. bacilli. † resistance to TMP-SMX.
Subacute/chronic	Anaerobic strep, Strep. milleri, Bacteroides sp., Enterobacteriaceae, M. tuberculosis	**Clinda** 450-900 mg IV q8h + **ceftriaxone**	**Cefoxitin** or **IMP** or **TC-CL** or **PIP-TZ** or **AM-SB** (Dosage, see footnote¹¹ page 25)	Intrapleural tissue plasminogen activator (t-PA) 10 mg + DNase 5 mg via chest tube twice daily for 3 days improved fluid drainage, reduced frequency of surgery, and reduced duration of the hospital stay; neither agent effective alone (N Engl J Med 365:518, 2011). Pro/con debate: Chest 145:14, 17, 20, 2014. Pleural biopsy with culture for mycobacteria and histology if TB suspected

25 Other options: (Tobra + aztreonam 50 mg per kg IV q8h); (IMP 15-25 mg per kg IV q6h + tobra); **CIP** commonly used in children, e.g., CIP IV/po q6h (or tobra).

*NOTE: All dosage recommendations are for adults (unless otherwise indicated) and assume normal renal function. § Alternatives consider allergy, PK compliance, local resistance, cost

Abbreviations on page 2.

TABLE 1 (42)

ANATOMIC SITE/DIAGNOSIS/ MODIFYING CIRCUMSTANCES	ETIOLOGIES (usual)	SUGGESTED REGIMENS*		ADJUNCT DIAGNOSTIC OR THERAPEUTIC MEASURES AND COMMENTS
		PRIMARY	ALTERNATIVE[1]	
LUNG—Other Specific Infections (continued)				
Human immunodeficiency virus (HIV+): See *SANFORD GUIDE TO HIV/AIDS THERAPY*				
CD4 T-lymphocytes <200 per mm³ or clinical AIDS Dry cough, progressive dyspnea, & diffuse infiltrate	Pneumocystis carinii most likely; also MTB, fungi, Kaposi's sarcoma. NOTE: AIDS pts may develop pneumonia due to DRSP or other pathogens—see next box below	Rx listed here is for severe pneumocystis; see Table 11A, page 123 for regimens for mild disease. **Prednisone first** (see Comment), then: **TMP-SMX** [V: 15 mg per kg per day div q8h (TMP 5 mg/kg q8h + TMP-SMX DS tabs q8h), total of 21 days	**Clinda** 600 mg IV q8h + **primaquine** (base) 30 mg po q24h) times 21 days. or **isethionate** 4 mg per kg per day (V) times 21 days. See Comment	**Diagnosis (induced sputum or bronchial wash)** for: histology or monoclonal antibody stains of BAL fluid. Beta-glucan serum levels in serum may be useful. Check LDH levels, usually elevated. **Prednisone** (before TMP-SMX or PCP po, 2OBr. Prednisone 40 mg po bid times 5 days, then 40 mg q24h po times 5 days, then 20 mg q24h po times 11 days. Drug should be given at initiation of anti-PCP rx; should be given at initiation of anti-PCP rx; should be given if pt's condition deteriorates. If PCP studies negative, consider bacterial pneumonia, Kaposi, histo, crypto, lymphoma. **Pentamidine not active vs. bacterial pathogens. NOTE: Pneumocystis resistant to TMP-SMX, albeit rare, does exist.**
Prednisone first if suspect pneumocystis (see Comment)				
CD4 T-lymphocytes normal Acute onset, purulent sputum & pulmonary infiltrates ± pleuritic pain. **Isolate pt until TBc excluded: Adults**	Strep. pneumoniae, H. influenzae, aerobic Gm-neg. bacilli (including P. aeruginosa), Legionella rare, MTB	Ceftriaxone 1 gm IV q24h (over age 65 1 gm IV q24h) + **azithro** Could use **Levo**, or **Moxi** IV as alternative (See Comment)		If Gram stain of TP-TZ, IMP, or MER. **AP-TC-CL, TP-TZ, IMP,** or **MER. Pos: Levo** 750 mg po/IV q24h; **Moxi** 400 mg po/IV q24h. Gati not available in US due to hypo- & hyperglycemic reactions
As above: Children	Same as adult with HIV + lymphoid interstitial pneumonia (LIP)	As for HIV + adults with pneumonia. If diagnosis is LIP, rx with steroids		In children with AIDS, LIP responsible for 1/3 of pulmonary complications, usually >1 yr of age. vs. PCP, which is seen at <1 yr of age. Clinically: clubbing, hepatosplenomegaly, salivary glands enlarged (take up gallium), lymphoproliferation.
LYMPH NODES (approaches below apply to lymphadenitis without an obvious primary source)				
Lymphadenitis, acute **Generalized**	Etiologies: EBV, early HIV infection, syphilis, toxoplasma, tularemia, Lyme disease, sarcoid, lymphoma, systemic lupus erythematosus, **Kikuchi-Fujimoto** disease and others. For differential diagnosis of fever and lymphadenopathy see NEJM 369:2333, 2013.			
Regional				
Cervical—see cat-scratch disease (CSD), below	CSD (B. henselae), Grp A strep, Staph. aureus, anaerobes, MTB (scrofula), M. avium, M. scrofulaceum, M. malmoense, toxo, tularemia	History & physical exam directs evaluation. If nodes fluctuant, aspirate and base rx on Gram & acid-fast stains. **Kikuchi-Fujimoto** disease causes fever and benign self-limited adenopathy; the etiology is unknown (CID 39:138, 2004).		
Inguinal				
Sexually transmitted	HSV, chancroid, syphilis, LGV			
Not sexually transmitted	GAS, SA, tularemia, CSD, Y. pestis (plague)	Consider bubonic plague & glandular tularemia.		
Axillary	GAS, SA, CSD, tularemia, Y. pestis, sporotrichosis	Consider bubonic plague & glandular tularemia.		
Extremity, with associated nodular lymphangitis	Sporotrichosis, leishmania, Nocardia brasiliensis, Mycobacterium marinum, Mycobacterium chelonae, tularemia	Treatment varies with specific etiology		A distinctive form of lymphangitis characterized by subcutaneous swellings along inflamed lymphatic channels. Primary site of skin invasion usually present; regional adenopathy variable.
Nocardia lymphadenitis & skin abscesses	N. asteroides, N. brasiliensis	**Sulfisoxazole** 2 gm po qid or **minocycline** 100-200 mg po bid		**Duration:** 3 mos. If immunocompetent; 6 mos. if immunocompromised (Ann Pharmacother 41:1694, 2007). **Linezolid:** 600 mg po bid reported effective
Cat-scratch disease— immunocompetent patient Axillary/epitrochlear nodes 46%, neck 26%, inguinal 17.5%. Ref: Ann Emerg Physician 83:152, 2011.	Bartonella henselae	**Azithro** dosage—**Adults** (>45.5 kg): 500 mg po x 1, then 250 mg/day x 4 days. **Children** (<45.5 kg): liquid azithro 10 mg/kg x 1, then 5 mg/kg per day x 4 days. Rx is controversial		No therapy, resolves in 2-6 mos. Needle aspiration relieves pain in suppurative nodes. Avoid I&D. **Clinical:** Approx. 10% nodes suppurate. Atypical presentation in ~5% pts. ise, hepatic/splenic granulomatosis, Parinaud's oculoglandular syndrome, CNS manifestations in 2% of pts (encephalitis, peripheral neuropathy, retinitis), FUO. **Dx:** Cat exposure. Positive IFA serology. Rarely need biopsy.

Abbreviations on page 2.   *NOTE: All dosage recommendations are for adults (unless otherwise indicated) and assume normal renal function. § Alternatives consider allergy, PK, compliance, local resistance, cost

TABLE 1 (43)

ANATOMIC SITE/DIAGNOSIS/ MODIFYING CIRCUMSTANCES	ETIOLOGIES (usual)	SUGGESTED REGIMENS*		ADJUNCT DIAGNOSTIC OR THERAPEUTIC MEASURES AND COMMENTS
		PRIMARY	ALTERNATIVE§	
MOUTH				
Aphthous stomatitis, recurrent	Etiology unknown	Topical steroids (Kenalog in Orabase) may ↓ pain and swelling. If AIDS, see SANFORD GUIDE TO HIV/AIDS THERAPY.		
Actinomycosis: "Lumpy jaw" after dental or jaw trauma	Actinomyces israeli	AMP 50 mg/kg/d IV div q6-8h x 4-6 wks, then Pen VK 2-4 gm/d x 3-6 mos	Ceftriaxone 2 gm IV q24h or Clinda 600-900 mg IV q8h or Doxy 100 mg IV (po bid) x 4-6 wks, then Pen VK 2-4 gm/d x 3-6 mos	Note: Metro not active vs. actinomyces. Ref: BMJ 343:d6099, 2011.
Buccal cellulitis Children <5 yrs	H. influenzae	Cefuroxime or ceftriaxone	AM-CL or TMP-SMX	With Hib immunization, invasive H. influenzae infections have ↓ by 95%. Now occurring in infants prior to immunization.
Candida Stomatitis ("Thrush")	C. albicans	Fluconazole	Echinocandin	See Table 11, page 114.
Herpetic stomatitis	Herpes simplex virus 1 & 2	See Table 14		
Submandibular space infection, bilateral (Ludwig's angina)	Oral anaerobes, facultative streptococci, S. aureus (rare)	PIP-TZ or TC-CL) or (Pen G IV + Metro IV)	Clinda 600 mg IV q6-8h (for Pen-allergic pt)	Ensure adequate airway and early surgical debridement. Add Vanco IV if gram-positive cocci on gram stain.
Ulcerative gingivitis (Vincent's angina or Trench mouth)	Oral anaerobes + vitamin deficiency	Pen G po/IV + Metro po/IV	Clinda	Replete vitamins (A-D). Can mimic scurvy. Severe form is NOMA (Cancrum oris) (Ln 368:147, 2006)
MUSCLE				
"Gas gangrene" Contaminated traumatic wound. Can be spontaneous without trauma.	C. perfringens, other histotoxic Clostridium sp.	(Clinda 900 mg IV q8h) + pen G 24 million units/day div. q4-6h IV	Ceftriaxone 2 gm IV q12h or erythro 1 gm q6h IV (not by bolus)	Surgical debridement primary therapy. Hyperbaric oxygen adjunctive: not recommended as efficacy debated and may delay surgical debridement. Clinda given to decrease toxin production. (CID 59:1147, 2014)
Pyomyositis	Staph. aureus, Group A strep, (rarely Gm-neg. bacilli), variety of anaerobic organisms	Nafcillin or oxacillin 2 gm IV q4h) or Cefazolin 2 gm IV q8h if MSSA	Vanco 15-20 mg/kg q8-12h if MRSA	Common in tropics; rare, but occurs, in temperate zones. Follows exercise or muscle injury, see Necrotizing fasciitis. Now seen in HIV/AIDS. Add metro if anaerobes suspected or proven.
PANCREAS: Review: NEJM 354:2142, 2006.				
Acute alcoholic (without necrosis) (idiopathic) pancreatitis	Not bacterial	None No necrosis on CT		1-9% become infected but prospective studies show no advantage of prophylactic antimicrobials. Observe for pancreatic abscesses or necrosis with newer therapy.
Post-necrotizing pancreatitis; infected pseudocyst; pancreatic abscess	Enterobacteriaceae, enterococci, S. aureus, S. epidermidis, anaerobes, candida	Need culture of abscess/infected pseudocyst to direct therapy; PIP-TZ is reasonable empiric therapy		Can often get specimen by fine-needle aspiration. Moxi, MER, IMP, ERTA are all options (AAC 56:6434, 2012).
Antimicrobial prophylaxis, necrotizing pancreatitis	As above	If > 30% pancreatic necrosis on CT scan (with contrast), initiate antibiotic therapy: IMP 0.5-1 gm IV q6h or MER 1 gm IV q8h. No need for empiric Fluconazole. If patient worsens PIP-TZ guided aspiration for culture & sensitivity. Controversial: Cochrane Database Sys Rev 2003: CD 002941. Gastroenterol 126:997, 2004; Ann Surg 245:674, 2007.		
PAROTID GLAND				
"Hot" tender parotid swelling	S. aureus, S. pyogenes, oral flora, & aerobic Gm-neg. bacilli (rare), mumps, rarely enterovirus/ influenza	Nafcillin or oxacillin 2 gm IV q4h or cefazolin 2 gm IV q8h if MSSA; vanco, metro or clinda for anaerobes		Predisposing factors: stone(s) in Stensen's duct, dehydration. Therapy depends on ID of specific etiologic organism.
"Cold" non-tender parotid swelling	Granulomatous disease (e.g., mycobacteria, fungi, sarcoidosis, Sjögren's syndrome), drugs (iodides, et al.), diabetes, cirrhosis, tumors			History/lab results may narrow differential; may need biopsy for diagnosis

Abbreviations on page 2.

*NOTE: All dosage recommendations are for adults (unless otherwise indicated) and assume normal renal function. § Alternatives consider allergy, PK, compliance, local resistance, cost

TABLE 1 (44)

ANATOMIC SITE/DIAGNOSIS/ MODIFYING CIRCUMSTANCES	ETIOLOGIES (usual)	SUGGESTED REGIMENS*		ADJUNCT DIAGNOSTIC OR THERAPEUTIC MEASURES AND COMMENTS
		PRIMARY	ALTERNATIVE§	
PERITONEUM/PERITONITIS: *Reference—CID 50:133, 2010*				
Primary (spontaneous bacterial peritonitis, SBP) *Hepatology 49:2087, 2009.* Dx: Pos. culture & ≥ 250 neutrophils/µL of ascitic fluid.	Enterobacteriaceae 63%, S. pneumo. 9%, enterococci 6–10%, anaerobes <1%. Extended β-lactamase (ESBL) positive Klebsiella species.	**Cefotaxime** 2 gm IV q8h (if life-threatening, q4h) or **TC-CL or PIP-TZ** [**ceftriaxone** 2 gm IV q24h) or **ERTA** 1 gm IV q24h **If resistant E. coli/Klebsiella species (ESBL+), then:** [**DORI, ERTA, IMP** or **MER**] or [**FQ: CIP, Levo, Moxi**] Check in vitro susceptibility. *(Dosage in footnote*).*		One-year **risk of SBP** in pts with ascites and cirrhosis is as high as 29% (*Gastro 104:1133, 1993*). Diagnosis of SBP: 30–40% of pts have neg. cultures of blood and ascitic fluid. % pos. cultures if in 10 mL of pt's ascitic fluid added to blood culture bottles (*JAMA 299:1166, 2008*). **Duration of rx unclear.** Treat for at least 5 days, perhaps longer if pt bacteremic (*Pharm & Therapeutics 34:204, 2009*). **IV albumin** (1.5 gm/kg day 1 & 1 gm/kg day 3) may ↓ frequency of renal impairment (p 0.002) & ↓ hospital mortality (p 0.01) (*NEJM 341:403, 1999*).
Prevention of SBP (*Amer J Gastro 104:993, 2009*): Cirrhosis & ascites *For prevention after UGI bleeding, see Liver, page 36*		**TMP-SMX-DS** 1 tab 5 days/wk or **CIP 750 mg** po q wk		**TMP-SMX**, ↓ peritonitis. O Cover both Gm-neg. aerobic & Gm-neg. anaerobic bacteria. Must "cover" both Gm-neg. aerobic & Gm-neg. anaerobic bacteria. Empiric coverage of MRSA, enterococci and candida not necessary unless culture indicates infection. Cover enterococci if valvular heart disease. **Drugs active only vs. anaerobic Gm-neg. bacilli:** metro. **Drugs active only vs. aerobic Gm-neg. bacilli:** aminoglycosides. P Ceph 2/3/4, aztreonam, AP Pen, CIP, Levo. **Drugs active vs. both aerobic/anaerobic Gm-neg. bacteria:** TC-CL, PIP-TZ, Dori, IMP, MER. Increasing resistance (R) of Bacteroides species (*Anaerobe 17:147, 2013; AAC 56:1247, 2012*) to:
Secondary (bowel perforation, ruptured appendix, ruptured diverticuli) *Ref: CID 50:133, 2010 (IDSA Guidelines)* **Antifungal rx?** No need if successful uncomplicated 1st surgery for viscus perforation. Treat for candida if: recurrent surg. perforation(s), anastomotic leaks, necrotizing pancreatitis, liver/pancreas transplant, pure peritoneal culture, candidemia (*Ln 2:1437, 1989*). Detection serum β-D-glucan antigen in serum of limited value due to low sensitivity/specificity and many false positives (*JCM 51:3478, 2013*).	Enterobacteriaceae, Bacteroides sp, enterococci, P. aeruginosa (3–15%). C. albicans (may contribute with recurrent perforation/multiple surgeries) If VRE documented, dapto. (*Int J Antimicrob Agents 32:369, 2008*).	**Mild-moderate disease—parenteral rx:** (e.g. focal periappendiceal peritonitis, peridiverticular abscess). **Usually need surgery for source control.** **PIP-TZ** 3.375 gm IV q6h or 4.5 gm IV q8h or 4-hr infusion of 3.375 gm q8h **TC-CL** 3.1 gm IV q6h OR **ERTA** 1 gm IV q24h OR **MOXI** 400 mg IV q24h **Severe life-threatening disease—ICU patient: Surgery for source control →** **IMP** 500 mg IV q6h or **MER** 1 gm IV q8h or **DORI** 1 gm IV q8h (1-hr infusion) or [(Ceftolozane-tazobactam 1.5 gm IV q8h or 500 mg IV q6h) + Metro 500 mg IV q6h] **Concomitant surgical management important.**	[**CIP** 400 mg IV q12h or **Levo** 750 mg IV q24h) + (**metro** 1 gm IV q12h)] or [(**metro** 1 gm q12h) + **metro** q24h] + (**metro** 1 gm IV q12h)] + **metro** Note: aminoglycoside (see Table 10A, page 11D) antimycobacterial due to increased mortality risk (FDA warning) **Severe life-threatening disease—ICU patient:** [**AMP** + **metro** + (**CIP** 400 mg IV q8h or **Levo** 750 mg IV q24h)] OR [**AMP** 2 gm IV q4–6h + **metro** 500 mg q6h + aminoglycoside (see Table 10D, page 110)]	metro, **PIP-TZ, TC-CL,** Cefotetan Clindamycin 135 % R Cefoxitin 1–30 5–30 13–87 Essentially no resistance of Bacteroides to: metro, **PIP-TZ, TC-CL, Carbapenems.** Case report of B. fragilis resistant to all drugs except minocycline, tigecycline & linezolid (*MMWR 62:694, 2013*). **Ertapenem** not active vs. P. aeruginosa/Acinetobacter species. If absence of ongoing fecal contamination, **aerobic culture** of peritoneal exudate/abscess may be of help in guiding specific therapy. Less need for aminoglycosides. **With severe pen allergy,** can "cover" Gm-neg. aerobes with **CIP** or **aztreonam. Remember DORI/IMP/MER are β-lactams.** IMP dose increased to 1 gm q8h if suspect P. aeruginosa and pt. is critically ill. Resistance to Moxi increasing. See *CID 59:698, 2014* (suscept. of anaerobic bacteria).

** Parenteral **IV therapy** for peritonitis: **TC-CL** 3.1 gm q6h, **PIP-TZ** 3.375 gm q6h or 4.5 gm q8h or 4-hr infusion of 3.375 gm q8h (*See Table 10*). **Dori** 500 mg IV q8h (1-hr infusion). **IMP** 0.5–1 gm q6h, **MER** 1 gm q8h, **Oflox** 400 mg q12h, **Levo** 750 mg q24h, **Moxi** 400 mg q24h). **AMP** 1 gm q6h, **aminoglycoside** (see Table 10D, page 110) **aminoglycoside** (see Table 10D, page 110), **cefotetan** 2 gm q8h, **P Ceph 3** (**cefotaxime** 2 gm q4–8h, **ceftizoxime** 1–2 gm q8h, **ceftriaxone** 2 gm q24h), **P Ceph 4 (cefepime** 2 gm q12h), **clinda** 600–900 mg q8h. **Metronidazole** 1 gm IV q8h (15 mg/kg) loading dose IV, then 7.5 mg/kg q6h, *(Some data supports once-daily dosing, see Table 10A, page 105)*, **AP Pen (ticarcillin** 4 gm q6h), **PIP** 4 gm q8h, **aztreonam** 2 gm q8h.)

*NOTE: All dosage recommendations are for adults (unless otherwise indicated) and assume normal renal function. § Alternatives consider allergy, PK, compliance, local resistance, cost

Abbreviations on page 2.

TABLE 1 (45)

ANATOMIC SITE/DIAGNOSIS/ MODIFYING CIRCUMSTANCES	ETIOLOGIES (usual)	SUGGESTED REGIMENS* PRIMARY	SUGGESTED REGIMENS* ALTERNATIVE§	ADJUNCT DIAGNOSTIC OR THERAPEUTIC MEASURES AND COMMENTS
PERITONEUM/PERITONITIS (continued)				
Abdominal actinomycosis	A. Israelii and rarely others	**AMP** 50 mg/kg/day IV div in 3-4 doses x 4-6 wks, then **Pen VK** 2-4 gm/day po	**Doxy** or **ceftriaxone** or **clinda**	Presents as mass +/- fistula tract after abdominal surgery; e.g., for ruptured appendix. Can use IV Pen G instead of AMP: 10-20 million units/day IV x 4-6 wks.
Associated with chronic ambulatory peritoneal dialysis (Adult doses; for peds see *Perit Dial Int* 20:S45, 2000). For empiric therapy, cloudy dialysate, dialysate WBC > 100 cell/µL with >50% neutrophils; normal = <8 cells/µL. Ref: *Perit Dial Int* 30:393, 2010.)	Gm+ 45%; Gm- 15%; Multiple 1%; Fungi 2%; Culture neg 20%.	**Empiric therapy**: Need activity vs. MRSA (**Vanco**) & aerobic gram-negative bacilli (**Ceftaz, CFP, Carbapenem, Gent**). Add **Vanco** if Grp empirical therapy. If culture shows Staph or other Gm+, start po **Vanco** (dosing). Use intraperitoneal dosing, unless bacteremia (rare). For bacteremia, IV dosing. For dosing detail, see *Table 19, page 214.*		**For diagnosis**: concentrate several hundred mL of removed dialysis fluid by centrifugation, Gram stain concentrate and then inject into aerobic/anaerobic blood culture bottles. **Positive Gram stain will guide initial therapy.** If culture shows yeast. **Remove catheter: if multiple Gm-neg, bacilli cultured, consider catheter-induced bowel perforation and need for catheter removal.** Other indications for catheter removal: relapsing/refractory peritonitis, fungal peritonitis, catheter tunnel infection.
PHARYNX				
Pharyngitis/Tonsillitis: "Strep throat"				
Exudative or Diffuse Erythema				
Associated cough, rhinorrhea, hoarseness and/or oral ulcers suggest viral etiology. IDSA Guidelines on Group A Strep, *CID* 55:1279, 2012; *CID* 53:686, 2012.	Group A, C, & G Strep; Fusobacterium (in research studies); EBV; Primary HIV; N. gonorrhoeae; Respiratory viruses	**For Strep pharyngitis:** (**Pen V** 10 days or **Benzathine Pen** 1.2 million units IM x 1 dose) OR **Cephalexin** or (**cefpodoxime** x 5 days) or **amoxicillin (adult and peds) doses** (Durations in adult and peds) FDA-approved).	**For Strep. pharyngitis: Pen allergic: Clinda** 300-450 mg po q8h x10 days are alternatives. **Clarithro** or **azithro** are alternatives. S. pyogenes resistance to these & reported (*EID* 18:1658, 2012). Sulfonamides and Tetracyclines have failed.	**Dx: Rapid Strep test.** If rapid test neg., do culture (*CID* 59:643, 2014). No need for post-treatment test of cure rapid strep test or culture. **Complications of Strep pharyngitis:** 1) Acute rheumatic fever 48° follows Grp A S. pyogenes infection, rare after Grp A/G/G infection. See footnote. For prevention, start treatment within 9 days of onset of symptoms. 2) Pediatric cases > 7 yrs at risk for post-streptococcal glomerulonephritis. 3) Children age < 7 yrs at risk for post-streptococcal glomerulonephritis. Pediatric autoimmune neuropsychiatric disorder associated with Grp A Strep (PANDAS) infection. 4) Peritonsillar abscess. Suppurative phlebitis are potential complications.
		Ceftriaxone 250 mg IM x 1 dose) or **Doxy** 100 mg po bid x 7 days	**FQs** not recommended due to resistance	Not effective for pharyngeal GC: spectinomycin, cefixime, cefpodoxime and cefuroxime. Ref: *MMWR* 61:590, 2012.
Gonococcal pharyngitis		**Ceftriaxone** 250 mg IM x 1 dose) or **Doxy** 100 mg po bid x 7 days		
Proven S. pyogenes recurrence	Proven S. pyogenes recurrence Grp A infections: 6 in 1 yr; 4 in 2 consecutive yrs	**Cefdinir** or **Cefpodoxime**	**AM-CL** or **Clinda**	Hard to distinguish true Grp A Strep infection from chronic Grp A Strep carriage and/or repeat viral infections.
		Tonsillectomy not recommended to decrease Strep infections		

[27] **Treatment of Group A, C, G and G strep:** Treatment durations are from approved package inserts. Subsequent studies indicate efficacy of shorter treatment courses. All po unless otherwise indicated. **PEDIATRIC DOSAGE: Benzathine penicillin** 25,000 units per kg IM to max. 1.2 million units; **Pen V** 25-50 mg per kg per day div. by q8h x 10 days; **amox** 1000 mg po once daily x 10 days; **cephalexin** 20 mg/kg/dose bid (max. 500 mg/dose) x10 days; **cefuroxime axetil** 20 mg per kg per day div. x 10 days; **cefpodoxime proxetil** 10 mg per kg. div. bid x 10 days; **cefdinir** 7 mg per kg po q24h x 10 days; **cefprozil** 15 mg per kg per day div. x 10 days; **cefadroxil** 30 mg/kg once daily x 10 days; **ADULT DOSAGE:** **clarithro** 15 mg per kg per day div. bid or 250 or 500 mg daily x 5 days; **azithro** 12 mg per kg once daily x 5 days; clinda 7 mg per kg per day div. q8h x 10 days; **cefpodoxime proxetil** 100 mg bid **Benzathine** penicillin 1.2 million units IM x 1; **Pen V** 500 mg bid or 250 mg tid x 10 days; **ceftibuten** 200 mg bid x 10 days; **cefuroxime axetil** 250 mg bid x 10 days; **cefpodoxime axetil** 250 mg bid x 5 days; **cefdinir** 300 mg q12h x 5-10 days or 600 mg q24h x10 days; **clarithro** 500 mg x 1 and then 250 mg q24h x 4 days; **azithro** 500 mg x 1 and then 250 mg q24h x 4 days increasing number of infections requiring Grp A strep eradication.

[28] Primary rationale for therapy is eradication of Group A strep (GAS) and prevention of acute rheumatic fever (ARF). Benzathine penicillin G has been shown in clinical trials to ↓ rate of ARF from 2.8 to 0.2%. This was associated with clearance of GAS on pharyngeal cultures (*CID* 19:1110, 1994). Subsequent studies have been based on cultures, not actual prevention of ARF. Treatment decreases duration of symptoms.

NOTE: All dosage recommendations are for adults (unless otherwise indicated) and assume normal renal function. § Alternatives consider allergy, PK, compliance, local resistance, cost

Abbreviations on page 2.

TABLE 1 (46)

ANATOMIC SITE/DIAGNOSIS/ MODIFYING CIRCUMSTANCES	ETIOLOGIES (usual)	SUGGESTED REGIMENS*		ADJUNCT DIAGNOSTIC OR THERAPEUTIC MEASURES AND COMMENTS
		PRIMARY	ALTERNATIVE†	
PHARYNX/Pharyngitis/Tonsillitis/Exudative or Diffuse Erythema (continued)				
Peritonsillar abscess – Sometimes a serious complication of exudative pharyngitis (Quinsy[1]) (JAC 68:1941, 2013)	F. necrophorum (44%) Grp A Strep (33%) Grp C/G Strep (9%) Strep anginosus grp	**Surgical drainage plus** PIP-TZ 3.375 gm IV q6h or (Metro 500 mg IV/po q6-8h + Ceftriaxone 2 gm IV q24h)	Pen allergic: Clinda 600-900 mg IV q6-8h	**Avoid macrolides: Fusobacterium is resistant.** Reports of beta-lactamase production by oral anaerobes (Anaerobe 9/105, 2003). See Jugular vein suppurative phlebitis below. See JAC 68:1941, 2013. Etiologies ref: CID 49:1467, 2009.
Other complications	See parapharyngeal space infection and jugular vein suppurative phlebitis (see next page)			
Membranous pharyngitis due to **Diphtheria** Respiratory isolation, nasal & pharyngeal cultures (special media), obtain antitoxin. **Place pt in respiratory droplet isolation.**	C. diphtheriae (human to human), C. ulcerans and C. pseudotuberculosis (animal to human) (rare)	**Treatment: antibiotics + antitoxin Antibiotic therapy: Erythro** 500 mg IV or OR **Pen G** 50,000 units/kg (max 1.2 million units) IV q12h. Can switch to Pen VK 250 mg po qid when able. Treat for 14 days	**Diphtheria antitoxin:** Horse serum. Obtain from CDC, +1 404-639-2889. Do scratch test before IV therapy. Dose depends on stage of disease: < 48hrs: 20,000-40,000 units; if NP membranes: 40,000-60,000 units: > 3 days & bull neck: 80,000-120,000 units	**Ensure adequate airway.** EKG & cardiac enzymes. F/U cultures 2 wks post-treatment to document cure. Then, diphtheria toxoid immunization. Culture contacts; treat contacts with either single dose of **Pen G** IM: 600,000 units if age < 6 yrs, 1.2 million units if age ≥ 6 yrs. If Pen-allergic, **Erythro** 500 mg po qid x 7-10 days. Assess immunization status of close contacts: toxoid vaccine as indicated; in vitro, C. diphtheriae suscept. to clarithro, azithro, clinda, FQs, TMP/SMX.
Vesicular, ulcerative pharyngitis (viral)	Coxsackie A9, B1-5, ECHO (multiple types), Enterovirus 71, Herpes simplex 1, 2	Antibacteria agents not indicated. For HSV-1, 2: **acyclovir** 400 mg tid po x 10 days.		Small vesicles posterior pharynx suggests enterovirus. Viruses are most common etiology of acute pharyngitis. Suspect viral if concurrent conjunctivitis, coryza, cough, &/or hoarseness.
Epiglottitis (Supraglottis): Concern in life-threatening obstruction of the airway				
Children	H. influenzae (rare), S. pyogenes, S. pneumoniae, S. aureus (includes MRSA), viruses	Peds dosage: (Cefotaxime 50 mg per kg IV q8h or ceftriaxone 50 mg per kg IV q12h) + Vanco	Peds dosage: Levo 10 mg/kg IV q24h + Clinda 7.5 mg/kg IV q8h	Have tracheostomy set "at bedside". **Levo** use in children is justified as emergency empiric therapy in pts with severe beta-lactam allergy. (Med Let Infect Dis Amer 53:275, 2006. Use of steroids is controversial; do not recommend.
Adults	Group A strep[1] H. influenzae (rare) & many others	Same regimens as for children.	Adult dosage: See footnote§	
Parapharyngeal space infection [Spaces include: sublingual, submandibular (Ludwig's angina), (see page 46) lateral pharyngeal, retropharyngeal, pretracheal] Poor dental hygiene, dental extractions, foreign bodies (e.g., toothpicks, fish bones) Ref: CID 49:1467, 2009	Polymicrobic: Strep sp., anaerobes, Eikenella corrodens; Anaerobes outnumber aerobes 10:1.	[(Clinda 600-900 mg IV q8h) or (pen G 24 million units/day by continuous infusion or div. q4-6h) + (cefotaxime 2 gm IV q4-8h or ceftriaxone 2 gm IV q24h)]	PIP-TZ 3.375 gm IV q6h or AM-SB 3 gm IV q6h	Close observation of airway, 1/3 require intubation. MRI or CT to identify abscess; surgical drainage. Metro may be given 1 gm IV q12h. complications: infection of carotid (rupture possible) & jugular vein phlebitis.
Jugular vein suppurative phlebitis (Lemierre's syndrome)[1] LnID 12:808, 2012.	Fusobacterium necrophorum in vast majority	PIP-TZ 4.5 gm IV q8h or IMP 500 mg IV q6h or (Metro 500 mg po/IV q6h + ceftriaxone 2 gm IV once daily)	Clinda 600-900 mg IV q8h **Avoid macrolides: fusobacterium are resistant**	Emboli: pulmonary and systemic common. Erosion into carotid artery can occur. Lemierre described F. necrophorum in 1936; other anaerobes & Gm-positive cocci are less common etiologies of suppurative phlebitis post-pharyngitis.
Laryngitis (hoarseness)	Viral (90%)	Not indicated		

29 Parapharyngeal space infection: **Ceftriaxone** 2 gm IV q24h; **cefotaxime** 2 gm IV q4-8h; **PIP-TZ** 3.375 gm IV q4-8h; **TC-CL** 3.1 gm IV q4-6h; **TMP-SMX** 8-10 mg per kg per day (based on TMP component) div q6h, q8h, or q12h; **Clinda** 600-900 mg IV q24h; **Levo** 750 mg IV q24h; **vanco** 15 mg/kg IV q12h.

Abbreviations on page 2.   *NOTE: All dosage recommendations are for adults (unless otherwise indicated) and assume normal renal function. § Alternatives consider allergy, PK, compliance, local resistance, cost

TABLE 1 (47)

ANATOMIC SITE/DIAGNOSIS/ MODIFYING CIRCUMSTANCES	ETIOLOGIES (usual)	SUGGESTED REGIMENS*		ADJUNCT DIAGNOSTIC OR THERAPEUTIC MEASURES AND COMMENTS
		PRIMARY	ALTERNATIVE§	
SINUSES, PARANASAL				
Sinusitis, acute (Ref: CID 54:e72, 2012). Guidelines: Pediatrics 132:e262 & 284, 2013 (American Academy of Pediatrics)				
Treatment goals: • Speed resolution • Prevent bacterial complications (see Comment) • Prevent chronic sinusitis • Avoid unnecessary use of antibiotics	S. pneumonia 33% H. influenza 32% M. catarrhalis 9% Anaerobes 6% Grp A strep 2% Viruses 15-18% S. aureus 10% (see Comment)	Most failures: obstruction of sinus ostia by inflammation from virus or allergy. Treatment: Saline irrigation **Antibiotics for bacterial sinusitis if:** 1) fever, pain, purulent nasal discharge; 2) still symptomatic after 10 days with no antibiotic; 3) clinical failure despite antibiotic therapy. **No penicillin allergy:** **Peds:** Amox 90 mg/kg/day divided q12h or **Amox-Clav** (Amox-Clav) suspension 90 mg/kg/day (Amox-Clav divided q12h. Treat for 10-14 days **Adult: Amox-Clav** 1000/62.5-2 tabs po bid x 5-7 days	**No penicillin allergy:** **Peds (if anaphylaxis):** **Clinda** 30-40 mg/kg/day divided tid or qid x 10-14 days **Peds (no anaphylaxis):** **Cefpodoxime** 10 mg/kg/day po div q12h **Adult (if anaphylaxis):** **Levo** or doxy **Adult (no anaphylaxis):** **Cefpodoxime** 200 mg po bid	**Treatment:** • **Clinda:** Haemophilus & Moraxella sp. are resistant; may need 2nd drug • Duration of rx: 5-7 days (IDSA Guidelines), 10-14 days (Amer Acad Ped Guidelines) • Adjunctive rx: 1) do not use topical decongestant for > 3 days; 2) no definite benefit from nasal steroids & antihistamines; saline irrigation may help. • Empiric rx does not target S. aureus: incidence same in pts & controls (CID 45:e121, 2007) Potential complications: transient hyposmia, orbital infection, epidural abscess, brain abscess, meningitis, cavernous sinus thrombosis. For other adult drugs and doses, see footnote[30].
Clinical failure after 3 days	As above, consider diagnostic tap/aspirate	**Mild/Mod. Disease: AM-CL-ER OR cefpodoxime, cefprozil or cefdinir** Treat 5-10 days. Adult doses in footnote[30]	**Severe Disease:** **Gati**[see footnote], **Gemi, Levo, Moxi**	
Diabetes mellitus with acute keto-acidosis; neutropenia; deferoxamine rx: Mucormycosis.	Rhizopus sp. (mucor), aspergillus	See Table 11, pages 113 & 123.		
Hospitalized + nasotracheal or nasogastric intubation	Gm-neg. bacilli 47% (pseudomonas, acinetobacter, E. coli common), Gm+ (S. aureus) 35%, yeasts 18%. Polymicrobial in 80%	Remove nasotracheal tube: if fever persists and ENT available, recommend sinus aspiration for C/S prior to empiric therapy **IMP** 0.5 gm IV q6h or **MER** 1 gm IV q8h. Add vanco for MRSA. If Gram stain suggestive.	**(Ceftaz** 2 gm IV q8h + **vanco)** or **(CFP** 2 gm IV q12h + **vanco)**	After 7 days of nasotracheal or nasogastric tubes, 95% have x-ray "sinusitis" (fluid in sinuses), but on transnasal puncture only 38% culture + (AJRCCM 150:776, 1994). For pts requiring mechanical ventilation with nasotracheal tube for ≥1 wk, bacterial sinusitis occurs in <10% (CID 27:851, 1998). May need fluconazole if yeast on Gram stain of sinus aspirate.
Sinusitis, chronic Adults **Defined:** (drainage, blockage, facial pain, ↓ sense of smell) + mucopurulence on endoscopy or CT scan changes) (Rhinology 50:1, 2012).	4 categories (alone or in combination): allergy, infection, dental, idiopathic	No persuasive evidence of benefit from antibiotics, but anti-inflammatory effect of anti-pseudomembrane steroid may help. Oral steroid (prednisone x 3-10 wks (Curr Opin Otolaryngol Head Neck Surg 21:61, 2013).	Otolaryngology consultation. In acute exacerbation, treat as acute bacterial disease, allergy ± polyps, occult immunodeficiency, and/or odontogenic disease (periodontitis in maxillary molars). If suspect allergy (Allergy 68:1, 2013), nasal inhalers may help; if allergic. Sinus irrigation may help.	Pathogenesis unclear and may be polyfactorial: damage to ostiomeatal complex during acute bacterial disease, allergy ± polyps, occult immunodeficiency, and/or odontogenic disease (periodontitis in maxillary molars). If suspect allergy (Allergy 68:1, 2013), nasal inhalers may help; if allergic. CT scan of maxillary bone if suspect odontogenic source.

[30] **Adult doses for sinusitis (all oral): AM-CL-ER** 2000/125 **mg** bid, **amox high-dose (HD)** 1 gm bid, **clarithro** 500 mg bid, **clarithro ext. release** 1 gm q24h, **doxy** 100 mg q24h, **respiratory FQs** (**Gati** 400 mg q24h)(NUS due to hypo/hyperglycemia), **Gemi** 320 mg q24h (not FDA indication but should work), **Levo** 750 mg q24h)(doxy), **Moxi** 400 mg q24h), **O Ceph** (**cefdinir** 300 mg q12h or 600 mg q24h), **cefpodoxime** 200 mg bid, **cefprozil** 250-500 mg bid, **cefuroxime** 250-500 mg bid). **TMP-SMX** double-strength (TMP 160 mg) q12h (results after 3- and 10-day rx similar).

Abbreviations on page 2.   *NOTE: All dosage recommendations are for adults (unless otherwise indicated) and assume normal renal function. § Alternatives consider allergy, PK, compliance, local resistance, cost

TABLE 1 (48)

ANATOMIC SITE/DIAGNOSIS/ MODIFYING CIRCUMSTANCES	ETIOLOGIES (usual)	SUGGESTED REGIMENS* PRIMARY	ALTERNATIVE§	ADJUNCT DIAGNOSTIC OR THERAPEUTIC MEASURES AND COMMENTS
SKIN See IDSA Guideline: CID 59:147, 2014.				
Acne vulgaris (Med Left Treatment Guidelines 11 (Issue 125):1, 2013).				
Comedonal acne: "blackheads", "whiteheads", earliest form, no inflammation	Excessive sebum production & gland obstruction. No Propionibacterium acnes	Once–q24h: Topical **tretinoin** (cream 0.025 or 0.05%) or (gel 0.01 or 0.025%).	All once–q24h: Topical **adapalene** 0.1% gel OR **azelaic acid** 20% cream or **tazarotene** 0.1% gel	Goal is prevention, ↓ number of new comedones and create an environment unfavorable to P. acnes. Adapalene causes less irritation than tretinoin. Azelaic acid less potent but less irritating than retinoids. **Tazarotene: Do not use in pregnancy.**
Mild inflammatory acne: small papules or pustules	Proliferation of P. acnes + abnormal desquamation of follicular cells	Topical **erythro** 3% + **benzoyl peroxide** 5%. bid	Can substitute **clinda** 1% gel for erythro	In random. controlled trial, topical benzoyl peroxide + erythro of equal efficacy to oral minocycline & tetracycline and not affected by antibiotic resistance of propionibacteria (Ln 364:2188, 2004).
Inflammatory acne: comedones, papules & pustules. Less common: deep nodules (cysts) Isotretinoin ref: JAMA 31: 2121, 2133; 2014.	Progression of above events. Also, drug induced, e.g., glucocorticoids, phenytoin, lithium, INH & others.	(Topical **erythro** 3% + **benzoyl peroxide** 5% bid) + oral antibiotic. See Comment for mild acne	Oral drugs: (**doxy** 50 mg bid) or (**minocycline** 50 mg bid). Others: **tetracycline**, **clinda**. Expensive extended release **once-daily minocycline** (Solodyn) 1 mg/kg/d	Systemic **isotretinoin** reserved for pts with severe widespread nodular cystic lesions that fail oral antibiotic rx; 4–5 mos. course of 0.1–1 mg per kg per day. Aggressive/violent behavior reported. **Teratogenic (Preg category X)**: contraception required. **Minocycline** side-effects: urticaria, vertigo, pigment deposition in skin or oral mucosa. Rare induced autoimmunity in children: fever, polyarthralgia, positive ANCA (J Peds 153:314, 2008).
Acne rosacea Ref: NEJM 352:793, 2005.	Skin mite. Demodex folliculorum (Arch Derm 146:896, 2010)	Facial erythema. Brimonidine gel (Mirvaso) applied to affected area bid (J Drugs Dermato 12:650, 2013)	Papulopustular rosacea: **Azelaic acid** gel bid, topical or **Metro** topical cream once daily or q24h	Avoid activities that provoke flushing, e.g., alcohol, spicy food, sunlight.
Anthrax, cutaneous **To report bioterrorism event: 770-488-7100;** For info: www.bt.cdc.gov Treat as inhalation anthrax if systemic illness. Refs: AJRCCM 184:1333, 2011 (Review); Pediatrics 133:e1411, 2014 (Clinical Prac. Guideline).	B. anthracis Spores are introduced into/under the skin by contact with infected animals/animal products. See Lung, page 41.	**Adults: CIP** 500 mg po q12h or **Doxy** 10 mg po q12h. **Children: CIP** 15 mg/kg (max dose 500 mg) po q12h or for pen-susceptible strain **Amox** 25 mg/kg (max dose 1 gm) po q8h For bioterrorism exposure, 3-dose series of Biothrax Anthrax Vaccine Adsorbed is indicated.		1. Duration of therapy 60 days for bioterrorism event because of potential inhalational exposure, 7-10 days for naturally acquired disease. 2. Consider alternative to Doxy for pregnancy. 3. Alternatives for adults: Levo 750 mg q24h or Moxi 400 mg q24h or Clinda 600 mg q8h or for pen-susceptible strains Amox 1 gm q8h or Pen VK 500 mg q6h 4. Alternatives for children: Doxy 2.2 mg/kg (max dose 100 mg) q12h (tooth staining likely with 60-day regimen age < 8 years) or Clindamycin 10 mg/kg (max dose 600 mg) q8h or Levo 8 mg/kg q12h (max dose 250 mg) if < 50 kg and 500 mg q24h if > 50 kg
Bacillary angiomatosis: For other Bartonella infections, see Cat-scratch disease lymphadenitis, page 45, and Bartonella systemic infections, page 57	Bartonella henselae and quantana	**Clarithro** 500 mg po bid or ext. release 1 gm po q24h or **azithro** 250 mg po q24h (see Comment)	**Erythro** 500 mg po bid or **doxy** 100 mg po bid or **doxy** 100 mg po bid + **RIF** 300 mg q12h	For AIDS pts, continue suppressive therapy until HIV treated and CD > 200 cells/μL for 6 mos.
In immunocompromised (HIV-1, bone marrow transplant) patients Also see SANFORD GUIDE TO HIV/AIDS THERAPY				

Abbreviations on page 2.   *NOTE: All dosage recommendations are for adults (unless otherwise indicated) and assume normal renal function. PK, compliance, local resistance, cost § Alternatives consider allergy, PK, compliance, local resistance, cost

TABLE 1 (49)

ANATOMIC SITE/DIAGNOSIS/ MODIFYING CIRCUMSTANCES	ETIOLOGIES (usual)	SUGGESTED REGIMENS*		ADJUNCT DIAGNOSTIC OR THERAPEUTIC MEASURES AND COMMENTS
		PRIMARY	ALTERNATIVE†	
SKIN (continued)				
Bite: Remember tetanus prophylaxis— See Table 20B, page 216 for rabies prophylaxis. Review: CMR 24:231, 2011. **Avoid primary wound closure.**				
Alligator (*Alligator mississipiensis*)	Gram negatives including Aeromonas hydrophila, Clostridia sp.	Severe wound: Surgical debridement + (**CIP** 400 mg IV /750 mg po bid or **Levo** 750 mg IV /750 mg po bid	Severe wound: Surgical debridement + (**TMP-SMX** 8-10 mg/kg/day IV q6h or q8h or **Cefepime** 2 gm IV q8h)	Oral flora of American alligator isolated: anaerobes, including Aeromonas hydrophila and Clostridia sp. *(S Med J 82:262, 1989).*
Bat, raccoon, skunk	Strep & staph from skin; rabies	**AM-CL** 875/125 mg po bid or 500/125 mg po tid	**Doxy** 100 mg po bid	In Americas, **anti-rabies rx indicated:** rabies immune globulin + vaccine. *(See Table 20B, page 216)* See EJCMID 18:918, 1999.
Camel	S. aureus, P. aeruginosa, Other Gm-neg bacilli	**Diclox** 250-500 mg po qid + **CIP** 750 mg po bid	**Cephalexin** 500 mg po qid + **CIP** 750 mg po bid	
Cat: 80% get infected, culture & treat empirically.	**Pasteurella multocida,** Streptococci, Staph. aureus, Neisseria, Moraxella	**AM-CL** 875/125 mg po bid or 500/125 mg po tid	**Cefuroxime axetil** 0.5 gm po q12h or **doxy** 100 mg po bid. **Do not use cephalexin.** Sens. to FQs in vitro.	**P. multocida resistant to dicloxacillin, cephalexin, clinda; many strains resistant to erythro** (most sensitive to azithro but no clinical data). P. multocida infection develops within 24 hrs. Observe for osteomyelitis. If culture + only for P. multocida, can switch to pen G,V or pen VK. See Dog Bite.
Cat-scratch disease, page 45				
Catfish sting	Toxins	See Comments		Presents as immediate pain, erythema and edema. Resembles strep cellulitis. May become secondarily infected; AM-CL is reasonable choice for prophylaxis.
Dog: Only 5% get infected; treat only if bite severe or bad co-morbidity (e.g. diabetes).	Pasteurella canis, S. aureus, Streptococci, Fusobacterium sp, Capnocytophaga canimorsus	**AM-CL** 875/125 mg po bid or 500/125 mg po tid	**Clinda** 300 mg po qid + FQ (adults) or **clinda** + TMP-SMX (children)	Consider rabies prophylaxis: rabies immune globulin + vaccine (see Table 20B). Capnocytophaga in splenectomized pts may cause local eschar, sepsis with DIC. **P. canis resistant to diclox, cephalexin, clinda. Eikenella resistant to diclox, cephalexin and FQs.**
Human For bacteriology, see CID 37:1481, 2003	Viridans strep 100%, Staph. epidermidis 53%, corynebacterium 41%, **Staph. aureus 29%, eikenella 15%,** bacteroides 82%, peptostrep 26%	**Early** (not yet infected): **AM-CL** 875/125 mg po bid times 5 days. **Later** (infected): (usually in 3-24 hrs) **AM-SB** 1.5 gm IV q6h or **cefoxitin** 2 gm IV q8h) or (**PIP-TZ** 3.375 gm IV q6h or 4.5 gm q8h or 4-hr infusion of 3.375 gm q8h)	Pen allergy: **Clinda** + (either **CIP** or **TMP-SMX**)	**Cleanse & debride. Rx most important.** Do not suture. For clenched fist injuries, x-rays should be obtained. Bites inflicted by hospitalized pts, consider aerobic Gm-neg. bacilli. **Eikenella resistant to clinda, nafcillin/oxacillin, metro, P Ceph 1, and erythro; susceptible to FQs and TMP-SMX.**
Leech (Medicinal) *(Ln 381:1686, 2013)*	Aeromonas hydrophila	**CIP** (400 mg IV or 750 mg po) bid	P Ceph 3 or TC-CL or AM-SB or IMP	Aeromonas found in GI tract of leeches. Some use prophylactic antibiotics when leeches used medicinally, but not universally accepted or necessary.
Pig (swine)	Polymicrobic: Gm+ cocci, Gm-neg. bacilli, anaerobes, Pasteurella sp.	**AM-CL** 875/125 mg po bid	**TMP-SMX DS** 1 tab po bid	Information limited but infection is common and serious (Ln 348:888, 1996).
Prairie dog	Monkeypox Microbiology	See Table 14A, page 166. **Acyclovir:** See Table 14B, page 166	No rx recommended	CID 20:421, 1995
Primate, non-human	Herpesvirus simiae			
Rat	Spirillum minus & Streptobacillus moniliformis	**AM-CL** 875/125 mg po bid	Doxy	Anti-rabies rx not indicated. Causes rat bite fever (Streptobacillus moniliformis). Pen. G or doxy, alternatively erythro or clinda. Can take weeks to respond after bite (Ln 364:448, 2004).
Seal	Marine mycoplasma	Tetracycline times 4 wks		
Snake: pit viper (Ref.: NEJM 347:347, 2002)	Pseudomonas sp., Enterobacteriaceae, Staph. epidermidis, Clostridium sp.		**Primary therapy is antivenom.** Ceftriaxone should be more effective	**Primary therapy is antivenom.** Penicillin generally used but would not be effective vs. organisms isolated. Tetanus prophylaxis indicated. Ref: CID 43:1309, 2006.

*NOTE: All dosage recommendations are for adults (unless otherwise indicated) and assume normal renal function. §Alternatives consider allergy, PK, compliance, local resistance, cost

Abbreviations on page 2

TABLE 1 (50)

ANATOMIC SITE/DIAGNOSIS/ MODIFYING CIRCUMSTANCES	ETIOLOGIES (usual)	SUGGESTED REGIMENS* PRIMARY	ALTERNATIVE†	ADJUNCT DIAGNOSTIC OR THERAPEUTIC MEASURES AND COMMENTS
SKIN/Bite (continued)				
Spider bite: Most necrotic ulcers attributed to spiders are probably due to another cause, e.g. cutaneous anthrax (Ln 364:549, 2004) or **MRSA infection** (spider bite painful; anthrax not painful.)				
Widow (Latrodectus)	Not infectious	None		May be confused with "acute abdomen" Diazepam or calcium gluconate helpful to control pain, muscle spasm; tetanus prophylaxis.
Brown recluse (Loxosceles) *NEJM 352:700, 2005*	Not infectious. "Overdiagnosed! Spider distribution limited to US Central & desert SW of US	Bite usually self-limited & self-healing. No therapy of proven efficacy.		Dapsone causes hemolysis (check for G6PD deficiency). Can cause hepatitis; baseline & weekly liver panels suggested.
Boils—Furunculosis—Subcutaneous abscesses in drug addicts ("skin poppers"). Carbuncles = multiple connecting furuncles; Emergency Dept. Perspective *(NEJM 370:1039, 2014)*				
Active lesions See Table 6, page 79	Staph. aureus, both MSSA & MRSA *IDSA Guidelines: CID 59:147, 2014, CID 59:147, 2014.*	**Boils and abscesses** – <5 cm, outpatient setting, no diabetes, immunosuppression, most will respond to simple I&D. For larger or multiple abscesses, systemic inflammatory response syndrome antibiotics may provide added benefit to I&D. Options include **TMP/SMX 1-2 DS bid** (higher dose if BMI > 40). **Clinda** 300-450 mg po bid or **Minocycline** 100 mg po bid, or **Doxy** 100 mg po bid (higher dose if BMI > 40), for 5-10 days.		Other options: **Linezolid** 600 mg po bid x 10 days; **Tedizolid** 200 mg po qd x 6 d; **Fusidic acid**NUS 250-500 mg po q8-12h ± **RIF** *(CID 42:394, 2006)*; **cephalexin** 500 mg po tid-qid or dicloxacillin 500 mg po tid-qid, only in low prevalence setting for MRSA. If dx uncertainty or for assessing adequacy of I&D, ultrasound is helpful *(NEJM 370:1039, 2014)*. **Note: needle aspiration is inadequate.**
To lessen number of furuncle recurrences—decolonization For surgical wounds, see Table 15B, page 193.	MSSA & MRSA. *IDSA Guidelines, CID 59:e10, 2014*	7-day therapy. **chlorhexidine** (2%) washes daily + mupirocin (2%) ointment anterior nares 2x daily + (**rifampin** 300 mg bid + **doxy** 100 mg bid)	**Mupirocin ointment** in anterior nares bid x 7 days + chlorhexidine (2%) washes daily x 7 days + **TMP-SMX DS** 1 tab po bid x 7 days	Optimal regimen uncertain. Can substitute bleach baths for chlorhexidine *(Inf Control Hosp Epidemiol 32:872, 2011)* but only modest effect *(CID 54:743, 2012; In vitro resistance of mupirocin & retapamulin roughly 10% (AAC 58:2878, 2014).*
Hidradenitis suppurativa Not infectious disease, but bacterial superinfection occurs	Lesions secondarily infected: S. aureus, Enterobacteriaceae, Pseudomonas, anaerobes	Clinda 1% topical cream **Adalimumab** 40 mg once weekly beneficial *(AnIM 157:846, 2012)*	Tetracycline 500 mg po bid x 3 months	Caused by keratinous plugging of apocrine glands of axillary, inguinal, perianal, perineal, infra-mammary areas. Other therapy: antiperspirants, loose clothing and anti-androgens. *Dermatol Clin 28:779, 2010.*
Burns. Overall management: *NEJM 350:810, 2004 – step-by-step case outline*				
Initial wound care Use burn unit, if available Topical rx options *(NEJM 359:1037, 2008; Clin Plastic Surg 36:597, 2009)*	Not infected Prophylaxis for potential pathogens: Gm-pos cocci Gm-neg bacilli Candida	Early excision & wound closure. Variety of skin grafts/substitutes. Shower hydrotherapy. Topical antimicrobials	Silver sulfadiazine cream 1% applied 1-2 daily. Minimal pain. Transient reversible neutropenia due to margination in burn – not marrow toxicity	Mafenide acetate cream is an alternative but painful to apply. Anti-tetanus prophylaxis indicated.
Burn wound sepsis Proposed standard def: *J Burn Care Res 28:776, 2007.* Need quantitative wound cultures	Strep. pyogenes, Enterobacter sp., S. aureus, S. epidermidis, E. faecalis, E. coli, P. aeruginosa, Fungi (rare). Herpesvirus (rare).	**Vanco** high dose to rapidly achieve trough concentration of 15-20 μg/mL + (**MER** 1 gm IV q8h or **cefepime** 2 gm IV q8h) + **Fluconazole** 6 mg/kg IV qd See Comments for alternatives		Vanco allergic/intolerant: **Dapto** 6-10 mg/kg IV qd If IgE mediated allergy to beta lactams: **Aztreonam** 2 gm IV q6h ESBL- or carbapenemase-producing MDR gm-neg bacilli: only option is **Colistin** *(CID 53:879, 2014)* or **(MER** or **IMP)**

Abbreviations on page 2.   *NOTE: All dosage recommendations are for adults (unless otherwise indicated) and assume normal renal function. †Alternatives consider allergy, PK, compliance, local resistance, cost

TABLE 1 (51)

ANATOMIC SITE/DIAGNOSIS/ MODIFYING CIRCUMSTANCES	ETIOLOGIES (usual)	SUGGESTED REGIMENS*		ADJUNCT DIAGNOSTIC OR THERAPEUTIC MEASURES AND COMMENTS
		PRIMARY	**ALTERNATIVE†**	
SKIN (continued)				
Cellulitis, erysipelas: NOTE: Consider diseases that masquerade as cellulitis. **Extremities, non-diabetic.** For diabetes, see below. Treatment guidelines: CID 59:147, 2014.	Streptococcus sp., Groups A, B, C & G. Staph. aureus, including MRSA (but rarely). Strept sp: No purulence. Staph sp.: Purulence.	**Inpatients: Elevate legs. Nafcillin** 2 million units IV q6h **or cefazolin** 1 gm IV q8h. If Pen-allergic: **Vanco** 15 mg/kg IV q12h. When afebrile: **Pen VK** 500 mg po qid x & hs. Total therapy: 10 days.	**Outpatient: Elevate legs. Pen VK** 500 mg po qid ac & hs. x 10 days. If Pen-allergic: **Azithro** 500 mg po x 1 dose, then 250 mg po once daily x 4 days (total 5 days). Rarely, **Linezolid** 600 mg bid (expensive) or **Tedizolid** 200 mg q24h†.	• Erysipelas: elevation, treat T. pedis if present. If no purulence, no need to cure. TMP-SMX may fail. • For pts unlikely to comply with hospitalization or multidose po regimen, could use long acting dalbavancin or oritavancin (both IV)(expensive). • If unsure as to presence of deep abscess, bedside ultrasound can help. If present: furunculosis (boils).
Facial, adult (erysipelas)	Strep. sp. (Grp A, B, C & G), Staph. aureus to include MRSA); S. pneumo	**Vanco** 15 mg/kg (actual wt) IV q8-12h (to achieve target trough concentration of 15-20 µg/mL).	**Dapto** 4 mg/kg IV q 24h **or Linezolid** 600 mg IV q12h	**Choice of empiric therapy must have activity vs. S. aureus. S. aureus** erysipelas of face can mimic streptococcal erysipelas of an extremity. Forced to treat empirically for MRSA until in vitro susceptibilities available.
Diabetes mellitus and erysipelas (See Foot, "Diabetic", page 16)	Strep. sp. (Grp A, B, C & G), Staph. aureus, Enterobacteriaceae; Anaerobes	**Early mild: TMP-SMX-DS** 1-2 tabs po bid + (**Pen VK** 500 mg po qid or **cephalexin** 500 mg po qid). **For severe disease: IMP, MER, ERTA** or **Dori** IV + (**Vanco** IV/po bid or **Linezolid** 600 mg IV/po bid or **Dosage: see page 16.**	For severe disease, use regimen that targets aerobic gram-neg bacilli & MRSA.	Prompt surgical debridement indicated to rule out necrotizing fasciitis and to obtain cultures. If septic, consider x-ray of extremity to demonstrate gas. **Prognosis dependent on blood supply: assess arteries.** See diabetic foot, page 16 for severe disease.
Erysipelas 2° to lymphedema (congenital = Milroy's disease); post-breast surgery with lymph node dissection	Streptococcus sp., Groups A, C, G	**Benzathine Pen G** 1.2 million units IM q4 wks **or azithro** 250 mg po qd	**Pen VK** 500 mg po bid or **azithro** 250 mg po qd	Benefit indicated only if pt is having frequent episodes of cellulitis. Benefit in controlled clinical trial (NEJM 368:1695, 2013).
Dandruff (seborrheic dermatitis)	Malassezia species	Ketoconazole shampoo 2% or selenium sulfide 2.5% (see page 10, chronic external otitis)		
Erythema multiforme	H. simplex type 1, mycoplasma. Strep. pyogenes, drugs (sulfonamides, phenytoin, penicillins)			Rx: Acyclovir if due to H. simplex (Dermatology 207:349, 2003).
Erythema nodosum	Sarcoidosis, inflammatory bowel disease, MTB, coccidioidomycosis, yersinia, sulfonamides, Whipple's disease.			Rx: NSAIDs; glucocorticoids if refractory. Identify and treat precipitant disease if possible.
Erythrasma	Corynebacterium minutissimum	Localized infection: Topical Clinda 2-3 x daily x 7-14 days	Widespread infection: Clarithro 500 mg po bid or Erythro 250 mg po bid x 14 days	Dx: Coral red fluorescence with Wood's lamp. If infection recurs, prophylactic bathing with anti-bacterial soap or wash with benzyl peroxide.
Folliculitis	S. aureus, candida, P. aeruginosa common	Usually self-limited, no Rx. Could use topical mupirocin for Staph and topical antifungal for Candida.		
Furunculosis	Staph. aureus	See Boils, page 53		
Hemorrhagic bullous lesions Hx of sea water-contaminated abrasion or eating raw seafood in cirrhotic pt.	**Vibrio vulnificus** (ICID 52:788, 2012; JAC 67:488, 2012)	**Ceftriaxone** 2 gm IV q24h + (**Doxy** or **Minocycline** 100 mg po/IV bid)	**CIP** 750 mg po bid or 400 mg IV bid	Wound infection in healthy hosts, but bacteremia mostly in cirrhotics. Pathogenesis: Open wound exposure to contaminated seawater. Can cause necrotizing fasciitis (JAC 67:488, 2012). Surgical debridement (Am J Surg 206:32, 2013).
Herpes zoster (shingles): See Table 14				

*NOTE: All dosage recommendations are for adults (unless otherwise indicated) and assume normal renal function. § Alternatives consider allergy, PK, compliance, local resistance, cost

TABLE 1 (52)

ANATOMIC SITE/DIAGNOSIS/ MODIFYING CIRCUMSTANCES	ETIOLOGIES (usual)	SUGGESTED REGIMENS* PRIMARY	SUGGESTED REGIMENS* ALTERNATIVE§	ADJUNCT DIAGNOSTIC OR THERAPEUTIC MEASURES AND COMMENTS
SKIN *(continued)*				
Impetigo—children, military "Honey-crust" lesions (non-bullous). Ecthyma is closely related. Causes "punched out" skin lesions.	**Group A strep impetigo** (rarely) Strept. sp. Groups B, C or G; crusted lesions can be Staph. aureus either as primary cause or Staph. aureus may be secondary colonizer.	Mupirocin ointment 2% tid or fusidic acid cream[xi.s] 2%, times 5 days or retapamulin ointment, 1% bid times 5 days *For dosages, see Table 10A for adults.*	No po antibiotic unless numerous and/or outbreak. MSSA: **Diclox** or **cephalexin**; MRSA: **Doxy, Clinda** or **TMP-SMX** *For dosages, see Table 10A for adults.*	In meta-analysis that combined strep & staph impetigo, mupirocin had higher cure rates than placebo. Mupirocin superior to oral erythro. Penicillin inferior to erythro. Few placebo-controlled trials. Ref.: *Cochrane Database Systemic Reviews, 2004(2): CD003261.* [40%] of USA-300 CA-MRSA isolates carry gene encoding resistance to Mupirocin (*Ln.367:731, 2006*) **Note:** While resistance to Mupirocin continues to evolve, over-the-counter triple antibiotic ointment (Neomycin, polymyxin B, Bacitracin) remains active in vitro (*DMID 54:63, 2006*). **Ecthyma:** Infection deeper into epidermis than impetigo. Military outbreaks reported: *CID 48: 1213 & 1220, 2009 (good images).*
Bullous (if ruptured, thin "varnish-like crust")	**Staph. aureus** MSSA & MRSA, strains that produce exfoliative toxin A.	**For MSSA: Dicloxacillin, oxacillin, cephalexin. AM-CL, clinda, TMP-SMX-DS** or **mupirocin ointment or retapamulin ointment**	**For MRSA: Mupirocin** ointment or po therapy with, **TMP-SMX-DS, minocycline, doxy, clinda**	
Infected wound, extremity —Post-trauma *(for bites, see page 52)* *for post-operative, see below*				
Mild to moderate, uncomplicated Debride wound, if necessary.	Polymicrobic: S. aureus (MSSA & MRSA), aerobic & anaerobic strep, Enterobacteriaceae, C. perfringens, tetani; if water exposure, Pseudomonas sp., Aeromonas sp., Acinetobacter in soldiers in Iraq. (*see CID 47:444, 2008*)	**TMP-SMX-DS** 1-2 tabs po bid or **clinda** 300–450 mg po bid *(see Comment)*	**Minocycline** 100 mg po bid or **linezolid** 600 mg po bid *(see Comment)* **— Gram stain negative**	**Culture & sensitivity, check Gram stain. Tetanus toxoid if indicated.** **Mild infection:** Suggested drugs focus on S. aureus & Strep species. If suspect Gm-neg bacilli, add **AM-CL-ER** 1000/62.5 two tabs po bid. If MRSA & erythro-resistant, may have inducible resistance to clinda. **Fever—sepsis:** Another alternative is **linezolid** 600 mg IV/po q12h. If Gm-neg & severe pen allergy, **CIP** 400 mg IV q12h (q8h if P. aeruginosa) or **Levo** 750 mg IV q24h. Why 1-2 **TMP-SMX-DS?** *See discussion in footnote 1 of Table 6 (MRSA)* **TMP-SMX** not predictably active vs. strep species.
Febrile with sepsis—hospitalized Debride wound, if necessary.		**TC-CL** or **PIP-TZ** or **DORI[NA]** or **IMP** or **MER** or **ERTA** (*Dosage, page 25*) + **vanco** 15-20 mg/kg q8-12h	(**Vanco** 15-20 mg/kg IV q8-12h or **dapto** 6 mg/kg IV q 24h or **ceftaroline** 600 mg IV q12h or **telavancin** 10 mg/kg IV q24h) + (**CIP** or **Levo** [—dose in Comment])	
Infected wound, post-operative—Gram stain positive cocci - see below				
Gram stain negative—Gram stain positive cocci - see below				
Surgery not involving GI tract Without sepsis (mild, afebrile) With sepsis (severe, febrile)	Staph. aureus, Group A, B, C or G strep sp.	**TMP-SMX-DS** 1 tab po bid --- **PIP-TZ** or (P **Ceph 3** + **metro**) or **MER**) + (**vanco** 1 gm IV q12h or **dapto** 6 mg/kg IV q 24h) if severely ill. **Mild infection: AM-CL-ER** 1000/62.5 mg 2 tabs po bid + **TMP-SMX-DS** 1-2 tabs po bid or cocci on Gram stain. *Dosages Table 10A & footnote 32, page 56*	**Clinda** 300–450 mg po tid --- **Dapto** 6 mg/kg IV q24h or **ERTA** or **PIP-TZ** or **TC-CL**) IV. Discussion on page 25. Why 1-2 **TMP-SMX-DS?** *See discussion in footnote 1 of Table 6 (MRSA).* **TMP-SMX** not predictably active vs. strep species.	Check Gram stain of exudate. If Gm-neg. bacilli, **add** β-lactam/β-lactamase inhibitor: **AM-CL-ER** or (**ERTA** or **PIP-TZ** or **TC-CL**) IV. Discussion on page 25. Why 1-2 **TMP-SMX-DS?** *See discussion in footnote 1 of Table 6 (MRSA).* **TMP-SMX** not predictably active vs. strep species.
Surgery involving GI tract (includes oropharynx, esophagus) or female genital tract—fever, neutrophilia	MSSA/MRSA, coliforms, bacteroides & other anaerobes			For all treatment options, see *Peritonitis, page 47.* Most important: Drain wound & get cultures. Can sub **linezolid** for vanco. Can sub **CIP** or **Levo** for β-lactams. Why 2 **TMP-SMX-DS?** *See discussion in footnote 1 of Table 6 (MRSA).*
Meleney's synergistic gangrene	*See Necrotizing fasciitis, page 56*			

Abbreviations on page 2.   *NOTE: All dosage recommendations are for adults (unless otherwise indicated) and assume normal renal function. § Alternatives consider allergy; PK, compliance, local resistance, cost*

TABLE 1 (53)

ANATOMIC SITE/DIAGNOSIS/ MODIFYING CIRCUMSTANCES	ETIOLOGIES (usual)	SUGGESTED REGIMENS*		ADJUNCT DIAGNOSTIC OR THERAPEUTIC MEASURES AND COMMENTS
		PRIMARY	ALTERNATIVE[1]	
SKIN/Infected wound, post-operative—Gram stain negative *(continued)*				
Infected wound, post-op, febrile patient—positive gram stain—positive cocci in clusters	S. aureus, possibly MRSA	**Do culture & sensitivity; open & drain wound** **Oral:** TMP-SMX-DS 1 tab po bid or **clinda** 300-450 mg po tid (see **Comment**)	**IV: Vanco** 15-20 mg/kg q8-12h or **dapto** 4-6 mg/kg IV q24h or **ceftaroline** 600 mg IV q12h or **televancin** 10 mg/kg IV q24h	Need culture & sensitivity to verify MRSA. Other po options for CA-MRSA include **minocycline** 100 mg po bid or **Doxy** 100 mg po bid (inexpensive) & **linezolid** 600 mg po q12h (expensive). If MRSA clinda-sensitive but erythro-resistant, watch out for inducible clinda resistance. Dalbavancin and oritavancin recently FDA approved for treatment of acute bacterial skin and skin structure infections.
Necrotizing fasciitis ("flesh-eating bacteria") Post-surgery, trauma, or streptococcal skin infections See *Gas gangrene, page 46*, & *Toxic shock, page 64*. Refs: *CID 59:147, 2014; NEJM 360:281, 2009.*	**5 types:** (1) Strep, Gp A, C, & (2) Clostridia sp. (3) polymicrobic: aerobic + anaerobic (if S. aureus + anaerobic strep = Meleney's synergistic gangrene) (4) Community-associated MRSA, (5) K. pneumoniae (CID 55:930 & 940, 2012)	For treatment of clostridia, see *Muscle, gas gangrene, page 46*. The terminology of **polymicrobic** wound infections is not precise: Meleney's synergistic gangrene, Fournier's gangrene, necrotizing fasciitis have common pathophysiology. **All require prompt surgical debridement + antibiotics.** Dx of necrotizing fasciitis req incision & probing. If no resistance to probing subcut with fascial plane involvement (fascial plane). diagnosis = necrotizing fasciitis = strep, clostridia, polymicrobial. **Need Gram stain/culture** to determine if etiology is strep, clostridia, polymicrobial. **Treatment: Pen G** if strep or clostridia; **DORI[NUS], IMP** or **MER** if polymicrobial; add **vanco OR dapto** if MRSA suspected. **NOTE:** If strep necrotizing fasciitis, reasonable to treat with penicillin & clinda; if clostridia ± gas gangrene, add clinda to penicillin (see page 46). MRSA ref: *NEJM 352:1445, 2005.* **See toxic shock syndrome, streptococcus, page 64.**		
Puncture wound—nail, toothpick Through tennis shoe: P. aeruginosa		Local debridement to remove foreign body & tetanus prophylaxis, no antibiotic therapy.		Osteomyelitis evolves in only 1-2% of plantar puncture wounds. Consider x-ray if chance of radio-opaque foreign body.
Staphylococcal scalded skin syndrome Ref: *PIDJ 19:819, 2000*	Toxin-producing S. aureus	**Nafcillin** or **oxacillin** 2 gm IV q4h (children: 150 mg/kg/day div. q6h) x 5-7 days for MSSA; **vanco** 15-20 mg/kg div q8h for MRSA (children 15-20 mg/kg div q6h) for MRSA		Toxin causes **intraepidermal split** and positive Nikolsky sign. Biopsy differentiates: drugs cause epidermal/dermal split, **called toxic epidermal necrolysis**—more serious.
Ulcerated skin lesions: Differential Dx.	Consider: anthrax, tularemia, insufficiency, venous stasis, and others.	P. aeruginosa (ecthyma gangrenosum), plague, blastomycosis, leishmania, YAWS, arterial		If ulcer clinically inflamed, treat IV with no topical rx. If not clinically inflamed, consider debridement, removal of foreign body, lessening direct pressure for weight-bearing limbs & leg edema (if no arterial insufficiency). Topical rx to reduce bacterial counts: silver sulfadiazine 1% or combination antibiotic ointment. **Chlorhexidine & povidone iodine may harm "granulation tissue"—Avoid.** If not inflamed, healing improved on bed: protein supplement, radiant heat, electrical stimulation (*AVM 159:09, 2013*).
Ulcerated skin: venous/arterial insufficiency; pressure with secondary infection (infected decubiti) Care of non-healing, non-infected ulcers (*AIM 159:ITC6, 2013*)	Polymicrobic: Streptococcus sp. (Groups A, C, G), enterococci, anaerobic strep, Enterobacteriaceae, Pseudomonas sp., Bacteroides sp., Staph. aureus	Severe local or possible bacteremia: **IMP** or **MER** or **DORI** or **TC-CL** or **PIP-TZ** or **ERTA**. If Gm-pos cocci on gram stain, add **Vanco**	**[CIP** or **Levo]** + **Metro]** or **[CFP** or **Ceftaz]** + **Metro]** If Gm-pos cocci on gram stain, add **Vanco** [5, 6, 7, 11, 14, 32]	
		Dosages, see footnotes[5, 6, 7, 11, 14, 32]		
Whirlpool: (Hot Tub) folliculitis	Pseudomonas aeruginosa	Usually self-limited, no antibiotic therapy.		Decontaminate hot tub: drain and chlorinate. Also associated with exfoliative beauty aids (loofah sponges).
Whirlpool: Nail Salon, soft tissue infection	Mycobacterium (fortuitum or chelonae)	**Minocycline, doxy** or **CIP**		Ref: *CID 38:38, 2004.*
SPLEEN. For post-splenectomy prophylaxis		Dosages from *Table 15A, page 192-193*; for *Septic Spleen Post-Splenectomy, see Table 1, pg 63.* Vaccines: *CID 58:309, 2014.*		
Splenic abscess Endocarditis, bacteremia	Staph. aureus, streptococci	**Nafcillin** or **oxacillin** 2 gm IV q4h or **cefazolin** 2 gm IV q8h if MSSA	**Vanco** 15-20 mg/kg IV q8-12h (to achieve target trough concentration of 15-20μg/mL)	Burkholderia (Pseudomonas) pseudomallei is common cause of splenic abscess in SE Asia. Presents with fever and LUQ pain. Usual treatment is antimicrobial therapy and splenectomy.
Contiguous from intra-abdominal site Immunocompromised	Polymicrobic Candida sp.	*Treat as Peritonitis, secondary, page 47* **Amphotericin B** (*Dosage, see Table 11, page 114*)	**Fluconazole, caspofungin**	

NOTE: All dosage recommendations are for adults (unless otherwise indicated) and assume normal renal function. PK, compliance, local resistance, cost

Abbreviations on page 2.

TABLE 1 (54)

ANATOMIC SITE/DIAGNOSIS/ MODIFYING CIRCUMSTANCES	ETIOLOGIES (usual)	SUGGESTED REGIMENS*		ADJUNCT DIAGNOSTIC OR THERAPEUTIC MEASURES AND COMMENTS
		PRIMARY	**ALTERNATIVE§**	
SYSTEMIC SYNDROMES (FEBRILE/NON-FEBRILE)				
Babesiosis, Lyme disease, & Anaplasma (Ehrlichiosis) have same reservoir & tick vector				
Babesiosis: Epidemiologic history crucial. see NEJM 366:2397, 2012. Do not use if asymptomatic, young, has spleen, and immunocompetent; can be fatal in lymphoma pts.	Etiol: B. microti et al. Vector: Usually Ixodes ticks Host: White-footed mouse & others	[(Atovaquone 750 mg po q12h) + (azithro 600 mg po day 1, then 500-1000 mg per day)] times 7-10 days]. If severe infection [clinda 650 mg IV/po q6h times 7 d + quinine 650 mg po tid times 7 d]. Ped. dosage: Clinda 20-40 mg per kg per day and quinine 25 mg per kg per day]. Exchange transfusion— See Comment		**Seven diseases where pathogen visible in peripheral blood smear:** African/American trypanosomiasis, babesiosis, bartonellosis, filariasis, malaria, relapsing fever (Borrelia), leishmaniasis. **Dx:** Giesa-stained blood smear; antibody test available. **Rx: Exchange transfusions successful adjunct if used early, in severe disease.** May need treatment for 6 or more wks if immunocompromised. Look for Lyme and/or Anaplasma co-infection.
Bartonella infections: Review EID 12:389, 2006				
Bacteremia, asymptomatic	B. quintana, B. henselae	**Doxy** 100 mg po/IV times 15 days		Can lead to endocarditis &/or trench fever: found in homeless, alcoholics, esp. if lice/leg pain. Often missed since asymptomatic.
Cat-scratch disease	B. henselae	**Azithro** 500 mg x 1 dose, then 250 mg/day po x 4 days.	**Azithro** 250 mg po once daily x 3 months	Or symptomatic only—see Lymphadenitis, page 45: usually lymphadenitis, hepatitis, splenitis, FUO, neuroretinitis, transverse myelitis, oculoglandular syndrome.
Bacillary angiomatosis; Peliosis hepatis—pts with AIDS MMWR 58:(RR-4):39, 2009; AAC 48:1921, 2004.	B. henselae, B. quintana	**Erythro** 500 mg qid or **Doxy** 100 mg po bid x 3 months or longer. If CNS involvement: **Doxy** 100 mg IV/po bid + **RIF** 300 mg po bid	**Azithro** 250 mg po once daily or longer	**Do not use:** TMP-SMX, CIP, Pen, Ceph. **Manifestations of Bartonella infections:** **Immunocompetent Patient:** Bacteremia/endocarditis/FUO/ encephalitis Cat scratch disease Vertebral osteo Trench fever Parinaud's oculoglandular syndrome **HIV/AIDS Patient:** Bacillary angiomatosis Bacillary peliosis Bacteremia/endocarditis/FUO
		Regardless of CD4 count, DC therapy after 3-4 mos. & observe. If no relapse, no suppressive rx. If relapse, **doxy, azithro** or **erythro** x 3 mos. Stop when CD4 >200 x 6 mos.		
Endocarditis (see page 28) (Circ 111:3167, 2005; AAC 48:1921, 2004)	B. henselae, B. quintana	Surgical removal of infected valve	If proven endocarditis: **Doxy** 100 mg IV/po bid x 6 wks + **Gent** 1 mg/kg IV q8h x 11 days	**Gentamicin toxicity:** If Gent toxicity, substitute Rifampin 300 mg IV/po bid x 14 days. Role of valve removal surgery to cure unclear. Presents as SBE. Diagnosis: ECHO, serology & PCR of resected heart valve.
		If suspect endocarditis: **Ceftriaxone** 2 gm IV once daily x 6 weeks + **Gent** 1 mg/kg IV q8h x 14 days + **Doxy** 100 mg IV/po bid x 6 wks.		
Oroya fever (acute) & Verruga peruana (chronic) (AAC 48:1921, 2004)	B. bacilliformis	**Oroya fever: CIP** 500 mg po bid or **Doxy** 100 mg po bid x 14 d. Alternative **Chloro** 500 mg IV/po q6h + another β-lactam. **Doxy** 100 mg po bid x 14 days	**Verruga peruana: RIF** 10 mg/kg po once daily x 14 d or **Streptomycin** 15-20 mg/kg IM/IV once daily x 10 days or **Azithro** 500 mg po q24h x 7 days	Oroya fever transmitted by sand-fly bite in Andes Mtns. Related Bartonella (B. rochalimae) caused bacteremia, fever and splenomegaly (NEJM 356:2346 & 2381, 2007). CIP and Chloro preferred due to prevention of secondary Salmonella infections.
Trench fever (FUO) (AAC 48:1921, 2004)	B. quintana	No endocarditis: **Doxy** 100 mg po bid x 4 wks. If endocarditis: **Doxy + Gentamicin** 3 mg/kg once daily for 1st 2 wks of therapy (AAC 48:1921, 2004).		Vector is body louse. Do not use: TMP-SMX, FQs, cefazolin or Pen

*NOTE: All dosage recommendations are for adults (unless otherwise indicated) and assume normal renal function. § Alternatives consider allergy, PK, compliance, local resistance, cost

TABLE 1 (55)

ANATOMIC SITE/DIAGNOSIS/ MODIFYING CIRCUMSTANCES	ETIOLOGIES (usual)	SUGGESTED REGIMENS*		ADJUNCT DIAGNOSTIC OR THERAPEUTIC MEASURES AND COMMENTS
		PRIMARY	ALTERNATIVE†	
SYSTEMIC SYNDROMES (FEBRILE/NON-FEBRILE) *(continued)*				
Ehrlichiosis³¹ CDC def is one of (1) 4x ↑ IFA antibody, (2) detection of Ehrlichia DNA in blood or CSF by PCR, (3) visible morulae in WBC and IFA ≥1:64. New species in WI, MN *(NEJM 365:422, 2011)*. **Human monocytic ehrlichiosis (HME)** *(MMWR 55(RR-4), 2006; CID 43:1089, 2006)*	Ehrlichia (Ehrlichia chaffeensis) (Lone Star tick is vector)	**Doxy** 100 mg po/IV bid times 7–14 days	**Tetracycline** 500 mg po qid times 7–14 days. Not in children or pregnancy	30 states, mostly SE of line from NJ to Ill. to Missouri to Oklahoma to Texas. History of outdoor activity and tick exposure. April–Sept. Fever, rash (36%), leukopenia and thrombocytopenia. Blood smears no help. PCR for early dx.
Human Anaplasmosis (formerly known as Human granulocytic ehrlichiosis)	Anaplasma (Ehrlichia) phagocytophilum (Ixodes sp. ticks are vector). Dog variant is Ehrlichia ewingii *(NEJM 341:148 & 195, 1999)*	**Doxy** 100 mg po bid or IV times 7–14 days	**Tetracycline** 500 mg po qid times 7–14 days. Not in children or pregnancy See Comment	Upper Midwest, NE, West Coast & Europe. H/O tick exposure. April–Sept. Febrile flu-like illness after outdoor activity. No rash. Leukopenia/ thrombocytopenia common. **Dx:** Up to 80% have + blood smear. Antibody test for confirmation. **Rx:** RIF active in vitro *(IDCNA 22:433, 2008)* but worry about resistance developing. Minocycline effective if doxy not available.
Lyme Disease (New York). NOTE: Think about concomitant tick-borne disease—e.g., babesiosis and ehrlichiosis. **Guidelines:** *CID 51:1, 2010; NEJM 370:1724, 2014.*				
Bite by *Ixodes*-infected tick in an endemic area — **Postexposure prophylaxis**	Borrelia burgdorferi **IDSA guidelines:** *CID 43:1089, 2006; CID 51:1, 2010*	If endemic area, if nymphal partially engorged deer tick: **doxy** 200 mg times 1 dose with food	If not endemic area, not engorged, not deer tick: No treatment	Prophylaxis study in endemic area: erythema migrans developed in 3% of the control group and 0.4% doxy group *(NEJM 345:79 & 133, 2001)*.
Early (erythema migrans) See Comment	Western blot diagnostic criteria **IgM**—Need 2 of 3 positive of kilodaltons (KD): 23, 39, 41 **IgG**—Need 5 of 10 positive of KD: 18, 21, 28, 30, 39, 41, 45, 58, 66, 93	**Doxy** 100 mg po bid, or **amoxicillin** 500 mg po tid or **cefuroxime axetil** 500 mg po bid. All regimens for 14–21 days. *AnIM 138:697, 2003)* See Comment *for peds doses*	**Cefuroxime axetil** 30 mg po bid for 14–21 days): **Amox** 50 mg per kg per day in 3 div. doses or **erythro** 30 mg per kg per day in 3 div. doses.	High rate of clinical failure with azithro & erythro *(Drugs 57:157, 1999)*. **Peds** (all po for 14–21 days): **Amox** 50 mg per kg per day in 3 div. doses or **cefuroxime axetil** 30 mg per kg per day in 2 div. doses or **erythro** 30 mg per kg per day in 3 div. doses.
Carditis See Comment	Interest in 2 tier diagnostic approach: 1) standard lyme ELISA & if positive; 2) C6 peptide ELISA, better sensitivity/specificity *(CID 57:333 & 341, 2013).*	**Ceftriaxone** 2 gm IV q24h) or (**cefotaxime** 2 gm IV q4h) or (**Pen G** 3 million units IV q4h) times 14–21 days	**Ceftriaxone** 2 gm IV q24h) 100 mg times bid times 14–21 days or **amoxicillin** 500 mg po times 14–21 days	Lesions usually homogeneous—not target-like *(AnIM 136:423, 2002)*. First degree AV block: Oral regimen. Generally self-limited. High degree AV block (PR >0.3 sec.): IV therapy—permanent pacemaker not necessary, but temporary pacing in 39% *(CID 53:996, 2014)*.
Facial nerve paralysis (isolated finding, early)		**Doxy** 100 mg po bid) or **amoxicillin** 500 mg po) tid times 14–21 days	**Ceftriaxone** 2 gm IV q24h times 14–21 days	LP suggested excluding central neurologic disease. If LP neg, oral regimen OK. If abnormal or not done, suggest parenteral Ceftriaxone.
Meningitis, encephalitis For encephalopathy, see Comment		**Ceftriaxone** 2 gm IV q24h times 14–28 days	(**Pen G** 20 million units IV (q4h in div. dose) or (**cefotaxime** 2 gm IV q8h) times 14–28 days	Encephalopathy: memory difficulty, depression, somnolence, or headache, CSF abnormalities. 89% had objective CSF abnormalities. 18/18 pts improved with ceftriaxone 2 gm per day times 30 days *(JID 180:377, 1999)*. No compelling evidence that prolonged treatment has any benefit in post-Lyme syndrome *(Neurology 69:91, 2007)*.
Arthritis		**Doxy** 100 mg po bid or **amoxicillin** 500 mg po tid, both times 30–60 days	**Ceftriaxone** 2 gm IV q24h) or (**pen G** 20-24 million units per day IV) times 14–28 days **If pen allergic: azithro** 500 mg po q24h times 7–10 days) or (**erythro** 500 mg po qid times 14–21 days)	Start with 1 mo of therapy. If only partial response, treat for a second mo.
Pregnancy		**Amoxicillin** 500 mg po tid times 21 days.	**If pen allergic: azithro** 500 mg po q24h times 7–10 days) or (**erythro** 500 mg po qid times 14–21 days)	No benefit from rx *(AJM 126:665, 2013; CID 51:1, 2010; AAC 58:6701, 2014; NEJM 345:85, 2001)*. Constructive review: CID 58:1267, 2014.
Post-Lyme Disease Syndromes		None indicated	Choice should not include doxy	No benefit from rx *(AJM 126:665, 2013; CID 51:1, 2010; AAC 58:6701, 2014; NEJM 345:85, 2001)*. Constructive review: CID 58:1267, 2014.

³¹ In endemic area (New York), high % of both adult ticks and nymphs were jointly infected with both Anaplasma (HGE) and B. burgdorferi *(NEJM 337:49, 1997)*.

Abbreviations on page 2.   *NOTE: All dosage recommendations are for adults (unless otherwise indicated) and assume normal renal function. § Alternatives consider allergy, PK, compliance, local resistance, cost

TABLE 1 (56)

ANATOMIC SITE/DIAGNOSIS/ MODIFYING CIRCUMSTANCES	ETIOLOGIES (usual)	SUGGESTED REGIMENS*		ADJUNCT DIAGNOSTIC OR THERAPEUTIC MEASURES AND COMMENTS
		PRIMARY	ALTERNATIVE§	

SYSTEMIC SYNDROMES (FEBRILE/NON-FEBRILE)/Spread by Infected TICK, FLEA, or LICE *(continued)*

ANATOMIC SITE/DIAGNOSIS/ MODIFYING CIRCUMSTANCES	ETIOLOGIES (usual)	PRIMARY	ALTERNATIVE§	ADJUNCT DIAGNOSTIC OR THERAPEUTIC MEASURES AND COMMENTS
Relapsing fever Louse-borne (LBRF)	Borrelia recurrentis Reservoir: human Vector: Louse pediculus humanus	Tetracycline 500 mg IV/po x 1 dose	Erythro 500 mg IV/po x 1 dose	Jarisch-Herxheimer (fever, ↑ pulse, ↑ resp., ↓ blood pressure) in most patients occurs in ~2 hrs (if present, treat/prevent). **Dx: Examine peripheral blood smear during fever for spirochetes.** Can relapse up to 10 times. Postexposure **doxy** pre-emptive therapy highly effective *(NEJM 355:148, 2006)*. *B. miyamotoi* ref: *EID 17:816, 2011*; Meningoencephalitis in lymphoma patient *(NEJM 368:240, 2013; ArM 159:21, 2013)*.
Tick-borne (TBRF)	No Amer: B. hermsii, B. turicata; Africa: B. hispanica, B. crocidurae, B. duttonii; Russia: B. miyamotoi	Doxy 100 mg po bid x 7–10 days	Erythro 500 mg po qid x 7–10 days	
Rickettsial diseases. Review—Disease in travelers *(CID 39:1493, 2004)*				
Spotted fevers (NOTE: Rickettsial pox not included)				
Rocky Mountain spotted fever (RMSF) *(LnID 7:724, 2008 and MMWR 55 (RR-4), 2007)*	R. rickettsii (Dermacentor tick vector)	Doxy 100 mg po/IV bid times 7 days or for ≥ 2 days after temp. normal. Do not use in pregnancy. Some suggest single 200 mg loading dose.	Chloro 50 mg/kg/day in 4 div doses. Use in pregnancy.	Fever, rash (88%), petechiae 40–50%. **Rash spreads from distal extremities to trunk.** Rash in < 50% pts in 1st 72 hrs. Dx: Immunohistology on skin biopsy; confirmation with antibody titers. Highest incidence in SE and South Central states; also seen in Oklahoma, S. Dakota, Montana. Cases reported from 42 U.S. states. **NOTE: Only 3–18% of pts present with fever, rash, and hx of tick exposure; many early deaths in children & empiric doxy reasonable** *(MMWR 49: 885, 2000)*.
NOTE: Can mimic ehrlichiosis. Pattern of rash important—see Comment				
Other spotted fevers, e.g., Rickettsial pox, African tick bite fever	At least 8 species on 6 continents *(CID 45 (Suppl 1) S39, 2007)*	Doxy 100 mg po bid times 7 days	Chloro 500 mg po/IV qid times 7 days; Children <8 y.o.: azithro or clarithro *(if mild disease)*	Clinical diagnosis suggested by: 1) fever, intense myalgia, headache; 2) exposure to mites or ticks; 3) localized eschar (tache noire) or rash. Definitive Dx: PCR of blood, skin biopsy or sequential antibody tests.
Typhus group—Consider in returning travelers with fever				
Louse-borne: epidemic typhus Ref: LnID 8:417, 2008	R. prowazekii (vector is body or head louse)	Doxy 100 mg po/IV bid times 7 days; single 200 mg dose 95% effective.	Chloro 500 mg IV/po bid times 5 days	**Brill-Zinsser disease** *(Ln 357:1198, 2001)* is a relapse of typhus acquired during WWII. Truncal rash (64%) spreads centrifugally—opposite of RMSF. Louse borne typhus is a winter disease. Diagnosis by serology. R. prowazekii found in flying squirrels in SE U.S. Deluxe dwelling of infected pt.
Murine typhus (cat flea typhus): EID 14:1019, 2008	R. typhi (rat reservoir and flea vector): CID 46:913, 2008	Doxy 100 mg IV/po bid times 7 days	Chloro 500 mg IV/po bid times 5 days	Rash in 20–54%, not diagnostic. Without treatment most pts recover in 2 wks. Faster recovery with treatment. Dx based on suspicion; confirmed serologically.
Scrub typhus	O. tsutsugamushi [rodent reservoir; vector is larval stage of mites (chiggers)]	Doxy 100 mg po/IV bid x 7 days. In pregnancy, Azithro 500 mg po single dose	Chloro 500 mg po/IV qid x 7 days	Asian rim of Pacific. Confirm with serology. If Doxy resistance suspected, alternatives are Doxy + RIF 900 or 600 mg once daily *(Ln 356:1057, 2000)* or Azithro 500 mg q24h *(AAC 58:1488, 2014)*.
Tularemia, typhoidal type Ref: bioterrorism, see JAMA 285:2763, 2001; LD Clin No Amer 22:489, 2008; MMWR 58:744, 2009.	Francisella tularensis. Vector depends on geography: ticks, biting flies, mosquitoes (identified)	Moderate/severe: [Gentamicin to tobra 5 mg per kg per day div q8h IV] or [Streptomycin 10 mg/kg IV/IM q12h]) X 10 days	Mild: CIP 400 mg IV (or 750 mg po) bid or Doxy 100 mg IV/po bid] x 14–21 days	Diagnosis: Culture on cysteine-enriched media & serology. Dangerous in the lab. Hematogenous meningitis is a complication; treatment = Streptomycin + Chloro 50-100 mg/kg/day IV in 4 divided doses *(Arch Neurol 66:523, 2009)*.

Abbreviations on page 2.

NOTE: All dosage recommendations are for adults (unless otherwise indicated) and assume normal renal function. § Alternatives consider allergy, PK, compliance, local resistance, cost

TABLE 1 (57)

ANATOMIC SITE/DIAGNOSIS/ MODIFYING CIRCUMSTANCES	ETIOLOGIES (usual)	SUGGESTED REGIMENS*		ADJUNCT DIAGNOSTIC OR THERAPEUTIC MEASURES AND COMMENTS
		PRIMARY	ALTERNATIVE§	
SYSTEMIC SYNDROMES (FEBRILE/NON-FEBRILE)				
Other Zoonotic Systemic Bacterial Febrile Illnesses: Obtain careful epidemiologic history				
Brucellosis Refs: NEJM 352:2325, 2005; CID 46:426, 2008; MMWR 57:603, 2008; BMJ 336:701, 2008; PLoS One 7:e32090, 2012.	B. abortus–cattle B. suis–swine B. melitensis–goats B. canis–dogs	**Non focal disease:** [**Doxy** 100 mg po bid x 6 wks + **Gent** 5 mg/kg once daily] for 1–7 days – – – – – – – – – – – – **Spondylitis, Sacroiliitis:** [**Doxy** + **Gent** (as above) + **RIF**] x min 3 mos – – – – – – – – – – – – **Neurobrucellosis:** [**Doxy** + **RIF** (as above) + **ceftriaxone** 2 gm IV q12h until CSF returned to normal (AAC 56:1523, 2012) **Endocarditis:** Surgery + [(**RIF** + **Doxy** + **TMP-SMX**) x 1-1/2 to 6 mos + **Gent** for 2-4 wks (CID 56:1407, 2013) **Pregnancy:** Not much data. **RIF** 900 mg po once daily x 6 wks	[**Doxy** 100 mg po bid + **RIF** 600-900 mg once daily) or **RIF** 600-900 mg once daily) – – – – – – – – – – – – [**CIP** 750 mg po bid + **RIF** 600-900 mg once daily) – – – – – – – – – – – – **RIF** 900 mg po once daily + **TMP-SMX** 5 mg/kg (TMP comp) po bid x 4 wks.	Bone involvement, esp. sacroiliitis in 20-30%. **Neurobrucellosis:** Usually meningitis. 1% of all pts with brucellosis. Role of corticosteroids unclear, not recommended. **Endocarditis:** Rare but most common cause of death. Need surgery + antimicrobials. **Pregnancy: TMP-SMX** may cause kernicterus if given during last week of pregnancy.
Leptospirosis (CID 36:1507 & 1514, 2003; LnID 3:757, 2003)	Leptospira—in urine of domestic livestock, dogs, small rodents	Severe illness: **Pen G** 1.5 million units IV q6h or **ceftriaxone** 2 gm q24h. Duration: 7 days Mild illness: [**Doxy** 100 mg IV/po q12h or **Levo** 500 mg po tid x 7 days		**Severity varies.** Varies from mild anicteric illness to severe icteric disease (Weil's disease) with renal failure and myocarditis. AST/ALT do not exceed 5x normal. **Rx:** Azithro 1 gm po, then 500 mg daily x 2 days; non-inferior to than, doxy in standard dose (AAC 57:3259, 2007). Jarisch-Herxheimer reaction can occur post-Pen therapy.
Salmonella bacteremia other than S. typhi–non-typhoidal)	Salmonella enteriditis— a variety of serotypes from animal sources	If NOT acquired in Asia: **Ceftriaxone** 2 gm iv q24h or **Azithro** 750 mg po q12h or q24h) **Levo** (See Comment) If acquired in Asia: **Ceftriaxone** 2 gm iv q24h or **Azithro** 1 gm po x 1 dose, then 500 mg once daily x5-7 days. Do NOT use FQs until susceptibility determined. (See Comment)		In vitro resistance to nalidixic acid indicates relative resistance to FQs. Bacteremia can infect any organ/tissue: look for infection of atherosclerotic aorta, osteomyelitis in sickle cell pts. Rx duration range 14 days (immunocompetent) to ≥6 wks of mycotic aneurism or endocarditis. **Alternative**, if susceptible: **TMP-SMX** 8-10 mg/kg/day (TMP comp) divided q6h CLSI has established new interpretive breakpoints for susceptibility to. Ciprofloxacin: susceptible strains, MIC < 0.06 µg/mL (CID 55:1107, 2012).

*NOTE: All dosage recommendations are for adults (unless otherwise indicated) and assume normal renal function. PK, compliance, local resistance, cost

§ Alternatives consider allergy,

TABLE 1 (58)

ANATOMIC SITE/DIAGNOSIS/ MODIFYING CIRCUMSTANCES	ETIOLOGIES (usual)	SUGGESTED REGIMENS* PRIMARY	SUGGESTED REGIMENS* ALTERNATIVE†	ADJUNCT DIAGNOSTIC OR THERAPEUTIC MEASURES AND COMMENTS
SYSTEMIC SYNDROMES (FEBRILE/NON-FEBRILE) (continued)				
Miscellaneous Systemic Febrile Syndromes				
Fever in Returning Travelers Etiology by geographic exposure & clinical syndrome (AnIM 158:456, 2013).	Dengue	Supportive care; See Table 14A, page 158 Diagnosis: peripheral blood smear		Average incubation period 4 days; serodiagnosis.
	Flavivirus			
	Plasmodia sp.	See Table 13A, page 145		See Table 13A, page 145
	Salmonella sp.	See Table 1, page 60		Average incubation 7-14 days; diarrhea in 45%
Kawasaki syndrome 6 weeks to 12 yrs of age, peak at 1 yr of age; 85% below age 5. Ref: Pediatrics 124:1, 2009.	Acute self-limited vasculitis with 1 temp., rash, conjunc-tivitis, stomatitis, cervical adenitis, red hands/feet & coronary artery aneurysms (25% if untreated)	**IVIG** 2 gm/kg IV over 8-12 hrs **ASA** 20-25 mg per kg qid THEN **ASA** 3-5 mg per kg per day po q24h times 6-8 wks	Instill febrile after 1st dose of IVIG, some give 2nd dose in Japan: **IVIG** + prednisolone 2 mg/kg/day. Continue steroid until CRP normal for 15 days (Lancet 379:1577, 2012).	IV gamma globulin (2 gm per kg over 10 hrs) in pts rx before 10th day of illness ↓ coronary artery lesions. See Table 14A, page 167 for IVIG adverse effects. In children, wait until 11+ months after IVIG before giving live virus vaccines.
Rheumatic Fever, acute Ref: Ln 366:155, 2005	Post-Group A strep pharyn-gitis (not Group B, C, or G)	(1) Symptom relief: **ASA** 80-100 mg per kg per day in children; 4-8 gm per day in adults. (2) Eradicate Group A strep: **Pen** times 10 days (see Pharyngitis, page 48). (3) Start prophylaxis; see below		Penicillin for 10 days prevents rheumatic fever even when started 7-9 days after onset of illness (see page 48).
Prophylaxis				
Primary prophylaxis: Treat S. pyogenes pharyngitis		**Benzathine pen G** 1.2 million units IM (see Pharyngitis, pg. 48)	**Penicillin V** 250 mg po bid or **sulfadiazine (sulfisoxazole)** 1 gm po q24h or **erythro** 250 mg po bid.	
Secondary prophylaxis (previous documented rheumatic fever)		**Benzathine pen G** 1.2 million units IM q3-4 wks (AAC 58:6735, 2014).	**Duration?** No carditis: 5 yrs or until age 21, whichever is longer; carditis without residual heart disease: 10 since last attack; carditis with residual valvular disease: 10 yrs since last episode or until age 40 whichever is longer (PEDS 96:758, 1995).
Typhoidal syndrome (typhoid fever) enteric fever Global susceptibility results: CID 50:241, 2010. Treatment: BMJ 338:b1159 & b1865, 2009.	Salmonella typhi, S. paratyphi A, B, C & S. choleraesuis. **NOTE: In vitro resistance to nalidixic acid predicts clinical failure of CIP (FQs).** Do not use empiric FQs if Asia-acquired infection. Need susceptibility results.	**If NOT acquired in Asia:** (Ceftriaxone 2 gm IV daily x7-14 d) or (Levo 750 mg po/IV q24h x 7-10 d) (See Comment) In children, azithro 10 mg/kg once daily x 7 days	**If acquired in Asia:** (Ceftriaxone 2 gm IV daily x 1 dose, then 500 mg po daily x 5-7 d) or (Chloro 500 mg IV q6h x 14 d) (See Comment) (AAC 51:819, 2007).	**Dexamethasone: Use in severely ill pts: 1st dose just prior to antibiotic, 3 mg/kg IV, then 1 mg/kg q6h x 8 doses. Complications:** perforation of terminal ileum &/or cecum, osteo, septic arthritis, **mycotic aneurysm**, meningitis, hematogenous pneumonia. FQs, including Gati, remain best treatment if isolate susceptible (BMJ 338:b1159 & 1865, 2009: LnID 11:445, 2011). CLSI has established new interpretive breakpoints for susceptibility to Ciprofloxacin: susceptible strains, MIC < 0.06 µg/mL (CID 55:1107, 2012).
Sepsis: Following suggested **empiric therapy assumes pt is bacteremic;** consider viral, fungal, rickettsial infections and pancreatitis (Intensive Care Medicine 34:17, 2008; IDC No Amer 22:1, 2008).				
Neonatal—early onset <1 week old	Group B strep, E. coli, kleb-siella, enterobacter, Staph. aureus (uncommon), listeria (rare in U.S.)	**AMP** 25 mg/kg IV q6h + **cefotaxime** 50 mg/kg IV q8h	**AMP** + **gent** 2.5 mg/kg IV/IM q12h) or (**AMP** + **ceftriaxone** 50 mg/kg IV/IM q24h)	Blood cultures are key but only 5–10% +. Discontinue antibiotics after 72 hrs if cultures and course do not support diagnosis. In Spain, listeria predominates; in S. America, salmonella. If Grp B Strep infection + severe beta-lactam allergy, alternatives include: erythro + clinda; report of clinda resistance at 38% & erythro resistance at 51% (AAC 56:739, 2012).
Neonatal—late onset 1-4 weeks old	As above + H influenzae & S. epidermidis	(**AMP** 25 mg/kg IV q6h + **cefotaxime** 50 mg/kg IV q8h) or (**AMP** + **ceftriaxone** 75 mg/kg IV q24h)	**AMP** + **gent** 2.5 mg/kg IV or IM	**If MSSA/MRSA** a concern, add vanco.

§ Alternatives consider allergy, PK, compliance, local resistance, cost

TABLE 1 (59)

ANATOMIC SITE/DIAGNOSIS/ MODIFYING CIRCUMSTANCES	ETIOLOGIES (usual)	SUGGESTED REGIMENS* PRIMARY	SUGGESTED REGIMENS* ALTERNATIVE§	ADJUNCT DIAGNOSTIC OR THERAPEUTIC MEASURES AND COMMENTS
SYSTEMIC SYNDROMES (FEBRILE/NON-FEBRILE)/Sepsis *(continued)*				
Child; not neutropenic	Strep. pneumoniae, Staph. aureus (MSSA & MRSA), H. influenzae now rare	Cefotaxime 50 mg/kg IV q8h or ceftriaxone 100 mg/kg IV q24h) + vanco 15 mg/kg q6h)	Aztreonam 7.5 mg/kg IV q8h + linezolid	Major concerns are S. pneumoniae & community-associated MRSA. Coverage for Gm-neg. bacilli included but H. influenzae infection now rare. Meningococcemia mortality remains high (Ln 356:961, 2000).
Adult; not neutropenic: NO HYPOTENSION but LIFE-THREATENING*—For Septic shock, see page 63	Aerobic Gm-neg. bacilli; S. aureus; streptococci; others	[(IMP or MER) + vanco] or (PIP-TZ + vanco) — If ESBL and/or carbapenemase-producing GNB. Empiric options pending culture results: **Low prevalence:** Vanco + PIP-TZ **High prevalence:** Colistin + (MER or IMP). See TABLE 5B, page 78	(Dapto 6 mg/kg IV q24h) + (cefepime or PIP-TZ or TC-CL)	Systemic inflammatory response syndrome (**SIRS**): 2 or more of the following: 1. Temperature >38°C or <36°C 2. Heart rate >90 beats per min. 3. Respiratory rate >20 breaths per min. 4. WBC >12,000 per mcL or >10% bands **Sepsis:** SIRS + a documented infection (+ culture). **Severe sepsis:** Sepsis + organ dysfunction (lactic acidosis, oliguria, ↓ mental status) hypoperfusion abnormalities (lactic acidosis, oliguria, ↓ mental status) or sepsis-induced hypotension (systolic BP <90 mmHg) **Septic shock:** Sepsis-induced hypotension not responsive to 500 mL IV fluid challenge - peripheral hypoperfusion.
If suspect biliary source (see Gallbladder pg. 17)	Enterococci + aerobic Gm-neg. bacilli	For Collistin combination dosing, see Table 10A, page 104. PIP-TZ or TC-CL	Ceftriaxone + metro (or CIP or Levo) + metro Dosages—footnote²	If enterococcus a concern, add ampicillin or vanco to metro regimens
If community-acquired pneumonia (see page 39 and following pages)	S. pneumoniae; MRSA, Legionella, Gm-neg. bacillus, others	(Levo or moxi) + (PIP-TZ) + Vanco	Aztreonam + (Levo or moxi) + linezolid	Many categories of CAP - see material beginning at page 39. Suggestions based on most severe forms of CAP., e.g., MRSA after influenza or Klebsiella pneumonia in alcoholics.
If illicit use IV drugs	S. aureus	Vanco if high prevalence of MRSA. Do NOT use empiric vanco + oxacillin pending organism ID. ... toxins (CA-MRSA (JID 195:202, 2007). Dosages—footnote32 page 13		In vitro nafcillin increased production of
If suspect intra-abdominal source	Mixture aerobic & anaerobic Gm-neg. bacilli	See secondary peritonitis, page 47		
If petechial rash	Meningococcemia	Ceftriaxone 2 gm IV q12h (until sure no meningitis), consider Rocky Mountain spotted fever—see page 59		
If suspect urinary source, e.g. pyelonephritis	Aerobic Gm-neg. bacilli & enterococci	See pyelonephritis, page 34		
Neutropenic: Child or Adult (absolute PMN count <500 per mm³) in cancer and transplant patients. **Guideline:** (CID 52:427, 2011 (inpatients); J Clin Oncol 31:794, 2013 (outpatients))				
Prophylaxis (J Clin Oncol 31:794, 2013)		In patients expected to have PMN < 100 for > 7 days consider Levo 500-750 mg po q24h. Acute leukemias undergoing intensive induction consider addition of Fluc 400 mg po q24h. In patients with AML or MDS who have prolonged neutropenia, consider Posa instead at 200 mg TID (N Engl J Med 356:348, 2007).		
Post-chemotherapy, impending neutropenia	Pneumocystis (PCP), Viridans strep	TMP-SMX (vs. PCP) + Acyclovir (vs. HSV/VZV) + pre-emptive monitoring for CMV + Posa (vs. mold)		In autologous HCT not active prophylaxis no CMV screening is recommended. Fluc OK with TMP-SMX and acyclovir.
Post allogeneic stem cell transplant	Aerobic Gm-neg. bacilli ↑ risk pneumovirus, herpes viruses, candida aspergillus			

P Ceph 3 (cefotaxime 2 gm IV q8h, use q4h if life-threatening; ceftizoxime 2 gm IV q4h; ceftriaxone 2 gm IV q12h), **AP Pen** (piperacillin 3 gm IV q12h; ticarcillin 3 gm IV q4h); **TC-CL** 3.1 gm IV q4h; **PIP-TZ** 3.375 gm IV q6h or 4-hr infusion of 3.375 gm q8h, see Table 10D (page 110). **AP Pen** 200 mg/kg/day divided q6h, **clinda** 900 mg IV q8h; **MER** 1 gm IV q8h; **ERTA** 1 gm IV q24h; **DORI** 500 mg IV q8h (1-hr infusion). **Nafcillin** or **oxacillin** 2 gm IV q4h, **aztreonam** 2 gm IV q8h, **metro** 1 gm loading dose then 0.5 gm q6h or 1 gm IV q12h; **vanco** loading dose 25-30 mg/kg IV, then 15-20 mg/kg IV q8-12h (dose in obese pt, see Table 17C, page 213), **cefepime** 2 gm IV q8h; **Cefepime** 2 gm IV q12h (q8h if neutropenic), **cefepime**^ab 2 gm IV q12h. **CIP** 400 mg IV q12h, **levo** 750 mg IV q24h; **linezolid** 600 mg IV q12h.

*NOTE: All dosage recommendations are for adults (unless otherwise indicated) and assume normal renal function. § Alternatives consider allergy, PK, compliance, local resistance, cost

Abbreviations on page 2.

TABLE 1 (60)

ANATOMIC SITE/DIAGNOSIS/ MODIFYING CIRCUMSTANCES	ETIOLOGIES (usual)	SUGGESTED REGIMENS*		ADJUNCT DIAGNOSTIC OR THERAPEUTIC MEASURES AND COMMENTS
		PRIMARY	ALTERNATIVE¹	
SYSTEMIC SYNDROMES (FEBRILE/NON-FEBRILE) Neutropenia *(continued)*				
Empiric therapy—febrile neutropenia (≥38.3°C for > 1 hr or sustained >38°C and absolute neutrophil count <500 cells/μL.)				(IDSA Guidelines: *CID 52:427, 2012*); *(Outpatients: J Clin Oncol 31:794, 2013)*.
Low-risk adults Anticipate < 7 days neutropenia, no co-morbid., can take po meds	Aerobic Gm-neg. bacilli, Viridans strep	**CIP** 750 mg po bid + **AM-CL** 875/125 mg po bid. Treat until absolute neutrophil count >1000 cells/μL		Treat as outpatients with 24/7 access to inpatient care if: no focal findings, no hypotension, no COPD, no fungal infection, age range 16-60 yrs, motivated and compliant pts & family. If pen allergy: can substitute clinda 300 mg po qid for AM-CL
High-risk adults and children Anticipate > 7 days prolonged neutropenia, active co-morbidities	**Aerobic Gm-neg. bacilli; to include P. aeruginosa; cephalosporin-resistant viridans strep; MRSA**	**Empiric therapy:** IMP or **MER; DORI** or **PIP-TAZO.** Consider addition of **Vanco** as below.	**Combination therapy.** If pt has severe sepsis/shock, consider add **Tobra** AND **Vanco AND Echinocandin** as below.	Increasing resistance of viridans streptococci to penicillins, cephalosporins & FQs *(CID 34:1469 & 1524, 2002)*. **What if severe IgE-mediated β-lactam allergy?** Aztreonam plus Tobra. Work-up should include blood, urine. CXR with additional testing based
		Dosages: **Footnote³⁰** *and Table 10B*		on symptoms. Low threshold for CT scan. If cultures remain neg, but pt
		Include empiric vanco if: Suspected CLABSI, severe mucositis, SSTI, PNA, or hypotension		afebrile, treat until absolute neutrophil count ≥ 500 cells/μL.
Persistent fever and neutropenia after 5 days of empiric antibacterial therapy—see *CID 52:427, 2011.*				
	Candida species, aspergillus, VRE, resistant GNB	Add either (**caspofungin** 70 mg IV day 1, then 50 mg IV q24h or **Micafungin** 100 mg IV q24h or **Anidulafungin** 200 mg IV x 1 dose, then 100 mg IV q24h) **OR voriconazole** 6 mg per kg IV q12h times 2 doses, then 4 mg per kg IV q12h		Conventional **ampho B** causes more fever & nephrotoxicity & lower efficacy than lipid-based ampho B; both **caspofungin & voriconazole** better tolerated & perhaps more efficacious than lipid-based ampho B *(NEJM 346:225, 2002 & 351:1391 & 1445, 2005)*.
Shock syndromes				
Septic shock: Fever & hypotension Bacteremic shock, endotoxin shock Goals: 1. Effective antibiotics 2. Fluid resuscitation 3. Vasoactive drugs , if needed 4. Source control Refs: *Chest 145:1407, 2014; NEJM 369:840, 2013; CCM 188:77, 2013*	Bacteremia with aerobic Gm-neg. bacteria or Gm + cocci	Lower mortality with **sepsis treatment "bundle"** *(AJRCCM 188:77, 2013)* • Blood cultures & serum lactate • Initiate effective antibiotic therapy: ○ No clear source & MDR GNB are rare: **PIP-TZ** + **Vanco** ○ No clear source but high prevalence of MDR GNB: **Colistin** + **MER** or **IMP** • IV crystalloid: 20-40 mL/kg for hypotension or elevated serum lactate *(AnIM 161:347 & 372, 2014)* • Attempt to identify & correct source of bacteremia • If hypotensive after fluids, nor-epinephrine • Monitor lactate, CVP (target ≥ 8 cm H2O) & central venous O2 sat (target ≥ 70%) • Low tidal volume (mL/kg) mechanical ventilation *(NEJM 369:2126, 2013)* • Transfuse if hematocrit < 30% *(NEJM 371:1381, 2014)* • See Comment for continuation		• Hydrocortisone in stress dose: 100 mg IV q8h if BP still low after fluids and vasopressor *(AR/JCCM 185:135, 2012)*. Benefit in pts with severe shock *(CCM 42:333, 2014)*. • Insulin Rx. Current target is glucose level of 140-180 mg/dL. Attempts at night control (80-110 mg/dL) resulted in excessive hypoglycemia *(NEJM 363:2540, 2010)*. • Impact of early effective antibiotic therapy *(CCM 38:1045 & 1211, 2010)*. • Bacteremia due to carbapenemase-producing K. pneumoniae: lowest mortality with combination rx: carbapenem + a polymyxin *(AAC 56:2322, 2014)*. • Number of pts needed to treat with appropriate antimicrobial rx to prevent one pt death reported as 4 *(CCM 42:2342 & 2444, 2014)*.
Septic shock: post-splenectomy or functional asplenia Asplenic pt care: *NEJM 371:349, 2014*	S. pneumoniae, N. meningitidis, H. influenzae, Capnocytophaga (DF-2)	No dog bite: **Ceftriaxone** 2 gm IV q24h (1 to 2 gm q12h if meningitis) Post-dog bite: **Pip-Tazo** 3.375 gm IV q6h OR **MER** 1 gm IV q8h + **Clinda** 900 mg IV q8h	No dog bite: (**Levo** 750 mg or **Moxi** 400 mg) once IV q24h	Howell-Jolly bodies in peripheral blood smear confirm absence of functional spleen. Often results in **symmetrical peripheral gangrene of digits** due to severe DIC. For prophylaxis, see Table 15A, page 192. Vaccines: *CID 58:309, 2014.*

Abbreviations on page 2

*NOTE: All dosage recommendations are for adults (unless otherwise indicated) and assume normal renal function. § Alternatives consider allergy, PK, compliance, local resistance, cost

TABLE 1 (61)

ANATOMIC SITE/DIAGNOSIS/ MODIFYING CIRCUMSTANCES	ETIOLOGIES (usual)	SUGGESTED REGIMENS* PRIMARY	ALTERNATIVE§	ADJUNCT DIAGNOSTIC OR THERAPEUTIC MEASURES AND COMMENTS
SYSTEMIC SYNDROMES (FEBRILE/NON-FEBRILE)/Shock syndromes				
Toxic shock syndrome, Clostridium sordellii				
Clinical picture: shock, capillary leak, hemoconcentration, leukemoid reaction, afebrile Ref: CID 43:1436 & 1447, 2006.	Clostridium sordellii–hemorrhagic & lethal toxins	Fluids, aq. **penicillin G** 18–20 million units per day div q4-6h + **clindamycin** 900 mg iv q8h. **Surgical debridement is key.**		Occurs in variety of settings that produce anaerobic tissue, e.g., illicit drug use, post-partum. Several deaths reported after use of abortifacient regimen of mifepristone (RU486) & misoprostol. (NEJM 363:2540, 2010). 2001-2005 standard medical abortion: po mifepristone & then vaginal misoprostol. Since 2006 switch to buccal, instead of vaginal misoprostol, plus prophylactic Doxy resulted in dramatic decrease in TSS (NEJM 361:145, 2009). Mortality nearly 100% if WBC >50,000/µL.
Toxic shock syndrome, staphylococcal. Review LnID 9:281, 2009				
Colonization by toxin-producing Staph. aureus of: vagina (tampon-assoc.), surgical/traumatic wounds, endometrium, burns	Staph. aureus (toxin-mediated)	**(Nafcillin** or **oxacillin** 2 gm IV q4h) or (if MRSA, **vanco** 15-20 mg/kg q8-12h) + **Clinda** 600-900 mg IV q8h (Dose in Comment)	**(Cefazolin** 1-2 gm IV q8h) or (if MRSA, **vanco** 15-20 mg/kg q8-12h OR **dapto** 6 mg/kg IV q24h) **Clinda** 600-900 mg IV q8h + **IVIG** (Dose in Comment)	**IVIG reasonable** (see Streptococcal TSS) — dose 1 gm per kg on day 1, then 0.5 gm per kg days 2 & 3 — antitoxin antibodies present. If suspect TSS, "turn off" toxin production with clinda; report of success with **linezolid** (JID 195:202, 2007). Exposure of MRSA to nafcillin increased toxin production in vitro (JID 195:202, 2007).
Toxic shock syndrome, streptococcal. NOTE: For Necrotizing fasciitis without toxic shock, see page 56. Ref: LnID 9:281, 2009.				
Associated with invasive disease, i.e., erysipelas, necrotizing fasciitis; secondary strep infection of varicella. ²Secondary reported (NEJM 335:547 & 590, 1996; CID 27:150, 1998).	Group A, B, C, & G Strep. pyogenes, Group B strep ref: EID 15:223, 2009.	**(Pen G** 24 million units per day IV in div. doses) + **clinda** 900 mg IV q8h) Prospective observational study (CID 59:358, 366 & 851, 2014) indicates: • Clinda decreases mortality • IVIG perhaps of benefit: 1 gm/kg day 1, then 0.5 gm/kg days 2,3 • High incidence of secondary cases in household contacts	**Ceftriaxone** 2 gm IV q24h + **clinda** 900 mg IV q8h	**Definition:** Isolation of Group A strep, hypotension and ≥2 of: renal impairment, coagulopathy, liver involvement, ARDS, generalized rash, soft tissue necrosis. Associated with invasive disease. **Surgery usually required.** Mortality with fasciitis 30–50%, myositis 80% even with early rx (CID 14:2, 1992). Clinda ↓ toxin production. Use of NSAID may predispose to TSS. For reasons unclear, pen G may fail in fulminant S. pyogenes infections (see JID 167:1401, 1993).
Toxin-Mediated Syndromes—no fever unless complicated				
Botulism (CID 41:1167, 2005. As biologic weapon: JAMA 285:1059, 2001: www.bt.cdc.gov)				
Food-borne Dyspnea at presentation bad sign (CID 43:1247, 2006)	Clostridium botulinum	For all types: Follow vital capacity, other supportive care. If no ileus, purge GI tract. Heptavalent equine serum antitoxin—CDC (see Comment)		**Equine antitoxin:** Heptavalent currently only antitoxin available (US) for non-infant botulism: CDC (+1 404-639-2206 M-F OR +1 404-639-2888 evenings/weekends). For infants, use Baby BIG (human botulism immune globulin): California Infant Botulism Treat & Prevent Program.
Infant (Adult intestinal botulism is rare variant: EIN 18:1, 2012).		Human botulinum immunoglobulin (BIG) IV, single dose. Call (+1) 510-540-2646. Do not use equine antitoxin.	No antibiotics: may lyse C. botulinum in gut and ↑ load of toxin	**Antimicrobials:** May make infant botulism worse. Untested in wound botulism. When used, pen G 10-20 million units per day usual dose. If complications (pneumonia, UTI) occur, avoid antimicrobials with assoc. neuromuscular blockade, i.e., aminoglycosides, tetracycline, polymyxins. **Differential dx:** Guillain-Barré, myasthenia gravis, tick paralysis, organo-phosphate toxicity, West Nile virus.
Wound		Debridement & anaerobic cultures. No proven value of local antitoxin. Role of antibiotics untested.	Trivalent equine antitoxin (see Comment)	Wound botulism can result from spore contamination of tar heroin. Ref: CID 31:1018, 2000. Mouse bioassay failed to detect toxin in 1/3 of patients (CID 48:1669, 2009).

Abbreviations on page 2.   *NOTE: All dosage recommendations are for adults (unless otherwise indicated) and assume normal renal function. § Alternatives consider allergy, PK, compliance, local resistance, cost

Abbreviations on page 2.

TABLE 1 (62)

ANATOMIC SITE/DIAGNOSIS/ MODIFYING CIRCUMSTANCES	ETIOLOGIES* (usual)	SUGGESTED REGIMENS*		ADJUNCT DIAGNOSTIC OR THERAPEUTIC MEASURES AND COMMENTS
		PRIMARY	ALTERNATIVE¹	

SYSTEMIC SYNDROMES/Toxin-Mediated Syndromes *(continued)*

ANATOMIC SITE/DIAGNOSIS/ MODIFYING CIRCUMSTANCES	ETIOLOGIES* (usual)	SUGGESTED REGIMENS* PRIMARY	ALTERNATIVE¹	ADJUNCT DIAGNOSTIC OR THERAPEUTIC MEASURES AND COMMENTS
Tetanus: Trismus, generalized muscle rigidity, muscle spasm. Ref: *AnIM* 154:329, 2011.	C. tetani–production of tetanospasmin toxin	**Six treatment steps:** 1–Urgent endotracheal intubation to protect the airway. Laryngeal spasm is common. Early tracheostomy. 2–Eliminate reflex spasms with diazepam, 20 mg/day IV or midazolam. Reports of benefit combining diazepam with magnesium sulfate (*Ln* 368:1436, 2006). Worst cases: need neuromuscular blockade with vecuronium. 3–Neutralize toxin: Human hyperimmune globulin IM: start tetanus immunization–no immunity from clinical tetanus. 4–Surgically debride infected source tissue. Start antibiotic: (**Pen G** 3 million units IV q12h or **Doxy** 100 mg IV q12h or **Metro** 1000 mg IV q12h) x 7–10 days. 5–Avoid light as may precipitate muscle spasms. 6–Use beta blockers, e.g., short acting esmolol, to control sympathetic hyperactivity.		

VASCULAR

ANATOMIC SITE/DIAGNOSIS/ MODIFYING CIRCUMSTANCES	ETIOLOGIES* (usual)	SUGGESTED REGIMENS* PRIMARY	ALTERNATIVE¹	ADJUNCT DIAGNOSTIC OR THERAPEUTIC MEASURES AND COMMENTS
IV line infection (See IDSA *Guidelines CID* 49:1, 2009). Heparin lock, midline catheter, **non-tunneled** central venous catheter (subclavian, internal jugular), peripherally inserted central catheter (PICC), dual lumen study found ↑ infection risk/thrombosis if femoral vein used, esp. if BMI >28.4 (*JAMA* 299:2413, 2008). *See Comment.*	Staph. epidermidis, Staph. aureus (MSSA/MRSA). **Diagnosis:** Fever & either + blood cult from line & peripheral vein **OR** >15 colonies on tip of removed line **OR** culture from catheter positive 2 hrs earlier than peripheral vein culture.	**Vanco** 15–20 mg/kg q8–12h. **Other alternatives—see Comment.** **(1)** If **S. aureus**, remove catheter. Can use TEE result to determine if 2 or 4 wks of therapy (*JAC* 57:1172, 2006). **(2)** If **S. epidermidis,** can try to "save" catheter. 80% cure after 7–10 days of therapy. With only systemic antibiotics, high rate of recurrence (*CID* 49:1187, 2009). If *leuconostoc* or *lactobacillus* are Vanco resistant; need Pen G, Amp or Clinda		For documented MSSA **nafcillin** or **oxacillin** 2 gm IV q4h or **cefazolin** 2 gm IV q8h, if no response to, or intolerant of, **vanco**, switch to **daptomycin** 6 mg per kg IV q24h. Culture removed catheter. With "roll" method, >15 colonies (*NEJM* 312:1142, 1985) suggests infection. Lines do not require "routine" changing when not infected. When infected, do not insert new catheter over a wire. Antimicrobial-impregnated catheters may ↓ infection risk; the debate is lively (*CID* 37:65, 2003 & 38:1287, 2004 & 39:1829, 2004). Are femoral lines more prone to infection than subclavian lines (*ICM* 40:2479, 2012); jugular lines? Meta-analysis found no difference (*CID* 49:1187, 2009). However, a number of confounders may influence conclusion (*AnIM* 157(10):JC5-5, 2012).
Tunnel type indwelling venous catheters and ports (Broviac, Hickman, Groshong, Quinton), dual lumen hemodialysis catheters (Permacath). For prevention, see below.	Staph. epidermidis, Staph. aureus, (Candida sp.). Rarely, leuconostoc or lacto-bacillus—both resistant to vanco (see *Table 2, page 68*)	**Vanco** 1 gm IV q12h or **IMP** or (**Cefepime** or **Ceftaz**) or (**Vanco** + **Pip-Tazo**) or (**Cefepime** or **Ceftaz**) + **Aminoglycoside**) *(Dosage in footnotes²⁸,³² , pages 47 and 13)*		If subcutaneous tunnel infected, very low cure rates; need to remove catheter. Beware of silent infection in clotted hemodialysis catheters. Indium scans detect. (*Am J Kid Dis* 40:832, 2002).
Impaired host (burn, neutropenic)	As above + Pseudomonas sp., Enterobacteriaceae, Corynebacterium jeikeium, aspergillus, rhizopus	if candida, **voriconazole** or an **echinocandin** (**anidulafungin, micafungin, caspofungin**) if clinically stable. Dosage: see *Table 11B, page 125.*		Usually have associated septic thrombophlebitis: biopsy of vein to rule out fungi. If fungal, surgical excision + amphotericin B. Surgical drainage, ligation or removal often indicated.
Hyperalimentation	As with tunnel, Candida sp. common (see *Table 11,* resistant Candida species)	**Vanco** 1 gm IV q12h **Fluconazole** 400 mg IV q24h		Remove venous catheter and discontinue antimicrobial agents if possible. Ophthalmologic consultation recommended. **Rx all patients with + blood cultures.** See *Table 11A, Candidiasis, page 114*
Intravenous lipid emulsion	Staph. epidermidis, Malassezia furfur			Discontinue intralipid

Abbreviations on page 2.

NOTE: All dosage recommendations are for adults (unless otherwise indicated) and assume normal renal function. PK: compliance, local resistance, cost

TABLE 1 (63)

ANATOMIC SITE/DIAGNOSIS/ MODIFYING CIRCUMSTANCES	ETIOLOGIES (usual)	SUGGESTED REGIMENS*		ADJUNCT DIAGNOSTIC OR THERAPEUTIC MEASURES AND COMMENTS
		PRIMARY	ALTERNATIVE‡	
Prevention of Infection of Long-Term IV Lines *CID 52:1087, 2011*	To minimize risk of infection: **Hand washing and**			**IV line "lock" solutions under study. No FDA-approved product.** Reports of the combination of TMP, EDTA & ethanol (*AAC 55:4430, 2011*). Trials to begin in Europe. Another report: lock soln of sodium citrate, methylene blue, methylparabens (*CCM 39:613, 2011*). Recent meeting abstracts support 70% ethanol.
	1. Maximal sterile barrier precautions during catheter insertion			
	2. Use >0.5% chlorhexidine prep with alcohol for skin antisepsis			
	3. If infection rate high despite # 1 & 2, use either chlorhexidine/silver sulfadiazine or minocycline/rifampin-impregnated catheters or "lock" solutions (see *Comment*)			
	4. If possible, use subclavian vein, avoid femoral vessels. Lower infection risk in jugular vs. femoral vein if BMI > 28.4 (*JAMA 299:2413, 2008*)			
Mycotic aneurysm	S. aureus (28-71%), S. epidermidis, Salmonella sp. (15-24%), M.Tbc., S. pneumonia, many others	**Vanco** (dose sufficient to achieve trough level of 15-20 μg/mL) + **(Ceftriaxone** or **CIP)**. Treatment is combination of antibiotic + surgical resection with revascularization.	**Dapto** could be substituted for Vanco. For GNB: **cefepime** or **carbapenems**. For MDR-GNB, **colistin** in combination therapy	No data for ceftaroline or telavancin. Best diagnostic imaging: CT angiogram. Blood cultures positive in 50-85%. **De-escalate to specific therapy when culture results known.** Treatment duration varies but usually 6 wks from date of definitive surgery.
Suppurative (Septic) Thrombophlebitis				
Cranial dural sinus:				
Cavernous Sinus	S. aureus (70%) Streptococcus sp. Anaerobes (rare) Mucormycosis (diabetes)	**Vanco** (dose for trough conc of 15-20 mcg/mL) + **Ceftriaxone** 2 gm IV q12h], add **Metro** 500 mg IV q8h if dental/sinus source	[**Dapto** 8-12 mg/kg IV q24h OR **Linezolid** 600 mg IV q12h), add **Metro** 500 mg IV q8h if dental/sinus source	• Diagnosis: CT or MRI • Treatment: 1) obtain specimen for culture; 2) empiric antibiotics; 3) may need adjunctive surgery; 4) heparin until afebrile, then coumadin for several weeks
Lateral Sinus: Complication of otitis media/mastoiditis	Polymicrobial (often) Aerobes Anaerobes S. aureus P. aeruginosa B. fragilis Other GNB	**Cefepime** 2 gm IV q8h + **Metro** 500 mg IV q8h + **Vanco** (dose for trough conc of 15-20 mcg/mL)	**Meropenem** 1-2 gm IV q8h + **Linezolid** 500 mg IV q12h	• Diagnosis: CT or MRI • Treatment: 1) consider radical mastoidectomy; 2) obtain cultures; 3) antibiotics; 4) anticoagulation controversial • Prognosis: favorable
Superior Sagittal Sinus: Complication of bacterial meningitis or bacterial frontal sinusitis	S. pneumoniae N. meningitides H. influenzae (rare) S. aureus (very rare)	As for meningitis: **Ceftriaxone** 2 gm IV q12h + **Vanco** (dose for trough conc of 15-20 mcg/mL) + **dexamethasone**	As for meningitis: **Meropenem** 1-2 gm IV q8h + **Vanco** (dose for trough conc of 15-20 mcg/mL) + **dexamethasone**	• Diagnosis: MRI • Prognosis: bad; causes cortical vein thrombosis, hemorrhagic infarcts and brainstem herniation. Anticoagulants not recommended

Abbreviations on page 2.   *NOTE: All dosage recommendations are for adults (unless otherwise indicated) and assume normal renal function. ‡ Alternatives consider allergy, PK, compliance, local resistance, cost*

TABLE 1 (64)

ANATOMIC SITE/DIAGNOSIS/ MODIFYING CIRCUMSTANCES	ETIOLOGIES (usual)	SUGGESTED REGIMENS*		ADJUNCT DIAGNOSTIC OR THERAPEUTIC MEASURES AND COMMENTS
		PRIMARY	ALTERNATIVE†	
VASCULAR/Suppurative (Septic) Thrombophlebitis (continued)				
Jugular Vein, Lemierre's Syndrome: Complication of pharyngitis, tonsilitis, dental infection, EBV	Fusobacterium necrophorum (anaerobe) Less often: Other Fusobacterium S. pyogenes Bacteroides sp.	(**Pip-Tazo** 3.375 gm IV q6h OR **Amp-Sulb** 3 gm IV q6h) x 4 weeks	[**Imipenem** 500 mg IV q6h OR **Metro** 500 mg IV q8h + **Ceftriaxone** 2 gm IV once daily] x 4 weeks. Another option: **Clinda** 600-900 mg IV q8h	• Diagnosis: Preceding pharyngitis and antibiotics therapy, persistent fever and pulmonary emboli • Imaging: Hi-res CT scan • Role of anticoagulants unclear
Pelvic Vein: Includes ovarian vein and deep pelvic vein phlebitis	Aerobic gram-neg bacilli Streptococcus sp. Anaerobes	Antibiotics + anticoagulation (heparin, then coumadin) Low prevalence of MDR GNB: **Pip-Tazo** 3.375 gm IV q8h or 4.5 gm IV q8h OR (**Ceftriaxone** 2 gm IV once daily + **Metro** 500 mg IV q8h)	High prevalence of MDR GNB: **Meropenem** 1 gm IV q8h. If severe beta-lactam allergy: (**CIP** 400 mg IV q12h + **Metro** 500 mg IV q8h)	• Diagnosis: ovarian vein infection presents 1 week post-partum with fever & local pain; deep pelvic vein presents 3-5 days post-delivery with fever but no local pain. CT or MRI may help. • Treat until afebrile for 48 hrs & WBC normal • Coumadin for 6 weeks
Portal Vein (Pylephlebitis): Complication of diverticulitis, appendicitis and (rarely) other intra-abdominal infection	Aerobic gram-neg bacilli: E. coli, Klebsiella & Proteus most common Other: aerobic/anaerobic streptococci, B. fragilis, Clostridia	Low prevalence of MDR GNB (<20%): **Pip-Tazo** 4.5 gm IV q8h OR (**CIP** 400 mg IV q12h + **Metro** 500 mg IV q8h)	High prevalence of MDR GNB (≥20%): If ESBL producer: **Meropenem** 1 gm IV q8h. If carbapenemase producer: **Colistin** + **Meropenem** (See Table 10A for dosing)	• Diagnosis: Pain, fever, neutrophilia in pt with intra-abdominal infection. • Abdominal CT scan • Pyogenic liver abscess is a complication • No anticoagulants unless hypercoagulable disease (neoplasm) • Surgery on vein not indicated

*NOTE: All dosage recommendations are for adults (unless otherwise indicated) and assume normal renal function. § Alternatives consider allergy, PK, compliance, local resistance, cost

Abbreviations on page 2.

TABLE 2 – RECOMMENDED ANTIMICROBIAL AGENTS AGAINST SELECTED BACTERIA

BACTERIAL SPECIES	ANTIMICROBIAL AGENT (See page 2 for abbreviations)		
	RECOMMENDED	ALTERNATIVE	ALSO EFFECTIVE[1] (COMMENTS)
Achromobacter xylosoxidans spp xylosoxidans (formerly Alcaligenes)	IMP, MER, DORI (no DORI for pneumonia)	TMP-SMX. Some strains susc. to ceftaz, PIP-TZ	Resistant to aminoglycosides, most cephalosporins & FQs.
Acinetobacter calcoaceticus—baumannii complex	If suscept: IMP or MER or DORI. For MDR strains: Colistin + (IMP or MER) (no DORI for pneumonia)	AM-SB used for activity of sulbactam (CID 51:79, 2010). Perhaps Minocycline IV	Resistant to aminoglycosides, FQs. Minocycline, effective against many strains (CID 51:79, 2010) (See Table 5A, pg 78)
Actinomyces israelii	AMP or Pen G	Doxy, ceftriaxone	Clindamycin, erythro
Aeromonas hydrophila & other sp.	CIP or Levo	TMP-SMX or (P Ceph 3, 4)	See AAC 56:1110, 2012.
Arcanobacterium (C.) haemolyticum	Erythro; azithro	Benzathine Pen G, Clinda	Sensitive to most drugs, resistant to TMP-SMX (AAC 38:142, 1994)
Bacillus anthracis (anthrax): inhalation	See Table 1, page 41		
Bacillus cereus, B. subtilis	Vancomycin, clinda	FQ, IMP	
Bacteroides sp., B. fragilis & others	Metronidazole or PIP-TZ	Dori, ERTA, IMP, MER, AM-CL	Increasing resistance to: clinda, cefoxitin, cefotetan, moxi. Ref: CID 59:698, 2014.
Bartonella henselae, quintana See Table 1, pages 30, 45, 51, 57	Varies with disease entity & immune status. See Table 1: Azithro, clarithro, erythro, doxy & in combination: RIF, gent, ceftriaxone. Not active: CIP, TMP-SMX, Pen, most cephalosporins, aztreonam		
Bordetella pertussis	Azithro or clarithro	TMP-SMX	See PIDJ 31:78, 2012.
Borrelia burgdorferi, B. afzelii, B. garinii (Lyme & relapsing fever)	See specific disease entity		
Brucella sp.	Drugs & duration vary with localization or non-localization. See specific disease entities. PLoS One 7:e32090, 2012.		
Burkholderia (Pseudomonas) cepacia	TMP-SMX or MER or CIP	Minocycline or chloramphenicol	(Usually resist to aminoglycosides, polymyxins) (AAC 37: 123, 1993 & 43:213, 1999; Inf Med 18:49, 2001) (Some resist to carbapenems) May need combo rx (AJRCCM 161:1206, 2000).
Burkholderia (Pseudomonas) pseudomallei Curr Opin Infect Dis 23:554, 2010; CID 41:1105, 2005	Initially, IV ceftaz or IMP or MER, then po (TMP-SMX + Doxy x 3 mos) ± Chloro (AAC 49:4010, 2005).		(Thai, 12–80% strains resist to TMP-SMX). FQ active in vitro. MER also effective (AAC 48: 1763, 2004)
Campylobacter jejuni	Azithro	Erythro or CIP	TMP-SMX, Pen & cephalosporins not active.
Campylobacter fetus	Gentamicin	IMP or ceftriaxone	AMP, chloramphenicol
Capnocytophaga ochracea (DF-1)	Dog bite: Clinda or AM-CL	Septic shock, post-splenectomy: PIP-TZ, Clinda, IMP, DORI, MER	FQ activity variable; aminoglycosides, TMP-SMX & Polymyxins have limited activity. LN ID 9:439, 2009.
Capnocytophaga canimorsus (DF-2)	Dog bite: AM-CL		
Chlamydophila pneumoniae	Doxy	Erythro, FQ	Azithro, clarithro
Chlamydia trachomatis	Doxy or azithro	Erythro	
Citrobacter diversus (koseri), C. freundii	Life threatening illness: IMP, MER, DORI	Non-life threatening illness: CIP or Gent	Emergence of resistance: AAC 52:995, 2007.
Clostridium difficile	Mild illness: Metronidazole (po)	Moderate/severe illness: Vancomycin (po) or Fidaxomicin (CID 51:1306, 2010).	See also Table 1, page 18 re severity of disease.
Clostridium perfringens	Pen G ± clindamycin	Doxy	Erythro, chloramphenicol, cefazolin, cefoxitin, AP Pen, carbapenems
Clostridium tetani	Metronidazole or Pen G	Doxy	Role of antibiotics unclear.
Corynebacterium. diphtheriae	Erythro + antitoxin	Pen G + antitoxin	RIF reported effective (CID 27:845, 1998)
Corynebacterium jeikeium	Vancomycin + aminoglycoside	Pen G + aminoglycoside	Many strains resistant to Pen (EJCMID 25:349, 2006).
Corynebacterium minutissimum	Clinda 1% lotion	Clarithro or Erythro	Causes erythrasma
Coxiella burnetii (Q fever) acute disease (CID 52:1431, 2011).	Doxy, FQ (see Table 1, page 31)	Erythro, Azithro, Clarithro	Endocarditis: doxy + hydroxychloroquine (JID 188:1322, 2003; LnID 3:709, 2003; LnID 10:527, 2010).
chronic disease, e.g., endocarditis	Doxy + hydroxy chloroquine	TMP-SMX, Chloro	

TABLE 2 (2)   69

BACTERIAL SPECIES	ANTIMICROBIAL AGENT (See page 2 for abbreviations)		
	RECOMMENDED	ALTERNATIVE	ALSO EFFECTIVE[1] (COMMENTS)
Ehrlichia chaffeensis, Ehrlichia ewubguum Anaplasrna (Ehrlichia) phagocytophillium	Doxy	RIF (CID 27:213, 1998), Levo (AAC 47:413, 2003).	CIP, ofloxa, chloramphenicol also active in vitro. Resist to clinda, TMP-SMX, IMP, AMP, erythro, & azithro (AAC 41:76, 1997).
Eikenella corrodens	AM-CL, IV Pen G	TMP-SMX, FQ	Resistant to clinda, cephalexin, erythro, metro, diclox
Elizabethkingae meningosepticum (formerly Chryseobacterium)	Levo or TMP-SMX	CIP, Minocycline	Resistant to Pen, cephalosporins, carbapenems, aminoglycosides and vancomycin (JCM 44:1181, 2006)
Enterobacter species	Recommended agents vary with clinical setting and degree and mechanism of resistance.		
Enterococcus faecalis	Highly resistant. See Table 5A, page 78		
Enterococcus faecium	Highly resistant. See Table 5A, page 78		
Erysipelothrix rhusiopathiae	Penicillin G or amox	P Ceph 3, FQ	IMP, AP Pen (vancomycin, APAG, TMP-SMX resistant)
Escherichia coli	Highly resistant. Treatment varies with degree & mechanism of resistance, see TABLE 5B.		
Francisella tularensis (tularemia) See Table 1, page 43	Gentamicin, tobramycin, or streptomycin	Mild infection: Doxy or CIP	Chloramphenicol, RIF. Doxy/chloro bacteriostatic → relapses CID 53:e133, 2011.
Gardnerella vaginalis (bacterial vaginosis)	Metronidazole or Tinidazole	Clindamycin	See Table 1, page 26 for dosage
Helicobacter pylori	See Table 1, pg 21		Drugs effective in vitro often fail in vivo.
Haemophilus aphrophilus (Aggregatibacter aphrophilus)	[(Penicillin or AMP) + gentamicin] or [AM- SB ± gentamicin]	(Ceftriaxone + Gent) or CIP or Levo	Resistant to vancomycin, clindamycin, methicillin
Haemophilus ducreyi (chancroid)	Azithro or ceftriaxone	Erythro, CIP	Most strains resistant to tetracycline, amox, TMP-SMX
Haemophilus influenzae Meningitis, epiglottitis, & other life-threatening illness	Cefotaxime, ceftriaxone	AMP if susceptible and ß-lactamase neg, FQs	Chloramphenicol (downgrade from 1st choice due to hematotoxicity).
non-life threatening illness	AM-CL, O Ceph 2/3		Azithro, clarithro, telithro
Klebsiella ozaenae/ rhinoscleromatis	CIP		Acta Otolaryngol 131:440, 2010.
Klebsiella species	Treatment varies with degree & mechanism of resistance, see TABLE 5B.		
Lactobacillus species	Pen G or AMP	Clindamycin	**May be resistant to vancomycin**
Legionella sp.	Levo or Moxi	Azithro	Telithro active in vitro.
Leptospira interrogans	Mild: Doxy or amox	Severe: Pen G or ceftriaxone	
Leuconostoc	Pen G or AMP	Clinda	**NOTE: Resistant to vancomycin**
Listeria monocytogenes	AMP + Gent for synergy	TMP-SMX	Erythro, penicillin G (high dose), APAG may be synergistic with ß-lactams. Meropenem active in vitro. **Cephalosporin-resistant!**
Moraxella (Branhamella) catarrhalis	AM-CL or O Ceph 2/3, TMP-SMX	Azithro, clarithro, dirithromycin, telithro	Erythro, doxy, FQs
Mycoplasma pneumoniae	Doxy	Azithro	Clindamycin & ß lactams NOT effective. Increasing macrolide resistance (JAC 68:506, 2013; AAC 58:1034, 2014).
Neisseria gonorrhoeae (gonococcus)	Ceftriaxone,	Azithro (high dose)	FQs and oral cephalosporins no longer recommended: high levels of resistance.
Neisseria meningitidis (meningococcus)	Ceftriaxone	Chloro, MER	Chloro-resist strains in SE Asia (NEJM 339:868, 1998) (Prophylaxis: pg 10)
Nocardia asteroides or **Nocardia brasiliensis**	TMP-SMX + IMP	Linezolid	Amikacin + (IMP or ceftriaxone or cefotaxime)(AAC 58:795, 2014).
Pasteurella multocida	Pen G, AMP, amox, cefuroxime, cefpodoxime	Doxy, Levo, Moxi, TMP-SMX	Resistant to cephalexin, oxacillin, clindamycin, erythro, vanco.
Plesiomonas shigelloides	CIP	TMP-SMX	AM-CL, Ceftriaxone & Chloro active. Resistant to: Amp, Tetra, aminoglycosides
Propionibacterium acnes (not acne)	Penicillin, Ceftriaxone	Vanco, Dapto, Linezolid	May be resistant to Metro.
Proteus sp, **Providencia sp**, Morganella sp. (Need in vitro susceptibility)	CIP, PIP-TZ; avoid cephalosporins	May need carbapenem if critically ill	Note: Proteus sp. & Providencia sp. have intrinsic resistance to Polymyxins.
Pseudomonas aeruginosa (ID Clin No Amer 23:277, 2009). Combination therapy? See Clin Micro Rev 25:450, 2012.	No in vitro resistance: AP Pen, AP Ceph 3, Dori, IMP, MER, tobramycin, CIP, aztreonam. For serious inf., use AP ß-lactam + (tobramycin or CIP)	For UTI, if no in vitro resistance, single drugs effective: AP Pen, AP Ceph 3, cefepime, IMP, MER, aminoglycoside, CIP, aztreonam	If resistant to all beta lactams, FQs, aminoglycosides: Colistin + MER or IMP. Do not use DORI for pneumonia.

TABLE 2 (3)

BACTERIAL SPECIES	ANTIMICROBIAL AGENT (See page 2 for abbreviations)		
	RECOMMENDED	**ALTERNATIVE**	**ALSO EFFECTIVE[1] (COMMENTS)**
Rhodococcus (C. equi)	Two drugs: Azithro, Levo or RIF	(Vanco or IMP) + (Azithro, Levo or RIF)	Vancomycin active in vitro; intracellular location may impair efficacy (CID 34:1379, 2002). Avoid Pen, cephalosporins, clinda, tetra, TMP-SMX.
Rickettsia species (includes spotted fevers)	Doxy	Chloramphenicol (in pregnancy), azithro (age < 8 yrs)	*See specific infections (Table 1).*
Salmonella typhi *(CID 50:241, 2010; AAC 54:5201, 2010; BMC ID 51:37, 2005)*	If FQ & nalidixic acid susceptible: CIP	Ceftriaxone, cefixime, azithro, chloro	Concomitant steroids in severely ill. Watch for relapse (1-6%) & ileal perforation. FQ resistance reported with treatment failures (AAC 52:1278, 2008).
Serratia marcescens	If no in vitro resistance: PIP-TZ, CIP, LEVO, Gent	If in vitro resistance: Carbapenem	Avoid extended spectrum Ceph if possible.
Shigella sp.	FQ or azithro	Ceftriaxone is alternative; TMP-SMX depends on susceptibility.	
Staph. aureus, methicillin-susceptible	Oxacillin/nafcillin	P Ceph 1, vanco, teicoplanin[NUS], clinda ceftaroline	ERTA, IMP, MER, BL/BLI, FQ, Pip-Tazo, linezolid, dapto, telavancin.
Staph. aureus, methicillin-resistant (health-care associated) *IDSA Guidelines: CID 52 (Feb 1):1, 2011.*	Vancomycin	Teicoplanin[NUS], TMP-SMX (some strains resistant), linezolid, daptomycin, telavancin	Fusidic acid[NUS]. >60% CIP-resistant in U.S. (Fosfomycin + RIF). Partially vancomycin-resistant strains (GISA, VISA) & highly resistant strains now described—see Table 6, pg 79.
Staph. aureus, methicillin-resistant [community- associated (CA-MRSA)]			CA-MRSA usually not multiply-resistant. Oft resist. to erythro & variably to FQ.
Mild-moderate infection	(TMP-SMX or doxy or mino)	Clinda (if D-test neg— see Table 5A & 6).	Vanco, teico[NUS], telavancin, daptomycin, ceftaroline can be used in pts requiring hospitalization
Severe infection	Vanco or teico[NUS]	Linezolid or daptomycin	*(see Table 6, pg 79)*. Also, ceftaroline.
Staph. epidermidis	Vancomycin ± RIF	RIF + (TMP-SMX or FQ), daptomycin (AAC 51:3420, 2007)	Cephalothin or nafcillin/oxacillin if sensitive to nafcillin/oxacillin but 75% are resistant. FQs. (See Table 5A).
Staph. haemolyticus	TMP-SMX, FQ, nitrofurantoin	Oral cephalosporin	Recommendations apply to UTI only.
Staph. lugdunensis	Oxacillin/nafcillin or penicillin G (if β-lactamase neg.)	P Ceph 1 or vancomycin or teico[NUS]	Approx. 75% are penicillin-susceptible.
Staph. saprophyticus (UTI)	Oral cephalosporin or AM-CL	FQ	Almost always methicillin-susceptible
Stenotrophomonas (Xanthomonas, Pseudomonas) maltophilia	TMP-SMX	TC-CL or FQ (AAC 58:176, 2014)	Minocycline, tigecycline, CIP, Ceftriaxone, moxifloxacin, ceftaz (LnID 9:312, 2009; JAC 62:889, 2008). [In vitro synergy (TC-CL + TMP-SMX) & (TC-CL + CIP), JAC 62:889, 2008].
Streptobacillus moniliformis	Penicillin G	Doxy	Maybe erythro, clinda, ceftriaxone
Streptococcus, anaerobic (Peptostreptococcus)	Penicillin G	Clindamycin	Doxy, vancomycin, linezolid, ERTA (AAC 51:2205, 2007).
Streptococcus anginosus group	Penicillin	Vanco or Ceftriaxone	Avoid FQs; macrolide resistance emerging
Streptococcus pneumoniae penicillin-susceptible	Penicillin G, Amox	Multiple agents effective, e.g., Ceph 2/3, Clinda	If meningitis, higher dose, see Table 1, page 9.
penicillin-resistant (MIC ≥2.0)	Vancomycin, Levo, ceftriaxone, Amox (HD), Linezolid		
Streptococcus pyogenes, (Grp A), **Streptococcus sp** (Grp B, C, G). Erysipelas, bacteremia	Penicillin G + Clinda	Pen (alone) or Clinda (alone)	JCM 49:439, 2011. Pockets of macrolide resistance
Index: Streptococcus sp (Grp A, B, C, G)			
Tropheryma whipplei	Doxy + Hydroxychloroquine	None	Clinical failures with TMP-SMX
Vibrio cholerae	Doxy, FQ	Azithro, erythro	Maybe CIP or Levo; some resistance.
Vibrio parahaemolyticus	Doxy	Azithro, CIP	If bacteremic, treat as for V. vulnificus
Vibrio vulnificus, alginolyticus, damsela	Doxy + ceftriaxone	Levo	CID 52:788, 2011
Yersinia enterocolitica	CIP or ceftriaxone	TMP-SMX; CIP (if bacteremic)	CIP resistance (JAC 53:1068, 2004), also resistant to Pen, AMP, erythro.
Yersinia pestis (plague)	Streptomycin or Gent	Doxy or CIP	Also Chloro, but potentially toxic.

[1] Agents are more variable in effectiveness than "Recommended" or "Alternative". Selection of "Alternative" or "Also Effective" based on in vitro susceptibility testing, pharmacokinetics, host factors such as auditory, renal, hepatic function, & cost.

TABLE 3 – SUGGESTED DURATION OF ANTIBIOTIC THERAPY IN IMMUNOCOMPETENT PATIENTS[1,2]

CLINICAL SITUATION	DURATION OF THERAPY
SITE — CLINICAL DIAGNOSIS	**(Days)**
Bacteremia Bacteremia with removable focus (no endocarditis)	10–14 (See Table 1)
Bone Osteomyelitis, adult; acute	42
adult; chronic	Until ESR normal (often > 3 months)
child; acute; staph. and enterobacteriaceae[3]	21
child; acute; strep, meningococci, haemophilus[3]	14
Ear Otitis media with effusion	<2 yrs: 10; ≥2 yrs: 5–7
Endo-cardium Infective endocarditis, native valve	
Viridans strep	14 or 28 (See Table 1, page 28)
Enterococci	28 or 42 (See Table 1, page 28)
Staph. aureus	14 (R-sided only) or 28 (See Table 1, page 29)
GI Bacillary dysentery (shigellosis)/traveler's diarrhea	3
Also see Table 1 — Typhoid fever (S. typhi): Azithro	5 (children/adolescents)
Ceftriaxone	14 [Short course † effective (AAC 44:450, 2000)]
FQ	5–7
Chloramphenicol	14
Helicobacter pylori	10–14. For triple-drug regimens, 7 days.
Pseudomembranous enterocolitis (C. difficile)	10
Genital Non-gonococcal urethritis or mucopurulent cervicitis	7 days doxy or single dose azithro
Pelvic inflammatory disease	14
Heart Pericarditis (purulent)	28
Joint Septic arthritis (non-gonococcal) Adult	14–28
Infant/child	Rx as osteomyelitis above.
	10-14 days of therapy sufficient (CID 48:1201, 2009), but not complete agreement on this (CID 48:1211, 2009).
Gonococcal arthritis/disseminated GC infection	7 (See Table 1, page 23)
Kidney Cystitis (bladder bacteriuria)	3 (Single dose extended-release cipro also effective) (AAC 49:4137, 2005)
Pyelonephritis	14 (7 days if CIP used; 5 days if levo 750 mg)
Lung Pneumonia, pneumococcal	Until afebrile 3–5 days (minimum 5 days).
Community-acquired pneumonia	Minimum 5 days and afebrile for 2-3 days (CID 44:S55, 2007; AJM 120:783, 2007).
Pneumonia, enterobacteriaceae or pseudomonal	21, often up to 42
Pneumonia, staphylococcal	21–28
Pneumocystis pneumonia (PCP) in AIDS;	21
other immunocompromised	14
Legionella, mycoplasma, chlamydia	7–14
Lung abscess	Usually 28–42[4]
Meninges[5] N. meningitidis	7
H. influenzae	7
S. pneumoniae	10–14
Listeria meningoencephalitis, gp B strep, coliforms	21 (longer in immunocompromised)
Multiple systems Brucellosis (See Table 1, page 60)	42 (add SM or gent for 1st 7–14 days) (PLoS One 7:e32092, 2012)
Tularemia (See Table 1, pages 45, 59)	7–14 (MMWR 58:744, 2009)
Muscle Gas gangrene (clostridial)	10
Pharynx Group A strep pharyngitis	10 O Ceph 2/3, azithromycin effective at 5 days (CID 55:1279, 2012)
Also see Pharyngitis, Table 1, page 48	
Diphtheria (membranous)	7–14
Carrier	7
Prostate Chronic prostatitis (TMP-SMX)	30–90
(FQ)	28–42
Sinuses Acute sinusitis	5–14[6]
Skin Cellulitis	Until 3 days after acute inflamm disappears
Systemic Lyme disease	See Table 1, page 58
Rocky Mountain spotted fever (See Table 1, page 59)	Until afebrile 2 days

[1] Early change from IV to po regimens (about 72 hrs) is cost-effective with many infections, i.e., intra-abdominal. There is emerging evidence that dc of antibiotic rx concomitant with normalization of serum procalcitonin level shortens treatment duration for pneumonia and peritonitis (JAMA 309:717, 2013).

[2] The recommended duration is a minimum or average time and should not be construed as absolute.

[3] These times are with proviso: sx & signs resolve within 7 days and ESR is normalized.

[4] After patient afebrile 4-5 days, change to oral therapy.

[5] In children relapses seldom occur until 3 days or more after termination of rx. For meningitis in children, see Table 1, page 8.

[6] Duration of therapy dependent upon agent used and severity of infection. Longer duration (10-14 days) optimal for beta-lactams and patients with severe disease. For sinusitis of mild-moderate severity shorter courses of therapy (5-7 days) effective with "respiratory FQs" (including gemifloxacin, levofloxacin 750 mg), azithromycin. Courses as short as 3 days reported effective for TMP-SMX and azithro and one study reports effectiveness of single dose extended-release azithro. Authors feel such "super-short" courses should be restricted to patients with mild-mod disease (Otolaryngol-Head Neck Surg 134:10, 2006).

TABLE 4 – COMPARISON OF ANTIBACTERIAL SPECTRA

Editorial Note: This table is not a source for making treatment decisions. Choice of antibacterial agent must be made in consideration of local/institutional patterns of organism susceptibility and drug resistance, as well as ability of the drug to achieve effective concentrations at the site of infection. Patterns vary considerably based on geography and temporal changes in patterns are continuous. These data are intended to convey a **generalized image** of susceptibility/resistance. These data reflect in vitro susceptibilities, package insert data and/or reports in the published literature. In vitro susceptibility is not a predictor of in vivo efficacy. **Drugs active in vitro, but not used clinically are indicated as: ‡** *See specific organism, syndrome or drug for treatment recommendations.*

Organisms	Penicillins — Penicillin G	Penicillin V	Antistaph. — Methicillin	Nafcillin/Oxacillin	Cloxacillin^NUS/Diclox.	Amino-Pen. — AMP/Amox	Amox/Clav	AMP-Sulb	Anti-Pseudo. — Ticarcillin	Ticar-Clav	Pip-Tazo	Piperacillin	Carbapenems — Doripenem	Ertapenem	Imipenem	Meropenem	Aztreonam	Fluoroquinolones — Ciprofloxacin	Ofloxacin	Peflox/Pruliflox	Levofloxacin	Moxifloxacin	Gemifloxacin	Gatifloxacin
GRAM-POSITIVE:																								
Strep, Group A, B, C, G	+	+	+	+	⊣	+	+	+	+	+	+	+	+	+	+	+	o	⊣	⊣	o	+	+	⊣	+
Strep. pneumoniae	+	+	+	+	+	+	+	+	+	+	+	+	+	+	+	+	o	⊣	⊣	o	+	+	+	+
Viridans strep	⊣	⊣	⊣	⊣	⊣	⊣	⊣	⊣	⊣	⊣	⊣	⊣	⊣	⊣	⊣	⊣	o	o	o	o	⊣	⊣	⊣	⊣
Strep anginosus gp	+	+	+	+	+	+	+	+	+	+	+	+	+	+	+	+	o	o	o	o	+	+	+	+
Enterococcus faecalis	⊣	⊣	o	o	o	+	+	+	o	o	+	+	+	o	+	⊣	o	⊣	⊣	+	⊣	⊣	+	⊣
Enterococcus faecium	o	o	o	o	o	o	o	o	o	o	o	o	o	o	o	o	o	o	o	+	o	⊣	⊣	+
Enterococci, vanco-resistant	o	o	o	o	o	o	o	o	o	o	o	o	o	o	o	o	o	o	o	o	+	⊣	+	+
Staph. aureus (MSSA)	o	o	+	+	+	o	+	+	o	+	+	o	+	+	+	+	o	+	+	+	+	+	⊣	+
Staph. aureus (MRSA)	o	o	o	o	o	o	o	o	o	o	o	o	o	o	o	o	o	o	o	o	⊣	⊣	⊣	⊣
Staph. aureus (CA-MRSA)	o	o	o	o	o	o	o	o	o	o	o	o	o	o	o	o	o	+	+	+	+	+	+	+
Staph. epidermidis	o	o	o	o	o	o	o	o	o	o	o	o	+	⊣	+	+	o	o	o	o	+	+	+	+
Corynebacterium jeikeium	o	o	o	o	o	o	o	o	o	o	o	o	o	o	o	o	o	o	o	o	o	o	o	o
Listeria monocytogenes	+	+	o	o	o	+	+	+	+	+	+	+	+	⊣	+	+	o	⊣	⊣	o	⊣	+	+	+
GRAM-NEGATIVE:																								
Neisseria gonorrhoeae	o	o	o	o	o	o	+	+	+	+	+	⊣	⊣	⊣	⊣	⊣	+	⊣	⊣	⊣	⊣	⊣	⊣	⊣
Neisseria meningitidis	+	+	o	o	o	+	+	+	+	+	+	⊣	⊣	⊣	⊣	⊣	+	+	+	⊣	+	+	+	+
Moraxella catarrhalis	o	o	o	o	o	o	+	+	⊣	+	+	⊣	+	+	+	+	+	+	+	+	+	+	+	+
Haemophilus influenzae	o	o	o	o	o	⊣	+	+	⊣	+	+	⊣	+	+	+	+	+	+	+	+	+	+	+	+
Escherichia coli	o	o	o	o	o	o	+	+	+	+	+	+	+	+	+	+	+	+	+	+	+	+	+	+
Klebsiella sp.	o	o	o	o	o	o	+	+	o	+	+	o	+	+	+	+	+	+	+	+	+	+	+	+
E. coli/Klebsiella sp, ESBL+	o	o	o	o	o	o	o	o	o	o	o	o	+	+	+	+	o	o	o	o	o	o	o	o
E. coli/Klebsiella sp, KPC+	o	o	o	o	o	o	o	o	o	o	o	o	o	o	o	o	o	o	o	o	o	o	o	o
Enterobacter sp.	o	o	o	o	o	o	o	o	+	+	+	+	+	⊣	+	+	+	+	+	+	+	+	+	+

+ = **usually susceptible**; ± = **variably susceptible/resistant**; O = **usually resistant**; blank = **no data**; ⊣ = **active in vitro, but not used clinically**

* Most strains ±, can be used in UTI, not in systemic infection

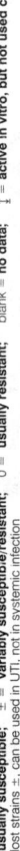

TABLE 4 (2)

Organisms	Pen V	Pen G	Methicillin	Nafcillin/Oxacillin	Cloxacillin^NUS/Diclox.	AMP/Amox	Amox/Clav	AMP-Sulb	Ticarcillin	Ticar-Clav	Pip-Tazo	Piperacillin	Doripenem	Ertapenem	Imipenem	Meropenem	Aztreonam	Ciprofloxacin	Ofloxacin	Peflox/Pruliflox	Levofloxacin	Moxifloxacin	Gemifloxacin	Gatifloxacin
Serratia sp.	0	0	0	0	0	0	0	0	0	+	+	+	+	+	+	+	+	+	+	+	+	+		+
Salmonella sp.	0	0	0	0	0	+	+	+	+	+	+	+	+	+	+	+	+	+	+	+	+	+		+
Shigella sp.	0	0	0	0	0	↕	+	+	+	+	+	+	+	+	+	+	+	+	+	+	+	+	+	+
Proteus mirabilis	0	0	0	0	0	↕	+	+	+	+	+	+	+	+	+	+	+	+	+	+	+	+		+
Proteus vulgaris	0	0	0	0	0	0	+	+	+	+	+	+	+	+	+	+	+	+	+	+	+	+		+
Providencia sp.	0	0	0	0	0	0	0	0	+	+	+	+	+	+	+	+	+	+	+	+	+	+		+
Morganella sp.	0	0	0	0	0	0	0	+	+	+	+	+	+	+	+	+	+	+	+	+	+	+		+
Citrobacter sp.	0	0	0	0	0	0	↕	+	+	+	↕	+	↕	+	↕	↕	+	↕	↕	0	↕	↕	↕	↕
Aeromonas sp.	0	0	0	0	0	0	0	+	0	0	+	0	+	0	+	+	0	+	+	+	+	+	+	0
Acinetobacter sp.	0	0	0	0	0	0	0	0	+	+	0	+	0	0	0	0	0	0	0	0	0	0		↕
Pseudomonas aeruginosa	0	0	0	0	0	0	0	0	+	+	+	+	+	0	+	+	+	+	+	+	+	+		+
Burkholderia cepacia	0	0	0	0	0	0	0	0	0	0	0	0	0	0	0	0	0	0	0		0	0		0
Stenotrophomonas maltophilia	0	0	0	0	0	0	0	0	0	0	0	0	0	0	0	0	0	0	0		↕	↕		↕
Yersinia enterocolitica	0	0	0	0	0	0	↕	↕	↕	+	↕	↕	+	+	+	↕	+	+	↕	+	+	+	↕	+
Pasteurella multocida	+	+	0	0	0	+	+	+	+	+	+	+	+	+	+	+	+	+	+	+	+	+		+
Legionella sp.																		+	+	+	+	+	+	+
Haemophilus ducreyi									0	0	↕	0	0	↕	0	0	0	0	↕		↕	↕		↕
MISC.:																								
Chlamydophila sp	0	0	0	0	0	0	0	0	0	0	0	0	0	0	0	0	0	0	↕		0	↕	0	↕
M. pneumoniae	0	0	0	0	0	0	0	0	0	0	0	0	0	0	0	0	0	0	+		+	+	+	+
ANAEROBES:																								
Actinomyces	↕	+	0	0	0	+	+	↕	0	+	+	0	+	+	+	+	0	0	↕		0	↕	0	+
Bacteroides fragilis	↕	0	0	0	0	0	+	+	0	+	+	+	+	+	+	+	0	0	0		+	↕	0	↕
Prevotella melaninogenica	0	+	0	0	0	+	+	+	+	+	+	+	↕	+	↕	↕	0	0	0		0	+		+
Clostridium difficile	↕	↕	0	0	0	0	+	↕	+	+	+	+	↕	↕	↕	↕	0	0	↕		0	+	0	0
Clostridium (not difficile)	+	↕	0	0	0	+	+	+	+	+	+	+	+	+	+	+	0	0	+		+	↕	0	+
Fusobacterium necrophorum	↕	↕	0	0	+	+	+	+	+	+	+	+	+	+	+	+	0	↕	↕		+	↕		
Peptostreptococcus sp.	+	+	+	+	+	+	+	+	+	+	+	+	+	+	+	+	0	↕	↕		+	+		+

+ = usually susceptible; ± = variably susceptible/resistant; 0 = usually resistant; blank = no data; ↕ = active in vitro, but not used clinically

TABLE 4 (3)

Organisms	1st Generation	2nd Generation			3rd/4th Generation (including anti-MRSA)						Oral Agents							
											1st Generation		2nd Generation			3rd Generation		
	Cefazolin	Cefotetan	Cefoxitin	Cefuroxime	Cefotaxime	Ceftizoxime	Ceftriaxone	Ceftaroline	Ceftazidime	Cefepime	Cefadroxil	Cephalexin	Cefaclor/Loracarbef	Cefprozil	Cefuroxime axetil	Cefixime	Ceftibuten	Cefpodox/Cefdinir/Cefditoren
GRAM-POSITIVE:																		
Strep, Group A, B, C, G	+	+	+	+	+	+	+	+	+	+	+	+	+	+	+	+	+	+
Strep. pneumoniae	+	+	+	+	+	+	+	+	+	+	+	+	+	+	+	+	+	+
Viridans strep	+	+	+	0	+	+	+	+	+	+	+	+	+	+	+	0	0	+
Enterococcus faecalis	0	0	0	0	0	0	0	±	0	0	0	0	0	0	0	0	0	0
Staph. aureus (MSSA)	+	+	+	+	+	+	+	+	+	+	+	+	+	+	+	+	+	+
Staph. aureus (MRSA)	0	0	0	0	0	0	0	+	0	0	0	0	0	0	0	0	0	0
Staph. aureus (CA-MRSA)	0	0	0	0	0	0	0	+	0	0	0	0	0	0	0	0	0	0
Staph. epidermidis	±	±	±	±	±	±	±	+	±	±	±	±	±	±	±	±	±	±
Corynebacterium jeikeium	0	0	0	0	0	0	0		0	0	0	0	0	0	0	0	0	0
Listeria monocytogenes	0	0	0	0	0	0	0		0	0	0	0	0	0	0	0	0	0
GRAM-NEGATIVE:																		
Neisseria gonorrhoeae	+	±	+	±	+	+	+	±	±	+	0	0	±	±	+	+	+	+
Neisseria meningitidis	0	±	±	+	+	+	+	+	±	+	0	0	±	±	+	+	+	+
Moraxella catarrhalis	±	+	+	+	+	+	+	+	+	+	±	±	+	+	+	+	+	+
Haemophilus influenzae	+	±	±	+	+	+	+	+	+	+	0	0	±	±	+	+	+	+
Escherichia coli	+	+	+	+	+	+	+	+	+	+	+	+	+	+	+	+	+	+
Klebsiella sp.	+	+	+	+	+	+	+	+	+	+	+	+	+	+	+	+	+	+
E. coli/Klebsiella sp. ESBL+	0	±	0	0	±	±	±	±	0	±	0	0	0	0	0	0	0	0
E. coli/Klebsiella sp. KPC+	0	0	0	0	0	0	0	0	0	0	0	0	0	0	0	0	0	0
Enterobacter sp. AmpC neg	0	0	0	±	+	+	+	+	±	+	0	0	0	0	±	+	+	+
Enterobacter sp. AmpC pos	0	0	0	0	±	±	±	±	±	+	0	0	0	0	0	±	±	±
Serratia sp.	0	0	0	0	+	+	+	+	+	+	0	0	0	0	0	+	+	+
Salmonella sp.					+	+	+	+	±	+			+	+	+	+	+	+
Shigella sp.	+				+	+	+	+	±	+			+	+	+	+	+	+
Proteus mirabilis	+	+	+	+	+	+	+	+	+	+	+	+	+	+	+	+	+	+
Proteus vulgaris	0	±	+	±	+	+	+	+	+	+	0	0	0	0	±	+	+	+
Providencia sp.	0	0	0	0	+	+	+	+	+	+	0	0	0	0	0	+	+	+
Morganella sp.	0	0	0	0	+	+	+	+	+	+	0	0	0	0	0	+	+	+
Citrobacter freundii	0	0	0	0	±	±	±	±	±	+	0	0	0	0	0	±	±	±
Citrobacter diversus	0	0	0	±	+	+	+	+	+	+	0	0	0	0	±	+	+	+
Citrobacter sp.	0	0	0	0	+	+	+	+	+	+	0	0	0	0	0	+	+	+
Aeromonas hydrophila	0	±	±	±	+	+	+	+	+	+	0	0	±	±	±	+	+	+

+ = usually susceptible;   ± = variably susceptible/resistant;   0 = usually resistant;   blank = no data;   ‡ = active in vitro, but not used clinically

TABLE 4 (4)

Organisms	CEPHALOSPORINS (including anti-MRSA)																	
	1st Gen.	2nd Generation			3rd/4th Generation (including anti-MRSA)						Oral Agents							
											1st Generation		2nd Generation			3rd Generation		
	Cefazolin	Cefotetan	Cefoxitin	Cefuroxime	Cefotaxime	Ceftizoxime	Ceftriaxone	Ceftaroline	Ceftazidime	Cefepime	Cefadroxil	Cephalexin	Cefaclor/Loracarbef	Cefprozil	Cefuroxime axetil	Cefixime	Ceftibuten	Cefpodox/Cefdinir/Cefditoren
Acinetobacter sp.	o	o	o	o	o	o	o		±	±	o	o	o	o	o	o	o	o
Pseudomonas aeruginosa	o	o	o	o	o	o	o	o	+	+	o	o	o	o	o	o	o	
Burkholderia cepacia	o	o	o	o	o	‡	o		+	‡	o	o	o	o	o	o		
Stenotrophomonas maltophilia	o	o	o	o	o	o	o		‡	o	o	o	o	o	o	o		
Yersinia enterocolitica	o	‡	o	‡	+	o	+	o	‡	+	o	o	o	o	o	+		
Legionella sp.		o	±	+	+	+	‡		‡	‡		o				+		
Pasteurella multocida	o	+		+	+	+	+		+	+	o	o	o	o	+	+		o
Haemophilus ducreyi					+	+	+		o				o	+	+	+	o	+
ANAEROBES:																		
Actinomyces	o	‡	‡	o	o	+	o	o	o	o	o		o	o	o	o	o	
Bacteroides fragilis		+	+		+	‡	o		+	o								
P. melaninogenica			+	+	o	+	o		+	o								
Clostridium difficile			o	‡	+	+	o		o	o								
Clostridium (not difficile)	o	+	+	+	+	+	‡		+	o				+	+	o		
Fusobacterium necrophorum				+		+	+							+	+	+		
Peptostreptococcus sp.		+	+	+	+	+	+		+	+		+	+	+	+	+	+	+

[1] Cefotetan is less active against B. ovatus, B. distasonis, B. thetaiotaomicron.

+ = usually susceptible; ± = variably susceptible/resistant; o = usually resistant; blank = no data; ‡ = active in vitro, but not used clinically

TABLE 4 (5)

Class	Antibiotic	Strep Group A,B,C,G	Strep. pneumoniae	Enterococcus faecalis	Enterococcus faecium	Enterococcus - vancomycin resistant	Staph. aureus (MSSA)	Staph. aureus (MRSA)	Staph. aureus (CA-MRSA)	Staph. epidermidis	C. jeikeium	L. monocytogenes	Neisseria gonorrhoeae	Neisseria meningitidis	Moraxella catarrhalis	Haemophilus influenzae	Aeromonas hydrophila	Escherichia coli	Klebsiella sp.	E. coli/Klebsiella sp. ESBL+	E. coli/Klebsiella sp. KPC+	Enterobacter sp.	Salmonella sp.
MISCELLANEOUS	Colistimethate (Colistin)	○	○	○	○	○	●	●	○	○	○		○	○				+	+	+	+		
MISCELLANEOUS	Linezolid	+	+	+	+	+	+	+	+	+	+	+		○	⊣	⊣		○	○	○	○	○	○
MISCELLANEOUS	Quinupristin-dalfopristin	+	+	○	+	↔	↔	+	+	+	+		↔	○	⊣			○	○	○	○	○	○
MISCELLANEOUS	Metronidazole	○	○	○	○	○	○	○	○	○	○		○	○	○	○	○	○	○				
MISCELLANEOUS	Rifampin	+	+	⊣	○	○	+	+	+	+	+		↔	+	⊣	+	○	○	○	⊣	○	○	
MISCELLANEOUS	Fosfomycin	+	+		○	+	+	+		○					+	⊣	+	+	+				
MISCELLANEOUS	Nitrofurantoin	+	+	+	⊣	○	+	+	+		○			+				+	⊣		○	⊣	⊣
	TMP-SMX	±[2]	+	↔[2]	○	○	○	+	+	+	⊣	○		⊣	↔	+	⊣	+	⊣	⊣	⊣	○	⊣
	Trimethoprim	+	+	⊣	○	○	⊣	⊣	+	+	○	+		○	⊣		+	⊣	⊣	○	⊣	⊣	
	Fusidic Acid[NUS]	⊣	⊣	+		○	+	+	+	+	+		+	+			○	○	○	○	○		
GLYCO-/LIPOGLYCO-/LIPO-PEPTIDES	Telavancin	+	+	+	⊣	○	+	+	+	⊣	+	+		○	○			○	○	○	○	○	
GLYCO-/LIPOGLYCO-/LIPO-PEPTIDES	Teicoplanin[NUS]	+	+	+	⊣	○	+	+	+	⊣	+	+		○	○			○	○	○	○	○	
GLYCO-/LIPOGLYCO-/LIPO-PEPTIDES	Vancomycin	+	+	+	⊣	○	+	+	+	+	+	+		○	○			○	○	○	○	○	
GLYCO-/LIPOGLYCO-/LIPO-PEPTIDES	Daptomycin	+[3]	+	+	+	+	+	+	+	+	⊣			○	○	○	○	○	○	○	○	○	
GLYCYL-CYCLINE	Tigecycline	+	+	+	+	+	+	+	+	+	+		↔		+	+	+	+	+	+	+	+	+
TETRA-CYCLINES	Minocycline	+	+	○	○	○	⊣	⊣	+	○	○	+	⊣	⊣	+	+	+	⊣	○	○		⊣	
TETRA-CYCLINES	Doxycycline	⊣	+	○	○	○	⊣	⊣	+	○	○	+	⊣	+	+	+	⊣	○	○		⊣		
KETOLIDE	Telithromycin	+	+	⊣	○	○	+	○	⊣	○	○	+		↔	↔	↔	○						
MACROLIDES	Clarithromycin	⊣	⊣	○	○	○	⊣	○	⊣	○	○	+		+	+	+	○						
MACROLIDES	Azithromycin	⊣	⊣	○	○	○	⊣	○	⊣	○	○	+		⊣	+	+	+	○					
MACROLIDES	Erythro	⊣	⊣	○	○	○	⊣	○	⊣	⊣	○	+		⊣	↔	↔	○						
	Clindamycin	+	+	○	○	○	+	○	●	⊣	○	○		○	○	○	○		○	○	○	○	
	Chloramphenicol	+	+	+	⊣	○	⊣	○	●	○	○		+	+	+	+	+	⊣	○	○	⊣		
AMINO-GLYCOSIDES	Amikacin	○	○	S	○	○	+	○	●		⊣	○	S		○	○	+	+	+	○	+		
AMINO-GLYCOSIDES	Tobramycin	○	○	S	○		+	○	●		⊣	○	S		○	○	+	+	+	○	+		
AMINO-GLYCOSIDES	Gentamicin	○	○	S	○		+	○	●		⊣	○	S		○	○	+	○	+	+	+	○	+

[2] Although active in vitro, TMP-SMX is not clinically effective for Group A strep pharyngitis or for infections due to E. faecalis.

[3] Although active in vitro, daptomycin is not clinically effective for pneumonia caused by strep pneumonia.

+ = usually susceptible; ± = variably susceptible; O = usually resistant/resistant; blank = no data; ⊣ = active in vitro, but not used clinically

Antimicrobials such as azithromycin have high tissue penetration & some such as clarithromycin are metabolized to more active compounds, hence in vivo activity may exceed in vitro activity.

** Vancomycin, metronidazole given po active vs C. difficile; IV vancomycin not effective. S = Synergistic with cell wall-active antibiotics.

TABLE 4 (6)

Organisms	Gentamicin	Tobramycin	Amikacin	Chloramphenicol	Clindamycin	Erythro	Azithromycin	Clarithromycin	Telithromycin	Doxycycline	Minocycline	Tigecycline	Daptomycin	Vancomycin	Teicoplanin[NUS]	Telavancin	Fusidic Acid[NUS]	Trimethoprim	TMP-SMX	Nitrofurantoin	Fosfomycin	Rifampin	Metronidazole	Quinupristin-dalfopristin	Linezolid	Colistimethate (Colistin)
	AMINO-GLYCOSIDES					**MACROLIDES**			**KETOLIDE**	**TETRACYCLINES**		**GLYCYLCYCLINE**	**GLYCO-/LIPOGLYCO-/LIPO-PEPTIDES**							**MISCELLANEOUS**						
Shigella sp.	+	+	+		0	0	0	0	0	±	±	+	0	0	0	0	0	±	±	+		0	0	0	0	
Serratia marcescens	+	+	+	+	0	0	0	0	0	0	0	+	0	0	0	0	0	0	±	0	+	0	0	0	0	+
Proteus vulgaris	+	+	+	0	0	0	0	0	0	0	0	±	0	0	0	0	0	0	0	0	+	0	0	0	0	0
Acinetobacter sp.	0	0	0	0	0	0	0	0	0	+	±	±	0	0	0	0	0	0	±	0	0	0	0	0	0	+
Pseudomonas aeruginosa	+	+	±	0	0	0	0	0	0	0	0	0	0	0	0	0	0	0	0	0	±	0	0	0	0	+
Burkholderia cepacia	0	0	0	+	0	0	0	0	0	±	+	±	0	0	0	0	0	+	+	0	0	S	0	0	0	0
Stenotrophomonas maltophilia	0	0	0	+	0	0	0	0	0	+	+	0	0	0	0	0	0	+	+	0	0	0	0	0	0	0
Yersinia enterocolitica	+	+	+	+	0	0	0	0	0	±	+	+	0	0	0	0	0	+	+	0	0	0	0	0	0	+
Francisella tularensis	+	+	+	+	0	0	0	0	0	±	+	±							±			S				
Brucella sp.	S	S		+	0	0	+	+	0	+	+							±	+			S				
Legionella sp.	S	S	S	+	0	±	+	+	↔	↔	↔	↔					±	↔	↔			↔		↔	↔	
Haemophilus ducreyi	±					+	+	+		↔	↔							+	+					+		±
Vibrio vulnificus	±			+		+	+			S	S	0						0	±					0		+
MISC.:																										
Chlamydophila sp.	0	0	0	+	±	+	+	+	+	+	+	+					+	↔	↔	0		↔	0		↔	
Rickettsia sp.	0	0	0	+		+	+	+	+	+	+	+					+					+				
Mycoplasma pneumoniae	0	0	0	+		±	+	+	+	+	+	+					+					+	0	±	±	
Mycobacterium avium	0	0	+			±	+	+		0	0	0					+	±	±			+				
ANAEROBES:																										
Actinomyces	0	0	0	+	±	±	+	+	+	+	+	+				+	+		0	0			0	±	±	
Bacteroides fragilis	0	0	0	+	±	+	+	+	+	H	H	+		+	+	+	+					↔	+	H	H	
Prevotella melaninogenica	0	0	0	+	+	H	+	+	+	H	H	+		+	+	+	+						+	H	↔	
Clostridium difficile	0	0	0	+	±	H	0	0		+	+	+		+	+	+	+		0	0		+	+	S	H	+
Clostridium (not difficile)[**]	0	0	0	+	H	H	+	+	+	+	+	+		+	+	+	+					+	+	H	H	H
Fusobacterium necrophorum	0	0	0	+	+	↔	+	+		+	+	+		+	+	+	+					+	+	↔	↔	+
Peptostreptococcus sp.	0	0	0	+	+	H	+	H	+	S	S	+		+	+	+	+	↔				H	H	↔	+	H

+ = usually susceptible;   ± = variably susceptible/resistant;   0 = usually resistant;   blank = no data;   ↕ = active in vitro, but not used clinically;   ↑ = active in vitro activity.
Antimicrobials such as azithromycin have high tissue penetration & some such as clarithromycin are metabolized to more active compounds, hence in vivo activity may exceed in vitro activity.
** Vancomycin, metronidazole given po active vs C. difficile; IV vancomycin not effective.   S = Synergistic with cell wall-active antibiotics.

TABLE 5A – TREATMENT OPTIONS FOR SYSTEMIC INFECTION DUE TO MULTI-DRUG RESISTANT GRAM-POSITIVE BACTERIA

ORGANISM	RESISTANT TO	PRIMARY TREATMENT OPTIONS	ALTERNATIVE TREATMENT OPTIONS	COMMENTS
Enterococcus sp.	Vancomycin, Ampicillin, Penicillin, Gentamicin	E. faecium: **Linezolid** 600 mg IV/po q12h x min 8 wks or **Quinu-dalfo** 7.5 mg/kg IV (central line) x min 8 wks. No clearly effective therapy. Can try **Daptomycin** 8-12 mg/kg IV q24h but monitor for emergence of resistance (NEJM 365:892, 2011; AAC 57:5013, 2013).	E. faecalis: (**Imipenem** 500 mg IV q6h + **Ampicillin** 2 gm IV q4h) x min 8 wks OR (**Ceftriaxone** 2 gm IV q12h + **Ampicillin** 2 gm IV q4h) x min 8 wks (CID 56:1261, 2013)	Daptomycin successful in single pts (AAC 56:6064, 2012); no activity against β-lactams and bacteriostatic with 40% relapse rate in endocarditis (AnIM 138:133, 2003). Meta-analysis: 30 day infection-related mortality higher with Dapto than Linezolid (AAC 58:734, 2014). Role of telavancin unclear.
Staphylococcus aureus (See also Table 6 for more details)	Vancomycin (VISA or VRSA) and all beta lactams (except Ceftaroline)	**Daptomycin** 6-12 mg/kg IV q24h or (**Daptomycin** 6-12 mg/kg IV q24h + **Ceftaroline** 600 mg IV q12h (AAC 56:5296, 2012).	**Telavancin** 10 mg/kg IV q24h or **Linezolid** 600 mg IV q8h	Confirm dapto susceptibility as VISA strains may be non-susceptible. If prior vanco therapy (or persistent infection on vanco) failure is significant chance of developing resistance to dapto (JAC 66:1696, 2011). Addition of an anti-staphylococcal beta-lactam (nafcillin or oxacillin) may restore susceptibility against Dapto-resistant MRSA (AAC 54:3161, 2010). Combination of Dapto + oxacillin has been successful in clearing refractory MRSA bacteremia (CID 53:158, 2011); Dapto + ceftaroline may also be effective.
Streptococcus pneumoniae	Penicillin G (MIC ≥ 4 µg/mL)	If no meningitis: **Cefotaxime** 2 gm IV once daily OR **Ceftaroline** 600 mg IV q12h OR **Linezolid** 600 mg IV/po q12h	Meningitis: **Vancomycin** 15 mg/kg IV q8h OR **Meropenem** 2 gm IV q8h	Ceftriaxone 2 gm IV q12h should also work for meningitis.

TABLE 5B: TREATMENT OPTIONS FOR SYSTEMIC INFECTION DUE TO SELECTED MULTI-DRUG RESISTANT GRAM-NEGATIVE BACILLI

The suggested treatment options in this Table are usually not FDA-approved. Suggestions are variably based on in vitro data, animal studies, and/or limited clinical experience.

ORGANISM	RESISTANT TO	PRIMARY TREATMENT OPTIONS	ALTERNATIVE TREATMENT OPTIONS	COMMENTS
Acinetobacter baumannii	All Penicillins, All Cephalosporins, Aztreonam, Carbapenems, Aminoglycosides and Fluoroquinolones	Combination therapy: **Polymyxin E (Colistin)** + (**Imipenem or Meropenem**) See Table 10A, page 104, for guidance on Colistin dosing.	**Minocycline** (IDCP 20:184, 2012) (in vitro synergy between minocycline and imipenem)	Refs: Int J Antimicrob Agts 37:244, 2011; BMC Inf Dis 11:109, 2011. Detergent effect of colistin reconstitutes antibiotic activity of carbapenems and other drugs. Do not use colistin as monotherapy. Colistin + Rifampin failed to influence infection-related mortality (CID 57:349, 2013).
Extended spectrum beta lactamase (ESBL) producing E. coli, Klebsiella pneumoniae, or other Enterobacteriaceae	All Cephalosporins, TMP-SMX, Fluoroquinolones, Aminoglycosides	**Imipenem** 500 mg IV q6h OR **Meropenem** 1 gm IV q8h OR **Doripenem** 500 mg IV q8h (CID 39:31, 2004) (Note: Dori is not FDA approved for treatment of pneumonia).	Perhaps high dose **Cefepime** 2 gm IV q12h (See Comment). **Polymyxin E (Colistin)** + (**MER or IMP**). For dosing, see Table 10A, page 104.	For UTI: Fosfomycin, nitrofurantoin (AAC 53:1278, 2009). Avoid PIP-TZ, even if susceptible in vitro (AAC 57:3402, 2013). Cefepime: outcome correlates with MIC. If MIC ≤ 1 µg/mL favorable result. If MIC 1-8 µg/mL unfavorable result (CID 56:488, 2013).
Carbapenemase producing aerobic gram-negative bacilli or P. aeruginosa	All Penicillins, Cephalosporins, Aztreonam, Carbapenems, Aminoglycosides, Fluoroquinolones	Combination therapy: **Polymyxin E (Colistin)** + (**MER or IMP**). See Table 10A, page 104, for guidance on Colistin dosing. See Comment.	Pneumonia: Inhaled **Colistin**[50a] 75 mg in 3-4 mL saline via nebulizer + **Colistin** (**MER or ERTA**) IMP	See Table 10A, page 104, for guidance on Colistin dosing. For inhalation dosing, see Table 10F. Anecdotal reports of successful dual carbapenem rx (MER + ERTA) for KPCs (JAC 69:1718, 2014).
Stenotrophomonas maltophilia	All beta-lactams except Ticar-Clav, Aminoglycosides, Fluoroquinolones	**TMP-SMX** 8-10 mg/kg/day IV divided q6h/q8h/q12h (based on TMP component)	**Ticar-Clav** 3.1 gm IV q4-6h	

TABLE 6 – SUGGESTED MANAGEMENT OF SUSPECTED OR CULTURE-POSITIVE COMMUNITY-ASSOCIATED METHICILLIN-RESISTANT S. AUREUS INFECTIONS

(See footnote[1] for doses)

IDSA Guidelines: CID 52 (Feb 1):1, 2011. With the magnitude of the clinical problem and a number of new drugs, it is likely new data will require frequent revisions of the regimens suggested. (See page 2 for abbreviations).
NOTE: Distinction between community and hospital strains of MRSA blurring.

CLINICAL ILLNESS	ABSCESS, NO IMMUNOSUPPRESSION, OUT-PATIENT CARE	PNEUMONIA	BACTEREMIA OR POSSIBLE ENDOCARDITIS OR BACTEREMIC SHOCK	TREATMENT FAILURE (See footnote[2])
Management Drug doses in footnote.	I&D alone may be sufficient, especially for boil or smaller abscess (e.g., < 5 cm). For larger abscesses, multiple lesions, systemic inflammatory response syndrome: I&D PLUS TMP-SMX 1 DS (2 DS if BMI > 40) po bid OR Clinda 300-450 mg tid (450 mg dose if BMI > 40) OR Doxy 100 mg po bid or Minocycline 100 mg po bid	Vanco IV or linezolid IV	Vanco 15-20 mg/kg IV q8-12h. Confirm adequate vanco troughs of 15-20 µg/mL. Switch to alternative regimen if vanco MIC > 2 µg/mL. Some reports of failure if vanco MIC = 2 µg/mL, but whether this is mediated by insensitivity to vancomycin per se or to other factor unclear (JID 204:340, 2011). If patient has slow response to vancomycin and isolate has MIC = 2, consider alternative therapy. Dapto 6 mg/kg IV q24h (FDA-approved dose but some authorities recommend 8-12 mg/kg for MRSA bacteremia)	Dapto 8-12 mg/kg IV q24h: confirm in vitro susceptibility as prior vanco therapy may select for daptomycin non-susceptibility (MIC >1 µg/mL) & some VISA strains are daptomycin non-susceptible. Use combination therapy for bacteremia or endocarditis: dapto + beta-lactam combination therapy (dapto 8-12 mg/kg IV q24h + (Nafcillin 2 gm IV q4h OR Oxacillin 2 gm IV q4h OR Ceftaroline 600 mg IV q8h) appears effective against MRSA strains as salvage therapy even if non-susceptible to dapto (Int J Antimicrob Agents, 42:450, 2013, AAC 54:3161, 2010; AAC 56:6192, 2013). Ceftaroline 600 mg IV q8h (J Antimicrob Chemother 67:1267, 2012; J Infect Chemother 19:42, 2013, Int J Antimicrob Agents 42:450, 2013, AAC 58:2541, 2014). Linezolid 600 mg IV/PO q12h (Linezolid is bacteriostatic and should not be used as a single agent in approved endovascular infection). Telavancin 10 mg/kg q24h IV (CID 52:31, 2011; AAC 58:2030, 2014).
Comments		Prospective study of Linezolid vs Vanco showed slightly higher cure rate with Linezolid, no difference in mortality (CID 54:621, 2012).		
	Patients not responding for complicated infection should be evaluated and switched to vancomycin.			
	Fusidic acid 500 mg tid (not available in the US) + rifampin also an option; do not use rifampin alone as resistance rapidly emerges.			

[1] Clindamycin: 300 mg po tid. Daptomycin: 6 mg/kg IV q24h is the standard, FDA-approved dose for bacteremia and endocarditis but 8-12 mg/kg q24h is recommended by some and for treatment failures. Doxycycline or minocycline: 100 mg po bid. Linezolid: 600 mg po/IV bid. Quinupristin-dalfopristin (Q-D): 7.5 mg per /kg IV q8h via central line. Rifampin: long serum half-life justifies dosing 600 mg q24h; however, frequency of nausea less with 300 mg po bid. TMP-SMX-SS: Standard (SS) is 80 mg TMP/400 mg per day. TMP-SMX-DS: Standard dose (DS) is 160 mg TMP and 800 mg SMX. The dose for treatment of CA-MRSA skin and soft tissue infections (SSTI) is 1 DS tablet twice daily. Vancomycin: 1 gm IV q12h; up to 45-60 mg/kg/day in divided doses may be required to achieve target concentrations of 15-20 mg/mL recommended for serious infections.

[2] The median duration of bacteremia in endocarditis is 7-9 days in patients treated with vancomycin (AnIM 115:674, 1991). Longer duration of bacteremia, greater likelihood of endocarditis (JID 190:1140, 2004). Definition of failure unclear. Unsatisfactory clinical response especially if blood cultures remain positive >4 days.

TABLE 7 – DRUG DESENSITIZATION METHODS

Penicillin. Oral route (Pen VK) preferred. 1/3 pts develep transient reaction, usually mild. **Perform in ICU setting. Discontinue β-blockers. Have IV line, epinephrine, ECG, spirometer available.**

Desensitization works as long as pt is receiving Pen; allergy returns after discontinuance. History of Steven-Johnson, exfoliative dermatitis, erythroderma are contraindications. Skin testing for evaluation of Pen allergy: Testing with major determinant (benzyl Pen polylysine) and minor determinants has negative predictive value (97-99%). Risk of systemic reaction to skin testing <1% (*Ann Allergy Asth Immunol 106:1, 2011*). General refs: *CID 35:26, 2002; Am J Med 121:572, 2008; Curr Clin Topics ID 13:131, 1993*.

- **Method:** Prepare dilutions using **Pen-VK** oral soln. 250 mg/5mL. Administer each dose @ 15 min intervals in 30 mL water/flavored bev. After Step 14 observe pt for 30 min, then give full therapeutic dose by route of choice. Ref: *Allergy, Prin & Prac, Mosby, 1993, pg. 1726*.

Step	Dilution (mg/mL)	mL Administered	Dose/Step mg	Dose/Step units	Cumulative Dose Given mg	Cumulative Dose Given units
1	0.5	0.1	0.05	80	0.05	80
2	0.5	0.2	0.1	160	0.15	240
3	0.5	0.4	0.2	320	0.35	560
4	0.5	0.8	0.4	640	0.75	1,200
5	0.5	1.6	0.8	1,280	1.55	2,480
6	0.5	3.2	1.6	2,560	3.15	5,040
7	0.5	6.4	3.2	5,120	6.35	10,160
8	5	1.2	6	9,600	12.35	19,760
9	5	2.4	12	19,200	24.35	38,960
10	5	4.8	24	38,400	48.35	77,360
11	50	1	50	80,000	98.35	157,360
12	50	2	100	160,000	198.35	317,360
13	50	4	200	320,000	398.35	637,360
14	50	8	400	640,000	798.35	1,277,360

Penicillin. Parenteral (Pen G) route. Follow procedures/notes under Oral (Pen-VK) route. Ref: *Allergy, Prin & Prac, Mosby, 1993, pg. 1726*.

- **Method:** Administer **Pen G** IM, IV or sc as follows:

Step	Dilution (units/mL)	mL Administered	Dose/Step (units)	Cumulative Dose Given (units)
1	100	0.2	20	20
2		0.4	40	60
3		0.8	80	140
4	1,000	0.2	200	340
5		0.4	400	740
6		0.8	800	1,540
7	10,000	0.2	2,000	3,540
8		0.4	4,000	7,540
9		0.8	8,000	15,540
10	100,000	0.2	20,000	35,540
11		0.4	40,000	75,540
12		0.8	80,000	155,540
13	1,000,000	0.2	200,000	355,540
14		0.4	400,000	755,540
15		0.8	800,000	1,555,540

Ceftriaxone. Ref: *Allergol Immunopathol (Madr) 37:105, 2009*.

- **Method:** Infuse **Ceftriaxone** IV @ 20 min intervals as follows:

Day	Dose (mg)
1	0.001, then 0.01, then 0.1, then 1
2	1, then 5, then 10, then 50
3	100, then 250, then 500
4	1000

Desensitization Methods for Other Drugs (References)

- **Imipenem-Cilastatin.** *Ann Pharmacother 37:513, 2003.*
- **Meropenem.** *Ann Pharmacother 37:1424, 2003.*
- **Metronidazole.** *Allergy Rhinol 5:1, 2014*
- **Daptomycin.** *Ann All Asthma Immun 100:87, 2008.*
- **Ceftazidime.** *Curr Opin All Clin Immunol 6(6): 476, 2006.*
- **Vancomycin.** *Intern Med 45:317, 2006.*
- General review, including desensitization protocols for Amp, CFP, CIP, Clarithro, Clinda, Dapto, Linezold, Tobra (*CID 58:1140, 2014*).

TMP-SMX. Perform in hospital/clinic. Refs: *CID 20:849, 1995; AIDS 5:311, 1991.*

- **Method:** Use **TMP-SMX** oral susp. (40 mg TMP/200 mg SMX)/5 mL. Take with 6 oz water after each dose. Corticosteroids, antihistaminics NOT used.

Hour	Dose (TMP/SMX) (mg)
0	0.004/0.02
1	0.04/0.2
2	0.4/2
3	4/20
4	40/200
5	160/800

TABLE 8 – RISK CATEGORIES OF ANTIMICROBICS IN PREGNANCY

Risk	Antibacterial	Antimycobacterial	Antifungal	Antiparasitic	Antiviral/Antiretroviral
B	Azithromycin, Aztreonam, Cephalosporins, Clindamycin, Daptomycin, Doripenem, Ertapenem, Erythromycin, Fidaxomicin, Fosfomycin, Meropenem, Metronidazole, Nitrofurantoin, Penicillins, Ortavancin, Polymyxin B, Quinu-Dalfo, Tinidazole	Rifabutin	Amphotericin B, Terbinafine	Mefloquine, Nitazoxanide, Praziquantel	**Antivirals:** Acyclovir, Famciclovir, Sofosbuvir, Telbivudine, Valacyclovir **ARVs:** Atazanavir, Didanosine, Dolutegravir, Emtricitabine, Enfuvirtide, Etravirine, Maraviroc, Nelfinavir, Nevirapine, Ritonavir, Saquinavir, Tenofovir
C	Chloramphenicol, Ciprofloxacin, Clarithromycin, Colistin, Dalbavancin, Gatifloxacin, Gemifloxacin, Imipenem, Levofloxacin, Linezolid, Moxifloxacin, Ofloxacin, Oritavancin, Polymyxin B, Rifaximin, Tedizolid, Telavancin, Telithromycin, Tedizolid, TMP-SMX, Vancomycin	Capreomycin, Dapsone, Isoniazid, Pyrazinamide, Rifampin	Anidulafungin, Caspofungin, Fluconazole (single dose), Flucytosine, Itraconazole, Ketoconazole, Micafungin, Posaconazole	Albendazole, Artemether/Lumefantrine, Atovaquone, Atovaquone/Proguanil, Chloroquine, Dapsone, Eflornithine, Ivermectin, Mebendazole, Pentamidine, Proguanil, Pyrimethamine/Sulfadoxine, Quinidine	**Antivirals:** Adefovir, Amantadine, Cidofovir, Entecavir, Foscarnet, Ganciclovir, Interferons, Oseltamivir, Rimantadine, Simeprevir, Valganciclovir, Zanamivir **ARVs:** Abacavir, Darunavir, Delavirdine, Fosamprenavir, Indinavir, Lamivudine, Lopinavir/r, Raltegravir, Stavudine, Tipranavir, Zalcitabine, Zidovudine
D	Amikacin, Gentamicin, Isepamicin, Minocycline, Netilmicin, Streptomycin, Tetracycline, Tigecycline, Tobramycin		Voriconazole, Fluconazole (other regimens)	Miltefosine	
X		Thalidomide		Quinine	Ribavirin
Other	Fusidic acid (none reported)	Clofazimine (avoid), Ethambutol (avoid), Ethionamide (do not use)			

FDA Pregnancy Categories: **A** = Adequate studies in pregnant women, no risk; **B** = Animal reproduction studies, no fetal risk; no controlled studies in pregnant women; **C** = Animal reproduction studies have shown fetal adverse effect; no controlled studies in humans; potential benefit may warrant use despite potential risk; **D** = Evidence of human fetal risk; potential benefit may warrant use despite potential risk; **X** = Animal and human studies demonstrate fetal abnormalities; risks in pregnant women clearly exceed potential benefits

TABLE 9A – SELECTED PHARMACOLOGIC FEATURES OF ANTIMICROBIAL AGENTS

For pharmacodynamics, see Table 9B; for Cytochrome P450 interactions, see Table 9C. Table terminology key at bottom of each page. Additional footnotes at end of Table 9A, page 92.

DRUG	REFERENCE DOSE (SINGLE OR MULTIPLE)	PREG RISK	FOOD REC (PO DRUGS)[1]	ORAL ABS (%)	PEAK SERUM CONC[2] (µg/mL)	PROTEIN BINDING (%)	VOLUME OF DISTRIBUTION (Vd)[3]	AVG SERUM T½ (hr)[4]	BILE PEN (%)[5]	CSF/ BLOOD[6] (%)	CSF PENETRATION[7]	AUC[8] (µg*hr/mL)	Tmax (hr)
AMINOGLYCOSIDES													
Amik, Gent, Kana, Tobra	See Table 10D	D			See Table 10D	0-10	0.26 L/kg	2.5	10-60	0-30	No		
Neomycin	po	D	Tab/soln ± food	<3	0								
BETA-LACTAMS													
Carbapenems													
Doripenem	500 mg IV	B			23 (SD)	8.1	16.8 L Vss	1	117 (0-611)	ND	ND	36.3	
Ertapenem	1 gm IV	B			154 (SD)	95	0.12 L/kg Vss	4	10	ND	ND	572.1	
Imipenem	500 mg IV	C			40 (SD)	15-25	0.27 L/kg	1	minimal	8.5	Possibly[9]	42.2	
Meropenem	1 gm IV	B			49 (SD)	2	0.29 L/kg	1	3-300	≈ 2	Possibly[9]	72.5	
Cephalosporins, IV, 1st gen													
Cefazolin	1 gm IV	B			188 (SD)	73-87	0.19 L/kg	1.9	29-300	1-4	No	236	
Cephalosporins, IV, 2nd gen													
Cefotetan	1 gm IV	B			158 (SD)	78-91	10.3 L	4.2	2-21			504	
Cefoxitin	1 gm IV	B			110 (SD)	65-79	16.1 L Vss	0.8	280	3	No		
Cefuroxime	1.5 gm IV	B			100 (SD)	33-50	0.19 L/kg Vss	1.5	35-80	17-88	Marginal	150	
Cephalosporins, IV, 3rd gen													
Cefotaxime	1 gm IV	B			100 (SD)	30-51	0.28 L/kg	1.5	15-75	10	Yes	70	
Ceftazidime	1 gm IV	B			69 (SD)	<10	0.24 L/kg Vss	1.9	13-54	20-40	Yes	127	
Ceftizoxime	1 gm IV	B			60 (SD)	30	0.34 L/kg	1.7	34-82			85	
Ceftriaxone	1 gm IV	B			150 (SD)	85-95	5.8-13.5 L	8	200-500	8-16	Yes	1006	
Cephalosporins, IV, 4th gen/anti-MRSA													
Cefepime	2 gm IV	B			164 (SD)	20	18 L Vss	2	10-20	10	Yes	284.8	
Ceftaroline	600 mg IV q12h	B			21.3 (SS)	20	20.3 L Vss	2.7		ND	ND	56.3 (12 hr)	
Ceftobiprole[NUS]	500 mg IV	B			33-34.2 (SD)	16	18 L Vss	2.9-3.3				116	
Cephalosporins, oral, 1st gen													
Cefadroxil	500 mg po	B	Cap/tab/susp ± food	90	16 (SD)	20	0.31 L/kg V/F	1.5	22			47.4	ND

Preg Risk: FDA risk categories: **A** = no risk in adequate human studies; **B** = animal studies suggest no fetal risk, but no adequate human studies, **C** = adverse fetal effects in animals, but no adequate studies in humans; potential benefit may warrant use despite potential risk, **D** = evidence of human risk, but potential benefit may warrant use despite potential risk **X** = evidence of human risk that clearly exceeds potential benefits; **Food Effect (PO dosing):** **+ food** = take with food, **no food** = take without food, **± food** = take with or without food; **Oral % AB** = % absorbed; **Peak Serum Level: SD** = after single dose, **SS** = steady state after multiple doses; **Volume of Distribution (Vd): V/F** = Vd/oral bioavailability, **Vss** = Vd at steady state; **Vss/F** = Vd at steady state/oral bioavailability; **CSF Penetration:** therapeutic efficacy comment based on dose, usual susceptibility of target organism & penetration into CSF; **AUC** = area under drug concentration curve; **24hr** = AUC 0-24; **Tmax** = time to max plasma concentration.

TABLE 9A (2) *(Footnotes at the end of table)*

DRUG	REFERENCE DOSE (SINGLE OR MULTIPLE)	PREG RISK	FOOD REC (PO DRUGS)[1]	ORAL ABS (%)	PEAK SERUM CONC[2] (µg/mL)	PROTEIN BINDING (%)	VOLUME OF DISTRIBUTION (Vd)[3]	AVG SERUM T½ (hr)[4]	BILE PEN (%)[5]	CSF/BLOOD[6] (%)	CSF PENETRATION[7]	AUC[8] (µg*hr/mL)	Tmax (hr)
BETA-LACTAMS, Cephalosporins, oral, 1st gen *(continued)*													
Cephalexin	500 mg po	B	Cap/tab/susp ± food	90	18 (SD)	5-15	0.38 L/kg V/F	1	216			29	1
Cephalosporins, oral, 2nd gen													
Cefaclor	500 mg po	B	Cap/susp ± food	93	13 (SD)	22-25	0.33 L/kg V/F	0.8				20.5	0.5-1.0
Cefaclor ER	500 mg po	B	Tab + food		8.4 (SD)	22-25		0.8	≥ 60			18.1	2.5
Cefprozil	500 mg po	B	Tab/cap/susp ± food	95	10.5 (SD)	36	0.23 L/kg Vss/F	1.5	≥ 60			25.7	1.5
Cefuroxime axetil	250 mg tab po	B	Susp + food, tab ± food	52	4.1 (SD)	50	0.66 L/kg V/F	1.5				12.9	2.5
Cephalosporins, oral, 3rd gen													
Cefdinir	300 mg po	B	Cap/susp ± food	25	1.6 (SD)	60-70	0.35 L/kg V/F	1.7				7.1	2.9
Cefditoren pivoxil	400 mg po	B	Tab + food	16	4 (SD)	88	9.3 L Vss/F	1.6				20	1.5-3.0
Cefixime	400 mg po	B	Tab/susp ± food	50	3-5 (SD)	65	0.93 L/kg V/F	3.1	800			25.8	4
Cefpodoxime proxetil	200 mg po	B	Tab + food, Susp ± food	46	2.3 (SD)	40	0.7 L/kg V/F	2.3	115			14.5	2-3
Ceftibuten	400 mg po	B	Cap/susp no food	80	15 (SD)	65	0.21 L/kg V/F	2.4				73.7	2.6
Monobactams													
Aztreonam	1 gm IV	B			90 (SD)	56	12.6 L Vss	2	115-405	3-52	ND	271	
Penicillins (natural)													
Benzathine Penicillin G	1.2 million units IM	B			0.15 (SD)								
Penicillin G	2 million units IV	B			20 (SD)	65	0.35 L/kg	0.5	500	5-10	Yes: Pen-sens S pneumo	20	
Penicillin V	500 mg po	B	Tab/soln no food	60-73	5-6 (SD)	65		0.5					
Penicillins (amino)													
Amoxicillin	500 mg po	B	Cap/tab/susp ± food	80	5.5-7.5 (SD)	17	0.36 L/kg	1.2	100-3000	13-14	Yes (IV only)	22	1-2
Amoxicillin ER	775 mg po	B	Tab + food		6.6 (SD)	20		1.2-1.5				29.8	3.1
Amox/Clav	875/125 mg po	B	Cap/tab/susp ± food	80/30-98	11.6/2.2 (SD)	18/25	0.36/0.21 (both L/kg)	1.4/1.1	100-3000			26.8/5.1	

Preg. Risk: FDA risk categories: A = no risk. **B** = No risk. **B** = No risk in animals – inadequate human studies. **C** = toxicity in animals – human studies. **D** = human risk, but benefit may outweigh risk. **X** = fetal abnormalities – risk > benefit. **Food Effect (PO dosing): + food** = take with food. **no food** = take without food. **± food** = take with or without food; **Oral % AB** = % absorbed; **Oral bioavailability. Vss/F** = Vd at steady state/oral bioavailability. **CSF Penetration:** therapeutic efficacy comment based on dose, usual susceptibility or target organism & penetration into CSF. **AUC** = area under drug concentration curve; **24hr** = AUC 0-24. **Tmax** = time to max plasma concentration. **Peak Serum Level: SD** = after single dose, **SS** = steady state after multiple doses; **Volume of Distribution (Vd): V/F** = Vd/oral bioavailability. **Vss/F** = Vd at steady state/oral bioavailability.

TABLE 9A (3) *(Footnotes at the end of table)*

DRUG	REFERENCE DOSE (SINGLE OR MULTIPLE)	PREG RISK	FOOD REC (PO DRUGS)[1]	ORAL ABS (%)	PEAK SERUM CONC[2] (µg/mL)	PROTEIN BINDING (%)	VOLUME OF DISTRIBUTION (Vd)[3]	AVG SERUM T½ (hr)[4]	BILE PEN (%)[5]	CSF/ BLOOD[6] (%)	CSF PENETRATION[7]	AUC[8] (µg*hr/mL)	Tmax (hr)
BETA-LACTAMS, Penicillins (amino) *(continued)*													
Amox/Clav ER	2 tabs [total 2000/125 mg]	B	Tab + food		17/2.1 (SD)	18/25		1.3/1.0				71.6/5.3	1.5/1.03
Ampicillin	2 gm IV	B			100 (SD)	18-22	0.29 L/kg	1.2	100-3000	13-14	Yes	120/71	
Amp/Sulb	3 gm IV	B			109-150/ 48-88 (SD)	28/38	0.29/0.3 (both L/kg)	1.2		ND	ND		
Penicillins (penicillinase-resistant)													
Cloxacillin[NUS]	500 mg po	B	Cap no food	50	7.5-14 (SD)	95	0.1 L/kg	0.5	5-8				1-1.5
Dicloxacillin	500 mg po	B	Cap no food	37	10-17 (SD)	98	0.1 L/kg	0.7					1-1.5
Nafcillin	500 mg IV	B			30 (SD)	90-94	27.1 L Vss	0.5-1	>100	9-20	Yes	18.1	
Oxacillin	500 mg IV	B	Cap no food	50	43 (SD)	90-94	0.4 L/kg	0.5-0.7	25	10-15	Yes		1-1.5
Penicillins (antipseudomonal)													
Pip/Tazo	3.375 gm IV	B			242/24 (SD)	16/48	0.24/0.4 (both L/kg)	1/1	>100	ND	ND	242/25	
Ticar/Clav	3.1 gm IV	B			330/8 (SD)	44/25	0.16/0.21 (both L/kg)	1.1/1.1	high	ND	ND	485/8.2	
FLUOROQUINOLONES[10]													
Ciprofloxacin	750 mg po q12h	C	Tab/susp ± food	70	3.6 (SS)	20-40	2.4 L/kg	4	2800-4500			31.6 (24 hr)	1-2
Ciprofloxacin	400 mg IV q12h	C			4.6 (SS)	20-40	2.4 L/kg	4	2800-4500	26	Inadequate for Strep	25.4 (24 hr)	
Ciprofloxacin	500 mg ER po q24h	C	Tab ± food		1.6 (SS)	20-40	2.4 L/kg	6.6				8 (24 hr)	1-4
Gemifloxacin	320 mg po q24h	C	Tab ± food	71	1.6 (SS)	55-73	2-12 L/kg Vss/F	7				9.9 (24 hr)	0.5-2.0
Levofloxacin	750 mg po/IV q24h	C	Tab ± food, soln no food	99	po 8.6, IV 12.1 (SS)	24-38	244 L Vss	7				po 90.7, IV 108 (24 hr)	po 1.6
Moxifloxacin	400 mg po/IV q24h	C	Tab ± food	89	4.2-4.6 (SS)	30-50	2.2 L/kg	10-14		>50	Yes *(CID 49:1080, 2009)*	po 48, IV 38 (24 hr)	po 1-3
Norfloxacin	400 mg po q12h	C	Tab no food	30-40	1.5 (400 mg SD)	10-15	1.7 L/kg	3-4	700		No	6.4 (400 mg)	1
Ofloxacin	400 mg po q12h	C	Tab ± food	98	4.6-6.2 (SS)	32	1-2.5 L/kg	7		ND		82.4 (24 hr)	1-2
Prulifloxacin[NUS]	600 mg po	C	Tab ± food	ND	1.6 (SD)	45	1231 L	10.6-12.1	ND	negligible		7.3	1

Preg Risk: FDA risk categories: A = no risk, **B** = No risk – human studies, **C** = toxicity in animals – inadequate human studies, **D** = human risk, but benefit may outweigh risk – risk > benefit; **Food Effect (PO dosing): + food** = take with food, **no food** = take without food, **± food** = take with or without food; **Oral % AB** = % absorbed; **Peak Serum Level; SD** = after single dose, **SS** = steady state after multiple doses; **Volume of Distribution (Vd): V/F** = Vd/oral bioavailability, **Vss** = Vd at steady state/oral bioavailability, **Vss/F** = Vd at steady state; **CSF Penetration:** therapeutic efficacy comment based on dose, usual susceptibility of target organism & penetration into CSF; **AUC** = area under drug concentration curve; **24hr** = AUC 0-24; **Tmax** = time to max plasma concentration.

TABLE 9A (4) (Footnotes at the end of table)

DRUG	REFERENCE DOSE (SINGLE OR MULTIPLE)	PREG RISK	FOOD REC (PO DRUGS)[1]	ORAL ABS (%)	PEAK SERUM CONC[2] (µg/mL)	PROTEIN BINDING (%)	VOLUME OF DISTRIBUTION (Vd)[3]	AVG SERUM T½ (hr)[4]	BILE PEN (%)[5]	CSF/ BLOOD[6] (%)	CSF PENETRATION[7]	AUC[8] (µg*hr/mL)	Tmax (hr)
GLYCOPEPTIDES, LIPOGLYCOPEPTIDES, LIPOPEPTIDES													
Dalbavancin	1 gm IV	C			280-300 (SD)	93-98	0.11 L/kg	147-258	ND	ND	ND	23,443	
Daptomycin	4-6 mg/kg IV q24h	B			58-99 (SS)	92	0.1 L/kg Vss	8-9	ND	0-8		494-632 (24 hr)	
Oritavancin	1200 mg IV	C			138 (SD)	85	87.6 L	245 (terminal)	ND	ND	ND	2800 (0-∞)	
Telavancin	10 mg/kg IV q24h	C			108 (SS)	90	0.13 L/kg	8.1	Low			780 (24 hr)	
Vancomycin	1 gm IV q12h	C			20-50 (SS)	<10-55	0.7 L/kg	4-6		7-14		300	
MACROLIDES, AZALIDES, LINCOSAMIDES, KETOLIDES													
Azithromycin	500 mg po	B	Tab/susp ± food	37	0.4 (SD)	7-51	31.1 L/kg	68	High			4,3	2.5
Azithromycin	500 mg IV	B			3.6 (SD)	7-51	33.3 L/kg	68	High			9.6 (24 hr, pre SS)	
Azithromycin ER	2 gm po	B	Susp no food	≈ 30	0.8 (SD)	7-51	31.1 L/kg	59	High!			20	5
Clarithromycin	500 mg po q12h	C	Tab/susp ± food	50	3-4 (SS)	65-70	4 L/kg	5-7	7000			20 (24 hr)	2.0-2.5
Clarithromycin ER	1 gm ER po q24h	C	Tab + food	≈ 50	2-3 (SS)	65-70							5-8
Clindamycin	150 mg po	B	Cap ± food	90	2.5 (SD)	85-94	1.1 L/kg	2.4	250-300		No	ND	0.75
Clindamycin	900 mg IV q8h	B			14.1 (SS)	85-94	1.1 L/kg	2.4	250-300		No	ND	
Erythromycin base, esters	500 mg po	B	Tab/susp no food, DR caps ± food	18-45	0.1-2 (SD)	70-74	0.6 L/kg	2.4		2-13	No		delay rel: 3
Erythromycin lactobionate	500 mg IV	B			3-4 (SS)	70-74	0.6 L/kg	2.4					
Telithromycin	800 mg po q24h	C	Tab ± food	57	2.3 (SS)	60-70	2.9 L/kg	10	7			12.5 (24 hr)	1
MISCELLANEOUS ANTIBACTERIALS													
Chloramphenicol	1 gm IV q6h	C	Cap ± food	High	18 (SS)	25-50	0.8 L/kg	4.1		45-89	Yes	ND	
Fosfomycin	3 gm po	B	Sachet ± food		26 (SD)	<10	136.1 L Vss/F	5.7				150	2
Fusidic acid[AUS]	500 mg po	C	Tab + food	91	30 (SD)	95-99	0.3 L/kg	5-15	100-200			315	2-4
Metronidazole	500 mg IV/po q6h	B	ER tab no food, tab/cap ± food	100	20-25 (SS)	20	0.6-0.85 L/kg	6-14	100	45-89	Yes	560 (24 hr)	ER 6,8, regular 1.6

Preg Risk: FDA risk categories: **A** = no risk, **B** = No risk in human studies, **C** = risk cannot be ruled out - human studies - inadequate human studies, **D** = human risk, but benefit may outweigh risk - risk > benefit; **Food Effect (PO dosing):** **+ food** = take with food, **no food** = take without food, **± food** = take with or without food; **Oral % AB** = % absorbed; **Peak Serum Level: SD** = after single dose, **SS** = steady state after multiple doses; **Volume of Distribution (Vd):** **V/F** = Vd/oral bioavailability; **Vss** = Vd at steady state; **Vss/F** = Vd at steady state/oral bioavailability; **CSF Penetration:** therapeutic, efficacy comment based on dose, usual susceptibility or target organism & penetration into CSF; **24hr** = AUC 0-24; **Tmax** = time to max plasma concentration.

TABLE 9A (5) *(Footnotes at the end of table)*

DRUG	REFERENCE DOSE (SINGLE OR MULTIPLE)	PREG RISK	FOOD REC (PO DRUGS)[1]	ORAL ABS (%)[2]	PEAK SERUM CONC[3] (μg/mL)	PROTEIN BINDING (%)	VOLUME OF DISTRIBUTION (Vd)[4]	AVG SERUM T½ (hr)[5]	BILE PEN (%)[6]	CSF/ BLOOD[6] (%)	CSF PENETRATION[7]	AUC[8] (μg·hr/mL)	Tmax (hr)
MISCELLANEOUS ANTIBACTERIALS *(continued)*													
Quinupristin-dalfopristin	7.5 mg/kg IV q8h	B			3.2/8 (SS)	ND	0.45/0.24 (both L/kg) Vss	1.5				21.6/31.8 (24 hr)	
Rifampin	600 mg po	C	Cap no food	70-90	4-32 (SD)	80	0.65 L/kg Vss	2-5	10,000	7-56	Yes	58	1.5-2
Rifaximin	200 mg po	C	Tab ± food	<0.4	0.004-0.01 (SD)	67.5		2-5			No	0.008	1
Trimethoprim	100 mg po	C	Tab ± food	80	1 (SD)	44	100-120 L/F	8-15				ND	1-4
TMP/SMX	160/800 mg po q12h	C	Tab/susp ± food	85	1-2/40-60 (SS)	44/70	100-120 L/ 12-18 L	11/9	100-200	50/40		ND	1-4
TMP/SMX	160/800 mg IV q8h	C			9/105 (SS)	44/70	100-120 L/ 12-18 L	11/9	40-70			ND	
OXAZOLIDINONES													
Linezolid	600 mg po/IV q12h	C	Tab/susp ± food	100	15-20 (SS)	31	40-50 L Vss	5		60-70	Yes (AAC 50.3971, 2006)	po 276, IV 179 (24 hr)	po 1.3
Tedizolid	200 mg po/IV q24h	C	Tab ± food	91	po 2.2, IV 3.0 (SS)	70-90	67-80 L Vss	12	ND	ND	ND	po 25.6, IV 29.2 (24 hr)	3
POLYMYXINS													
Colistin (polymyxin E)	150 mg IV	C			5-7.5 (SD)	≈ 50	0.34 L/kg	colistimethate 1.5-2, colistin >4	0	26	No	31.7	2
Polymyxin B	0.45-3.4 mg/kg/day IV	C			2.8 (avg conc at SS)	60	ND	4.5-6 (old data)			No	66.9 (24 hr)	
TETRACYCLINES, GLYCYLCYCLINES													
Doxycycline	100 mg po	D	Tab/cap/susp + food	100	1.5-2.1 (SD)	93	53-134 L Vss	18	200-3200	26	No	31.7	2
Minocycline	200 mg po	D	Cap/tab ± food	ND	2.0-3.5 (SD)	76	80-114 L Vss	16	200-3200		No	48.3	2.1
Tetracycline	250 mg po	D	Cap no food	ND	1.5-2.2 (SD)	ND	1.3 L/kg	6-12	200-3200	7	No	30	2-4
Tigecycline	50 mg IV q12h	D			0.63 (SS)	71-89	7-9 L/kg	42	138	5.9-10.6	No	4.7 (24 hr)	
ANTIFUNGALS (POLYENES)													
Ampho B deoxycholate	0.4-0.7 mg/kg IV q24h	B			0.5-3.5 (SS)		4 L/kg	24		0	No	17 (24 hr)	
Ampho B lipid complex (ABLC)	5 mg/kg IV q24h	B			1-2.5 (SS)		131 L/kg	173			No	14 (24 hr)	
Ampho B liposomal	5 mg/kg IV q24h	B			83 (SS)		0.1-0.4 L/kg Vss	6.8				555 (24 hr)	

Preg Risk: FDA risk categories: A = no risk. **B** = No risk. **C** = toxicity in animals - inadequate human studies. **D** = human risk, but benefit may outweigh risk - risk > benefit. **Food Effect (PO dosing): ± food** = take with or without food. **no food** = take without food. **+ food** = take with food. **Oral AB** = % absorbed. **Peak Serum Level: SD** = after single dose, **SS** = steady state after multiple doses. **Volume of Distribution (Vd): V/F** = Vd/oral bioavailability. **Vss** = Vd at steady state. **Vss/F** = Vd at steady state/oral bioavailability. **CSF Penetration:** therapeutic efficacy comment based on dose, usual susceptibility or target organism & penetration into CSF; **AUC** = area under drug concentration curve; **24hr** = AUC 0-24; **Tmax** = time to max plasma concentration.

TABLE 9A (6) (Footnotes at the end of table)

DRUG	REFERENCE DOSE (SINGLE OR MULTIPLE)	PREG RISK	FOOD REC (PO DRUGS)[1]	ORAL ABS (%)	PEAK SERUM CONC[2] (µg/mL)	PROTEIN BINDING (%)	VOLUME OF DISTRIBUTION (Vd)[3]	AVG SERUM T½ (hr)[4]	BILE PEN (%)[5]	CSF/BLOOD[6] (%)	CSF PENETRATION[7]	AUC[8] (µg·hr/mL)	Tmax (hr)
ANTIFUNGALS (ANTIMETABOLITES)													
Flucytosine	2.5 gm po	C	Cap ± food	78-90	30-40 (SD)	ND	0.6 L/kg	3-5		60-100	Yes	ND	2
ANTIFUNGALS (AZOLES)													
Fluconazole	400-800 mg po/IV	C	Tab/susp ± food	90	6.7-14 (SD)	10	50 L V/F	20-50		50-94	Yes		po: 1-2
Itraconazole	200 mg oral soln po q24h	C	Cap/tab ± food, soln no food	55+	Itra 2.0, OH-Itra 2.0 (SS)	99.8	796 L	35	ND	0		Itra 29.3, OH-Itra 45.2 (24 hr)	Itra 2.5, OH-Itra 5.3
Ketoconazole	200 mg po	C	Tab ± food	75	1-4 (SD)	99	1.2 L/kg	6-9		<10	No	12	1-2
Posaconazole	200 mg po susp	C	Susp + food		0.2-1.0 (SD)	98-99	226-295 L	20-66			Yes (JAC 56:745, 2005)	15.1	3-5
Posaconazole	300 mg tab po q24h	C	Tab + food	54	2.1-2.9 (SS)	98-99	226-295 L	20-66				37.9-51.6	3-5
Posaconazole	300 mg IV q24h	C			3.3 (SS)	98-99	226-295 Vss	20-66				36.1	1.5
Voriconazole	200 mg po q12h	D	Tab/susp no food	96	3 (SS)	58	4.6 L/kg Vss	variable		22-100	Yes (CID 37:728, 2003)	39.8 (24 hr)	1-2
ANTIFUNGALS (ECHINOCANDINS)													
Anidulafungin	100 mg IV q24h	C			7.2 (SS)	>99	30-50 L	26.5			No	112 (24 hr)	
Caspofungin	50 mg IV q24h	C			9.9 (SD)	97	9.7 L Vss	9-11			No	87.3 (24 hr)	
Micafungin	150 mg IV q24h	C			16.4 (SS)	>99	0.39 L/kg	15-17			No	167 (24 hr)	
ANTIMYCOBACTERIALS													
First line, tuberculosis													
Ethambutol	25 mg/kg po	C	Tab + food	80	2-6 (SD)	10-30	6 L/kg Vss/F	4		10-50	No	29.6	2-4
Isoniazid (INH)	300 mg po	C	Tab/syrup no food	100	3-5 (SD)	<10	0.6-1.2 L/kg	0.7-4		up to 90	Yes	20.1	1-2
Pyrazinamide	20-25 mg/kg po	C	Tab ± food	95	30-50 (SD)	5-10	9.3 L/kg Vss	10-16		100	Yes	500	2
Rifabutin	300 mg po	B	Cap ± food	20	0.2-0.6 (SD)	85	9.3 L/kg Vss	32-67	300-500	30-70	ND	8.6	2.5-4.0
Rifampin	600 mg po	C	Cap no food	70-90	4-32 (SD)	80	0.65 L/kg Vss	2-5	10,000	7-56	Yes	58	1.5-2
Rifapentine	600 mg po q72h	C	Tab ± food	ND	15 (SS)	98	70 L	13-14	ND	ND	ND	320 (72 hr)	4.8
Streptomycin	15 mg/kg IM	D			25-50 (SD)	0-10	0.26 L/kg	2.5	ND	0-30	No		

Preg Risk: FDA risk categories: **A** = no risk, **B** = No risk - human studies, **C** = toxicity in animals - inadequate human studies, **D** = human risk, but benefit may outweigh risk, **X** = fetal abnormalities - risk > benefit; **Food Effect (PO dosing): + food** = take with food, **no food** = take without food, **± food** = take with or without food; **Oral % AB** = % absorbed; oral bioavailability; **V/F** = Vd/oral bioavailability; **Vss/F** = Vd at steady state/oral bioavailability; **CSF Penetration:** therapeutic efficacy comment based on dose, usual susceptibility or target organism & penetration into CSF. **AUC** = area under drug concentration curve; **24hr** = AUC 0-24; **Tmax** = time to max plasma concentration.

Peak Serum Level: SD = after single dose; **SS** = steady state after multiple doses. **Vss** = Vd at steady state; **Vss/F** = Vd at steady state/oral bioavailability.

TABLE 9A (T) *(Footnotes at the end of table)*

DRUG	REFERENCE DOSE (SINGLE OR MULTIPLE)	PREG RISK	FOOD REC (PO DRUGS)[1]	ORAL ABS (%)	PEAK SERUM CONC[2] (µg/mL)	PROTEIN BINDING (%)	VOLUME OF DISTRIBUTION (Vd)[3]	AVG SERUM T½ (hr)[4]	BILE PEN (%)[5]	CSF/BLOOD[6] (%)	CSF PENETRATION[7]	AUC[8] (µg*hr/mL)	Tmax (hr)
Second line, tuberculosis													
Amikacin	15 mg/kg IM	D		ND	25-50 (SD)	0-10	0.26 L/kg	2.5	10-60	0-30	No	ND	
Bedaquiline	400 mg po qd	B	Tab + food	ND	3.3 (week 2)	>99	≈ 60 x total body water Vss	24-30 (terminal 4-5 mo)	ND	ND	ND	22 (24 hr) after 8 wk	5
Capreomycin	15 mg/kg IM	C		ND	25-35 (SD)	ND	ND	2-5	ND	<10	No	ND	1-2
Cycloserine	250 mg po	C	Cap no food	70-90	4-8 (SD)	<20	0.4 L/kg	10	ND	54-79	Yes	110	1-2
Ethionamide	500 mg po	C	Tab ± food	90	2.2 (SD)	10-30	0.47 L/kg	1.9	ND	≈ 100	Yes	10.3	1.5
Kanamycin	15 mg/kg IM	D		ND	25-50 (SD)	0-10	80 L	2.5	10-60	0-30	No	ND	
Para-aminosalicylic acid (PAS)	4 g po	C	Granules + food	ND	20 (SD)	50-73	0.26 L/kg	0.75-1.0	ND	10-50	Marginal	108	8
ANTIPARASITICS (ANTIMALARIALS)													
Artemether/lumefantrine	4 tabs (80 mg/480 mg)	C	Tab + food	ND	Art 0.06-0.08, DHA 0.09-0.1, Lum 7.4-9.8 (SD)	Art 95.4, DHA 47-76, Lum 99.7	ND	Art 1.6-2.2, DHA 1.6-2.2, Lum 101-119				Art 0.15-0.26, DHA 0.29, Lum 158-243	Art 1.5-2, Lum 6-8
Atovaquone	750 po bid	C	Susp + food	47	24 (SS)	99.9	0.6 L/kg Vss	67	ND	<1	No	801 (750 mg x1)	17
Mefloquine	1.25 gm po	B	Tab + food		0.5-1.2 (SD)	98	20 L/kg	13-24 days	ND				
Proguanil[11]	100 mg po	C	Tab + food		ND	75	1600-2600 L V/F	12-21	ND				
Quinine	648 mg po	C	Cap + food	76-88	3.2 (SD)	69-92	2.5-7.1 L/kg V/F	9.7-12.5	ND	2-7	No	28 (12 hr)	2.8
ANTIPARASITICS (OTHER)													
Albendazole	400 mg po	C	Tab + food	ND	0.5-1.6 (sulfoxide)	70	ND	8-12	ND	ND	ND	ND	2-5 (sulfoxide)
Dapsone	100 mg po q24h	C	Tab ± food	70-100	1.1 (SS)	70	1.5 L/kg	10-50	ND	ND	ND	ND	2-6
Ivermectin	12 mg po tid	C	Tab no food	60	0.05-0.08 (SD)	93	3-3.5 L/kg	20	ND	ND	ND	ND	4
Miltefosine	50 mg po	D	Cap + food	ND	76 (after 23 days)	95	ND	7-31 days	ND	ND	ND	486	2-8
Nitazoxanide	500 mg po	B	Tab/susp + food	ND	9-10 (SD)	99	ND	0.8-1.5	ND	ND	ND	41.9 (Tizox)	1-4 (Tizox)
Praziquantel	20 mg/kg po	B	Tab + food	80	0.2-2.0 (SD)	80	8000 L V/F	0.8-1.5	ND	ND	ND	1.51	1-3

Preg Risk: FDA risk categories: A = no risk - human studies, **B** = No risk - human studies, **C** = toxicity in animals - inadequate human studies, **D** = human risk, but benefit may outweigh risk, **X** = fetal abnormalities - risk > benefit. **Food Effect: (PO Drugs): + food** = take with food, **no food** = take without food, **± food** = take with or without food. **Oral % AB** = % absorbed; **Peak Serum Level: SD** = after single dose, **SS** = steady state after multiple doses; **Volume of Distribution (Vd): V/F** = Vd/oral bioavailability, **Vss** = Vd at steady state. **Vss/F** = Vd at steady state/oral bioavailability. **CSF Penetration:** therapeutic efficacy comment based on dose, usual susceptibility of target organism & penetration into CSF; **AUC** = area under drug concentration curve, **24hr** = AUC 0-24, **Tmax** = time to max plasma concentration.

TABLE 9A (8) *(Footnotes at the end of table)*

DRUG	REFERENCE DOSE (SINGLE OR MULTIPLE)	PREG RISK	FOOD REC (PO DRUGS)[1]	ORAL ABS (%)	PEAK SERUM CONC[2] (µg/mL)	PROTEIN BINDING (%)	VOLUME OF DISTRIBUTION (Vd)[3]	AVG SERUM T½ (hr)[4]	BILE PEN (%)[5]	CSF/BLOOD[6] (%)	CSF PENETRATION[7]	AUC[8] (µg*hr/mL)	Tmax (hr)
ANTIVIRALS (HEPATITIS B, C)													
Adefovir	10 mg po	C	Tab ± food	59	0.02 (SD)	≤4	0.37 L/kg Vss	7.5	ND	ND	ND	0.22	1.75
Dasabuvir	250 mg po q12h	?	Tab ± food	ND	0.03-3.1 (10-1200 mg SD)	ND	ND	5-8	ND	ND	ND	ND	3
Entecavir	0.5 mg po q24h	C	Tab/soln no food	100	4.2 µg/mL (SS)	13	>0.6 L/kg V/F	128-149	ND	ND	ND	0.14	0.5-1.5
Ledipasvir + Sofosbuvir	(90 mg + 400 mg) po q24h	B	Tab ± food	ND	0.3 (SS)	>99.8	ND	47	ND	ND	ND	7.3 (24hr)	4-4.5
Ombitasvir (with Paritaprevir/RTV)	25 mg po q24h	?	Tab + food	ND	0.56 (SS)	ND	ND	28-34	ND	ND	ND	0.53 (24 hr)	4-5
Paritaprevir/RTV (with Ombitasvir)	150 mg (+ RTV 100 mg) po q24h	?	Tab + food	ND	ND	ND	ND	5.8	ND	ND	ND	ND	4,3
Ribavirin	600 mg po	X	Tab/cap/soln + food	64	0.8 (SD)	minimal	2825 L V/F	44	ND	ND	ND	25,4	2
Simeprevir	150 mg po	C	Cap ± food	ND	ND	>99.9	ND	41	ND	ND	ND	57.5 (24 hr)	4-6
Sofosbuvir	400 mg po q24h	B	Tab ± food	ND	0.6 (SS)	61-65	ND	0.5-0.75	ND	ND	ND	0.9 (24 hr)	0.5-2
Telbivudine	600 mg po q24h	B	Tab/soln ± food	ND	3.7 (SS)	3,3	>0.6 L/kg V/F	40-49	ND	ND	ND	26.1 (24 hr)	2
ANTIVIRALS (HERPESVIRUS)													
Acyclovir	400 mg po bid	B	Tab/cap/susp ± food	10-20	1.21 (SS)	9-33	0.7 L/kg	2.5-3.5	ND	ND	ND	7.4 (24 hr)	1.5-2
Cidofovir (w/probenecid)	5 mg/kg IV	C	Probenecid: ± food		19.6 (SD)	<6	0.41 L/kg Vss	2.2	ND	0	No	40.8	1,1
Famciclovir	500 mg po	B	Tab ± food	77	3-4 (SD)	<20	1.1 L/kg (Penciclovir)	2-3 (Penciclovir)	ND			8.9 (Penciclovir)	0.9 (Penciclovir)
Foscarnet	60 mg/kg IV	C			155 (SD)	4	0.46 L/kg	<1	No			2195 µM*hr	
Ganciclovir	5 mg/kg IV	C			8.3 (SD)	1-2	0.7 L/kg Vss	3.5				24,5	
Valacyclovir	1 gm po	B	Tab ± food	55	5.6 (SD)	13-18	0.7 L/kg	3				19.5 (Acyclovir)	
Valganciclovir	900 mg po q24h	C	Tab/soln + food	59	5.6 (SS)	1-2	0.7 L/kg	4				29.1 (Ganciclovir)	1-3 (Ganciclovir)

Preg Risk: FDA risk categories: **A** = no risk, **B** = No risk - human studies, **C** = toxicity in animals - inadequate human studies, **D** = human risk, but benefit may outweigh risk - risk > benefit; **X** = fetal abnormalities - risk > benefit. **Food Effect (PO dosing):** **+ food** = take with food, **no food** = take without food, **± food** = take with or without food. **Oral %** = % absorbed; **Peak Serum Level, SD** = after single dose. **SS** = steady state after multiple doses; **Volume of Distribution (Vd): V/F** = Vd/oral bioavailability, **Vss** = Vd at steady state, **Vss/F** = Vd at steady state/oral bioavailability; **CSF Penetration:** therapeutic efficacy comment based on dose, usual susceptibility of target organism & penetration into CSF; **AUC** = area under drug concentration curve; **24hr** = AUC 0-24, **Tmax** = time to max plasma concentration.

TABLE 9A (9) *(Footnotes at the end of table)*

DRUG	REFERENCE DOSE (SINGLE OR MULTIPLE)	PREG RISK	FOOD REC (PO DRUGS)[1]	ORAL ABS (%)	PEAK SERUM CONC[2] (µg/mL)	PROTEIN BINDING (%)	VOLUME OF DISTRIBUTION (Vd)[3]	AVG SERUM T½ (hr)[4]	BILE PEN (%)[5]	CSF/BLOOD[6] (%)	CSF PENETRATION[7]	AUC[8] (µg*hr/mL)	Tmax (hr)
ANTIVIRALS (INFLUENZA)													
Oseltamivir	75 mg po bid	C	Cap/susp ± food	75	carboxylate 0.35 (SS)	3	carboxylate 23-26 L	carboxylate 6-10				carboxylate 5.4 (24 hr)	
Peramivir	600 mg IV				35-45 (SD)	<30	ND	7.7-20.8	ND		ND	90-95	
Rimantadine	100 mg po q12h	C	Tab ± food	75-93	0.4-0.5 (SS)	40	17-19 L/kg	25	ND	ND	ND	3.5	6

DRUG	REFERENCE DOSE (SINGLE OR MULTIPLE)	PREG RISK	FOOD REC (PO DRUGS)	ORAL ABS (%)	PEAK SERUM CONC (µg/mL)	PROTEIN BINDING (%)	VOLUME OF DISTRIBUTION (Vd)	AVG SERUM T½ (hr)	INTRACEL L T½ (HR)	CPE[12]	CSF/BLOOD (%)	AUC (µg*hr/mL)	Tmax (hr)
ANTIRETROVIRALS (NRTIs)													
Abacavir (ABC)	600 mg po q24h	C	Tab/soln ± food	83	4.3 (SS)	50	0.86 L/kg	1.5	20.6	3	36	12 (24 hr)	1.3
Didanosine enteric coated (ddI)	400 mg EC po q24h	B	Cap no food	30-40	ND	<5	308-363 L	1.6	25-40	2	ND	2.6	2
Emtricitabine (FTC)	200 mg po q24h	B	Cap/soln ± food	cap 93, soln 75	1.8 (SS)	<4	ND	10	39	3	ND	10 (24 hr)	1-2
Lamivudine (3TC)	300 mg po q24h	C	Tab/soln ± food	86	2.6 (SS)	<36	1.3 L/kg	5-7	18	2	ND	11 (300 mg x1)	ND
Stavudine (d4T)	40 mg po bid (pt ≥60 kg)	C	Cap/soln ± food	86	0.54 (SS)	<5	46 L	1.2-1.6	3.5	2	20	2.6 (24 hr)	1
Tenofovir (TDF)	300 mg po q24h	B	Tab ± food	39 w/food	0.3 (300 mg x1)	<7	1.2-1.3 L/kg Vss	17	>60	1	ND	2.3 (300 mg x1)	1
Zidovudine (ZDV)	300 mg po bid	C	Tab/cap/syrup ± food	60	1-2 (300 mg x1)	<38	1.6 L/kg	0.5-3	11	4	2	2.1 (300 mg x1)	0.5-1.5

Preg Risk: FDA risk categories: A = no risk. **B** = No risk – human studies. **C** = toxicity in animals – inadequate human studies. **D** = human risk, but benefit may outweigh risk. **X** = fetal abnormalities – risk > benefit; **Food Effect (PO dosing): + food** = take with food. **no food** = take without food. **± food** = take with or without food; **Oral % AB** = % absorbed; **Peak Serum Level: SD** = after single dose, **SS** = steady state after multiple doses; **Volume of Distribution (Vd): V/F** = Vd/oral bioavailability. **Vss** = Vd at steady state. **Vss/F** = Vd at steady state/oral bioavailability. **AUC** = area under drug concentration curve; **24hr** = AUC 0-24; **Tmax** = time to max plasma concentration. **CSF Penetration: therapeutic:** therapeutic plasma concentration. efficacy comment based on dose, usual susceptibility or target organism & penetration into CSF.

TABLE 9A (10) *(Footnotes at the end of table)*

DRUG	REFERENCE DOSE (SINGLE OR MULTIPLE)	PREG RISK	FOOD REC (PO DRUGS)	ORAL ABS (%)	PEAK SERUM CONC (µg/mL)	PROTEIN BINDING (%)	VOLUME OF DISTRIBUTION (Vd)	AVG SERUM T½ (hr)	INTRACEL L T½ (HR)	CPE12	CSF/BLOOD (%)	AUC (µg*hr/mL)	Tmax (hr)
ANTIRETROVIRALS (NNRTIs) *(cont'd)*													
Delavirdine (DLV)	400 mg po tid	C	Tab ± food	85	19 (SS)	98	ND	5.8	ND	3	ND	180 µM*hr (24 hr)	1
Efavirenz (EFV)	600 mg po q24hr	D	Cap/tab no food	42	4.1 (SS)	99	252 L V/F	40-55	ND	3	ND	184 µM*hr (24 hr)	3-5
Etravirine (ETR)	200 mg po bid	B	Tab + food	ND	0.3 (SS)	99.9	ND	41	ND	2	ND	9 (24 hr)	2.5-4.0
Nevirapine (NVP)	200 mg po bid	B	Tab/susp ± food	>90	2 (200 mg x1)	60	1.21 L/kg Vss	25-30	ND	4	63	110 (24 hr)	4
Rilpivirine (RPV)	25 mg po qd	B	Tab ± food	ND	0.1-0.2 (25 mg x1)	99.7	152 L	45-50	ND	1	ND	2.4 (24 hr)	4-5
ANTIRETROVIRALS (PIs)													
Atazanavir (ATV)	400 mg po q24hr	B	Cap/powder + food	Good	2.3 (SS)	86	88.3 L V/F	7	ND	2	ND	22.3 (24 hr)	2.5
Darunavir (DRV)	600 mg (+ RTV 100 mg) po bid	B	Tab + food	82	3.5 (SS)	95	2 L/kg	15	ND	3	ND	116.8 (24 hr)	2.5-4.0
Fosamprenavir (FPV)	700 mg (+RTV 100 mg) po bid	C	Tab ± food; susp: adult no peds +	ND	6 (SS)	90	ND	7.7	ND	3	ND	79.2 (24 hr)	2.5
Indinavir (IDV)	800 mg (+ RTV 100 mg) po bid	C	Boosted cap + food	65	9 (SS)	60	ND	1.2-2.0	ND	4	11	92.1 µM*hr (24 hr)	0.8
Lopinavir/RTV (LPV/r)	400 mg/100 mg po bid	C	Tab ± food, soln + food	ND	9.6 (SS)	98-99	ND	LPV 5-6	ND	3	ND	LPV 186 (24 hr)	LPV 4
Nelfinavir (NFV)	1250 mg po bid	B	Tab/powder + food	20-80	3-4 (SS)	98	2-7 L/kg V/F	3.5-5	ND	1	0	53 (24 hr)	ND
Ritonavir (RTV)	Boosting dose varies	B	Cap/soln + food	65	11.2 (600 mg SS)	98-99	0.41 L/kg V/F	3-5	ND	1	ND	ND	soln 2-4
Saquinavir (SQV)	1 gm (+RTV 100 mg) po bid	B	Tab/cap + food	4 (SQV alone)	0.37 (SS)	97	700 L Vss	1-2	ND	1	ND	29.2 (24 hr)	ND
Tipranavir (TPV)	500 mg (+RTV 200 mg) po bid	C	Cap/soln + food	Low	47-57 (SS)	99.9	7.7-10 L	5.5-6	ND	1	ND	1600 µM*hr (24 hr)	3

Preg Risk: FDA risk categories: A = no risk, **B** = No risk — human studies, **C** = toxicity in animals - inadequate human studies, **D** = human risk, but benefit may outweigh risk, **X** = fetal abnormalities - risk > benefit; **Food Effect (PO dosing): + food** = take with food, **no food** = take without food, **± food** = take with or without food; **Oral % AB** = % absorbed; **Peak Serum Level**: **SD** = after single dose, **SS** = steady state after multiple doses; **Volume of Distribution (Vd): V/F** = Vd/oral bioavailability, **Vss** = Vd at steady state, **Vss/F** = Vd at steady state/oral bioavailability, **CSF Penetration**: time to max plasma concentration. **SS** = steady state after multiple doses; **Volume of Distribution (Vd): V/F** = Vd/oral bioavailability, **Vss** = Vd at steady state, **Vss/F** = Vd at steady state/oral bioavailability, **CSF Penetration**: time to max plasma concentration. **24hr** = AUC 0-24; **Tmax** = time to max plasma concentration. efficacy comment based on dose, usual susceptibility or target organism & penetration into CSF, **AUC** = area under drug concentration curve; **24hr** = AUC 0-24; **Tmax** = time to max plasma concentration.

TABLE 9A (11) *(Footnotes at the end of table)*

DRUG	REFERENCE DOSE (SINGLE OR MULTIPLE)	PREG RISK	FOOD REC (PO DRUGS)	ORAL ABS (%)	PEAK SERUM CONC (µg/mL)	PROTEIN BINDING (%)	VOLUME OF DISTRIBUTION (Vd)	AVG SERUM T½ (hr)	INTRACEL LT½ (HR)	CPE[12]	CSF/BLOOD (%)	AUC (µg*hr/mL)	Tmax (hr)
ANTIRETROVIRALS (INSTIs)													
Dolutegravir (DTG)	50 mg po q24h	B	Tab ± food	ND	3.67 (SS)	>99	17.4 L V/F	14	ND	4	ND	53.6 (24 hr)	2-3
Elvitegravir (EVG) (part of Stribild)	150 mg po q24h	C	Tab + food	ND	1.7 (SS)	98-99	ND	12.9	ND	ND	ND	23 (24 hr)	4
Raltegravir (RAL)	400 mg po bid	C	Tab/susp ± food	ND	11.2 µM (SS)	83	287 L Vss/F	9	ND	3	ND	28.7 µM*hr (12 hr)	3
ANTIRETROVIRALS (FUSION/ENTRY INHIBITORS)													
Enfuvirtide (ENF, T20)	90 mg sc bid	B		84 (sc % ab)	5 (SS)	92	5.5 L Vss	3.8	ND	1	ND	97.4 (24 hr)	4-8
Maraviroc (MVC)	300 mg po bid	B	Tab ± food	33	0.3-0.9 (SS)	76	194 L	14-18	ND	3	ND	3 (24 hr)	0.5-4.0

[1] Refers to adult oral preparations unless otherwise noted.
[2] SD = after a single dose, SS = at steady state
[3] V/F = Vd/oral bioavailability, Vss/F = Vd at steady state; Vss/F = Vd at steady state/oral bioavailability
[4] Assumes CrCl >80 mL/min
[5] Peak concentration in blip/peak concentration in serum) x100. If blank, no data.
[6] CSF concentrations with inflammation
[7] Judgment based on drug dose and organism susceptibility. CSF concentration ideally ≥ 10x MIC.
[8] AUC = area under serum concentration vs. time curve; 12 hr = AUC 0-12, 24 hr = AUC 0-24
[9] Concern over seizure potential (see Table 10B)
[10] Take all oral FDs 2-4 hours before sucralfate or any multivalent cation (calcium, iron, zinc).
[11] Given with atovaquone as Malarone for malaria prophylaxis
[12] CPE (CNS Penetration Effectiveness) value: 1 = low penetration, 2-3 = intermediate penetration, 4 = highest penetration (Letendre et al., CROI 2010, abs #430)

Preg Risk: FDA risk categories: A = no risk. **B** = No risk – human studies. **C** = toxicity in animals - inadequate human studies. **D** = human risk - inadequate human studies. **X** = fetal abnormalities – risk > benefit; **Food Effect (PO dosing): + food** = take with food. **no food** = take without food. **± food** = take with or without food; **Oral % AB** = % absorbed; **Peak Serum Level; SD** = after single dose. **SS** = steady state after multiple doses; **Volume of Distribution (Vd): V/F** = Vd/oral bioavailability. **Vss** = Vd at steady state/oral bioavailability. **CSF Penetration:** therapeutic efficacy comment based on dose, usual susceptibility or target organism & penetration into CSF; **AUC** = area under drug concentration curve; **24hr** = AUC 0-24; **Tmax** = time to max plasma concentration.

TABLE 9B - PHARMACODYNAMICS OF ANTIBACTERIALS*

BACTERIAL KILLING/PERSISTENT EFFECT	DRUGS	THERAPY GOAL	PK/PD MEASUREMENT
Concentration-dependent/Prolonged persistent effect	Aminoglycosides; daptomycin; ketolides; quinolones; metro	High peak serum concentration	24-hr AUC*/MIC
Time-dependent/No persistent effect	Penicillins; cephalosporins; carbapenems; monobactams	Long duration of exposure	Time above MIC
Time-dependent/Moderate to long persistent effect	Clindamycin; erythro/azithro/clarithro; linezolid; tetracyclines; vancomycin	Enhanced amount of drug	24-hr AUC/MIC

* Adapted from Craig, WA: IDC No. Amer 17:479, 2003 & Drusano, G.L: CID 44:79, 2007

TABLE 9C- ENZYME -AND TRANSPORTER- MEDIATED INTERACTIONS OF ANTIMICROBIALS

DRUG	ISOZYME/TRANSPORTER THAT DRUG IS A SUBSTRATE OF	INHIBITED BY DRUG	INDUCED BY DRUG	IMPACT ON SERUM DRUG CONCENTRATIONS*
Antibacterials				
Azithromycin	PGP	PGP (weak)		mild ↑
Chloramphenicol		2C19, 3A4		↑
Ciprofloxacin		1A2; 3A4 (minor)		↑
Clarithromycin	3A4	3A4, PGP, OAT		↑
Erythromycin	3A4, PGP	3A4, PGP, OAT		↑
Levofloxacin		OCT		↑
Metronidazole		2C9		↑
Nafcillin			2C9 (?), 3A4	mild ↑
Norfloxacin		1A2 (weak)		↑
Oritavancin		2C9 (weak), 2C19 (weak)	2D6 (weak), 3A4 (weak)	mild ↑ or ↓
Quinupristin-Dalfopristin		3A4		
Rifampin	PGP	OAT	1A2, 2B6, 2C8, 2C9, 2C19, 2D6 (weak), 3A4, PGP	↓
Telithromycin		3A4, PGP (?)		↑
TMP/SMX	SMX: 2C9 (major), 3A4	TMP: 2C8; SMX: 2C9		↑
Trimethoprim		2C8		↑
Antifungals				
Fluconazole		2C9, 2C19, 3A4		↑
Itraconazole	3A4	3A4, PGP		↑
Ketoconazole	3A4	3A4, PGP		↑
Posaconazole	PGP	3A4, PGP		↑
Terbinafine		2D6		↑
Voriconazole	2C9, 2C19, 3A4	2C9, 2C19, 3A4		↑

TABLE 9C (2)

DRUG	Substrate	Inhibits	Induces	Impact
Antimycobacterials (Rifampin listed above)				
Bedaquiline	3A4			
Isoniazid (INH)	2E1	2C19, 3A4		
Rifabutin	3A4		3A4	↑
Rifapentine			2C9, 3A4	↑ ↓
Thalidomide	2C19			→
Antiparasitics				
Artemether/Lumefantrine	3A4 (Art, Lum)	2D6 (Lum)	3A4 (Art)	↑ or ↓
Chloroquine	2C8, 2D6	2D6		↑
Dapsone	3A4			
Halofantrine	3A4	2D6		↑
Mefloquine	3A4, PGP	PGP		↑
Praziquantel	3A4			
Proguanil	2C19 (→cycloguanil)			
Tinidazole	3A4			
Antivirals (hepatitis C)				
Boceprevir	3A4, PGP	3A4		↑
Dasabuvir	3A4, PGP, OATP1B1	2C8, UGT1A1, OATP1B1, OATP1B3		↑
Ledipasvir	PGP, BCRP	PGP, BCRP		↑
Ombitasvir	3A4, PGP	2C8, UGT1A1		↑
Paritaprevir	2C8, 2D6, 3A4, PGP	UGT1A1, OATP1B1		↑
Simeprevir	3A4, PGP, OAT	1A2 (weak), 3A4, PGP, OAT		↑
Sofosbuvir	PGP, BCRP			
Telaprevir	3A4, PGP	3A4, PGP		↑
Antiparasitics				
Artemether/Lumefantrine	3A4 (Art, Lum)	2D6 (Lum)	3A4 (Art)	↑ or ↓

TABLE 9C (3)

DRUG	Substrate	Inhibits	Induces	Impact
Antiretrovirals				
Atazanavir	3A4	1A2, 2C8, 3A4, UGT1A1		↑
Cobicistat (part of Stribild)	2D6, 3A4	2D6, 3A4, PGP, BCRP, OATP1B1, OATP1B3		↑
Darunavir	3A4	3A4		↑
Delavirdine	2D6, 3A4	2C9, 2C19, 3A4		↑
Dolutegravir	3A4, UGT1A1			↑
Efavirenz	2B6, 3A4	2B6, 2C9, 2C19	2C19, 3A4	↑ or ↓
Elvitegravir (part of Stribild)	CYP3A4, UGT1A1/3	PGP (weak)	2C9 (weak)	mild ↑ or ↓
Etravirine	2C9, 2C19, 3A4	2C9, 2C19 (weak)	3A4	↑ or ↓
Fosamprenavir	3A4	2C19, 3A4		↑
Indinavir	3A4, PGP	3A4, PGP		↑
Lopinavir	3A4	3A4		↑
Maraviroc	3A4, PGP	2D6		↑ or ↓
Nelfinavir	2C19, 3A4, PGP	3A4, PGP	3A4	↑
Nevirapine	2B6, 3A4		3A4	↓
Raltegravir	UGT			
Rilpivirine	3A4			
Ritonavir	3A4, PGP	2D6, 3A4, PGP	long term (?): 1A2, 2B6, 2C9, 3A4, PGP	↑ or ↓
Saquinavir	3A4, PGP	3A4, PGP	3A4, PGP (weak)	↑
Tipranavir	3A4, PGP	1A2, 2C9, 2C19, 2D6		↑ or ↓

*Refers to serum concentrations of companion drugs that may be affected by the listed antimicrobial. ↑=increase, ↓=decrease, blank=no drugs should be affected

TERMINOLOGY:
BCRP = breast cancer resistance protein
CYP450 nomenclature, e.g. 3A4: 3 = family, A = subfamily, 4 = gene
OAT = organic anion transporter
OATP = organic anion transporter polypeptide
OCT = organic cation transporter
PGP = P-glycoprotein
UGT = uridine diphosphate glucuronosyltransferase

REFERENCES:
Hansten PD, Horn JR. The Top 100 Drug Interactions: A Guide to Patient Management. Freeland (WA): H&H Publications, 2014; primary literature, package inserts.

TABLE 10A – ANTIBIOTIC DOSAGE* AND SIDE-EFFECTS

CLASS, AGENT, GENERIC NAME (TRADE NAME)	USUAL ADULT DOSAGE*	ADVERSE REACTIONS, COMMENTS (See Table 10B for Summary)
NATURAL PENICILLINS		**Allergic reactions a major issue.** 10% of all hospital admissions give history of pen allergy; but only 10% have allergic reaction if given penicillin. Why? Possible reasons: inaccurate history, waning immunity with age, aberrant response during a viral illness (e.g., ampicillin given during infectious mono). **Benzathine Pen** could be reaction to procaine.
Benzathine penicillin G (Bicillin L-A)	600,000–1.2 million units IM q2–4 wks	**Most serious reaction is immediate IgE IM (procaine) or IV (anaphylaxis).** Incidence anaphylaxis 0.6%, fatal 0.1–0.6%. IgE-mediated reactions: urticaria, angioedema, laryngeal edema, bronchospasm, abdominal pain with emesis, or hypotension. All appear within 4 hrs. Can form IgE antibody against either the beta-lactam ring or the R-group side chain. **Morbilliform rash after 72 hrs is not IgE-mediated and not serious.**
Penicillin G	Low: 600,000–1.2 million units IM per day High: ≥20 million units IV q24h (=12 gm) div q4h	
Penicillin V (250 & 500 mg caps)	0.25–0.5 gm po bid, tid, qid before meals & at bedtime. Pen V preferred over Pen G for oral therapy due to greater acid stability.	**Serious late allergic reactions:** Coombs-positive hemolytic anemia, neutropenia, serum sickness, interstitial nephritis, hepatitis, eosinophilia, drug fever. **Cross-allergy to cephalosporins and carbapenems** varies from 0-11%. One factor is similarity, or lack of similarity, of side chains. For pen desensitization, see Table 7. For skin testing, suggest referral to allergist. High **CSF** concentrations cause seizures. Reduce dosage with renal impairment, see Table 17A. Allergy refs: *AIM 121:572, 2008; NEJM 354:601, 2006; CID 59:1113, 2014; JAC 69:20-43, 2014.*
PENICILLINASE-RESISTANT PENICILLINS		
Dicloxacillin (Dynapen) (250 & 500 mg caps)	0.125–0.5 gm po q6h before meals	Blood levels ~2 times greater than cloxacillin so preferred for po therapy. Acute hemorrhagic cystitis reported.
Flucloxacillin x,β (Floxapen, Lutropin, Stapholi)	0.25–0.5 gm po q6h 1–2 gm IV q4h	Acute abdominal pain with GI bleeding without antibiotic-associated colitis also reported. Cholestatic hepatitis occurs in 1:15,000 exposures: more frequently in age > 55 yrs, females and therapy > 2 wks duration. Can appear wks after end of therapy and take wks to resolve (*JAC 66:1431, 2011*). **Recommendation: use only in severe disease.**
Nafcillin (Unipen, Nallil)	1–2 gm IV/IM q4h. Due to > 90% protein binding, need 12 gm/day for bacteremia.	Extravasation can result in tissue necrosis. With dosages of 200–300 mg per kg per day hypokalemia may occur. **Reversible neutropenia (WBC <1000 per mm³), occasionally WBC <1000 per mm³,** usually after 2 wks of rx.
Oxacillin (Prostaphlin)	1–2 gm IV/IM q4h. Due to > 90% protein binding, need 12 gm/day for bacteremia.	**Hepatic dysfunction with ≥12 gm per day.** LFTs usually 12-24 days after start of rx, reversible. In children, more rash and liver toxicity as compared to nafcillin (*CID 34:50, 2002*).
AMINOPENICILLINS		
Amoxicillin (Amoxil, Polymox)	250 mg–1 gm po tid	IV available in UK & Europe. IV amoxicillin rapidly converted to ampicillin. Rash with infectious mono—*see Ampicillin.*
Amoxicillin extended release (Moxatag)	One 775 mg tab po once daily	Increased risk of cross-allergenicity with oral cephalosporins with identical side-chains: cephadroxil, cefprozil. Allergic reactions, C. difficile associated diarrhea, false positive test for urine glucose with clinitest.
Amoxicillin-clavulanate (Augmentin) AM-CL Extra-strength peds suspension (ES-600) AM-CL-ER—extended release adult: tabs	See Comment for adult products Peds Extra-Strength susp: 600/42.9 per 5 mL Dose: 90/6.4 mg/kg div bid. For adult formulations, see Comments IV amox-clav available in Europe	With bid regimen, less clavulanate & less diarrhea. IV available in pts with immediate allergic reaction to AM-CL, ½ due to Clav component (*J Allergy Clin Immunol 125:502, 2010*). Positive blood tests for 1,3-beta D-glucan with IV AM-CL (*NEJM 354:2834, 2006*). Hepatotoxicity linked to clavulanic acid. AM-CL causes 13-23% of drug induced liver injury. Onset delayed. Usually mild; rare liver failure (*JAC 66:1431, 2011*). **Comparison of Augmentin dosage regimens:**
		Augmentin 500/125 1 tab po tid
		Augmentin 875/125 1 tab po bid
		Augmentin-XR 1000/62.5 2 tabs po bid
Ampicillin (Principen) (250 & 500 mg caps)	0.25–0.5 gm po q6h. 50–200 mg/kg IV/day.	A maculopapular rash occurs (not urticarial), **not true penicillin allergy,** in 65–100% pts with infectious mono, 90% with chronic lymphocytic leukemia, and 15–20% pts taking allopurinol. EBV-associated rash does not indicate permanent allergy; post-EBV no rash when challenged. Increased risk of true cross-allergenicity with oral cephalosporins with identical side chains: cefaclor, cephalexin, loracarbef.

*NOTE: all dosage recommendations are for adults (unless otherwise indicated) & assume normal renal function.
(See page 2 for abbreviations)

TABLE 10A (2)

CLASS, AGENT, GENERIC NAME (TRADE NAME)	USUAL ADULT DOSAGE*	ADVERSE REACTIONS, COMMENTS *(See Table 10B for Summary)*
AMINOPENICILLINS *(continued)*		
Ampicillin-sulbactam (Unasyn)	**1.5–3 gm IV q6h; for Acinetobacter: 3 gm (Amp 2 gm/Sulb 1 gm) IV q4h**	Supplied in vials: ampicillin 1 gm, sulbactam 0.5 gm or amp 2 gm, sulbactam 1 gm. AM-SB is not active vs pseudomonas. Total daily dose sulbactam ≤4 gm. Increasing resistance of aerobic gram-negative bacilli. Subactam doses up to 9–12 gm/day evaluated *(J Infect 56:432, 2008)*. See also *CID 50:133, 2010.*
EXTENDED SPECTRUM PENICILLINS. NOTE: Platelet dysfunction may occur with any of the antipseudomonal penicillins, esp. in renal failure.		
Piperacillin (Hard to find PIP alone; usually PIP-TZ)	**3–4 gm IV q4–6h (max 24 gm/day). For urinary tract infection: 2 gm IV q6h.** See Comment	1.85 mEq Na+ per gm. See PIP-TZ comment on extended infusion. For P. aeruginosa infections: 3 gm IV q4h. Associated with bleeding due to impaired platelet aggregation *(JID 155:1242, 1987; J Lab Clin Med 108:217, 1986)*.
ANTIPSEUDOMONAL PENICILLINS		
Piperacillin-tazobactam (PIP-TZ) (Zosyn). Prolonged infusion dosing, see Comment and Table 10E. Obesity dosing, see Table 17C.	**Formulations:** PIP-TZ: 2/0.25 gm (2.25 gm) PIP-TZ: 3/0.375 gm (3.375 gm) PIP-TZ: 4/0.5 gm (4.5 gm) **Standard Dose (no P. aeruginosa): 3.375 gm IV q6h or 4.5 gm IV q8h Standard Dose for P. aeruginosa: 3.375 gm IV q4h or 4.5 gm IV q6h**	Based on PK/PD studies, there is emerging evidence in support of **prolonged infusion** of PIP-TZ: initial "loading" dose of 4.5 gm over 30 min, then, 4 hrs later, start 3.375 gm IV over 4 hrs q 8h (CrCl> 20) or 3.375 gm IV over 4 hrs q12h (CrCl<20) *(CID 44:357, 2007; AAC 54:460, 2010).* • P. aeruginosa pneumonia: PIP-TZ or CIP or Tobra. If dosed correctly, no need for dual therapy. Misc: Assoc. false-pos galactomannan test for aspergillus, thrombocytopenia *(PLoS One 8(11):e81477).* In critically ill pts, may contribute to thrombocytopenia *(PLoS One 8(11):e81477)*, page 213.
Temocillin[NUS]	**2 gm IV q12h.**	Semi-synthetic penicillin stable in presence of classical & ESBLs plus AmpC beta-lactamases. Source: www.eumedica.be
Ticarcillin disodium (Ticar)	**3 gm IV q4–6h.**	Coagulation abnormalities common with large doses, interferes with platelet function, ↑ bleeding times; may be clinically significant in pts with renal failure. (4.5 mEq Na+ per gm)
Ticarcillin-clavulanate (Timentin)	**3.1 gm IV q4–6h.**	Supplied in vials: ticarcillin 3 gm, clavulanate 0.1 gm per vial. 4.5–5 mEq/L Na+ per gm. Diarrhea due to clavulanate. Rare reversible cholestatic hepatitis secondary to clavulanate. (4.5 mEq Na+ per gm) Stenotrophomonas maltophilia.
CARBAPENEMS. Review: AAC 55:4943, 2011. **NOTE: Cross allergenicity: In studies of pts with history of Pen-allergy but no confirmatory skin testing, 0–11% had allergic reactions with cephalosporin therapy** *(JAC 54:1155, 2004).* **In better studies, pts with positive skin tests for Pen allergy were given Carbapenem: no reaction in 99%** *(J Allergy Clin Immunol 124:167, 2009).* Of 112 pts with IgE-mediated reaction to ceph; 2 suffered rash & 1 an IgE reaction when given a carbapenem *(CID 59:1113, 2014).*		
Doripenem (Doribax) Ref: CID 49:291, 2009. For prolonged infusion dosing, see Table 10E	**500 mg IV q8h (1-hr infusion).** For prolonged infusion see Table 11. Do not use for pneumonia	Most common adverse reactions (≥5%): Headache, nausea, diarrhea, rash & phlebitis. Seizure reported in post-marketing surveillance. Can lower serum valproic acid levels. Adjust dose if renal impairment. Somewhat more stable in solution than IMP or MER *(JAC 65:1023, 2010; CID 49:291, 2009).* FDA safety announcement (01/05/12): Trial of Dori for the treatment of VAP stopped early due to safety concerns. Compared to IMP, patients treated with Dori were observed to have excess mortality and poorer cure rate. **NOTE: Dori is not approved to treat any type of pneumonia.**
Ertapenem (Invanz)	**1 gm IV/IM q24h.**	**Dori is not approved for doses greater than 500 mg q8h. Lidocaine** diluent for IM use; ask about lidocaine allergy. Standard dosage may be inadequate in obesity (BMI ≥40). Reports of DRESS (drug rash eosinophilia systemic symptoms) Syndrome. Visual hallucinations reported *(NZ Med J 122:76, 2009).* No predictable activity vs. P. aeruginosa
Imipenem + cilastatin (Primaxin) Ref: JAC 58:916, 2006	**0.5 gm IV q6h; for P. aeruginosa: 1 gm q6h (see Comment).**	For infection due to P. aeruginosa, increase dosage to 3 or 4 gm per day div. q6h or q8h. Continuous infusion of carbapenems may be more efficacious & safer *(AAC 49:1881, 2005).* **Seizures:** In meta-analysis, risk of seizure low but greatest with carbapenems among beta-lactams. No diff between IMP and MER *(JAC 69:2043, 2014).* Cilastatin blocks enzymatic degradation of Imipenem in lumen of renal proximal tubule & also prevents tubular toxicity.

(See page 2 for abbreviations)

*NOTE: all dosage recommendations are for adults (unless otherwise indicated) & assume normal renal function.

TABLE 10A (3)

CLASS, AGENT, GENERIC NAME (TRADE NAME)	USUAL ADULT DOSAGE*	ADVERSE REACTIONS, COMMENTS (See Table 10B for Summary)
CARBAPENEMS (continued)		
Meropenem (Merrem)	**0.5–1 gm IV q8h. Up to 2 gm IV q8h for meningitis. Prolonged infusion** in critically ill: If CrCl ≥ 50: 2 gm (over 3 hr) q8h If CrCl 30-49: 1 gm (over 3 hr) q8h If CrCl 10-29: 1 gm (over 3 hr) q12h (Inten Care Med 37:632, 2011)	**Seizures:** In meta-analysis, risk of seizure low but greatest with carbapenems among beta-lactams. No diff between IMP and MER (JAC 69:2043, 2014). Comments: Does not require a dehydropeptidase inhibitor (cilastatin). Activity vs aerobic gm-neg. slightly ↑ over IMP, activity vs staph & strep slightly ↓; anaerobes: B. ovatus, B. distasonis more resistant to meropenem.
MONOBACTAMS		
Aztreonam (Azactam)	1 gm q8h–2 gm q6h.	Can be used in pts with allergy to penicillins/cephalosporins. Animal data and a letter raise concern about cross-reactivity with ceftazidime as **side-chains of aztreonam and ceftazidime are identical.** AEs:
Aztreonam for inhalation (Cayston)	75 mg inhaled tid x 28 days. Use bronchodilator before each inhalation.	Improves respiratory symptoms in CF pts colonized with P. aeruginosa. Alternative to inhaled Tobra. AEs: bronchospasm, cough, wheezing. So far, no emergence of other resistant pathogens. Ref: Chest 135:1223, 2009.
CEPHALOSPORINS (1st parenteral, then oral drugs). NOTE: Prospective data demonstrate correlation between use of cephalosporins (esp. 3rd generation) and ↑ risk of C. difficile toxin-induced diarrhea. Drug may also ↑ risk of colonization with vancomycin-resistant enterococci. See Oral Cephalosporins, page 99, **for important note on cross-allergenicity.**		
1st Generation, Parenteral		
Cefazolin (Ancef, Kefzol)	1-1.5 gm IV/IM q8h, occasionally 2 gm IV q8h for serious infections, e.g., MSSA bacteremia (max. 12 gm/day)	Do not give into lateral ventricles—seizures! No activity vs. MRSA.
2nd Generation, Parenteral (Cephamycins): May be active in vitro vs. ESBL-producing aerobic gram-negative bacilli. Do not use as there are no clinical data for efficacy.		
Cefotetan (Cefotan)	1–3 gm IV/IM q12h. (max. dose not > 6 gm q24h).	Increasing resistance of B. fragilis, Prevotella bivia, Prevotella disiens (most common in pelvic infections); do not use for intra-abdominal infections. Methyltetrazole (MTT) side chain can inhibit vitamin K activation. Avoid alcohol-disulfiram reaction.
Cefoxitin (Mefoxin)	1 gm q6h–2 gm IV/IM q6-8h.	Increasing resistance of B. fragilis isolates.
Cefuroxime (Keturox, Ceftin, Zinacef)	0.75–1.5 gm IV/IM q8h.	Improved activity against H. influenzae compared with 1st generation cephalosporins. See Cefuroxime axetil for oral preparation.
3rd Generation, Parenteral—Use correlates with ↑ incidence of C. difficile toxin diarrhea, all are inactivated by ESBLs and amp C cephalosporinase from aerobic gram-negative bacilli.		
Cefoperazone-sulbactam[NUS] (Sulperazon)	Usual dose (Cefoperazone comp) 1-2 gm IV q12h; if larger doses, do not exceed 4 gm/day of sulbactam.	In SE Asia & China-assoc. diarrhea and/or selection of vancomycin-resistant E. faecium. Other uses due to broad spectrum of activity. Possible clotting problem due to side-chain.
Cefotaxime (Claforan)	1 gm q8-12h to 2 gm q4h.	Maximum daily dose: 12 gm; give as 4 gm IV q8h. Similar to ceftriaxone but, unlike ceftriaxone, but, requires multiple daily doses.
Ceftazidime (Fortaz, Tazicef)	**Usual dose: 1–2 gm IV/IM q8-12h. Prolonged infusion: total daily dose divided q8h:** initial dose: 15 mg/kg over 30 min, then immediately begin: If CrCl > 50: 6 gm (over 24 hr) daily If CrCl 31-50: 4 gm (over 24 hr) daily If CrCl 16-30: 2 gm (over 24 hr) daily If CrCl 10-30: 2 gm (over 24 hr) daily (AAC 59:5639, 2015, CID 56:272, 2013; Drugs 37:418, 2009)	Often used in healthcare-associated infections, where P. aeruginosa is a consideration. Use may result in ↑ incidence of C. difficile-assoc. diarrhea and/or selection of vancomycin-resistant E. faecium. Risk of cross-allergenicity with aztreonam (same side chain).
Ceftizoxime (Cefizox)	From **1-2 gm IV q8-12h** up to **2 gm IV q4h.** Commonly used IV dosage in adults: 1-2 gm IV q8-12h.	Maximum daily dose: 12 gm. Can give as 4 gm IV q8h.
Ceftriaxone (Rocephin)	P-2 gm once daily For serious meningitis: **2 gm q12h.** Can give IM in 1% lidocaine.	**"Pseudocholelithiasis"** ↓ 2° to sludge in gallbladder by ultrasound (50%), symptomatic (9%) (NEJM 322:1821, 1990). More likely with 22 gm per day or with ↓ in total parenteral nutrition and not eating (AnIM 115:712, 1991). Clinical significance still unknown in children (JID 17:366, 1995) and gallstone pancreatitis (Ln 177:662, 1998). In pilot study, 2 gm once daily by continuous infusion superior to 2 gm bolus once daily (JAC 59:285, 2007). For Ceftriaxone Desensitization, see Table 7, page 80.

*NOTE: all dosage recommendations are for adults (unless otherwise indicated) & assume normal renal function.

(See page 2 for abbreviations)

TABLE 10A (4)

CLASS, AGENT, GENERIC NAME (TRADE NAME)	USUAL ADULT DOSAGE*	ADVERSE REACTIONS, COMMENTS *(See Table 10B for Summary)*
CEPHALOSPORINS (1st parenteral, then oral drugs) *(continued)*		
Other Generation, Parenteral:	**All are substrates for ESBLs & amp C cephalosporinase for aerobic gram-negative bacilli. Cefepime penetrates to target faster than other cephalosporins.**	
Cefepime (Maxipime) Obesity dosing, see Table 17C	Active vs P. aeruginosa and some strains of Enterobacter, Citrobacter resistant to 3rd generation cephalosporins. Active vs MSSA like other 3rd generation cephalosporins. Not "porin-dependent". Neutropenia after 14 days rx *(Scand J Infect Dis 42:156, 2010).*	
	Usual dose: 1-2 gm IV q8-12h.	**FDA Safety warning (June 2012):** risk of non-convulsive status epilepticus, especially in pts with renal insufficiency when doses not adjusted. Seizure activity resolved after drug discontinuation and/or hemodialysis in the majority of pts. Postulated mechanism: binding to GABA receptors *(Scand J Infect Dis 46:272, 2014; Crit Care 17:R264, 2013).*
	Initial dose: 15 mg/kg (over 30 min, then immediately begin. If CrCl > 60, 8.6 gm (over 24 hr) daily If CrCl 30-60, 4 gm (over 24 hr) daily If CrCl 11-29, 1.25 gm (over 24 hr) daily	
Cefpirome[NUS] (HR 810)	**1-2 gm IV q12h**	Similar to cefepime: ↑ activity vs enterobacteriaceae, P. aeruginosa, Gn + organisms. Anaerobes less active than cefoxitin, more active than cefotax or ceftaz.
Ceftaroline fosamil (Teflaro)	**600 mg IV q12h (1-hr infusion)** Pneumonia/bacteremia 600 mg IV q8h[NUS] See Comment	**Avid binding to PBP 2a; active vs. MRSA.** Inactivated by Amp C & ↑ ESBL enzymes. Approved for MRSA skin and skin structure infections and used for MRSA pneumonia and bacteremia, but not approved indications *(J Infect Chemother 19:42, 2013).* Active in vitro vs. VISA, VRSA. Refs: CID 52:1156, 2011; Med Lett 53:5, 2011. Used successfully for bacteremia and bone/joint infections, but NA *(AAC 58:2541, 2014).*
Ceftobiprole[NUS]	**0.5 gm IV q8h for mixed gm-neg & gm-pos infections. 0.5 gm IV q12h for gm-pos infections**	Infuse over 1 hr. Active vs. P. aeruginosa similar to cefepime. Cross-reaction in penicillin-allergic pts. Decreased efficacy w/ CrCl 30-50 mL/min.
Ceftolozane-tazobactam (Zerbaxa)	**1.5 gm (1/0.5 gm) IV q8h for gm-neg complicated UTI & complicated intra-abdominal infections** (add Metro 500 mg IV q8h) infection	Ref. Clin Microbiol Infections 13(Suppl 2):17 & 25, 2007. Active vs. MRSA.
Oral Cephalosporins		**Cross-Allergenicity:** Patients with a history of IgE-mediated allergic reactions to penicillin (e.g., bronchospasm anaphylaxis, angioneurotic edema, immediate urticaria) should not receive a cephalosporin. If the history is a "measles-like" rash to penicillin, available data suggest a 5–10% risk of rash in such patients, there is no enhanced risk of anaphylaxis.
1st Generation, Oral		
Cefadroxil (Duricef) (500 mg caps, 1 gm tabs)	**0.5–1 gm po q12h.**	Most patients with a history of penicillin allergy can be given a cephalosporin *(Ann Allergy Asthma Proc 26:135, 2006).* If positive Pen G skin test, only 2% given a cephalosporin will react. Can predict with cephalosporin skin testing, but not easily available *(An Int Med 141:16, 2004; AJM 125:572, 2008).*
Cephalexin (Keflex) (250 & 500 mg tabs)	**0.25–1 gm po q6h (max 4 gm/day).**	• IgE antibodies against either drug structure or side chains: 80% pts lose IgE over 10 yrs post-reaction *(J Aller Clin Immunol 103:918, 1999).* Amox, Cefadroxil, Cefprozil have similar side chains; Amp, Cefaclor, Cephalexin, Cephedrine have similar side chains.
2nd Generation, Oral		• If Pen/Ceph skin test not available or clinically no time, proceed with cephalosporin if history does not suggest IgE-mediated reaction, prior reaction more than 10 yrs ago or cephalosporin side chain differs from implicated Pen.
Cefaclor (Ceclor, Raniclor) (250 mg caps)	**0.25–0.5 gm po q8h.**	Any of the cephalosporins can result in C. difficile toxin-mediated diarrhea.
Cefprozil (Cefzil) (250 & 500 mg tabs)	**0.25–0.5 gm po q12h.**	The incidence of C. difficile toxin diarrhea is summarized in Table 10B.
Cefuroxime axetil[NUS] (Ceftin) (250 & 500 mg tabs)	**0.125–0.5 gm po q12h.**	There are a few drug-specific adverse effects, e.g.: **Cefdinir:** Drug-iron complex causes red stools in 1% of pts. **Cefditoren pivoxil:** Hydrolysis yields pivalate. Pivalate absorbed (70%) & becomes pivaloylcarnitine which is renally excreted: 39–63% ↓ in serum carnitine concentrations. Carnitine involved in fatty acid (FA) metabolism & FA transport into mitochondria. Effect on FA metabolism might result in clinically significant carnitine deficiency or those in whom protein is strict-like in nutrition. Avoid if milk allergy (not same as lactose intolerance). Need gastric acid for optimal absorption.
3rd Generation, Oral		
Cefdinir (Omnicef) (300 mg cap)	**300 mg po q12h or 600 mg po q24h.**	
Cefditoren pivoxil (Spectracef) (200 mg tab)	**400 mg po bid.**	**Cefpodoxime:** Milk and antacids decrease absorption. Also contains caseinate (milk protein); avoid if milk allergy (not same as lactose intolerance).
Cefixime (Suprax) (400 mg tab)	**0.4 gm po q12-24h.**	**Cefpodoxime:** There are rare reports of acute liver injury, bloody diarrhea, pulmonary infiltrates with eosinophilia.
Cefpodoxime proxetil (Vantin) (100 & 200 mg tabs)	**0.1–0.2 gm po q12h.**	**Cephalexin:** Can cause false-neg. urine dipstick test for leukocytes.
Ceftibuten (Cedax) (400 mg cap)	**0.4 gm po q24h.**	

(See page 2 for abbreviations)

NOTE: all dosage recommendations are for adults (unless otherwise indicated) & assume normal renal function.

TABLE 10A (5)

CLASS, AGENT, GENERIC NAME (TRADE NAME)	USUAL ADULT DOSAGE* —See Table 10D, page 110, and Table 17A, page 205	ADVERSE REACTIONS, COMMENTS (See Table 10B for Summary)
AMINOGLYCOSIDES AND RELATED ANTIBIOTICS—See Table 10D, page 110, and Table 17A, page 205		
GLYCOPEPTIDES, LIPOGLYCOPEPTIDES, LIPOPEPTIDES		
Dalbavancin (Dalvance)	1000 mg IV over 30 min; one week later, 500 mg IV over 30 min. Avoid use with saline, drug may precipitate out of solution.	If CrCl<30: 750 mg IV initial dose, then one week later 375 mg IV. **Hemodialysis:** Dose as for normal renal function
Daptomycin (Cubicin) Ref. on resistance *CID 50:S10, 2010.* Case series success in treating right- & left-sided endocarditis with higher dose of 8-10 mg/kg/day (*JAC 68:936 & 2921, 2013).*	**Skin/soft tissue infections: 4 mg per kg IV over 2 or 30 minutes q24h** **Bacteremia/right-sided endocarditis:** **6 mg per kg IV over 2 or 30 minutes q24h;** up to 12 mg/kg/day IV q24h under study **Morbid obesity:** base dose on total body weight (*AAC 51:2741, 2007*). For other dosing recommendations, see *Table 17C, page 213.* Dapto + ceftaroline may work as salvage therapy in pts with refractory MRSA bacteremia (*AAC 57:66, 2013; AAC 56:5296, 2012*)	Red man syndrome can occur with rapid infusion. No activity vs. VRE. No drug-drug interactions. **Pneumonia:** Dapto should not be used to treat pneumonia unless hematogenous in origin and is FDA approved for right-sided endocarditis (*CID 55:1538, 2012; CID 59:1-2 & 1673, 2014*) with or without septic embolization/hematogenous pneumonia due to S. aureus. **Dapto Resistance:** Can occur de novo, after or during Vanco therapy, & during Dapto therapy (*CID 50:S10/oj S1; CID 50:S409 & JAC 51:1-2/1-5:10*). **Potential muscle toxicity:** At 4 mg per kg dose, 1 CPK in 2.8%, dapto pts & 1.8% comparator-treated pts. Risk increases if min conc ≥24.3 mg/L (*CID 50:1568, 2010*). Suggest weekly CPK; CPK exceeds 10x normal level or if symptoms of myopathy and CPK > 1,000. Package insert: stop statins during dapto rx. Dapto interferes with prothrombin reagents, & artificially prolongs the PT [*Blood Coag & Fibrinolysis 19:32, 2008*]. **NOTE:** Dapto well-tolerated in healthy volunteers given up to 12 mg/kg q24h x 14d (*AAC 50:3245, 2006*) and in pts given mean dose of 8 mg/kg/day (*CID 49:177, 2009*). **Immune thrombocytopenia** reported (*AAC 56:6430, 2012*). Reversible neutropenia with long-term use reported (*CID 56:1353, 2013*). **Eosinophilic pneumonia/chronic steroid-dep pneumonia** reported (*CID 50:737, 2010; CID 60:e3, 2010*).
Oritavancin (Orbactiv)	**1200 mg IV over 3 hr x 1 dose.** Dilute in D5W; do not use saline	Artificially increases PT & INR x 24 hr & aPTT x 48 hr. **Drug-drug interactions with warfarin:** 1 warfarin serum levels. No adjustment of renal or hepatic insuff. Not removed by hemodialysis. Acute urticarial rxs reported (*CID 56:1639, 2012*). Hypersensitivity: Fever (at 3 mg/kg 2.2%, at 24 mg per kg 8.2%), skin reactions 2.4%. Marked ↓ platelets (high dose ≥15 mg/kg per day). Red neck syndrome less common than with vancomycin.
Telavancin (Vibativ) Lipoglycopeptide *Med Lett 52:1, 2010.*	10 mg/kg IV q24h If CCr > 50 mL/min. Infuse each dose over 1 hr. Adjust dose if wt ≥30% over IBW, see *Table 10D.*	**Avoid during pregnancy: teratogenic in animals.** Do pregnancy test before therapy. Adverse events: **dysgeusia (taste) 33%,** nausea 27%, vomiting 14%, headache 14%; ↑ creatinine (3.1%); foamy urine; flushing if infused rapidly. **Evidence of renal injury** in 3% telavancin vs. 1% vanco. In practice, renal injury reported in 1/3 of 21 complicated pts (*JAC 67:723, 2012*). Interferes with PT, aPTT & INR for 18 hrs post-infusion.
Teicoplanin[NUS] (Targocid)	**For septic arthritis—maintenance dose 12 mg/kg per day, S. aureus endocarditis—12 mg/kg per day, higher doses required (12 mg/kg q12h times 4 loading doses, then 12 mg/kg q24h)**	
Vancomycin (Vancocin) Guidelines *Ref. CID 49:325, 2009.* See Comments for po dose. Continuous infusion dosing, see *Table 10E*	**For septic arthritis—maintenance dose 12 mg/kg per day, S. aureus endocarditis—12 mg/kg per day, higher doses required (12 mg/kg q12h times 4 loading doses, then 12 mg/kg q24h)** **Initial doses based on actual wt, including for obese patients.** Subsequent doses adjusted based on measured trough serum levels. **For critically ill pts, give loading dose of 25-30 mg/kg IV then 15-20 mg/kg IV q8-12h.** Target trough level is 15-20 μg/mL. For individual doses over 1 gm, infuse over ≥ 1.5-2 hrs. **Morbid obesity (actual BMI ≥40):** Loading dose 25-30 mg/kg (actual wt) IV, then 15-20 mg/kg (actual wt) IV q8-12h. If CrCl ≤50 mL/min & pt not critically ill: 30 mg/kg/day divided q8-12h—no dose over 2 gm. Infuse doses of 1 gm or more over 1.5-2 hrs. Check trough levels. **Morbid obesity if critically ill:** see above. Loading dose 25-30 mg/kg, then 15-20 mg/kg q8-12h. Infuse over 1.5-2 hrs. **Limit maximal single dose to 2 gm.** Oral tabs for C. difficile: 125 mg po q6h Generic drug now available	Vanco treatment failure of MRSA bacteremia associated with Vanco trough concentration <15 μg/mL & MIC > 1 μg/mL (*CID 52:975, 2011*). IDSA/ASHP/SIDP guideline support target trough 15-20 μg/mL (*AJHP 82:e18, 2011*). Pertinent Issues: • MIC values vary with method used, so hard to be sure/compare (*JCM 49:269, 2011*). • Max Vanco MIC for S. aureus is 2 μg/mL; Vanco dose >3 gm/day IV, AUC/MIC > 400 in 86% Vanco trough 35%) of 25%. With MIC for vanco MIC = 2 & 4 gm/day IV, AUC/MIC > 400 in only 57% (nephrotoxicity risk 35%) (*CID 52:969, 2011*). • Higher Vanco doses assoc with nephrotoxicity, causal relation uncertain; other factors: renal disease, other nephrotoxic drugs, ICU stay, duration of therapy, etc. (*CID 52:e18, 2011; AJM 123:182e1, 2010*). If clinically failing Vanco (regardless of MIC) or AUC/MIC), consider other drugs active vs. MRSA: ceftaroline, daptomycin, linezolid, telavancin. (see *Table 5A for MDR options*). **PO vanco for C. difficile colitis: 125 mg po q6h.** Commercial oral formulation expensive. Can compound po vanco from IV formulation: 5 g, IV Vanco powder + 47.5 mL sterile H₂O 0.2 gm saccharin, 0.05 gm stevia powder, 40 mL glycerin and then enough cherry syrup to yield 100 mL = 50 mg vanco/mL. Oral dose = 2.5 mL q6h po (*Am J Health Syst Pharm 66:642, 2009*). Another recipe uses 50 mg/mL concentration of 10-20 μg/mL. **Nephrotoxicity:** Risk increases with dose and duration, reversible. (*AAC 57:734, 2013*). **Red Neck Syndrome:** consequence of rapid infusion with non-specific histamine release. **Other adverse effects:** rash, immune thrombocytopenia (*NEJM 356:904, 2007*); fever, neutropenia, and rare report of dose-dependent decrease in platelet count (*JAC 67:672, 2012*). **IgA bullous dermatosis** (*CID 38:e42, 2004*). **Obesity dosing:** Frequent under dosing. (*AJM 127:1095, 2014*). **Obesity** see page 213. For CrCl calculation for morbidly obese patient see *Table 10D for AI options*.

TABLE 10A (6)

CLASS, AGENT, GENERIC NAME (TRADE NAME)	USUAL ADULT DOSAGE*	ADVERSE REACTIONS, COMMENTS *(See Table 10B for Summary)*
CHLORAMPHENICOL, CLINDAMYCIN(S), ERYTHROMYCIN GROUP, KETOLIDES, OXAZOLIDINONES, QUINUPRISTIN-DALFOPRISTIN		
Chloramphenicol (Chloromycetin)	50-100 mg/kg/day po/IV div q6h (max 4 gm/day)	No oral drug distrib in U.S. Hematologic (↓ RBC −1/3 pts, aplastic anemia 1:21,600 courses). Gray baby syndrome in premature infants, anaphylactoid reactions, optic atrophy or neuropathy (very rare), drug paresthesias, minor disulfiram-like reactions.
Clindamycin (Cleocin)	0.15-0.45 gm po q6h. 600-900 mg IV/IM q8h.	Based on number of exposed pts, these drugs are the most frequent cause of **C. difficile toxin-mediated diarrhea.** In most severe form can cause pseudomembranous colitis/toxic megacolon. Available as caps, IV soln, topical (for acne) & intravaginal suppositories & cream. **Used to inhibit synthesis of toxic shock syndrome toxins.**
Lincomycin (Lincocin)	0.6 gm IV/IM q8h.	Risk of C. difficile colitis. Rarely used.
Erythromycin Group (Review drug interactions before use)		**Motilin:** activates myenteric/jejunal receptors that initiate peristalsis. Erythro (E) and E esters activate motilin receptors and cause uncoordinated peristalsis with resultant anorexia, nausea or vomiting. Less binding and GI distress with azithromycin.
Azithromycin (Zithromax) Azithromycin ER (Zmax)	**po preps:** Tabs 250 & 600 mg. Peds suspension: 100 & 200 mg per 5 mL. Adult ER suspension: 2 gm. Dose varies with indication, see Table 1, page 17). acute exacerbations chronic bronchitis (page 37), Comm-acq pneumonia (pages 39–40) & sinusitis (page 50). IV: 0.5 gm per day.	Erythro IV can be assoc with QTc prolongation. No peristalsis benefit vs IV (JAC 59:347, 2001). Infantile hypertrophic pyloric stenosis (J Ped 139:380, 2001). Systemic erythro in 1° 2 wks of life associated with **infantile hypertrophic pyloric stenosis** (J Ped 139:380, 2001). **Frequent drug-drug interactions:** see Table 22, page 218. Major concern is prolonged QTc interval on EKG. **Prolonged QTc:** Erythro, clarithro & azithro all increase risk of ventricular tachycardia via increase in QTc interval. Can be congenital or acquired (NEJM 358:169, 2008). Two studies show variable degree of increased risk of CV death among azithro recipients: presumably from prolonged QTc (NEJM 366:1881, 2012; NEJM 366:1665 & 1704, 2013). Caution if positive family history of sudden cardiac death, electrolyte abnormalities or concomitant drugs that prolong QTc.
Erythromycin Base and esters (Erythrocin) IV name: E. lactobionate	0.25 gm q6h–0.5 gm po/IV q6h; 15–20 mg/kg up to 4 gm IV q24h. Infuse over 30+ min.	Refs on risk of CV death with azithro use: NEJM 366:1881, 2012; NEJM 368:1704, 2013. ↑ **risk QTc >500 msec. Risk amplified by other drugs** (macrolides, antiarrhythmics, & drug-drug interactions (see FDA, page 1/3 for list) www.crdrugs.org & www.qtdrugs.org). Cholestatic hepatitis in approx. 1:1000 adults (not children) gm E estolate.
Clarithromycin (Biaxin) or clarithro extended release (Biaxin XL)	0.5 gm po q12h. **Extended release:** Two 0.5 gm tabs po per day.	**Drug-drug interactions of note:** Erythro or clarithro with statins: high statin levels, rhabdomyolysis (Ann Int Med 158:869, 2013); concomitant clarithro & colchicine (gout) can cause fatal colchicine toxicity (pancytopenia, renal failure) (CID 41:291, 2005). Concomitant clarithro & Ca++ channel blockers increase risk of hypotension, kidney injury (JAMA 310:2544, 2013).
Fidaxomicin (Dificid) (200 mg tab)	**One 200 mg tab** po bid x 10 days with or without food	**Transient reversible tinnitus or deafness** with ≥4 gm per day of erythro IV in pts with renal or hepatic impairment. Reversible sensorineural hearing loss with Azithro (J Otolaryngol 36:257, 2007). Dosages of oral erythro preparations expressed as base equivalents. Variable amounts of erythro esters required to achieve same free erythro serum level. Azithromycin reported to exacerbate symptoms of myasthenia gravis. Approved for C. difficile toxin-mediated diarrhea, including hypervirulent NAP-1/B1/027 strains. Minimal GI absorption (high fecal concentrations. Limited activity vs. normal bowel flora. In trial vs. po Vanco, lower relapse rate vs. non-NAP1 strains than Vanco (NEJM 364:422, 2011). Despite absence of GI absorption, 3 pts developed allergic reactions; known macrolide allergy in 3 of 12 (CID 58:537, 2014).
Ketolide: Telithromycin (Ketek) (Med Lett 46:66, 2004; Drug Safety 31:561, 2008)	Two 400 mg tabs po q24h. 300 mg tabs available.	Drug warnings: acute liver failure & serious liver injury post treatment. (AnIM 144:415, 447, 2006). **Uncommon: blurred vision 2° slow accommodation; may cause exacerbation of myasthenia gravis (Black Box Warning: Contraindicated in this disorder).** Liver, eye and myasthenia complications may be due to inhibition of nicotinic acetylcholine receptor at neuromuscular junction (AAC 54:5399, 2010). Potential QTc prolongation (Table 22, pages 218–219) (NEJM 355:2260, 2006).

(See page 2 for abbreviations)   ***NOTE:** all dosage recommendations are for adults (unless otherwise indicated) & assume normal renal function.*

TABLE 10A (7)

CLASS, AGENT, GENERIC NAME (TRADE NAME)	USUAL ADULT DOSAGE*	ADVERSE REACTIONS, COMMENTS (See Table 10B for Summary)
CHLORAMPHENICOL, CLINDAMYCIN(S), ERYTHROMYCIN GROUP, KETOLIDES, OXAZOLIDINONES, QUINUPRISTIN-DALFOPRISTIN (continued)		
Tedizolid phosphate (Sivextro) Ref: CID 58(Suppl 1):S1557, 2014.	**200 mg IV/po once daily.** Infuse IV over 1 hr.	**IV dose reconstituted in 250 mL of normal saline;** incompatible with lactated ringers due to absence of solubility in presence of divalent cations. SST clinical trial result (LnID 14:696, 2014; JAMA 309:559 & 609, 2013). Excreted by liver. No adjustment for renal insufficiency. Weak inhibitor of monoamine oxidase , hence risk of serotonin syndrome, but low risk based on in vitro, animal & human study (AAC 57:3060, 2013).
Linezolid (Zyvox) (600 mg tab) Review JAC 66(Suppl 1):S1557, 2014.	**PO or IV dose: 600 mg q12h.** Available as 600 mg tabs, oral suspension (100 mg per 5 mL, & IV solution. Special populations Refs: Renal insufficiency (J Infect Chemother 17:70, 2011); Liver transplant (CID 42:434, 2006); Cystic fibrosis (AAC 48:281, 2004); Burns (J Burn Care Res 31:207, 2010); Obesity clinical failure with standard dose in 265 kg patient (Ann Pharmacother 47:e25, 2013).	**Reversible myelosuppression:** thrombocytopenia, anemia, & neutropenia reported. Most often after >2 wks of therapy. **Lactic acidosis; peripheral neuropathy, optic neuropathy:** After 4 or more wks of therapy. Data consistent with time & dose-dependent inhibition of intramitochondrial protein synthesis (CID 42:1111, 2006; AAC 50:2042, 2006; Pharmacotherapy 27:771, 2007). Neuropathy not reversible. **Inhibitor of monoamine oxidase:** risk of severe hypertension if taken with foods rich in tyramine. Avoid concomitant pseudoephedrine, phenylpropanolamine, and caution with SSRIs. **Serotonin syndrome** (fever, agitation, mental status changes, tremors). Risk with concomitant SSRIs (CID 42:1578 and 43:180, 2006). Actual incidence seems low (JAC 67:494, 2012; AAC 57:5901, 2013). Other adverse effects: black hairy tongue and acute interstitial nephritis (IDCP 17:61, 2009). **Rhabdomyolysis:** a case of this entity, probably related to linezolid, was reported in a patient receiving linezolid as a component of multi-drug therapy for XDR tuberculosis (CID 54:1624, 2012). **Resistance** Linezolid resistant S. epidermidis and MRSA due to other mobile gene that methylates ribosomal target of linezolid or primarily, to mutation of the 23S rRNA binding site (JAC 68:4, 2013).
Quinupristin + dalfopristin (Synercid) (CID 36:473, 2003)	**7.5 mg per kg IV q8h via central line**	Venous irritation (5%), none with central venous line. Asymptomatic ↑ in unconjugated bilirubin. **Arthralgia** 2%–50% (CID 36:476, 2003). **Note:** E. faecium susceptible, E. faecalis resistant. **Drug-drug interactions:** Cyclosporine, nifedipine, midazolam, many others—see Table 22.
TETRACYCLINES		
Doxycycline (Vibramycin, Doryx, Monodox, Adoxa, Periostat) (20, 50, 75, 100 mg tab)	**0.1 gm po/IV q12h**	Similar to other tetracyclines. ↑ nausea on empty stomach. Erosive esophagitis, esp. if taken at bedtime; **take with lots of water.** Phototoxicity & photo-onycholysis occur but less than with tetracycline. Deposition in teeth less. Can be used in patients with renal failure. Comments: Effective in treatment and prophylaxis for malaria, leptospirosis, typhus fevers.
Minocycline (Minocin, Dynacin) (50, 75, 100 mg cap; 45, 90, 135 mg ext rel tab; IV prep)	**200 mg po/IV loading dose, then 100 mg po/IV q12h** IV minocycline available.	Comments: More effective than other tetracyclines vs staph and in prophylaxis of meningococcal disease. P. acnes: many resistant to other tetracyclines, not to mino. Active vs Nocardia asteroides, Mycobacterium marinum and marine/actobacter isolates (J Ped 153:314, 2008). Active vs. tetra-4), anaphylactoid reaction (rare), deposits in teeth, negative N balance, hepatotoxic, enamel ageness, GI (ow 19%; tetra-4), anaphylactoid reaction (rare), deposits in teeth, negative N balance, hepatotoxic, enamel ageness, pseudotumor cerebri/encephalopathy. Outdated drug: Fanconi syndrome. See drug-drug interactions, Table 22.
Tetracycline, Oxytetracycline (Sumycin) (250, 500 mg cap) (CID 36:462, 2003)	**0.25–0.5 gm po q6h, 0.5–1 gm IV q12h**	**Contraindicated in pregnancy, hepatotoxicity in pregnancy; transplacental; fetus.** **Pregnancy:** IV dosage over 2 gm per day may be associated with fatal hepatotoxicity. (Ref: JAC 66:1431, 2011). Derivative of tetracycline. High incidence of nausea (25% & vomiting (20%) but only 1% of this discontinued therapy. Pregnancy Category D. Do not use in children under age 18. Like other tetracyclines, may cause photosensitivity, pseudotumor cerebri, pancreatitis, a catabolic state (elevated BUN) and may cause hyperpigmentation (CID 45:136, 2007).
Tigecycline (Tygacil) Meta-analysis & editorial: Ln ID 11:804 & 834, 2011. Also CID 54:1699 & 1710, 2012.	**100 mg IV initially, then 50 mg IV q12h with po food. If possible to decrease risk of nausea.**	**Tetracycline, minocycline, & tigecycline** associated with acute pancreatitis (Int J Antimicrob Agents, 34:486, 2009). **Black Box Warning:** Increased mortality (4.0%) in pts treated with tigecycline. Ref: Diagn Micro Infec Dis 64:40, 2010. Black Box Warning—meta-analysis of clinical trials showed all-cause mortality higher in pts treated with tigecycline (2.5%) vs. 1.8% in comparators. Cause of mortality risk difference of 0.6% (95% CI 0.1, 1.2) not established. Tigecycline should be reserved for use in situations when alternative treatments are not suitable (FDA MedWatch Sep 27, 2013). Poor result due to low serum levels (AAC 57:1756, 2013).

If severe liver dis. (Child Pugh C): 100 mg IV initially, then 25 mg IV q12h

---

[1] **SSRI** = selective serotonin reuptake inhibitors, e.g., fluoxetine (Prozac).
(See page 2 for abbreviations)   *NOTE: all dosage recommendations are for adults (unless otherwise indicated) & assume normal renal function.

TABLE 10A (8)

CLASS, AGENT, GENERIC NAME (TRADE NAME)	USUAL ADULT DOSAGE*	ADVERSE REACTIONS, COMMENTS (See Table 10B for Summary)
FLUOROQUINOLONES (FQs): All can cause false-positive urine drug screen for opiates (*Pharmacother 26:435, 2006*). Toxicity review: *Drugs Aging 27:193, 2010.*		
Ciprofloxacin (Cipro) and Ciprofloxacin-extended release (Cipro XR, Proquin XR) (100, 250, 500, 750 mg tab; 500 mg ext rel tab)	Usual Parenteral Dose: **400 mg IV q12h.** For P. aeruginosa: **400 mg IV q8h.** Uncomplicated Urethritis/cystitis (Oral) Dose: **250 mg po bid or CIP XR 500 mg po once daily.** Other Indications (Oral): **500-750 mg po bid**	**FQs are a common precipitant of C. difficile toxin-mediated diarrhea.** **Children:** No FQ approved for use under age 16 based on joint cartilage injury in immature animals. Articular SEs in children 1.5–3%. Use of FQs in children may be justified... Pathogenesis believed to involve FQ chelation of Mg^{++} and damaging chondrites (*AAC 51:1022, 2007; Int J Antimicrob Agents 33:194, 2009*). No evidence of cartilage damage with Levo in children (*Pediatrics 134:e146, 2014*). **CNS toxicity:** Poorly understood. Varies: lightheadedness, confusion, seizures. May be aggravated by NSAIDs. Peripheral neuropathy occurs: rapid onset, potentially permanent injury Phototoxicity & skin rash: with some FQs, incidence of rash with ≤5 days of therapy only 1.5%. Frequency highest females; <2 age 40, treated 14 days (22.6%) in men, age 40, treated 14 days, frequency 7.7%. Mechanism unclear. Indication to D/C therapy. Ref: Diag Micro Infect Dis 68: 140, 2010. **Hypoglycemia/hyperglycemia (Dysglycemia):** Increased risk, esp. of hypoglycemia in diabetic pts from any of the marketed FQs (*CID 57:971, 2013*). (*PLoS One 8(1):e81477*). Thrombocytopenia in critically ill... Opiate screen false-positives: FQs can cause false-positive urine drug assay for opiates (*Ann Pharmacotherapy 38:1525, 2004*). Photosensitivity: See Table 10C, page 109. Rarely, retinal detachment (*JAMA 307:1414, 2012*). QT_c **(corrected QT) interval prolongation:** ↑ QT_c (>500 msec or >60 msec from baseline) is considered possible with any FQ. ↑ QT_c can lead to torsades de pointes and ventricular fibrillation. Overall risk is 4.7/10,000 person yrs (*CID 55:1457, 2012*). Risk low with current marketed drugs. Risk ↑ in women, ↓ K^+, ↓ mg++, bradycardia. (Refs: *CID 43:1603, 2006*). Major problem is ↑ risk with concomitant drugs.
Gatifloxacin (Tequin)^ILS See comments	**200-400 mg IV/po q24h.** (See comment) Ophthalmic solution (Zymar)	
Gemifloxacin (Factive) (320 mg tab)	**320 mg po q24h.**	

Avoid concomitant drugs with potential to prolong QTc such as (see *www.qtdrugs.org*; *www.torsades.org*):

Antiarrhythmics:	Anti-infectives:	CNS Drugs:	Misc:
Amiodarone	Azoles (not posa)	Fluoxetine	Dolasetron
Disopyramide	Clarithro/erythro	Haloperidol	Droperidol
Dofetilide	FQs (not CIP)	Phenothiazines	Fosphenytoin
Flecainide	Halofantrine	Pimozide	Indapamide
Ibutilide	NNRTIs	Quetiapine	Methadone
Procainamide	Pentamidine	Risperidone	Naratriptan
Quinidine, quinine	Protease Inhibitors	Sertraline	Salmeterol
Sotalol	Telavancin	Tricyclics	Sumatriptan
	Telithromycin	Venlafaxine	Tamoxifen
Anti-Hypertensives:		Ziprasidone	Tizanidine
Bepridil			
Isradipine			
Nicardipine			
Moexipril			

CLASS, AGENT, GENERIC NAME (TRADE NAME)	USUAL ADULT DOSAGE*	ADVERSE REACTIONS, COMMENTS
Levofloxacin (Levaquin) (250, 500, 750 mg tab)	**250-750 mg po/IV q24h.** For most indications, 750 mg q24h. Po therapy: avoid concomitant dairy products, multivitamins, iron, antacids due to chelation by multivalent cations & interference with absorption. No dose adjustment for morbid obesity.	**Tendinopathy:** Over age 60, approx. 2–6% of all Achilles tendon ruptures attributable to use of FQ (*AJM 163:1801, 2003*). ↑ risk with concomitant steroid, renal disease or post-transplant (heart, lung, kidney) (*CID 36:1404, 2003*). **Chelation:** Risk of ↓ absorption of FQ. Do not take with milk or cation-containing solutions (Ca^{++}, Mg^{++}, Fe^{++}, Zn^{++}). Avoid dairy products, multivitamins (*Clin Pharmacol Ther 40 (Suppl 1):33, 2001*).
Moxifloxacin (Avelox) (400, 250, 750 mg tab)	**400 mg po/IV q24h.** Note: no need to increase dose for morbid obesity (*JAC 66:2330, 2011*). Ophthalmic solution (Vigamox)	**Allergic Reactions:** Rare (1:50,000). IgE-mediated: urticaria, anaphylaxis. 3 pts with Moxi had immediate reactions but tolerated CIP (*Ann Pharmacofher 44:740, 2010*). **Myasthenia gravis:** Any of the FQs may exacerbate muscle weakness in pts. with myasthenia gravis. **Retinal detachment:** Association with FQs in 2 studies (*JAMA 307:1414, 2012*) but not in 2 other studies (*JAMA 310:2184, 2013; JACS 29:2253, 2014*).
Ofloxacin (Floxin)	**200-400 mg po bid** Ophthalmic solution (Ocuflox)	

*NOTE: all dosage recommendations are for adults (unless otherwise indicated) & assume normal renal function.

TABLE 10A (9)

CLASS, AGENT, GENERIC NAME (TRADE NAME)	USUAL ADULT DOSAGE*	ADVERSE REACTIONS, COMMENTS (See Table 10B for Summary)
FLUOROQUINOLONES (FQs) (continued)		
Prulifloxacin Ref: Drugs 64:2221, 2004.	Tablets: 250 and 600 mg. Usual dose: **600 mg po once daily**	Not available in the U.S.
POLYMYXINS (POLYPEPTIDES)	**Note: Proteus sp., Providencia sp., Serratia sp.,**	**B. cepacia are intrinsically resistant to polymyxins.** Review: CID 59:88, 2014.
Polymyxin B (Poly-Rx) 1 mg = 10,000 international units of Colistin base Avoid monotherapy, see Colistin.	Doses based on actual body weight. **LOADING DOSE:** 2.5 mg/kg IV over 2 hrs. **MAINTENANCE DOSE:** 12 hrs later 1.5 mg/kg over 1 hr, then repeat q12h. Combination therapy with carbapenem suggested to increase efficacy and reduce risk of resistance. No dose reduction for renal insufficiency. **Intrathecal therapy for meningitis:** 5 mg/day into CSF x 3-4 days, then 5 mg every other day x 2 or more weeks.	**Adverse effects: Neurologic:** rare but serious is neuromuscular blockade; other, circumoral paresthesias, extremity numbness, blurred vision, drowsy, irritable, ataxia, can manifest as respiratory arrest (Chest 141:515, 2012). **Renal:** reversible acute tubular necrosis. Renal injury in 42% (Polymyxin B) vs. 60% (Colistin) (CID 57:1300, 2013). PK study showed no need to reduce dose for renal insufficiency (CID 57:524, 2013). Polymyxin B preferred over Colistin when urgent need to quickly achieve therapeutic serum levels.

Colistin, Polymyxin E (Colymycin)
 	
All doses are based on mg of Colistin base.
 	
Calculated doses are higher than the package insert dosing; need to avoid underdosage in the critically ill.
 	
Do not use as monotherapy (combine with carbapenem or rifampin)
 	
Dosing formula based on PK study of 105 pts (AAC 55:3284, 2011). Loading dose (AAC 53:3430, 2009). PK/PD studies (AAC 54:3783, 2010 (in vitro), JAC 65:1984, 2010 (in vivo)). **Recommendations are evolving, see Sanford Guide digital editions for most current information and dosing calculator.**
	• **Severe Systemic Infection:**
	  LOADING DOSE: 3.5 (targeted average serum steady state level) x 2 x body weight in kg (lower of ideal or actual body weight) IV. This will often result in a loading dose of over 300 mg (4 million units). First maintenance dose is given 12 hrs. later.
	  MAINTENANCE DOSE: Formula for calculating the daily maintenance dosage:
	  = 3.5 (the desired serum steady state concentration) x [(1.5 x CrCln) +30] = total daily dose. Divide and give q8h or maybe q12h. The maximum suggested daily dose is 475 mg.
	  • **NOTE:** CrCln is the Creatinine Clearance (CrCln) normalized (n) for Body Surface Area (BSA) such that the CrCln = CrCl x BSA in m²/1.73 m².
	• *Combination therapy is recommended for all pts.*
	• **Colistin** (as above) + (**IMP** or **MER**) or **RIF**) (based on IBW)
	• **Intrathecal or intraventricular for meningitis:** 10 mg/day
	• *Inhalation therapy:* 50-75 mg in 3-4 mL of Saline via nebulizer 2-3x/day
		• **GNB Resistance:** Some sp. are intrinsically resistant: Serratia sp. Providencia sp., B. cepacia. In vitro and in animal models, gram-negative bacilli quickly become resistant: concomitant Tigecycline or Minocycline may attenuate risk of resistance (JAC 60:421, 2007). Synergy with Rifampin or Tigecycline unpredictable. The greater the resistance of GNB to Colistin, the greater the susceptibility to beta-lactams (AM-SB, PIP-TZ, extended spectrum Ceph.) maybe carbapenems).
		• **Caveat:** higher doses of colistin (> 5 mg/kg of ideal body weight per day) are associated with increased risk of nephrotoxicity and should be reserved for critically ill patients (Clin Infect Dis 53:879, 2011).
		• **Bactericidal activity concentration dependent** but no post-antibiotic effect; do not dose once daily.
		• **Nephrotoxic:** exact risk unclear, but increased by concomitant nephrotoxins (IV contrast), hypotension, maybe Rifampin. Reversible.
		• **Neurotoxicity:** Frequent: circumoral paresthesia, vertigo, abnormal vision, confusion, ataxia. Rare: neuromuscular blockade with respiratory failure.
		• **Caution:** Some colistimethate products are expressed in IUs. To convert IUs to mg of colistin base: 1,000,000 IUs colistimethate = 30 mg colistin base. See CID 58:139, 2014.
		  colistimethate = 80 mg colistimethate base = 30 mg colistimethate.
		• Colistin preferred over Polymyxin B for treatment of UTIs.

*NOTE: all dosage recommendations are for adults (unless otherwise indicated) & assume normal renal function.

*See page 2 for abbreviations)

(See page 2 for abbreviations)

TABLE 10A (10)

CLASS, AGENT, GENERIC NAME (TRADE NAME)	USUAL ADULT DOSAGE*	ADVERSE REACTIONS, COMMENTS *(See Table 10B for Summary)*
MISCELLANEOUS AGENTS		
Fosfomycin (Monurol) (3 gm packet)	**3 gm with water po times 1 dose.** For emergency use: single patient IND for IV use. From FDA, 1-888-463-6332.	Diarrhea in 9% compared to 6% of pts given nitrofurantoin and 2.3% given TMP-SMX. Available outside U.S., IV & PO, for treatment of multi-drug resistant bacteria. For MDR-GNB: 6-12 gm/day IV divided q6-8h. Ref: *Int J Antimicrob Ag 37:415, 2011.*
Fusidic acid^NUS (Fucidin, Taksta)	**500 mg po tid (Denmark & Canada)** US: loading dose of 1500 mg po bid x 1 day, then 600 mg po bid	Activity vs. MRSA of importance. Approved outside the U.S.; currently in U.S. clinical trials. Ref for proposed US regimen: *CID 52 (Suppl 7):S520, 2011.*
Methenamine hippurate (Hiprex, Urex) Methenamine mandelate (Mandelamine)	**1 gm po bid** **1 gm po qid**	Nausea and vomiting, skin rash or dysuria. Overall ~3%. Methenamine requires (pH ≤5) urine to liberate formaldehyde. Useful in suppressive therapy after infecting organisms cleared; do not use for pyelonephritis. *Comment:* Do not force fluids; may dilute formaldehyde. Of no value in pts with chronic Foley. If urine pH >5.0, co-administer ascorbic acid (1-2 gm) to acidify the urine; cranberry juice (1200-4000 mL per day) has been used, results ±. Do not use concomitantly with sulfonamides (precipitate), or in presence of renal or severe hepatic dysfunction.
Metronidazole (Flagyl) (250, 375, 500 mg tab/cap) Ref.: *Activity vs. B. fragilis Still drug of choice (CID 50 (Suppl 1):S16, 2010).*	Anaerobic infections: **usually IV, 7.5 mg per kg (~500 mg) q6h (not to exceed 4 gm q24h).** With long T½, can use 15 mg per kg q12h. If life-threatening, use loading dose of IV 15 mg per kg. **Oral dose: 500 mg qid; extended release tabs** available 750 mg	**Common AEs:** nausea (12%), metallic taste, "furry tongue," vaginal & urethral burning. Disulfiram-like reaction (N/V, flushing, tachycardia, dyspnea). Neurologic AEs with high dose/long Rx: peripheral, autonomic and optic neuropathy (*J Child Neurol 21:429, 2006*). Aseptic meningitis, encephalopathy, seizures & reversible cerebellar lesion reported (*NEJM 346:68, 2002*). Also: topical & vaginal gels. Can use IV soln as enema for *C. diff* colitis. Resistant anaerobic organisms: Actinomyces, Peptostreptococci. Once-daily IV dosing of 1,500 mg: rational based on long serum T½; standard in Europe; supportive retrospective studies in adults with intra-abdominal infections (*JAC 19:410, 2007*).
Nitazoxanide	See *Table 13B, page 154*	Absorption ↑ with meals, chronic active liver disease.
Nitrofurantoin macrocrystals (Macrobid, Macrodantin, Furadantin) (25, 50, 100 mg caps)	Active UTI. **Furadantin/Macrodantin 50-100 mg po qid x 5-7 days OR Macrobid 100 mg po bid x 5-7 days** Dose for long-term UTI suppression: **50-100 mg at bedtime**	Nausea & vomiting, much reduced at pH 8 or over. Nausea and vomiting. **Neurologic:** headache, nystagmus, polyneuropathy (with chronic rx), acute ARDS type, **chronic peripheral neuropathy, pancreatitis. Pulmonary reactions** (with chronic rx): acute ARDS type, **chronic desquamative interstitial pneumonia with fibrosis.** Intrahepatic cholestasis & **hepatitis** similar to chronic active hepatitis. Hemolytic anemia in G6PD deficiency. Drug rash, eosinophilia, systemic symptoms (DRESS). Hypersensitivity syndrome reported (*Neth J Med 67:147, 2009*). Concern that efficacy may be reduced and AEs increased with CrCl under 40 mL/min. Should not be used in infants <1 month of age. Birth defects: increased risk reported (*Arch Ped Adolesc Med 163:978, 2009*).
Rifampin (Rimactane, Rifadin) (150, 300 mg cap)	**300 mg po/IV bid or 600 mg po/IV qd.** Rapid selection of resistant bacteria if used as monotherapy	Causes orange-brown discoloration of sweat, urine, tears, contact lens. **Many important drug-drug interactions,** see *Table 22.* Immune complex flu-like syndrome: fever, headache, myalgias, arthralgia—especially with intermittent rx. Thrombocytopenia, vasculitis reported (*C Ann Pharmacother 42:727, 2008*). Can cause interstitial nephritis. Risk-benefit of adding RIF to standard therapies for S. aureus endocarditis (*AAC 52:2463, 2008*). *See also, Antimycobacterial Agents, Table 12B, page 140.*
Rifaximin (Xifaxan) (200, 550 mg tab)	Traveler's diarrhea: **200 mg tab po tid times 3 days.** Hepatic encephalopathy: **550 mg tab po bid.** C. diff diarrhea as "chaser": **400 mg po bid**	For traveler's diarrhea & hepatic encephalopathy (*AAC 54:3618, 2010; NEJM 362:1071, 2010*). In general, adverse events equal to or less than placebo.
Sulfonamides [e.g., sulfisoxazole (Gantrisin), sulfamethoxazole (Gantanol, Truxazole), sulfadiazine]	Dose varies with indications. *See Nocardia & Toxoplasmosis*	**CNS:** fever, headache, dizziness; **Derm:** mild rash to life threatening Stevens-Johnson syndrome, toxic epidermal necrolysis, photosensitivity; **Hem:** agranulocytosis, aplastic anemia. **Cross-allergenicity:** other sulfa drugs, sulfonylureas, diuretics, crystalluria (esp. sulfadiazine–need ≥ 1500 mL po fluid/day); **Other:** serum sickness, hemolysis if G6PD def, polyarteritis, SLE reported.
Tinidazole (Tindamax)	Tabs 250, 500 mg. Dose for giardiasis: **2 gm** po times 1 with food.	**Adverse reactions:** metallic taste 3.7%, nausea 3.2%, anorexia/vomiting 1.5%. All higher with multi-day dosing. Avoid alcohol during & for 3 days after last dose, can cause disulfiram reaction, flushing, N/V, tachycardia.
Trimethoprim (Trimpex, Proloprim, and others) (100, 200 mg tab)	**100 mg po q12h or 200 mg po q24h.**	**CNS:** drug fever, aseptic meningitis; **Derm:** rash (3-7% at 200 mg/day), photoxicity, Stevens-Johnson syndrome (rare), toxic epidermal necrolysis (rare); **Hem:** neutropenia, thrombocytopenia, methemoglobinemia. **Renal:** ↑K+, ↓Na+, ↑Cr; Hem: neutropenia, thrombocytopenia, methemoglobinemia.

(See page 2 for abbreviations)   *NOTE: all dosage recommendations are for adults (unless otherwise indicated) & assume normal renal function.

TABLE 10A (11)

CLASS, AGENT, GENERIC NAME (TRADE NAME)	USUAL ADULT DOSAGE*	ADVERSE REACTIONS, COMMENTS (See Table 10B for Summary)
MISCELLANEOUS AGENTS (continued)		
Trimethoprim (TMP)–Sulfamethoxazole (SMX) (Bactrim, Septra, Sulfatrim, Cotrimoxazole) Single-strength (SS) is 80 TMP/400 SMX, double-strength (DS) 160 TMP/800 SMX	**Standard po rx: 1 DS tab bid. P. carinii:** see Table 11A, page 123. **IV rx** (base on TMP component): standard 8–10 mg per kg IV per day divided q6h, q8h, or q12h. **For shigellosis:** 2.5 mg per kg IV q6h.	Adverse reactions in 10%. GI: nausea, vomiting, anorexia. Skin: Rash, urticaria, photosensitivity. More serious (1–10%): **Stevens-Johnson syndrome & toxic epidermal necrolysis.** Skin reactions may represent toxic metabolites of SMX rather than allergy (Ann Pharmacotherapy 32:381, 1998). Daily ascorbic acid 0.5–1.0 gm may promote detoxification (JAIDS 36:1041, 2004). Rare hypoglycemia, esp. AIDS pts (LnID 6:178, 2006). **Sweet's Syndrome** can occur. TMP competes with creatinine for tubular secretion; serum creatinine can ↑. TMP also blocks distal renal tubule secretion of K⁺. ↑ serum K⁺ in 21% of pts (AnIM 124:316, 1996). Risk of hyperkalemia increased 7x if concomitant ACE inhibitor (Arch Int Med 170:1045, 2010). Discussion of renal injury (JAC 67:1271, 2012). TMP one etiology of **aseptic meningitis.** Report of psychosis during treatment of PCP (JAC 66:1117, 2011). TMP-SMX contains sulfites and may trigger asthma in sulfite-sensitive pts. Frequent drug cause of thrombocytopenia. No cross allergenicity with other sulfonamide non-antibiotic drugs (NEJM 349:1628, 2003). **For TMP-SMX desensitization, see Table 7, page 80.**
Topical Antimicrobial Agents Active vs. S. aureus & Strep. pyogenes (CID 49:1541, 2009). Review of topical antiseptics, antibiotics (CID 49:1541, 2009).		
Bacitracin (Baciguent)	20% bacitracin zinc ointment; apply 1–5 x/day	Active vs. staph, strep & clostridium. Contact dermatitis occurs. Available without prescription.
Fusidic acid¹ⁿᵃ ointment	**2% ointment, apply tid**	Available in Canada and Europe (Leo Laboratories). Active vs. S. aureus & S. pyogenes.
Mupirocin (Bactroban)	**Skin cream or ointment 2%: Apply tid** times 5 days. **Nasal ointment 2%: apply bid** times 5 days.	Skin cream: itch, burning, stinging 1–1.5%; Nasal: headache 9%, rhinitis 6%, respiratory congestion 5%. Not active vs. enterococci or gm-neg bacteria. Summary of resistance: AAC 58:740, 2014. If large amounts used in azotemic pts, can accumulate polyethylene glycol (CID 49:1541, 2009).
Polymyxin B—Bacitracin (Polysporin)	5000 units/gm; 400 units/gm. Apply 1–4x/day	Polymyxin active vs. some gm-neg bacteria but not Proteus sp.. Serratia sp. or gm-pos bacteria. See Bacitracin comment above. Available without prescription.
Polymyxin B—Bacitracin—Neomycin (Neosporin, triple antibiotic ointment (TAO))	5000 units/gm; 400 units/gm; 3.5 mg/gm. Apply 1–3x/day	See Bacitracin and polymyxin B comments above. Neomycin active vs. gm-neg bacteria and staphylococci; not active vs. streptococci. Contact dermatitis incidence 1%; risk of nephro- & oto-toxicity if absorbed. TAO spectrum broader than mupirocin and active mupirocin-resistant strains (DMID 54:63, 2006). Available without prescription.
Retapamulin (Altabax)	1% ointment; apply bid 5, 10 & 15 gm tubes.	Microbiologic success in 90% S. aureus infections and 97% of S. pyogenes infections (J Am Acd Derm 55:1003, 2006). Package insert says **do not use for MRSA** (not enough pts in clinical trials). Active vs. some mupirocin-resistant S. aureus strains.
Silver sulfadiazine	1% cream, apply once or twice daily.	A sulfonamide but the active ingredient is released silver ions. Activity vs. gram-pos & gram-neg bacteria (including P. aeruginosa). Often used to prevent infection in pts with 2nd/3rd degree burns. Rarely, may stain into the skin.

(See page 2 for abbreviations)   *NOTE: all dosage recommendations are for adults (unless otherwise indicated) & assume normal renal function.

TABLE 10B – SELECTED ANTIBACTERIAL AGENTS—ADVERSE REACTIONS—OVERVIEW

Adverse reactions in individual patients represent all-or-none occurrences, even if rare. After selection of an agent, the physician should read the manufacturer's package insert [statements in the product labeling (package insert) must be approved by the FDA]. **For unique reactions, see the individual drug** (Table 10A) For drug-drug interactions, see Table 22.
Numbers = frequency of occurrence (%); + = occurs, incidence not available; 0 = not reported; R = rare, defined as <1%.
NOTE: Important reactions in bold print. A blank means no data found. Any antibacterial can precipitate C. difficile colitis.

ADVERSE REACTIONS (AR) For unique ARs, see individual drug, Table 10A		PENICILLINASE-RESISTANT ANTI-STAPH PENICILLINS			AMINOPENICILLINS				AP PENS				CARBAPENEMS				MONOBACTAMS	AMINOGLYCOSIDES	MISC.	
	Penicillin G, V	Dicloxacillin	Nafcillin	Oxacillin	Amoxicillin	Amox-Clav	Ampicillin	Amp-Sulb	Piperacillin	Pip-Taz	Ticarcillin	Ticar-Clav	Doripenem	Ertapenem	Imipenem	Meropenem	Aztreonam	Amikacin, Gentamicin, Kanamycin, Netilmicin[NUS], Tobramycin	Linezolid	Tedizolid
Rx stopped due to AR						2-4.4			3.2	3.2			3.4	1-5		1.2	<1			0.5
Rash	3	4	4	4	5	3	5	2	1	4	3	2	1-5	+	+	+	2		2	
+ Coombs	3	R	R	R	+	+	+	+	+	+	R	+	+	1	2	2	R			
Neutropenia	R	0	+	R	+	+	+	+	6	+	+	+	R	1	+	+	8		1.1	0.5
Eosinophilia	+	+	22	22	2	R	22	22	+	+	R	R	R	+	+	+	+			
Thrombocytopenia	R	R	R	R	R	R	R	R	+	+	R	R	+				R		3	2.3
Nausea/vomiting		+	0	0	2	3	3	2	2	7	+	1	4-12	3	2	4	R		6/4	8/3
Diarrhea		+	0	0	5	9	10	2	2	11	3	5	6-11	6	2	5	2		8.3	10
↑LFTs	R	R	22	+	R	+	R	6	+	+	+	+	6	6	4	4	2		5-10	6
↑BUN, Cr	R	0	0	0	R	R	R	R	+	0	0	R	0		+	0	0	5-25		
Seizures	R	0	0	+	0	R	R	R	R	R	R	+	See footnote[1]		R	+	+			
Ototoxicity	0	0	0	0	0	0	0	0	0	0	0	0	0	0	R	0	0	3-14		
Vestibular	0	0	0	0	0	0	0	0	0	0	0	0	0	0	0	0	0	4-6		

[1] **All β-lactams in high concentration can cause seizures.** In rabbit, IMP 10x more neurotoxic than benzyl penicillin (JAC 22:687, 1988). In clinical trial of IMP for pediatric meningitis, trial stopped due to seizures in 7/25 IMP recipients; hard to interpret as purulent meningitis causes seizures (PIDJ 10:122, 1991). Risk with IMP ↓ with careful attention to dosage (Epilepsia 42:1590, 2001).
Postulated mechanism: Drug binding to GABA$_A$ receptor. IMP binds with greater affinity than MER.
Package insert, percent seizures: ERTA 0.5, IMP 0.4, MER 0.7. However, in 3 clinical trials of MER for bacterial meningitis, no drug-related seizures (Scand J Inf Dis 31:3, 1999; Drug Safety 22:191, 2000).
In meta-analysis, seizure risk low but greatest with carbapenems vs. other beta-lactams. No difference in incidence between IMP & MER (JAC 69:2043, 2014).

TABLE 10B (2)

CEPHALOSPORINS/CEPHAMYCINS

ADVERSE REACTIONS (AR) — For unique ARs, see individual drug, Table 10A	Rx stopped due to AR	Rash	+ Coombs	Neutropenia	Eosinophilia	Thrombocytopenia	↑PT/PTT	Nausea/vomiting	Diarrhea	↑LFTs	Hepatic failure	↑BUN, Cr	Headache
Cefazolin	1	+	3	+	+		++	1	4	1	0	+	0
Cefotetan		+	+		+		1	4			0	0	
Cefoxitin		2	2	2	3				+		0		3
Cefuroxime		R	R	R	7		R	R	R	4	0		
Cefotaxime		2	6	6	1		R	1	1	0	0		
Ceftazidime		2	4	1	8		+	1	6	R	0	R	
Ceftizoxime		2		+	4	+	R		4	0	0	1	
Ceftriaxone		2	R	2	6	+	+	R	3	3	0	0	R
Cefepime	1.5		14	1		+		1	1	0	0	0	2
Ceftaroline	2.7	3	9.8				4/2	5	2				2
Ceftobiprole[NUS]		2.7		+	+			9.8	9.1/4.8	<2	R	R	4.5
Cefaclor / Cef.ER / Loracarbef[NUS]	R	1		+	+	2		2	1–4	3		+	3
Cefadroxil		+		+	+				+				
Cefdinir	3	R		R	R			15	1	R		R	2
Cefixime		1		R	R	R		7	16	R		+	R
Cefpodoxime	2.7	1	R	R	3			4	7	4		+	4
Cefprozil	2	1	+	R	2	+		4	3	2		R	2
Ceftibuten	2	1	R		5	R		2	3	R		R	R
Cefditoren pivoxil	2	2	R	R	R			6/1	1.4			R	2
Cefuroxime axetil	2.2	R	R	R	1			3	4	2		R	R
Cephalexin		1		3	9						+	+	+

OTHER AGENTS

ADVERSE REACTIONS (AR) — For unique ARs, see individual drug, Table 10A	Rx stopped due to AR	Rash	Nausea/vomiting	Diarrhea	↑LFTs	↑BUN, Cr	Headache
Vancomycin		3				0	5
TMP-SMX	+	+	+	3	+		+
Tigecycline	5	2.4	30/20	13	4	2	3.5
Tetracycline/Doxy/Mino	+	+	+	+	+		+
Telavancin	4		27/14	7		3	3.1
Rifampin	+	R	+	+	+	+	+
Quinupristin-dalfopristin		R		R	2		
Metronidazole	12		12	+			+
Daptomycin	3	2.8	6.3	5	R		
Dalbavancin	2.7	4	6.3	4.4	0.8	R	
Polymyxin B & E (Colistin)	+	+	7			++	
Clindamycin	+	+	+	7	+	0	+
Chloramphenicol	+	+	+		+		+

MACROLIDES / FLUOROQUINOLONES

ADVERSE REACTIONS (AR) — For unique ARs, see individual drug, Table 10A	Rx stopped due to AR	Rash	Nausea/vomiting	Diarrhea	↑LFTs	↑BUN, Cr	Dizziness, light headedness	Headache
Erythromycin	3	+	25	8	+			2
Clarithromycin, Reg. & ER	3	3	3	3–6	R	R	4	2
Azithromycin, Reg. & ER	5	R	3	5	R	R	R	R
Ofloxacin	4	2	2	4	R		3	1
Moxifloxacin	3.8	R	7/2	5	R		2	
Levofloxacin	4.3	2	7/2	5	0.1–1	0	0.8	6
Gemifloxacin	2.2	1–22[a]	2.7	3.6	1.5		3	1.2
Gatifloxacin[NUS]	2.9	R	8/<3	4		R	3	4
Ciprofloxacin / Cipro XR	3.5	R	5	2	R	R	R	1

[a] Highest frequency: females <40 years of age after 14 days of rx, with 5 days or less of Gemi, incidence of rash <1.5%.

TABLE 10C – ANTIMICROBIAL AGENTS ASSOCIATED WITH PHOTOSENSITIVITY

The following drugs (listed alphabetically) are known to cause photosensitivity in some individuals. Note that photosensitivity lasts for several days after the last dose of the drug, at least for tetracyclines. There is no intent to indicate relative frequency or severity of reactions. *Ref: Drug Saf 34:821, 2011.*

DRUG OR CLASS	COMMENT
Azole antifungals	Voriconazole, Itraconazole, Ketoconazole, but not Fluconazole
Cefotaxime	Manifested as photodistributed telangiectasia
Ceftazidime	Increased susceptibility to sunburn observed
Dapsone	Confirmed by rechallenge
Efavirenz	Three reports
Flucytosine	Two reports
Fluoroquinolones	Worst offenders have halogen atom at position 8 (Lomefloxacin, Sparfloxacin)
Griseofulvin	Not thought to be a potent photosensitizer
Isoniazid	Confirmed by rechallenge
Pyrazinamide	Confirmed by rechallenge
Quinine	May cross-react with quinidine
Saquinavir	One report
Tetracyclines	Least common with Minocycline
Trimethoprim	Alone and in combination with Sulfamethoxazole

TABLE 10D – AMINOGLYCOSIDE ONCE-DAILY AND MULTIPLE DAILY DOSING REGIMENS

(See Table 17A, page 205, if estimated creatinine clearance <90 mL per min.)

- General Note: dosages are given as once daily dose (OD) and multiple daily doses (MDD).

- For **calculation of dosing weight** in non-obese patients use **Ideal Body Weight (IBW)**:

  Female: 45.5 kg + 2.3 kg per inch over 60 inch height = dosing weight in kg.

  Male: 50 kg + 2.3 kg per inch over 60 inch height = dosing weight in kg.

- **Adjustment for calculation of dosing weight in obese patients** (actual body weight (ABW) is ≥30% above IBW): IBW + 0.4 (ABW minus IBW) = adjusted weight (*Pharmacotherapy 27:1081, 2007; CID 25:112, 1997*).

- If CrCl <90, *use doses in Table 17A, page 205.*

- If CrCl >90 mL/min, use doses in this table.

- **For non-obese patients, calculate estimated creatinine clearance (CrCl) as follows:**

$$\text{CrCl in mL/min for men} = \frac{(140 \text{ minus age})(\text{IBW in kg})}{72 \times \text{serum creatinine}}$$

Multiply by 0.85 for women (estimated)

- **For morbidly obese patients, calculate estimated creatinine clearance (CrCl) as follows:**

$$\frac{(137 \text{ minus age}) \times [(0.285 \times \text{wt in kg}) + (12.1 \times \text{ht in meters}^2)]}{51 \times \text{serum creatinine}} = \text{CrCl (obese male)}$$

$$\frac{(146 \text{ minus age}) \times [(0.287 \times \text{wt in kg}) + (9.74 \times \text{ht in meters}^2)]}{60 \times \text{serum creatinine}} = \text{CrCl (obese female)}$$

DRUG	MDD AND OD IV REGIMENS/ TARGETED PEAK (P) AND TROUGH (T) SERUM LEVELS	COMMENTS. For more data on once-daily dosing, see AAC 55:2528, 2011 and Table 17A, page 204
Gentamicin (Garamycin), **Tobramycin** (Nebcin)	MDD: 2 mg per kg load, then 1.7 mg per kg q8h P 4–10 mcg per mL, T 1–2 mg per mL OD: 5.1 (7 if critically ill) mg per kg q24h P 16–24 mcg per mL, T <1 mcg per mL	All aminoglycosides have potential to cause tubular necrosis and renal failure, deafness due to cochlear toxicity, vertigo due to damage to vestibular organs, and rarely neuromuscular blockade. Risk minimal with oral or topical application due to small % absorption unless tissues altered by disease.
Kanamycin (Kantrex), **Amikacin** (Amikin), **Streptomycin**	MDD: 7.5 mg per kg q12h P 15–30 mcg per mL, T 5–10 mcg per mL OD: 15 mg per kg q24h P 56–64 mcg per mL, T <1 mcg per mL	Risk of nephrotoxicity ↑ with concomitant administration of cyclosporine, vancomycin, ampho B, radiocontrast. Risk of nephrotoxicity ↓ by concomitant AP Pen and perhaps by once-daily dosing method (especially if baseline renal function normal).
Netilmicin[NUS]	MDD: 2 mg per kg q8h P 4–10 mcg per mL, T 1–2 mcg per mL OD: 6.5 mg per kg q24h P 22–30 mcg per mL, T <1 mcg per mL	In general, same factors influence risk of ototoxicity. **NOTE: There is no known method to eliminate risk of aminoglycoside nephro/ototoxicity. Proper Rx attempts to ↓ the % risk.** The clinical trial data of OD aminogly-cosides have been reviewed extensively by meta-analysis (*CID 24:816, 1997*).
Isepamicin[NUS]	Only OD: Severe infections 15 mg per kg q24h, less severe 8 mg per kg q24h	**Serum levels:** Collect peak serum level (PSL) exactly 1 hr after the start of the infusion of the 3rd dose. In critically ill pts, PSL after the 1st dose as volume of distribution and renal function may change rapidly.
Spectinomycin (Trobicin)[NUS]	2 gm IM times 1–gonococcal infections	Other dosing methods and references: For once-daily 7 mg per kg per day of gentamicin—Hartford Hospital method (may under dose if <7 mg/kg/day dose), see *AAC 39:650, 1995*.
Neomycin–oral	Prophylaxis GI surgery: 1 gm po times 3 with erythro, see *Table 15B, page 193* For hepatic coma: 4–12 gm per day po	One in 500 humans (Europe) have mitochondrial mutation that predicts cochlear toxicity (*NEJM 360:640 & 642, 2009*). Aspirin supplement (3 gm/day) attenuated injury from gentamicin (*NEJM 354:1856, 2006*). Vestibular injury usually bilateral & hence no vertigo but imbalance & oscillopsia (*Med J Aust 196:701, 2012*).
Tobramycin—inhaled (Tobi): See *Cystic fibrosis, Table 1, page 44 & Table 1OF, page 112*. Adverse effects few: transient voice alteration (13%) and transient tinnitus (3%).		
Paromomycin—oral: *See Entamoeba and Cryptosporidia, Table 13A, page 143.*		

TABLE 10E: PROLONGED OR CONTINUOUS INFUSION DOSING OF SELECTED BETA LACTAMS

Based on current and rapidly changing data, it appears that prolonged or continuous infusion of beta-lactams is at least as successful as intermittent dosing. Hence, this approach can be part of stewardship programs as supported by recent publications.

Antibiotic stability is a concern. Factors influencing stability include drug concentration, IV infusion diluent (e.g. NS vs. D5W), type of infusion device, and storage temperature (Ref: P&T 36:723, 2011). Portable pumps worn close to the body expose antibiotics to temperatures closer to body temperature (37°C) than to room temperature (around 25°C). Carbapenems are particularly unstable and may require wrapping of infusion pumps in cold packs or frequent changes of infusion bags or cartridges.

A meta-analysis of observational studies found reduced mortality among patients treated with extended or continuous infusion of carbapenems or piperacillin-tazobactam (pooled data) as compared to standard intermittent regimens. The results were similar for extended and continuous regimens when considered separately. There was a mortality benefit with piperacillin-tazobactam but not carbapenems (CID 56:272, 2013). The lower mortality could, at least in part, be due to closer professional supervision engendered by a study environment. On the other hand, a small prospective randomized controlled study of continuous vs. intermittent pip-tazo, ticar-clav, and meropenem found a higher clinical cure rate and a trend toward lower mortality in the continuous infusion patients (CID 56:236, 2013).

DRUG/METHOD	MINIMUM STABILITY	RECOMMENDED DOSE	COMMENTS
Cefepime (Continuous)	@ 37°C: 8 hours @ 25°C: 24 hours @ 4°C: ≥24 hours	Initial dose: 15 mg/kg over 30 min, then immediately begin: • If CrCl > 60: 6 gm (over 24 hr) daily • If CrCl 30-60: 4 gm (over 24 hr) daily • If CrCl 11-29: 2 gm (over 24 hr) daily	CrCl adjustments extrapolated from prescribing information, not clinical data. Refs: JAC 57:1017, 2006; Am. J. Health Syst. Pharm. 68:319, 2011.
Ceftazidime (Continuous)	@ 37°C: 8 hours @ 25°C: 24 hours @ 4°C: ≥24 hours	Initial dose: 15 mg/kg over 30 min, then immediately begin: • If CrCl > 50: 6 gm (over 24 hr) daily • If CrCl 31-50: 4 gm (over 24 hr) daily • If CrCl 10-30: 2 gm (over 24 hr) daily	CrCl adjustments extrapolated from prescribing information, not clinical data. Refs: Br J Clin Pharmacol 50:184, 2000; IJAA 17:497, 2001; AAC 49:3550, 2005; Infect 37: 418, 2009; JAC 68:900, 2013.
Doripenem (Prolonged)	@ 37°C: 8 hours (in NS) @ 25°C: 24 hours (in NS) @ 4°C: 24 hours (in NS)	• If CrCl ≥ 50: 500 mg (over 4 hr) q8h • If CrCl 30-49: 250 mg (over 4 hr) q8h • If CrCl 10-29: 250 mg (over 4 hr) q12h	Based on a single study (Crit Care Med 36:1089, 2008).
Meropenem (Prolonged)	@ 37°C: <4 hours @ 25°C: 4 hours @ 4°C: 24 hours	• If CrCl ≥ 50: 2 gm (over 3 hr) q8h • If CrCl 30-49: 1 gm (over 3 hr) q8h • If CrCl 10-29: 1 gm (over 3 hr) q12h	Initial 1 gm dose reasonable but not used by most investigators. Ref: Intens Care Med 37:632, 2011.
Pip-Tazo (Prolonged)	@ 37°C: 24 hours @ 25°C: 24 hours @ 4°C: no data	Initial dose: 4.5 gm over 30 min, then 4 hrs later start: • If CrCl ≥ 20: 3.375 gm (over 4 hr) q8h • If CrCl < 20: 3.375 gm (over 4 hr) q12h	Reasonable to begin first infusion 4 hrs after initial dose. Refs: CID 44:357, 2007; AAC 54:460, 2010. See CID 56:236, 245 & 272, 2013. In obese patients (> 120 kg), may need higher doses: 6.75 gm or even 9 gm (over 4 hrs) q8h to achieve adequate serum levels of tazobactam (Int J Antimicrob Agts 41:52, 2013).
Vancomycin (Continuous)	@ 37°C: 48 hours @ 25°C: 48 hours @ 4°C: 58 days (at conc 10 µg/mL)	Loading dose of 15-20 mg/kg over 30-60 minutes, then 30 mg/kg by continuous infusion over 24 hrs. No data on pts with renal impairment.	Adjust dose to target plateau concentration of 20-25 µg/mL. Higher plateau concentrations (30-40 µg/mL) achieved with more aggressive dosing increase the risk of nephrotoxicity (Ref: Clin Micro Inf 19:E98, 2013). Continuous infusion may reduce risk of Vanco nephrotoxicity (CCM 42:2527 & 2635, 2014).

TABLE 10F: INHALATION ANTIBIOTICS

Introductory remarks: There is interest in inhaled antimicrobials for several patient populations, such as those with bronchiectasis due to cystic fibrosis or as a result of other conditions. Interest is heightened by growing incidence of infection due to multi-drug resistant Gram-negative bacilli. Isolates of *P. aeruginosa, A. baumannii,* or *Klebsiella* species susceptible only to colistin are of special concern.

There are a variety of ways to generate aerosols for inhalation: inhalation of dry powder, jet nebulizers, ultrasonic nebulizers, vibrating mesh nebulizers. The vibrating mesh inhalers generate fine particle aerosols with enhanced delivery of drug to small airways *(Cochrane Database of Systematic Reviews 4:CD007639, 2013). Review: Curr Opin Infect Dis 26:538, 2013.*

Inhaled DRUG	DELIVERY SYSTEM	DOSE	COMMENT
Amikacin + Ceftazidime	Vibrating plate nebulizer	AMK: 25 mg/kg once daily x 3 days Ceftaz: 15 mg/kg q3h x 8 days	Radiographic and clinical cure of *P. aeruginosa* ventilator-associated pneumonia (VAP) similar to IV AMK/Ceftaz, including strains with intermediate resistance *(AJRCCM 184:106, 2011).*
Aztreonam (Cayston)	Altera vibrating mesh nebulizer	75 mg tid x 28 days (every other month)	Improves pulmonary function, reduces bacterial load, reduces frequency of exacerbations, and improves symptoms in cystic fibrosis (CF) pts *(Exp Opin Pharmacother 14:2115, 2013).* Cost per treatment cycle about $6670.
Colistin	Various (see comment)	Various (see comment)	Much variability and confusion in dosing. Nebulized colistimethate (CMS) 1-2 million U (33-66 mg colistin base) effective for CF *(Exp Opin Drug Deliv 9:333, 2012).* Adjunctive role for VAP still unclear *(CID 43:S89, 2006; CID 51:1238, 2010).* "High-dose" nebulized CMS (400 mg q8h) via vibrating-mesh nebulizer effective for VAP due to multidrug-resistant *P. aeruginosa* and *A. baumannii (Anesth 117:1335, 2012).* Efficacy of adding inhaled colistin to IV colistin for VAP due to GNB susceptible only to colistin was studied. Colistin: 1 million IU q8h (as CMS) nebulized with either jet or ultrasonic nebulizer. Higher cure rate with combined inhaled plus IV colistin as compared to IV colistin alone *(Chest 144: 1768, 2013).*
Fosfomycin + Tobramycin (FTI) 4:1 wt/wt	eFlow vibrating mesh nebulizer	FTI 160/40 or 80/20 bid x 28 days	Both doses maintained improvements in FEV₁ following a 28-day inhaled aztreonam run-in (vs. placebo) in CF patients with *P. aeruginosa.* FTI 80/20 better tolerated than 160/40 *(AJRCCM 185:171, 2012).*
Levofloxacin	eFlow vibrating mesh nebulizer	240 mg bid x 28 days	Reduced sputum density of *P. aeruginosa,* need for other antibiotics, and improved pulmonary function compared to placebo in CF pts *(AJRCCM 183:1510, 2011).*
Liposomal Amikacin	PARI LC STAR jet nebulizer	500 mg qd x 28 days (every other month)	Company reports Phase 3 study in CF pts with *P. aeruginosa* has met primary endpoint of non-inferiority compared to TOBI for FEV₁ improvement. Insmed website: *http://investor.insmed.com/releasedetail.cfm?ReleaseID=774638.* Accessed November 30, 2013.
Tobramycin (TOBI, Bethkis)	PARI LC PLUS jet nebulizer	300 mg bid x 28 days (every other month)	Cost: about $6700 for one treatment cycle *(Med Lett 56:51, 2014)*
Tobramycin (TOBI Podhaler)	28 mg dry powder caps	4 caps (112 mg) bid x 28 days (every other month)	Improvement in FEV₁, similar to Tobra inhaled solution in CF patients with chronic *P. aeruginosa* but more airway irritation with the powder. Cost of one month treatment cycle about $6700 *(Med Lett 56:51, 2014).*

TABLE 11A – TREATMENT OF FUNGAL INFECTIONS—ANTIMICROBIAL AGENTS OF CHOICE*

TYPE OF INFECTION/ORGANISM/ SITE OF INFECTION	ANTIMICROBIAL AGENTS OF CHOICE		COMMENTS
	PRIMARY	ALTERNATIVE	
Aspergillosis (A. fumigatus most common, also A. flavus and others) (See NEJM 360:1870, 2009; Chest 146:1358, 2014).			
Allergic bronchopulmonary aspergillosis (ABPA) Clinical manifestations: wheezing, pulmonary infiltrates, bronchiectasis & fibrosis. Airway colonization assoc. with ↑ blood eosinophils, ↑ serum IgE, ↑ specific serum antibodies.	Acute asthma attacks associated Rx of ABPA: **Corticosteroids** with ABPA.	For failures try **Itra** 200 mg po bid times 16 wks or longer	Itra decreases number of exacerbations requiring corticosteroids with improved immunological markers, improved lung function & exercise tolerance (IDSA Guidelines updated CID 46:327, 2008).
Allergic fungal sinusitis: relapsing chronic sinusitis; nasal polyps without bony invasion; asthma, eczema or allergic rhinitis; ↑ IgE levels and isolation of Aspergillus sp. or other dematiaceous sp. (Alternaria, Cladosporium, etc.)	**Rx controversial:** systemic corticosteroids + surgical debridement (relapse common).	**Itra** 200 mg po bid times 12 mos or fluconn nasal spray.	Controversial area.
Aspergilloma (fungus ball)	No Rx required or surgical resection. Efficacy of antimicrobial agents not proven.		Aspergillus may complicate pulmonary sequestration.
Invasive, pulmonary (IPA) or **extrapulmonary:** Post-chemotherapy and post-chemotherapy in neutropenic pts (PMN <500 per mm³) but may also be present with neutrophil recovery. Common pneumonia in transplant recipients. Usually a late (≥100 days) complication in allogeneic bone marrow & liver transplantation. High mortality (CID 44:531, 2007). **Typical x-ray/CT lung lesions** (halo sign, cavitation, or macronodules) (CID 44:373, 2007). An immunologic test that detects circulating **galactomannan antigen** is available for dx of invasive aspergillosis (Lancet ID 4:349, 2005). Serum galactomannan relatively insensitive; antifungal rx may decrease sensitivity (CID 40:1762, 2005). Improved sensitivity when performed on BAL fluid. (Am J Respir Crit Care Med 177:27, 2008). **False-pos. tests occur with serum from pts receiving PIP-TZ, Amox-Clav** & with other beta lactams, infection with other fungi, & some blood product conditioning fluid (CID 55:e22, 2012). **Better diagnostic strategy:** combination of serum galactomannan & aspergillus PCR (not routinely available) (LnID 13:519, 2013). **Beta D-Glucan:** in fungal cell wall. Can detect with immunoassay. Many false positives + low sensitivity (JCM 51:3478, 2013).	**Primary therapy** (See CID 46:327, 2008): **Voriconazole 6 mg/kg IV q12h on day 1; then either (4 mg/kg IV q12h) or (200 mg po q12h for body weight ≥40 kg, but 100 mg po q12h for body weight <40 kg (use actual wt). Goal trough (day 4): 1.0–5.5 mg/L associated with improved response rates and reduced adverse effects (Clin Infect Dis 55:1080, 2012).** **Alternative therapies:** **Liposomal ampho B** (L-AMB) 3-5 mg/kg/day IV; OR **Ampho B lipid complex** (ABLC) 5 mg/kg/day IV; OR **Caspofungin** 70 mg/day (JAC 64-840, 2009– based on PK/PD study): 50 mg/day thereafter; OR **Micafungin**^NAI 100 mg bid (JAC 64-840, 2009– based on PK/PD study): OR **Posaconazole**^NAI 200 mg qid, then 400 mg bid after stabilization of disease; OR **Itraconazole** capsules 600 mg/day for 3 days, then 400 mg/day (or 2.5 mg/kg of oral solution once daily).		**Voriconazole** more effective than ampho B. Vori, both a substrate and an inhibitor of CYP2C19, CYP2C9, and CYP3A4, has potential for deleterious drug interactions (e.g., with protease inhibitors). Review concomitant meds. Measure serum level with prolonged therapy or for patients with possible drug-drug interactions. In patients with CrCl <50 mL/min, po may be preferred due to concerns for nephrotoxicity of IV vehicle in renal dysfunction. (Clin Infect Dis 54:913, 2012). **Ampho B: not recommended except as a lipid formulation,** either L-AMB or ABLC. 10 mg/kg and 3 mg/kg doses of L-AMB are equally efficacious with greater toxicity of higher dose (CID 2007; 44:1289–97). One comparative trial found greater toxicity with ABLC than with L-AMB: 34.6% vs 9.4% adverse events and 21.2% vs 2.8% nephrotoxicity (Cancer 112:1282, 2008). Vori preferred as primary therapy. **Caspo:** ~50% response rate in IPA. Licensed for salvage therapy. **Micafungin:** Favorable responses to micafungin as a single agent in 6/12 patients in a primary therapy group and 9/22 in the salvage therapy group (J Infect 53; 337, 2006). **Posaconazole:** 42% response rate in open-label trial of patients refractory/intolerant to conventional therapy (Clin Infect Dis 44:2, 2007). Concern for cross-resistance with azole-non-responders. Measurement of serum concentrations advisable. **Itraconazole:** Itraconazole formulated as capsules, oral solution in hydroxypropyl-beta-cyclodextrin (HPCD), and parenteral solution in HPCD as a solubilizer; and parenteral formulation not licensed for treatment of invasive aspergillosis. 2.5 mg/kg oral solution provides dose equivalent to 400 mg capsules. Measurements of plasma concentrations recommended during oral therapy of invasive aspergillosis: target troughs concentrations > 0.25 mcg/ml. Itraconazole is a substrate of CYP3A4 and non-competitive inhibitor of CYP3A4 with potential for significant drug-drug interactions. Do not use for azole-non-responders. **Combination therapy:** Suggested benefit from combining Vori or Ampho B with an echinocandin, but, to date, no clear clinical benefit (CID 59:1437, 2014).

See page 2 for abbreviations. All dosage recommendations are for adults (unless otherwise indicated) and assume normal renal function

TABLE 11A (2)

TYPE OF INFECTION/ORGANISM/ SITE OF INFECTION	ANTIMICROBIAL AGENTS OF CHOICE		COMMENTS
	PRIMARY	ALTERNATIVE	
Aspergillosis (continued)			
Blastomycosis (CID 46: 1801, 2008) (Blastomyces dermatitidis) Cutaneous, pulmonary or extrapulmonary.	**LAB** 3-5 mg/kg per day, OR **Ampho B** (0.7-1 mg/kg) per day, for 1-2 weeks, **then Itra** oral soln 200 mg tid for 3 days followed by Itra 200 mg tid for 6-12 months	**Itra** oral soln 200 mg tid for 3 days then once or twice per day for 6-12 months for mild to moderate disease: OR **Flu** 400-800 mg per day for those intolerant to Itra.	Serum levels of **Itra** should be determined after 2 weeks to ensure adequate drug exposure. Flu less effective than Itra or posa but once or twice per day. It is unclear but active in vitro. Can look for Blastomyces in antigen in urine as aid to diagnosis.
Blastomycosis: CNS disease (CID 50:797, 2010)	**LAB** 5 mg/kg per day for 4-6 weeks, followed by **Flu** 800 mg per day	**Itra** oral soln 200 mg bid or tid; OR **Vori** 200-400 mg q12h	Flu and vori have excellent CNS penetration, to counterbalance their slightly reduced activity compared to Itra. Treat for at least 12 months and until CSF has normalized. Monitor serum Itra levels to assure adequate drug concentrations. More favorable outcome with Voriconazole (CID 50:797, 2010).
Candidiasis: Candida is a common cause of nosocomial bloodstream infection. C. albicans & non-albicans species show ↓ susceptibility to antifungal agents (esp. fluconazole). In immunocompromised pts where antifungal prophylaxis (esp. fluconazole) is widely used. Oral, esophageal, or vaginal candidiasis is a major manifestation of advanced HIV & represents common AIDS-defining diagnosis. See CID 48:503, 2009 for updated IDSA Guidelines.			
Candidiasis: Bloodstream infection			
Bloodstream: non-neutropenic patient Remove all intravascular catheters if possible; replace catheters at a new site (not over a wire). Higher mortality associated with delay in therapy (CID 43:25, 2006).	**Caspofungin** 70 mg IV loading dose, then 50 mg IV daily; OR **Micafungin** 100 mg IV daily; OR **Anidulafungin** 200 mg IV loading dose then 100 mg IV daily. Note: Reduce **Caspo** dose for renal impairment	**Fluconazole** 800 mg (12 mg/kg) loading dose, then 400 mg daily IV OR Lipid-based ampho B 3-5 mg/kg IV daily; OR **Ampho B** 0.7 mg/kg IV daily; OR **Voriconazole** 400 mg (6 mg/kg) IV twice daily for 2 doses then 200 mg q12h.	**Echinocandin** is recommended for empiric therapy, particularly for patients with recent azole exposure or with moderately severe or severe illness, hemodynamic instability. An echinocandin should be used for treatment of Candida glabrata unless susceptibility to fluconazole or voriconazole has been confirmed. Echinocandin preferred empiric therapy in centers with high prevalence of non-albicans candida species. Echinocandin vs. polyenes or azole associated with better survival (Clin Infect Dis 54:1110, 2012). A double-blind randomized trial of anidulafungin (n=127) and fluconazole (n=118) showed an 88% microbiologic response rate (119/135 candida species) with anidulafungin vs a 76% (99/130 candida species) with fluconazole (p=0.02) (NEJM 356: 2472, 2007). Fluconazole is not recommended for empiric therapy, but could be considered recommended for patients with mild-to-moderate illness, hemodynamically stable, with no recent azole exposure. Fluconazole not recommended for treatment of documented C. krusei; use an echinocandin or voriconazole or posaconazole (note: echinocandins have better in vitro activity than either vori or posa against C. glabrata). Fluconazole recommended for treatment of Candida parapsilosis because of reduced susceptibility of this species to echinocandins. Transition from echinocandin to fluconazole for stable patients with Candida albicans or other azole-susceptible species. **Voriconazole** with little advantage over fluconazole (more drug-drug interactions) except for oral step-down therapy of Candida krusei or voriconazole-susceptible Candida glabrata. Recommended **duration of therapy** is 14 days after last positive blood culture. Duration of systemic therapy should be extended to 4-6 weeks for eye involvement
	Funduscopic examination within first week of therapy to exclude ophthalmic involvement. Ocular disease present in ~15% of patients with candidemia, but endophthalmitis is uncommon (~2%) (CID 53:262, 2011). Intraocular injections of ampho B required for endophthalmitis as echinocandins have poor penetration into the eye. For **septic thrombophlebitis**, catheter removal and incision and drainage and resection of the vein, as needed, are recommended; duration of therapy at least 2 weeks after last positive blood culture.		

See page 2 for abbreviations. All dosage recommendations are for adults (unless otherwise indicated) and assume normal renal function

TABLE 11A (3)

TYPE OF INFECTION/ORGANISM/ SITE OF INFECTION	ANTIMICROBIAL AGENTS OF CHOICE		COMMENTS
	PRIMARY	ALTERNATIVE	
Candidiasis: Bloodstream Infection *(continued)*			
Bloodstream: neutropenic patient Remove all intravascular catheters if possible; replace catheters at a new site (not over a wire).	**Caspofungin** 70 mg IV loading dose, then 50 mg IV daily, 35 mg for moderate hepatic insufficiency; OR **Micafungin** 100 mg IV daily; OR **Anidulafungin** 200 mg IV loading dose then 100 mg IV daily; OR **Lipid-based ampho B** 3–5 mg/kg IV daily.	**Fluconazole** 800 mg (12 mg/kg) loading dose, then 400 mg daily IV or PO; OR **Voriconazole** 400 mg (6 mg/kg) IV twice daily for 2 doses then 200 mg (3 mg/kg) IV q12h.	**Duration of therapy** in absence of metastatic complications is for 2 weeks after last positive blood culture, resolution of signs, and resolution of neutropenia. Perform funduscopic examination after recovery of white count as signs of ophthalmic involvement may not be seen during neutropenia. *See comments above for recommendations concerning choice of specific agents.*
Candidiasis: Bone and joint infections			
Osteomyelitis	**Fluconazole** 400 mg (6 mg/kg) daily IV or PO; OR **Lipid-based ampho B** 3–5 mg/kg daily for several weeks, then oral fluconazole.	**Caspo. Mica** or **Anidula** or **ampho B** 0.5–1 mg/kg daily for several weeks then oral **fluconazole.**	Treat for a total of 6–12 months. **Surgical debridement** often necessary; **remove hardware** whenever possible.
Septic arthritis	**Fluconazole** 400 mg (6 mg/kg) daily IV or PO; OR **Lipid-based ampho B** 3–5 mg/kg daily for several weeks, then oral fluconazole.	**Caspo. Mica** or **Anidula** or **ampho** B 0.5–1 mg/kg IV daily for several weeks then oral fluconazole.	**Surgical debridement** in all cases; removal of prosthetic joints whenever possible. Treat for at least 6 weeks and indefinitely if retained hardware.
Candidiasis: Cardiovascular infections			
Endocarditis *(See Eur J Clin Microbiol Infect Dis 27:519, 2008)*	**Caspofungin** 50–150 mg/day IV; OR **Micafungin** 100–150 mg/day IV; OR **Anidulafungin** 100–200 mg/day IV; OR **Lipid-based ampho B** 3–5 mg/kg IV daily + **5-FC** 25 mg/kg po qid.	**Ampho** B 0.6–1 mg/kg IV daily + **5-FC** 25 mg/kg po qid	Consider use of higher doses of echinocandins for endocarditis or other endovascular infections. Can switch to **fluconazole 400–800 mg orally in stable patients** with negative blood cultures and fluconazole susceptible organism. *See Med 90:237, 2011.* Valve replacement strongly recommended, particularly if prosthetic valve endocarditis. Duration of therapy not well defined, but treat for at least 6 weeks after valve replacement and longer in those with complications (e.g., perivalvular or myocardial abscess, extensive disease, delayed resolution of candidemia). Long-term (life-long?) suppression with fluconazole 400–800 mg daily for native valve endocarditis and no valve replacement; life-long suppression for prosthetic valve endocarditis if no valve replacement.
Myocarditis	**Lipid-based ampho B** 3–5 mg/kg IV daily OR **Fluconazole** 400–800 mg (6–12 mg/kg) daily IV or PO; OR **Caspo. Mica** or **Anidula** *(see endocarditis).*		Can switch to **fluconazole 400–800 mg orally in stable patients** with negative blood cultures and fluconazole susceptible organism. Recommended duration of therapy is for several months.

See page 2 for abbreviations. All dosage recommendations are for adults (unless otherwise indicated) and assume normal renal function

TABLE 11A (4)

TYPE OF INFECTION/ORGANISM/ SITE OF INFECTION	ANTIMICROBIAL AGENTS OF CHOICE		COMMENTS
	PRIMARY	ALTERNATIVE	
Candidiasis: Cardiovascular Infections *(continued)*			
Pericarditis	**Lipid-based ampho B** 3-5 mg/kg daily; OR **Fluconazole** 400-800 mg (6-12 mg/kg) daily IV or po; OR **An echinocandin IV** *(see endocarditis)*		**Pericardial window or pericardiectomy** also is recommended. Can switch to **fluconazole 400-800 mg orally in stable patients** with negative blood cultures and fluconazole susceptible organism. Recommended duration of therapy is for several months.
Candidiasis: Mucosal, esophageal, and oropharyngeal			
Candida esophagitis Primarily encountered in HIV-positive patients Dysphagia or odynophagia predictive of esophageal candidiasis.	**Fluconazole** 200-400 (3-6 mg/kg) mg IV/po daily; OR **echinocandin (caspofungin** 50 mg IV daily; OR **micafungin** 150 mg IV daily; OR **anidulafungin** 200 mg IV loading dose then 100 mg IV daily); OR **Ampho B** 0.5 mg/kg IV daily.	An azole (**itraconazole** solution 200 mg daily; OR **posaconazole** suspension 400 mg bid for 3 days then 400 mg daily or **voriconazole** IV/po 200 mg q12h.	**Duration of therapy** 14-21 days. IV echinocandin or ampho B for patients unable to tolerate oral therapy. For fluconazole refractory disease, itra (80% will respond), posa, vori, an echinocandin, or ampho B. Echinocandins associated with higher relapse rate than fluconazole. ART recommended. Suppressive therapy with fluconazole 200 mg po 3x/wk until CD4 > 200/mm³.
Oropharyngeal candidiasis Non-AIDS patient	**Clotrimazole troches** 10 mg 5 times daily; OR **Nystatin suspension** or pastilles po qid; OR **Fluconazole** 100-200 mg daily.	**Itraconazole** solution 200 mg daily; OR **posaconazole** suspension 400 mg bid for 3 days then 400 mg daily; or **voriconazole** 200 mg q12h; OR an echinocandin (**caspofungin** 70 mg IV loading then 50 mg IV daily; or **micafungin** 100 mg IV daily; or **anidulafungin** 200 mg IV loading dose then 100 mg IV daily); OR **Ampho B** 0.3 mg/kg daily.	**Duration of therapy** 7-14 days. Clotrimazole or nystatin recommended for mild disease; fluconazole preferred for moderate-to-severe disease. Alternative agents reserved for refractory disease.
AIDS patient	**Fluconazole** 100-200 mg po daily for 7-14 days.	Same as for non-AIDS patient for 7-14 days.	ART in HIV-positive patients. Suppressive therapy until CD4 > 200/mm³, but if required fluconazole 100 mg po thrice weekly. Oral itra, posa, or vori for 28 days for fluconazole-refractory disease. IV echinocandin also an option. Dysphagia or odynophagia predictive of esophageal candidiasis.

See page 2 for abbreviations. All dosage recommendations are for adults (unless otherwise indicated) and assume normal renal function

TABLE 11A (5)

TYPE OF INFECTION/ORGANISM/ SITE OF INFECTION	ANTIMICROBIAL AGENTS OF CHOICE		COMMENTS
	PRIMARY	ALTERNATIVE	
Candidiasis: Mucosal, esophageal, and oropharyngeal *(continued)*			
Vulvovaginitis **Non-AIDS Patient**	**Topical azole therapy: Butoconazole 2% cream** (5 gm) q24h at bedtime x 3 days or 2% cream SR 5 gm x 1; OR **Clotrimazole 100 mg vaginal tabs** (2 at bedtime x 3 days) or 1% cream (5 gm) at bedtime times 7 days (14 days may ↑ cure rate) or 100 mg vaginal tab x 7 days or 500 mg vaginal tab x 1; OR **Miconazole 200 mg vaginal suppos** (1 at bedtime x 3 days) or 100 mg vaginal suppos q24h x 7 days or 2% cream (5 gm) at bedtime x 7 days; OR **Terconazole 80 mg vaginal tab** (1 at bedtime x 3 days) or 0.4% cream (5 gm) at bedtime x 7 days or 0.8% cream 5 gm intravaginal q24h x 3 days; or ticoconazole 6.5% vag. ointment x 1 dose. **Oral therapy:** **Fluconazole** 150 mg po x 1, OR **Itraconazole** 200 mg po bid x 1 day.		**Recurrent vulvovaginal candidiasis:** fluconazole 150 mg weekly for 6 months.
AIDS Patient	Topical **azoles** (clotrimazole, buto, mico, tico, or tercon) x3–7d; OR Topical **nystatin** 100,000 units/day as vaginal tablet x14d; OR Oral **flu** 150 mg x1 dose.		For recurrent disease 10-14 days of topical azole or oral flu 150 mg, then **flu** 150 mg po weekly for 6 mos.
Candidiasis: Other infections			
CNS Infection	**Lipid-based ampho B** 3-5 mg/kg IV daily ± 5-FC 25 mg/kg po qid	**Fluconazole** 400–800 mg (6–12 mg/kg) IV or po.	Removal of **intraventricular devices** recommended. Flu 400-800 mg as step-down therapy in the stable patient and in patient intolerant of ampho B. Experience too limited to recommend echinocandins at this time. **Treatment duration** for several weeks until resolution of CSF, radiographic, and clinical abnormalities.
Cutaneous *(including paronychia. Table 1, page 27)*	Apply topical ampho B, clotrimazole, econazole, miconazole, or nystatin 3-4 x daily for 7–14 days. Ciclopirox olamine 1% cream/lotion; apply topically bid x 7–14 days.		
Endophthalmitis /Chorioretinitis • Occurs in 10% of candidemia, thus ophthalmological consult for all pts • Diagnosis: typical white exudates on retinal exam and/or positive vitrectomy culture • Chorioretinitis accounts for 85% of ocular disease while endophthalmitis occurs in only 15% (*Clin Infect Dis* 53:262, 2011).	Chorioretinitis or Endophthalmitis: Lipid-based **Amphotericin B** 3-5 mg/kg daily + **Flucytosine** 25 mg/kg po/IV q12 OR **Voriconazole** 6 mg/kg po/IV q12 x 2 doses and then 4 mg/kg po/IV q12. Consider intravitreal **Amphotericin B** 5-10 mcg in 0.1 mL or intravitreal **Voriconazole** 100 mcg in 0.1 mL for sight threatening disease.	Chorioretinitis or Endophthalmitis: **Fluconazole** 6-12 mg/kg IV daily (poor activity against C. glabrata or C. krusei) and consider intravitreal **Amphotericin B** 5-10 mcg in 0.1 mL for sight-threatening disease. Consider vitrectomy in advanced disease. *Clin Infect Dis* 52:648, 2011.	**Duration of therapy:** 4-6 weeks or longer, based on resolution determined by repeated examinations. Vitrectomy may be necessary for those with vitritis or endophthalmitis (*Br J Ophthalmol* 92:466, 2008; *Pharmacotherapy* 27:1711, 2007).

See page 2 for abbreviations. All dosage recommendations are for adults (unless otherwise indicated) and assume normal renal function

TABLE 11A (6)

TYPE OF INFECTION/ORGANISM/ SITE OF INFECTION	ANTIMICROBIAL AGENTS OF CHOICE		COMMENTS
	PRIMARY	ALTERNATIVE	
Candidiasis: Other infections (continued)			
Neonatal candidiasis	Ampho B 1 mg/kg IV daily; OR Fluconazole 12 mg/kg IV daily.	Lipid-based ampho B 3-5 mg/kg IV daily.	**Lumbar puncture** to rule out CNS disease, **dilated retinal examination**, and **intravascular catheter removal** strongly recommended. Lipid-based ampho B used only if there is no renal involvement. Echinocandins considered 3rd line therapy. **Duration of therapy is at least 3 weeks.**
Peritonitis (Chronic Ambulatory Peritoneal Dialysis) See Table 19, page 214.	Fluconazole 400 mg po q24h x 2-3 wks; or **caspofungin** 70 mg IV on day 1 followed by 50 mg IV q24h for 14 days; or **micafungin** 100 mg IV q24h for 14 days.	Ampho B, continuous intraperitoneal dosing at 1.5 mg/L of dialysis fluid times 4-6 wks.	Remove cath immediately or if no clinical improvement in 4-7 days.
Candidiasis: Urinary tract infections			
Cystitis **Asymptomatic** See CID 52:s427, 2011; CID 52:s452, 2011.	If possible, remove catheter or stent. **No therapy indicated except in patients at high risk for dissemination or undergoing a urologic procedure.**		**High risk patients** (neonates and neutropenic patients) should be managed as outlined for treatment of bloodstream infection. For patients undergoing urologic procedures, flu 200 mg (3 mg/kg) IV/po daily or ampho B 0.5 mg/kg IV daily (for flu-resistant organisms) for several days pre- and post-procedure.
Symptomatic	Fluconazole 200 mg (3 mg/kg) IV/po daily for 14 days.	Ampho B 0.5 mg/kg IV daily (for fluconazole resistant organisms) for 7-10 days.	Concentration of echinocandins is low; case reports of efficacy versus azole resistant organisms (Can J Infect Dis Med Microbiol 18:149, 2007; CID 44:e46, 2007). Persistent candiduria in immunocompromised pt warrants ultrasound or CT of kidneys to rule out fungus ball.
Pyelonephritis	Fluconazole 200-400 mg (3-6 mg/kg) once daily orally.	Itraconazole: 200-400 mg oral soln q24h or 400 mg pulse therapy once daily for 1 week of each month for 6-12 months (or until response)*. Ampho B 0.5 mg/kg daily IV ± 5-FC 25 mg/kg po qid.	**Treat for 2 weeks.** For suspected disseminated disease treat as if bloodstream infection is present.
Chromoblastomycosis (Clin Exp Dermatol, 34:849, 2009). (Cladophialophora, Phialophora, or Fonsecaea). Cutaneous (usually feet, legs); raised scaly lesions, most common in tropical areas	If lesions small & few, **surgical excision or cryosurgery with liquid nitrogen.** If lesions chronic, extensive, burrowing: **itraconazole.**	Itraconazole: 200-400 mg oral soln q24h or 400 mg pulse therapy once daily for 1 week of each month for 6-12 months (or until response)*.	**Terbinafine[NM]** 500-1000 mg once daily alone or in combination with **itraconazole** (800 mg/d) po may be effective. Anecdotal report of efficacy of topical imiquimod 5%: 5x/wk (CID 58:1734, 2014).

See page 2 for abbreviations. All dosage recommendations are for adults (unless otherwise indicated) and assume normal renal function

TABLE 11A (7)

TYPE OF INFECTION/ORGANISM/ SITE OF INFECTION	ANTIMICROBIAL AGENTS OF CHOICE		COMMENTS
	PRIMARY	ALTERNATIVE	
Coccidioidomycosis (Coccidioides immitis) (IDSA Guidelines 2005: CID 41:1217, 2005; see also Mayo Clin Proc 83:343, 2008)			
Primary pulmonary (San Joaquin or Valley Fever): **For pts at low risk of persistence/complication**	Antifungal rx not generally recommended. Treat if fever, wt loss and/or fatigue that does not resolve within 4-8 wks		Uncomplicated pulmonary in normal host common in endemic areas (Emerg Infect Dis 12:958, 2006) Influenza-like illness of 1-2 wks duration.
Primary pulmonary in pts with ↑ risk for complications or dissemination. Rx indicated: • Immunosuppressive disease, post-transplantation, hematological malignancies or therapies (steroids, TNF-α antagonists) • Pregnancy in 3rd trimester. • Diabetes • F antibody >1:16 • Pulmonary infiltrates	**Mild to moderate severity** (EID 20:983, 2014): Itraconazole solution 200 mg po q12h OR **Fluconazole** 400 mg po q24h for 3-12 mos **Locally severe or disseminated disease** **Ampho B** 0.6-1 mg/kg per day x 7 days then 0.8 mg/kg every other day OR **liposomal ampho B** 3-5 mg/kg/d IV, until clinical improvement (usually several wks or longer in disseminated disease), followed by **itra** or **flu** for at least 1 year. Some use combination of Ampho B & Flu for progressive severe disease; controlled series lacking.		Itra may have slight advantage esp. in soft tissue infection. Relapse rates after rx 40%. Relapse rate 1 if f CF titer 1:256. Following CF titers after completion of rx important; rising titer warrants retreatment. **Post rx** without warning/evidence useful in 73% of pts with refractory non-meningeal cocci (Chest 132:952, 2007). Not frontline therapy. Treatment of pediatric cocci to include salvage therapy with Vori & Caspo (CID 56:1573, 1579 & 1587, 2013).
• Dissemination (identification of spherules or culture of organism from ulcer, joint effusion, pus from subcutaneous abscess or bone biopsy, etc.)	**Consultation with specialist recommended:** surgery may be required. Suppression in HIV+ patients until CD4 >250 & infection controlled: flu 200 mg/day po or itra oral soln 200 mg po bid (Mycosis 46:42, 2003).		
Meningitis: occurs in 1/3 to 1/2 of pts with disseminated coccidioidomycosis			
Adult (CID 42:103, 2006)	**Fluconazole** 400-1,000 mg po q24h indefinitely OR **Fluconazole** (po) (Pediatric dose not established, 6 mg per kg q24h used)	**Ampho B** IV as for pulmonary (above) + 0.1-0.3 mg daily intra-thecal (intraventricular) via reservoir device. **OR itra** oral soln 400-800 mg q24h **OR voriconazole** (see Comment)	80% relapse rate, **continue flucon indefinitely. Voriconazole** successful in high doses (6 mg/kg IV q12h) followed by oral suppression (200 mg po q12h)
Child (Cryptococcus neoformans, C. gattii)			
Cryptococcosis (IDSA Guideline: CID 50:291, 2010. **Non-meningeal (non-AIDS)** Risk 57% in the transplant & those receiving other forms of immunosuppressive agents (EID 13:953, 2007).	**Fluconazole** 400 mg/day IV or po for 8 wks to 6 mos **For more severe disease:** **Ampho B** 0.5-0.8 mg/kg per day IV until response then change to **fluconazole** 400 mg po q24h for 8-10 wks course	**Itraconazole** 200-400 mg po solution q24h for 6-12 mos OR (**Ampho B** 0.3 mg/kg per day IV + **flucytosine** 37.5 mg/kg times 6 wks (use ideal body wt)	**Flucon alone 90%** effective for meningeal and non-meningeal forms. Fluconazole as effective as ampho B. Addition of interferon-γ (IFN-γ) b 50 mcg per M² subcut. 3x per wk x 9 wks) to liposomal ampho B assoc. with response in pt failing antifungal rx (CID 38: 910, 2004). Posaconazole 400-800 mg also effective in a small series of patients (CID 45:562, 2007; Chest 132:952, 2007)
Meningitis (non-AIDS)	**Ampho B** 0.5-0.8 mg/kg per day IV + **flucytosine** 37.5 mg/kg (use 25 mg/kg) po q6h until pt afebrile & cultures neg (~6 wks) (NEJM 301:126, 1979), then stop ampho B/flucyt, start **fluconazole** 200 mg po q24h (AnIM 113:183, 1990). OR **Fluconazole** 400 mg po q24h x 8-10 wks (less severe ill pt). Some recommend fluconazole for 2 yrs to reduce relapse rate (CID 28:297, 1999). Some recommend Ampho B plus fluconazole as induction Rx. Studies underway.		**If CSF opening pressure ≥25 cm H₂O, repeat LP ± drain fluid to control pressure.** **C. gattii** meningitis reported in the Pacific Northwest (EID 13:42, 2007); severity of disease and prognosis appear to be worse than with C. neoformans; initial therapy with **ampho B + flucytosine** recommended. C. gattii less susceptible to flucon than C. neoformans (Clin Microbiol Int 14:727, 2008). Outcomes in non AIDS and non-AIDS cryptococcal meningitis improved with Ampho B + 5-FC induction therapy for 14 days in those with neurological abnormalities or high organism burden (PLoS ONE 3:e2870, 2008).

See page 2 for abbreviations. All dosage recommendations are for adults (unless otherwise indicated) and assume normal renal function

TABLE 11A (8)

TYPE OF INFECTION/ORGANISM/ SITE OF INFECTION	ANTIMICROBIAL AGENTS OF CHOICE		COMMENTS
	PRIMARY	ALTERNATIVE	
Cryptococcosis *(continued)*			
HIV+/AIDS: Cryptococcemia and/or Meningitis			
Treatment See *Clin Infect Dis 50:291, 2010 (IDSA Guidelines).* ↓ with ARV but still common presenting OI in newly diagnosed AIDS pts. Cryptococcal infection may be manifested by positive blood culture or positive serum cryptococcal antigen (CRAG; >95% sens). CRAG no help in monitoring response to therapy. With ARV, symptoms of acute meningitis may return: immune reconstitution inflammatory syndrome (IRIS). ↑ CSF pressure (**> 250 mm H₂O**) associated with high mortality, lower with CSF removal. If frequent LPs not possible, ventriculoperitoneal shunts an option *(Surg Neurol 63:529 & 531, 2005).*	**Ampho B** 0.7 mg/kg IV q24h + **flucytosine** 25 mg/kg po q6h for at least two weeks or longer until CSF is sterilized. *See Comment.* **Then** **Consolidation therapy:** Fluconazole 400-800 mg po q24h to complete a 10-wks course then suppression *(see below).* Deferring ART for 5 wks after initiation cryptococcal meningitis therapy significantly improved survival as compared to starting ART during the first 2 wks *(NEJM 370:2487, 2014).*	**Amphotericin B** IV or **liposomal ampho B** IV + **fluconazole** 400 mg po or IV daily. OR **Amphotericin B** 0.7 mg/kg IV q24h alone, **OR Fluconazole** ≥ 800 mg/day (1200 mg preferred) (po or IV) **plus flucytosine** 25 mg/kg po q6h for 4-6 weeks.	Outcome of treatment: treatment failure associated with dissemination of infection & high serum antigen titer, indicative of high burden of organisms and lack of 5FC use during inductive Rx, abnormal neurological evaluation & underlying hematological malignancy. Mortality rates still high, particularly in those with concomitant pneumonia *(Postgrad Med 121:107, 2009).* Early Dx essential for improved outcome *(PLOS Medicine 4:e47, 2007).* Ampho B + 5FC treatment ↓ crypto CFUs more rapidly than ampho + flu or ampho + 5FC + flu. Ampho B 1 mg/kg/d alone much more rapidly fungicidal in vivo than flu 400 mg/d *(CID 45:76&81, 2007).* Use of lipid-based ampho B associated with lower mortality compared to ampho B deoxycholate in solid organ transplant recipients *(CID 48:1566, 2009).* Monitor 5-FC levels: peak 70-80 mg/L, trough 30-40 mg/L. Higher levels assoc. with bone marrow toxicity. No difference in outcome if given IV or po *(AAC 51:1038, 2007).* Failure of flu may rarely be due to resistant organism, especially if burden of organism high at initiation of Rx. Although 200 mg qd = 400 mg qd of flu, median survival 76 & 82 days respectively, authors prefer 400 mg po qd *(BMC Infect Dis 6:118, 2006).* Trend toward improved outcomes with fluconazole 400-800 mg combined with ampho B versus ampho B alone in AIDS patients *(CID 48:1775, 2009).* Role of the azoles uncertain: successful outcomes were observed in 14/29 (48%) subjects treated with posaconazole *(JAC 56:745, 2005).* Voriconazole also may be effective. **When to initiate antiretroviral therapy (ART)?** Defer ART to allow for 5 weeks of anti-fungal treatment. When ART was started 1-2 weeks after diagnosis of cryptococcal meningitis mortality was increased when compared to initiation of ART > 5 weeks after diagnosis *(NEJM 370:2487, 2014).*
Suppression (chronic maintenance therapy) Discontinuation of antifungal rx can be considered among pts who remain asymptomatic, with CD4 >100-200/mm³ for ≥6 months. Some perform a lumbar puncture before discontinuation of maintenance rx. Reappearance of pos. serum CRAG may predict relapse	**Fluconazole** 200 mg/day po [If CD4 count rises > 100-200/mm³ with effective antiretroviral rx. See www.hivatis.org. Authors would dc suppressive rx. Some authorities recommend dc suppressive rx only dc if CSF culture negative.]	**Itraconazole** 200 mg po q12h if flu intolerant or failure. No data on Vori for maintenance.	Itraconazole less effective than fluconazole & not recommended because of higher relapse rate (23% vs 4%). Recurrence rate of 0.4 to 3.9 per 100 patient-years with discontinuation of suppressive therapy in 100 patients on ARV with CD4 >100 cells/mm³.

See page 2 for abbreviations. All dosage recommendations are for adults (unless otherwise indicated) and assume normal renal function

TABLE 11A (9)

TYPE OF INFECTION/ORGANISM/ SITE OF INFECTION	ANTIMICROBIAL AGENTS OF CHOICE		COMMENTS
	PRIMARY	**ALTERNATIVE**	
Dermatophytosis			
Onychomycosis (Tinea unguium) (primarily cosmetic) **Laser rx FDA approved:** modestly effective, expensive (Med Lett 55:15, 2013)/(NEJM 360:2108, 2009) Ref: Am J Clin Derm 15:17, 2014; BMJ 348:g1800, 2014; Clinics Derm 31:544, 2013	**Fingernail Rx Options:** **Terbinafine**[1] 250 mg po q24h (children <20 kg: 67.5 mg/day, 20–40 kg: 125 mg/day; >40 kg: 250 mg/day) x 6 wks (79% effective)[NAI] OR **Itraconazole** 200 mg po bid x 1 wk/mo x 2 mos.[NAI] OR **Itraconazole** 200 mg po q24h x 3 mos.[NAI] OR **Fluconazole** 150–300 mg po q wk x 3–6 mos.[NAI]		**Toenail Rx Options:** **Terbinafine**[1] 250 mg po q24h (children <20 kg: 67.5 mg/day, 20–40 kg: 125 mg/day; >40 kg: 250 mg/day) x 12 wks (76% effective)[NAI] OR **Itraconazole** 200 mg po q24h x 3 mos (59% effective)[NAI] OR **Efinaconazole** 10% solution applied to nail once daily for 48 wks (25–54% effective)[NAI] OR **Itraconazole** 200 mg po bid x 1 wk/mo x 4 mos. (63% effective)[NAI] OR **Fluconazole** 150–300 mg po q wk x 6–12 mos (48% effective)[NAI] OR topical **Tavaborole** (Kerydin) or topical **efinaconazole** (Jublia). Duration of therapy for T. tonsurans; treat for approx. twice as long for M. canis. All agents with similar cure rates (60–100%) in clinical studies. Addition of topical ketoconazole or selenium sulfate shampoo reduces transmissibility (Int J Dermatol 39:261, 2000).
Tinea capitis ("ringworm")[1] (Trichophyton tonsurans, Microsporum canis, N. America, other sp. elsewhere) (PIDJ 18:191, 1999)	**Terbinafine**[1] 250 mg po q24h x 2–4 wks (adults), 5 mg/kg/day x 4 wks (children)	**Itraconazole**[1] 5 mg/kg per day x 2 wks. OR **Fluconazole** 6 mg/kg q wk x 8–12 wks.[NAI] Cap at 150 mg per day for adults **Griseofulvin:** adults 500 mg q24h x 6-8 wks, children 10–20 mg/kg per day until hair regrows.	**Keto** po often effective in severe recalcitrant infection. Follow for hepatotoxicity, many drug-drug interactions.
Tinea corporis, cruris, or pedis (Trichophyton rubrum, T. mentagrophytes, Epidermophyton floccosum) "Athlete's foot, jock itch", and ringworm	**Topical rx:** Generally applied 2x/day. Available as creams, ointments, sprays, by prescription & over the counter. Apply 2x/day for 2–3 wks. Recommend: Lotrimin Ultra or Lamisil AT; contain butenafine & terbinafine—both are fungicidal	**Terbinafine** 250 mg po q24h x 2 wks[NAI] OR **ketoconazole** 200 mg po q24h x 4 wks OR **fluconazole** 150 mg po q wk for 2–4 wks[NAI] **Griseofulvin:** adults 500 mg po q24h times 4–6 wks, children 10–20 mg/kg per day. Duration: 2–4 wks for corporis, 4–8 wks for pedis.	**Keto** (po) times 1 dose was 97% effective in 1 study. Another alternative: **Selenium sulfide** (Selsun), 2.5% lotion, apply as lather, leave on 10 min then wash off, 1/day x 7 day or 3-5/wk times 2-4 wks
Tinea versicolor (Malassezia furfur or Pityrosporum obiculare) Rule out erythrasma—see Table 1, page 54	**ketoconazole** (400 mg po single dose)[NAI] or (200 mg q24h) x 7 days) or (2% cream 1x q24h x 2 wks)	**Fluconazole** 400 mg po single dose of **itraconazole** 400 mg po q24h x 3–7 days	
Fusariosis Third most common cause of invasive mold infections, after Aspergillus and Mucorales and related molds, in patients with hematologic malignancies (Mycoses 52:197, 2009). Pneumonia, skin infections, bone and joint infections, and disseminated disease occur in severely immunocompromised patients. In contrast to other molds, blood cultures are frequently positive. Fusarium solani, F. oxysporum, F. verticillioides and F. moniliforme account for approx. 90% of isolates (Clin Micro Rev 20: 695, 2007) Frequently fatal, outcome depends on decreasing the level of immunosuppression.	**ketoconazole** (400 mg po q24h x 7 days)[NAI] or (200 mg q24h) x 7 days) or (2% cream 1x q24h x 2 wks)	**Posaconazole** 400 mg po bid with meals (if not taking meals, 200 mg qid); OR **Voriconazole** IV 6 mg per kg q12h times 1 day; then 4 mg per kg q12h; PO: 400 mg q12h, then 200 mg q12h. See comments. **Lipid-based ampho B** 5–10 mg/kg/d IV; OR **Ampho B** 1–1.5 mg/kg/d IV.	**Surgical debridement** for localized disease. Fusarium spp. resistance to most antifungal agents, including echinocandins. F. solani and F. verticillioides typically are resistant to azoles. F. oxysporum and F. moniliforme may be susceptible to voriconazole and posaconazole. Role of combination therapy not well defined but case reports of response (Mycoses 50: 227, 2007). Given variability in susceptibilities can consider combination therapy with vori and ampho B awaiting speciation. Outcome dependent on reduction or discontinuation of immuno-suppression. Duration of therapy depends on response; long-term suppressive therapy for patients remaining on immunosuppressive therapy.

[1] **Serious but rare cases of hepatic failure** have been reported in pts receiving terbinafine & should not be used in those with chronic or active liver disease (see Table 11B, page 127).

[2] Use of itraconazole has been associated with myocardial dysfunction and with onset of congestive heart failure.

See page 2 for abbreviations. All dosage recommendations are for adults (unless otherwise indicated) and assume normal renal function

TABLE 11A (10)

TYPE OF INFECTION/ORGANISM/ SITE OF INFECTION	ANTIMICROBIAL AGENTS OF CHOICE		COMMENTS
	PRIMARY	ALTERNATIVE	
Histoplasmosis (Histoplasma capsulatum): See *IDSA Guideline: CID 45:807, 2007*. Best diagnostic test is urinary, serum, or CSF histoplasma antigen. MiraVista Diagnostics (1-866-647-2847)			
Acute pulmonary histoplasmosis	**Mild to moderate disease, symptoms <4 wks:** No rx. If symptoms last over one month: **itraconazole** oral soln 200 mg po tid for 3 days then once or twice daily for 6-12 wks.	**Ampho B** for patients at low risk of nephrotoxicity. Check for drug drug interactions.	
	Moderately severe or severe: Liposomal ampho B, 3-5 mg/kg/d IV or **ABLC** 5 mg/kg/d IV or ampho B 0.7-1.0 mg/kg/d for 1-2 wks, then **itra** 200 mg tid for 3 days, then bid for 12 wks. + **methylprednisolone** 0.5-1 mg/kg/d for 1-2 wks.		
Chronic cavitary pulmonary histoplasmosis	**itra** oral soln 200 mg po tid for 3 days then once or twice daily for at least 12 mos (some prefer 18-24 mos)		Document therapeutic itraconazole blood levels at 2 wks. Relapses occur in 9-15% of patients.
Mediastinal lymphadenitis, mediastinal granuloma, pericarditis; and rheumatologic syndromes	**Mild cases:** Antifungal therapy not indicated. Nonsteroidal anti-inflammatory drug for pericarditis or rheumatologic syndromes. If no response to non-steroidals, **Prednisone** 0.5-1.0 mg/kg/d tapered over 1-2 weeks for 1) pericarditis with hemodynamic compromise, 2) lymphadenitis with obstruction or compression syndromes, or 3) severe rheumatologic syndromes.		
	itra 200 oral soln mg po once or twice daily for 6-12 wks for moderately severe to severe cases, or if prednisone is administered.		
Progressive disseminated histoplasmosis	**Mild to moderate disease: itra** 200 mg po tid for 3 days then bid for at least 12 mos.		Check itra blood levels to document therapeutic concentrations. Check for itra drug-drug interactions.
	Moderately severe to severe disease: Liposomal ampho B, 3 mg/kg/d or **ABLC** 5 mg/kg/d for 1-2 weeks then **itra** 200 mg tid for 3 days, then bid for at least 12 mos.	**Ampho B** 0.7-1.0 mg/kg/d may be used for patients at low risk of nephrotoxicity. Confirm therapeutic itra blood levels. Azoles are teratogenic; itra should be avoided in pregnancy; use a lipid ampho formulation. Urinary antigen levels useful for monitoring response to therapy and relapse
CNS histoplasmosis	**Liposomal ampho B,** 5 mg/kg/d, for a total of 175 mg/kg over 4-6 wks, then **itra** 200 mg 2-3x a day for at least 12 mos. Vori likely effective for CNS disease or itra failures. (*Arch Neurology* 57:1235, 2006).		Monitor CNS histo antigen, monitor itra blood levels. PCR may be better for Dx than histo antigen. Absorption of itra (check levels) and CNS penetration may be an issue; case reports of success with Fluconazole (*Braz J Infect Dis* 12:555, 2008) and Posaconazole (*Drugs* 65:1553, 2005) following Ampho B therapy
Prophylaxis (immunocompromised patients)	**itra** 200 mg po daily. Check for itra drug-drug interactions.		Consider primary **prophylaxis in HIV-infected** patients with < 150 CD4 cells/mm³ in high prevalence areas. Secondary prophylaxis (i.e. suppressive therapy) indicated in HIV-infected patients with < 150 CD4 cells/mm³ and other immunocompromised patients in who immunosuppression cannot be reversed

See page 2 for abbreviations. All dosage recommendations are for adults (unless otherwise indicated) and assume normal renal function

TABLE 11A (11)

TYPE OF INFECTION/ORGANISM/ SITE OF INFECTION	ANTIMICROBIAL AGENTS OF CHOICE		COMMENTS
	PRIMARY	**ALTERNATIVE**	
Madura foot (See *Nocardia* & *Scedosporium*) **Mucormycosis**, & other related species—*Rhizopus, Rhizomucor, Lichtheimia (CID 54:1629, 2012)*. Rhinocerebral, pulmonary due to angioinvasion with tissue necrosis. Key to successful rx: early dx with symptoms suggestive of sinusitis, abnormal facial pain or numbness); think mucor with palatal ulcers &/or black eschars, onset unilateral blindness in immunocompromised or diabetic pt. Rapidly fatal without rx. Dx by culture of tissue or stain: wide ribbon-like, non-septated with variation in diameter & right angle branching. Diabetics are predisposed to mucormycosis due to microangiopathy & ketoacidosis. Iron overload/deferoxamine doses stimulates fungal growth.	**Liposomal ampho B** 5-10 mg/kg/day; OR **Ampho B** 1-1.5 mg/kg/day.	**Posaconazole** 400 mg po bid with meals (if not taking meals, 200 mg po qid)[vii].	**Ampho B** (ABLC) monotherapy relatively ineffective with 20% success rate vs 69% for other polyenes (*CID 47:364, 2008*). Complete or partial response rate 60-80% in **posaconazole salvage protocols** (*JAC 61; Suppl 1: i35, 2008*). Resistant to **voriconazole**: prolonged use of voriconazole prophylaxis predisposes to mucormycosis infections. Total duration of therapy based on response: continue therapy until 1) resolution of clinical signs and symptoms of infection, 2) resolution or stabilization of radiographic abnormalities; and 3) resolution of underlying immunosuppression. Posaconazole for secondary prophylaxis for those on immunosuppression therapy (*CID 48:1743, 2009*).
Paracoccidioidomycosis (South American blastomycosis) *P. brasiliensis (Dermatol Clin 26:257, 2008; Expert Rev Anti Infect Ther 6:251, 2008)*. Important cause of death from fungal infection in HIV-infected patients in Brazil (*Mem Inst Oswaldo Cruz 104:513, 2009*).	**TMP/SMX** 800/160 mg bid-tid for 30 days, then 400/80 mg/day indefinitely (up to 3-5 years); OR **Itraconazole** oral sol'n (100 or 200 mg orally daily)	**Ketoconazole** 200-400 mg daily for 6-18 months; OR **Ampho B** total dose > 30 mg/kg	Improvement in > 90% pts on itra or keto.[viii] **Ampho B** reserved for severe cases and for those intolerant to other agents. TMP-SMX suppression life-long in HIV+. Check for itra or keto drug-drug interactions.
Penicilliosis (*Penicillium marneffei*) Common disseminated fungal infection in AIDS pts in SE Asia (esp. Thailand & Vietnam).	**Ampho B** 0.5-1 mg/kg per day times 2 wks followed by **itraconazole** 400 mg/day for 10 wks followed by **itraconazole** oral soln 200 mg/day **indefinitely for HIV-infected pts.**	For less sick patients **itra** oral soln 200 mg po tid x 3 days, then 200 mg po bid x 12 wks, then 200 mg po bid[ix] (Oral soln better absorbed)	3rd most common OI in AIDS following TBc and crypto-coccal meningitis. Prolonged fever, lymphadenopathy, hepatomegaly. Skin nodules are umbilicated (mimic cryptococcal infection or molluscum contagiosum). *CID 43:1060, 2006.* Preliminary data suggests vori effective: *CID 43:1060, 2006.*
Lobomycosis (keloidal blastomycosis)/*P. loboi*	Surgical excision, clofazimine or itraconazole.		
Phaeohyphomycosis, Black molds, Dematiaceous fungi (*See Clin Microbiol Rev. 77:527, 2014*). Opportunistic infection in immunocompromised hosts (e.g., HIV/AIDS, transplants). Most often presents with skin and soft tissue infection or mycetoma but can cause disease in bone and joint, brain abscess, endocarditis, and disseminated disease. Most clinically relevant species are within the genera of Exophiala, Phialophora, Bipolaris, Cladosporium, Cyphellophora, Fonsecaea, Phialophora, and Rhinocladiella.	**Surgery + itraconazole** oral soln 400 mg/day po, duration not defined, probably 6 mo[viii]	**Voriconazole** 6 mg/kg po bid x 1 day and then 4 mg/kg po bid or Posaconazole (suspension) 400 mg po bid	Both Vori and Posa have demonstrated efficacy (*Med Mycol 48:769, 2010; Med Mycol 43:91, 2005*), often in addition to surgical therapy. Consider obtaining anti-fungal susceptibility testing.
Pneumocystis pneumonia (PCP) caused by **Pneumocystis jiroveci**. *Ref: JAMA 301:2578, 2009.* **Not acutely ill,** able to take po meds. PaO₂ >70 mmHg. Diagnosis: sputum PCR. Serum Beta-D Glucan may help; reasonable sensitivity & specificity, but also many false positives (*JCM 51:3478, 2013*).	**TMP-SMX-DS**, 2 tabs po q8h x21 days OR (**Dapsone** 100 mg po q24h + **trimethoprim** 5 mg/kg po bid x21 days) NOTE: Concomitant use of corticosteroids usually reserved for sicker pts with PaO₂ <70 (see below)	**Clindamycin** 300-450mg po q6h + **primaquine** 15 mg base po q24h) x21 days OR **Atovaquone** suspension 750 mg po bid with food x21 days	Mutations in gene of enzyme target (dihydropteroate synthetase) of sulfamethoxazole identified. Unclear whether mutations result in resist to TMP-SMX or dapsone + TMP (*EID 10:1721, 2004*). Dapsone ref: *CID 27:191, 1998.* **After 21 days, chronic suppression in AIDS pts (see below—post-treatment suppression).**

See page 2 for abbreviations. All dosage recommendations are for adults (unless otherwise indicated) and assume normal renal/renal function

TABLE 11A (12)

TYPE OF INFECTION/ORGANISM/ SITE OF INFECTION	ANTIMICROBIAL AGENTS OF CHOICE		COMMENTS
	PRIMARY	ALTERNATIVE	
Pneumocystis pneumonia (PCP) *(continued)*			
Acutely ill, poxn not possible: PaO2 <70 mmHg. Still unclear whether antiretroviral therapy (ART) should be started during treatment of PCP (CID 46: 634, 2008).	**Prednisone** (15–30 min. before **TMP-SMX**): **40 mg po bid** times 5 days, then **20 mg po q24h** times 11 days] + **TMP-SMX** (15 mg of TMP component per kg per day IV div. q6–8h times 21 days)	**Prednisone** as in primary rx PLUS [Clinda 600 mg IV q8h] q24h)] times 21 days OR **Pentamidine** 4 mg per kg per day IV times 21 days. **Caspofungin** active in animal models, CID 38:1445, 2003	**After 21 days, chronic suppression in AIDS pts** (see post-treatment suppression). **PCP can occur in absence of HIV infection & steroids** (CID 25:215 & 219, 1997). Wait 4–8 days before declaring treatment failure& switching to clinda + primaquine or pentamidine (AIDS 48:63, 2008); or adding dapsone to caspofungin (Transplant 84:685, 2007).
	Can substitute IV prednisone (reduce dose 25%) for po prednisone		
Primary prophylaxis and post-treatment suppression	**TMP-SMX-DS or -SS**, 1 tab po q24h; or 1 DS 3x/wk) OR (**dapsone** 100mg [po q24h] DC when CD4 >200 X3 mos. (*NEJM 344:159, 2001*)	[**Pentamidine** 300mg/4ml sterile water by aerosol q4wks) OR (**dapsone** 200 mg po + **pyrimethamine** 75mg po + folinic acid 25mg po)—**all once a week**) or **atovaquone** 1500 mg po q24h with food.	TMP-SMX-DS regimen provides cross-protection vs toxo and other bacterial infections. Dapsone + pyrimethamine protects vs toxo. Atovaquone suspension 1500 mg once daily as effective as daily dapsone (NEJM 339:1889, 1998) or inhaled pentamidine (JID 180:369, 1999).
Scedosporium species (Scedosporium apiospermum [Pseudallescheria boydii] and S. prolificans) Infection by inhalation or inoculation of skin. Normal hosts often have cutaneous disease. Immunocompromised hosts can have pulmonary colonization –> invasive disease in lung or skin –> disseminated disease.	*Scedosporium apiospermum:* **Voriconazole** 6 mg/kg PO/IV q12h on day 1, then 4 mg/kg q12h. Surgical debridement and reduction of immunosuppression, consider addition of Voriconazole as above although usually usually resistant.	**Posaconazole** 400 mg po bid with meals (may be less active)	Surgical debridement should be considered in most cases. S. apiospermum is resistant Amphotericin B and Scedosporium prolificans is resistant to all antifungal agents. Synergy with Terbinafine and echinocandins have been reported in vitro although clinical data is limited (CID 48:1257, 2009). S. prolificans osteomyelitis responded to miltefosine in a case report. Consider susceptibility testing. Treatment guidelines/review: Clin Microbiol Infect 3:27, 2014. Clin Microbiol Rev 21:157, 2008.
Sporotrichosis *IDSA Guideline: CID 45:1255, 2007.*			
Cutaneous/Lymphocutaneous	**Itraconazole** oral soln po 200 mg/day po for 2–4 wks after all lesions resolved, usually 3–6 mos.	If no response, **itra** 200 mg po bid or **terbinafine** 500 mg po bid or **SSKI** 5 drops po tid & increase to 40–50 drops tid	Fluconazole 400–800 mg daily only if no response to primary or alternative suggestions. Pregnancy or nursing: local hyperthermia *(see below).*
Osteoarticular	**Itra** oral soln 200 mg po bid x 12 mos.		After 2 wks of therapy, document adequate serum levels of itraconazole.
Pulmonary	**Severe**: [**lipid ampho B** 3.5 mg/kg IV or **standard ampho B** 0.7–1 mg/kg IV once daily until response, then **itra** 200mg po bid. Total of 12 mos.	**Less severe:** **itraconazole** 200 mg po bid x total 12 mos.	After 2 weeks of therapy document adequate serum levels of itra. Surgical resection plus ampho B for localized pulmonary disease.
Meningeal or Disseminated	**Lipid ampho B** 5 mg/kg IV once daily x 4–6 wks, then—if better— **itra** 200 mg po bid for total of 12 mos.	AIDS/Other immunosuppressed pts: chronic therapy with **itra** oral soln 200 mg po once daily.	After 2 weeks of therapy document adequate serum levels of itra.
Pregnancy and children	Pregnancy: Cutaneous—local hyperthermia. Severe: **lipid ampho B** 3–5 mg/kg IV once daily. **Avoid itraconazole.**	**Children:** Cutaneous: **Itra** 6–10 mg/kg (max of 400 mg) daily. Alternative is **SSKI** 1 drop tid increasing to max of 1 drop/kg or 40–50 drops tid/day, whichever is lowest.	For children with disseminated sporotrichosis: Standard ampho B 0.7 mg/kg IV once daily & after response, Itra 6–10 mg/kg po daily (max 400 mg) once daily.

See page 2 for abbreviations. All dosage recommendations are for adults (unless otherwise indicated) and assume normal renal function

TABLE 11B – ANTIFUNGAL DRUGS: DOSAGE, ADVERSE EFFECTS, COMMENTS

DRUG NAME, GENERIC (TRADE) / USUAL DOSAGE	ADVERSE EFFECTS/COMMENTS
Non-lipid amphotericin B **deoxycholate** (Fungizone) 0.5–0.7 mg/kg IV per day as single infusion **ampho B predictably not active vs.** Aspergillus terreus & Candida lusitaniae & Aspergillus terreus (TABLE 11C, page 128)	**Admin:** Ampho B is a colloidal suspension that must be prepared in electrolyte-free D5W at 0.1 mg/mL to avoid precipitation. No need to protect suspensions from light. Febrile reactions cause chills/fever, myalgia, anorexia, nausea, rarely hypotension. Postulated due to proinflammatory cytokines, doesn't appear 1 hr infus. Febrile reactions (severe dyspnea, pulm infiltrates) (drug-related) assoc with rapid infus. **Infusion duration usu. 4+ hrs.** No difference found in 1 vs 4 hr infus. except chills/fever occurred sooner with 1 hr infus. Febrile reactions (severe dyspnea, etc.) appear to histamine release (Pharmaco' 23:966, 2003). Rare pulmonary reactions (severe dyspnea, hypoxemia) esp. with rapid infus. **Severe rigors respond to meperidine (25–50 mg).** With repeat doses, slow infusion rate, premed. with diphenhydramine, hydrocortisone (25–50 mg) and heparin (1000 units) had no influence on rigors (Bl/ Haematol 14:403, 2000). Corticosteroids, NSAIDs or high-dose steroids may prove efficacious but their use may risk worsening infection under rx. Fall in serum bicarbonate (may proceed to renal tubular acidosis), ↓ in age. **Toxicity:** Major concern is nephrotoxicity (i.e., NSAIDs). Manifest initially by kaliuresis and **hypokalemia**, then fall in serum bicarbonate (may proceed to renal tubular acidosis), ↓ in renal erythropoietin and anemia, and rising BUN/serum creatinine. Hypomagnesemia may occur. Hypomagnesemia recur. Can reduce risk of renal injury by **(a)** pre- & post-infusion hydration with 500 mL saline **(if clinical status allows salt load)**, **(b)** avoidance of other nephrotoxins, (e.g, radiocontrast, aminoglycosides, cis-platinum), **(c)** use of lipid prep of ampho B.
Lipid-based ampho B products[1]: **Amphotericin B lipid complex (ABLC)** (Abelcet); 5 mg/kg per day as single infusion	**Admin:** Consists of ampho B complexed with 2 lipid bilayer ribbons. Compared to standard ampho B; larger volume of distribution, rapid blood clearance and high tissue concentrations (liver, spleen, lung). Dosage: **5 mg/kg once daily;** infuse at 2.5 mg/kg per hr; adult and ped. dose the same. Saline pre- and post-dose lessens toxicity. Do NOT use an in-line filter. **Toxicity:** Fever and chills 14–18%, nausea 9%, vomiting 8%; serum creatinine ↑ in 11%, renal failure 5%, anemia 4%; ↓ K 5%; rash 4%. A fatal fat embolism following ABLC infusion (Exp Mol Path 177:246, 2004). Majority of pts tolerant of liposomal ampho B. Can tolerate ABLC (CID 56:701, 2013). Do not dilute with saline or mix with other drugs or electrolytes.[2]
Liposomal amphotericin B[1], **LAB**, AmBisome); 3–5 mg/kg IV per day as single infusion. Approved in lipid form (CID 56:701, 2013).	**Admin:** Consists of vesicular bilayer liposome with ampho B intercalated within the membrane. Dosage: **3–5 mg/kg per day** IV as single dose infused over a period of approx. 120 min. If tolerated, infusion time reduced to 60 min (drug footnote[2]). Saline pre- and post-dose lessens toxicity. **Toxicity** (AE): Gen less than with standard ampho B. Nephrotoxicity 18.7% vs 33.7% for ampho B; chills 47% vs 75%, vomiting 31.8% vs 43.9%, rash 24% for both; ↓ Ca 18.4% vs 20.9%, ↓ K 20.9% vs 25.6%, ↓ mg 20.4% vs 25.6%. Acute reactions common with liposomal ampho B, 20–40%, 86% occur within 5 min of infusion, incl chest pain, dyspnea, hypoxia or severe abdom, flank or leg pain; reaction abated at end of 4 hr infusion. All responded to diphenhydramine (1 mg/kg) & interruption of infusion. Reactions may be due to complement activation by liposome (CID 36:1213, 2003).
Caspofungin (Cancidas) 70 mg IV on day 1, followed by 50 mg IV q24h (reduce to 35 mg IV q24h with moderate hepatic insufficiency)	An echinocandin that inhibits synthesis of β-(1,3)-D-glucan. Fungicidal against candida (MIC <2 mcg/mL) including those resistant to other antifungals & active against aspergillus (MIC 0.4–2.7 mcg/mL). Approved indications: empirical rx for febrile, neutropenic pts; rx of candidemia, candida intraabdominal abscesses, peritonitis, & pleural space infections, esophageal candidiasis; & invasive aspergillosis in pts refractory to or intolerant of other therapies. Serum levels on inc. dosages = peak 12, trough 1.3 (24 hrs) mcg/mL. **Toxicity:** remarkably non-toxic. Most common adverse effect: pruritus at infusion site & headache, fever, chills, vomiting, & diarrhea assoc with infusion. ↑ serum creatinine in 8% on caspo vs 21% short-course ampho B in 422 pts with candidemia (Ln, Oct 12, 2005, online). Drug metab in liver & dosage ↓ 35 mg in moderate hepatic insuff. See Table 22, page 218 for drug-drug interactions, esp. cyclosporine (hepatic toxicity) & tacrolimus (drug level monitoring recommended (Pharmacother 24:1408, 2004). **No drug in CSF, urine or vitreous humor of the eye.**
Micafungin (Mycamine) 50 mg IV q24h for prophylaxis post-bone marrow stem cell (trans; 100 mg IV q24h candidemia, 150 mg IV q24h candida esophagitis.	Approved for rx of esophageal candidiasis & prophylaxis against candida infections in HSCT recipients. Active against most strains of candida sp. & aspergillus sp but not as effective vs ampho B for non-albicans species such as C. glabrata & C. krusei. No antagonism seen when combo with other antifungal drugs. No dosage adjust for severe renal failure or moderate hepatic impairment. Watch for drug-drug interactions with sirolimus or nifedipine. Micafungin well tolerated & common adverse events incl nausea 2.8%, vomiting 2.4%, headache 2.4%. Transient ↑ LFTs, BUN, creatinine reported; rare cases of significant hepatitis & renal insufficiency. See CID 42:1171, 2006. **No drug in CSF or urine.**

---

[1] Published data from patients intolerant of or refractory to conventional ampho B deoxycholate. **None of the lipid ampho B preps has shown superior efficacy compared to ampho B in prospective trials (except liposomal ampho B in prospective bone marrow stem cell trans; 100 mg for prophylaxis against candida such as C. glabrata & C. krusei. No dosage adjust for severe renal failure vs ampho B in prospective trials except liposomal ampho B.** Dosage equivalency has not been established (CID 36:1500, 2003).

[2] Comparisons between Abelcet & AmBisome suggest higher infusion-assoc. toxicity (rigors) & febrile episodes (70% vs 36%) but higher frequency of mild hepatic toxicity with AmBisome (59% vs 38%, p=0.05). Mild elevations in serum creatinine were observed in 1/3 of both (Bl/ Hemat 103:198, 1998; Focus on Fungal Inf #9, 1999; Bone Marrow Tx 20:39, 1997; CID 26:1383, 1998).

[3] HSCT = hematopoietic stem cell transplant.

See page 2 for abbreviations. All dosage recommendations are for adults (unless otherwise indicated) and assume normal renal function

TABLE 11B (2)

DRUG NAME, GENERIC (TRADE/USUAL DOSAGE)	ADVERSE EFFECTS/COMMENTS
Anidulafungin (Eraxis) For Candidemia; 200 mg IV on day 1 followed by 100 mg/day IV. Esophageal candida: 100 mg IV x 1, then 50 mg IV once/d.	An echinocandin with antifungal activity (cida) against candida sp. including ampho B- & triazole-resistant strains. FDA approved for treatment of esophageal candidiasis (EC), candidemia, and other complicated Candida infections. Effective in clinical trials of esophageal candidiasis & in 1 trial was superior to fluconazole in rx of invasive candidiasis/candidemia in 245 pts (75.6% vs 60.2%). Like other echinocandins, remarkably non-toxic; most common side-effects: nausea, vomiting, ↓ K & headache in 11–13% of pts. No dose adjustments for renal or hepatic insufficiency. See CID 43:215, 2006. **No drug in CSF or urine.**
Fluconazole (Diflucan) 100 mg tabs 150 mg tabs 200 mg tabs 400 mg IV Oral suspension: 50 mg per 5 mL	IV=oral dose because of excellent bioavailability. **Pharmacology:** absorbed po, water solubility enables IV. For peak serum levels (see Table 9A, page 87). T½ 30hr (range 20-50 hr). 12% protein bound. **CSF levels 50-90% of serum in normals,** ↑ in meningitis. No effect on mammalian steroid metabolism. **Drug-drug interactions common,** see Table 22. Side-effects overall 16% [more common in HIV+ pts (21%)]. Nausea 3.7%, headache 1.9%, skin rash 1.8%, abdominal pain 1.7%, vomiting 1.7%, diarrhea 1.5%. ↑ SGOT 20%. Alopecia (scalp, pubic crest) in ≥400 mg po q24h after median of 3 mos (reversible in approx. 6mo). Rare: severe hepatotoxicity (CID 41:301, 2005), exfoliative dermatitis. **Note: Candida krusei and Candida glabrata resistant to Flu.**
Flucytosine (Ancobon, 5-FC) 500 mg tabs	AEs: Overall 30%. GI 6% (diarrhea, anorexia, nausea, vomiting); hematologic 22% [leukopenia, thrombocytopenia, when serum level >100 mcg/mL. (esp. in azotemic pts)], hepatotoxicity (asymptomatic ↑ SGOT, reversible), skin rash 7%, aplastic anemia (rare—2 or 3 cases). False ↑ in serum creatinine on EKTACHEM analyzer.
Griseofulvin (Fulvicin, Grifulvin, Grisactin) 500 mg, susp 125 mg/mL	Photosensitivity, urticaria, GI upset, fatigue, leukopenia (rare). Interferes with warfarin drugs. Increases blood and urine porphyrins, should not be used in patients with porphyria. Minor disulfiram-like reactions. Exacerbation of systemic lupus erythematosus.
Imidazoles, topical For vaginal and/or skin use	Not recommended in 1st trimester of pregnancy. Local reactions: 0.5-1.5%: dyspareunia, mild vaginal or vulvar erythema, burning, pruritus, urticaria, rash. Rarely similar symptoms in sexual partner.
Itraconazole (Sporanox) 100 mg cap – – – – – – – – 10 mg/mL oral solution – – – – – – – – IV usual dose 200 mg bid x 4 doses followed by 200 mg q24h for a max of 14 days	**Itraconazole tablet & solution forms not interchangeable, solution preferred.** Many authorities recommend measuring drug serum concentration after 2 wks to ensure satisfactory absorption. To obtain highest plasma concentration, tablet is given with food & acidic drinks (e.g., cola) while solution is taken in fasted state; under these conditions, the peak conc. of capsule is approx. 3 mcg/mL & of solution 5.4 mcg/mL. **Peak plasma concentrations after IV injection (200 mg) compared to oral capsule (200 mg): 2.8 mcg/mL (on day 7 of rx) vs 2 mcg/mL (on day 36 of rx).** Protein-binding for both preparations is over 99%, which explains virtual absence of penetration into CSF (not use to treat meningitis). Adverse effects: dose-related nausea 10%, diarrhea 8%, vomiting 5%, & abdominal discomfort 5.7%. Allergic rash 8.6%, ↑ bilirubin 6%, edema 3.5%, & hepatitis 2.7% reported. ↑ doses may produce hypokalemia 8% & blood pressure 3.2%. Delirium, peripheral neuropathy & tremor reported (J Neur Neurosurg Psych 81:327, 2010). **Reported to produce impairment in cardiac function.** Severe liver failure req transplant in pts receiving pulse rx for onychomycosis: FDA reports 24 cases with 11 deaths out of 50 mil people who received the drug prior to 2001. Other concern, as with fluconazole and ketoconazole, is **drug-drug interactions;** see Table 22. Some can be life-threatening.
Ketoconazole (Nizoral) 200 mg tab	**Gastric acid required for absorption**—cimetidine, omeprazole, antacids block absorption. In achlorhydria, dissolve tablet in 4 mL 0.2N HCl, drink with a straw. Coca-Cola ↑ absorption by 65%. CSF levels 'none'. **Drug-drug interactions important,** see Table 22. **Some interactions can be life-threatening. Dose-dependent nausea and vomiting.** Liver toxicity of hepatocellular type reported in about 1:10,000 exposed pts—usually after several days to weeks of exposure. At doses of ≥800 mg/day serum testosterone and plasma cortisol levels fall. With high doses, adrenal (Addisonian) crisis reported.
Miconazole (Monistat IV) 200 mg—not available in U.S.	IV miconazole indicated in patient critically ill with Scedosporium (Pseudallescheria boydii) infection. Very toxic due to vehicle needed to get drug into solution. Less effective than imidazoles and triazoles. PO: large doses give occasional GI distress and diarrhea.
Nystatin (Mycostatin) 30 gm cream 500,000 units oral tab	Topical: virtually no adverse effects.

See page 2 for abbreviations. All dosage recommendations are for adults (unless otherwise indicated) and assume normal renal function

TABLE 11B (3)

DRUG NAME, GENERIC (TRADE)/USUAL DOSAGE	ADVERSE EFFECTS/COMMENTS
Posaconazole (*Noxafil*) Suspension (40 mg/mL): **400 mg po bid with meals (if not taking meals, 200 mg po tid (with food)** for prophylaxis. Delayed-release tablets (100 mg): 300 mg bid x 1 day and then 300 mg daily for prophylaxis. Intravenous formulation: 300 mg IV bid x 1 day, then 300 mg daily (prophylaxis). Takes 7–10 days to achieve steady state. No IV formulation.	An oral triazole with activity against a wide range of fungi refractory to other antifungal rx including: aspergillosis, mucormycosis (variability by species), fusariosis, Scedosporium (Pseudallescheria), phaeohyphomycosis, histoplasmosis, refractory candidiasis, refractory cryptococcosis, & refractory chromoblastomycosis. Approved for prophylaxis of invasive aspergillus and candidiasis. Clinical response in 75% of 176 AIDS pts with azole-refractory oral/esophageal candidiasis. Posaconazole has similar toxicities as other triazoles: nausea 9%, vomiting 6%, abd. pain 5%, headache 5%, diarrhea, ↑ ALT, AST, & rash (3% each). In pts for >6 mos., serious side-effects have included adrenal insufficiency (AAC 53:24, 2009). **100 mg delayed-release tablets:** loading dose of 300 mg (three 100 mg delayed-release tablets) twice daily on the first day, followed by a once-daily maintenance dose of 300 mg (three 100 mg delayed-release tablets) starting on the second day of therapy. Approved for prophylaxis only and not treatment. Tablets allow patients to achieve better levels than the suspension. Treatment dose unknown but prophylactic dose often achieves therapeutic levels. The tablet and solution are not interchangeable. Intravenous formulation: 300 mg IV daily after a loading dose at 300 mg IV daily x 1 day. Consider therapeutic drug monitoring with a goal trough of > 0.7 for prophylaxis and > 1.0 for treatment. *JAC 69:1162, 2014.*
Terbinafine (*Lamisil*) 250 mg tab	In pts given terbinafine for onychomycosis, rare cases (8) of idiosyncratic & symptomatic hepatic injury & more rarely liver failure leading to death or liver transplant. The drug is **not recommended** for pts with **chronic or active liver disease;** hepatotoxicity may occur in pts with or without pre-existing disease. Pretreatment serum transaminases (ALT & AST) advised & alternate rx used for those with abnormal serum transaminases. Pts started on terbinafine should be warned about symptoms suggesting liver dysfunction (persistent nausea, anorexia, fatigue, vomiting, RUQ pain, jaundice, dark urine or pale stools). If symptoms develop, drug should be discontinued & liver function immediately evaluated. In controlled trials, changes in ocular lens and retina reported—clinical significance unknown. Major drug-drug interaction is 100%. ↑ in rate of clearance by rifampin, inhibits CYP3A4 (*see Table 22*). % with AE, terbinafine vs placebo: nausea/diarrhea 2.6–5.6 vs 2.9; rash 5.6 vs 2.7; taste abnormality 2.8 vs 0.7. Inhibits CYP2D6 enzymes (*see Table 22*). An acute generalized exanthematous pustulosis and subacute cutaneous lupus erythematosus reported.
Voriconazole (*Vfend*) IV: **Loading dose 6 mg per kg q12h times 1 day, then 4 mg per kg q12h IV** for invasive aspergillus & serious mold infections; **3 mg per kg IV q12h** for serious candida infections. **Oral: >40 kg body weight:** 400 mg po q12h, then 200 mg po q12h. **<40 kg body weight:** 200 mg po q12h, then 100 mg po q12h **Take oral dose 1 hour before or 1 hour after eating.** Oral suspension (40 mg per mL). Oral suspension dosing: Same as for oral tabs. Reduce to ½ maintenance dose for moderate hepatic insufficiency	A triazole with activity against Aspergillus sp. **including Ampho resistant strains of A. terreus.** Active vs Candida sp. (including krusei), Fusarium sp. & various molds. Steady state serum levels reach 2.5–4 mcg per mL. Up to 20% of patients with subtherapeutic levels with oral administration; check levels for suspected treatment failure. In life threatening infections, serum levels may be required to achieve target steady-state drug concentrations. Pts started on terbinafine should be warned about symptoms 1–6 mcg/mL. **Toxicity** similar to other azoles including uncommon serious hepatic toxicity (hepatitis, cholestasis & fulminant hepatic failure. Liver function tests should be monitored during rx & drug dc'd if abnormalities develop. Photosensitivity is common and can be severe. Many reports of associated skin cancers. Strongly recommend sun protective measures. *CID 58:997, 2014* & hallucinations & anaphylactoid infusion reactions with fever and hypertension. 1 case of QT prolongation with ventricular tachycardia in a 15 y/o pt with ALL reported. **Approx. 21% experience a transient** visual change (often in first dose of rx or within 30 min) after (altered/enhanced visual perception", blurred or colored visual change, photophobia) within 30–60 min after start of drug. **Do not drive at night.** Persistent visual changes occur rarely. Cause unknown. In patients with CrCl <50 per min, IV vehicle (SBECD-sulfobutylether-B cyclodextrin) may accumulate but not obviously toxic (*CID 54:913, 2012*). Hallucinations, hypoglycemia, electrolyte disturbance & pneumonitis attributed to ↑ drug concentrations. Potential for drug-drug interactions high—*see Table 22.* **With prolonged use, fluoride in drug can cause a painful periostitis.** *(CID 59:1237, 2014).* **NOTE: Not in urine in active form. No activity vs. mucormycosis.**

See page 2 for abbreviations. All dosage recommendations are for adults (unless otherwise indicated) and assume normal renal function

TABLE 11C – AT A GLANCE SUMMARY OF SUGGESTED ANTIFUNGAL DRUGS AGAINST TREATABLE PATHOGENIC FUNGI

Microorganism	Antifungal[1,2,3,4]					
	Fluconazole[5]	Itraconazole	Voriconazole	Posaconazole	Echinocandin[6]	Amphotericin
Candida albicans	+++	+++	+++	+++	+++	++
Candida dubliniensis	+++	+++	+++	+++	+++	++
Candida glabrata	±	±	++	++	+++	++
Candida tropicalis	+++	+++	+++	+++	+++	++
Candida parapsilosis[7]	+++	+++	+++	+++	++ (higher MIC)	++
Candida krusei	-	++	++	++	+++	++
Candida guilliermondii	-/±	++	+++	+++	++ (higher MIC)	++
Candida lusitaniae	+	+	++	++	++	-[8]
Cryptococcus neoformans	+++	+++	+++	+++	-	+++
Aspergillus fumigatus[9]	-	++	+++	+++	++	+++
Aspergillus flavus[9]	-	++	+++	+++	++	++ (higher MIC)
Aspergillus terreus	-	++	+++	+++	++	-
Fusarium sp.	-	±	++	++	-	++ (lipid formulations)
Scedosporium apiospermum (Pseudallescheria boydii)	-		++	++	-	-
Scedosporium prolificans[10]	-	-	±	±	-	-
Trichosporon spp.	±	-	++	++	-	+
Mucormycosis (e.g. Mucor, Rhizopus, Lichtheimia)	-	-	-	++	-	++ (lipid formulations)
Dematiaceous molds[11] (e.g., Alternaria, Bipolaris, Curvularia, Exophiala)	-	++	++	++	+	+
Dimorphic Fungi						
Blastomyces dermatitidis	++	+++	++	++		+++
Coccidioides immitis/posadasii	+++	+++	++	+++		+++
Histoplasma capsulatum	+	+++	++	++		+++
Sporothrix schenckii	-	++	-	+		+++

- = no activity; ± = possibly activity; + = active (least active clinically), 3rd line therapy (least active clinically)

++ = Active, 2nd line therapy (less active clinically); +++ = Active, 1st line therapy (usually active clinically)

1 Minimum inhibitory concentration values do not always predict clinical outcome.
2 Echinocandins, voriconazole, posaconazole and polyenes have poor urine penetration.
3 During severe immune suppression, success requires immune reconstitution.
4 **Flucytosine** has activity against Candida sp., Cryptococcus sp., and dematiaceous molds, but is primarily used in combination therapy.
5 For infections secondary to Candida sp., patients with prior triazole therapy have higher likelihood of triazole resistance.
6 Echinocandin pharmacodynamics, see JAC 65:1108, 2010.
7 Successful treatment of infections from Candida parapsilosis requires removal of foreign body or intravascular device.
8 Treatment failures reported, even for susceptible strains.
9 Lipid formulations of amphotericin may have greater activity against A. fumigatus and A. flavus (+++).
10 Scedosporium prolificans is poorly susceptible to single agents and may require combination therapy (e.g. addition of terbinafine).
11 Infections from mucormycosis, some Aspergillus sp. and dematiaceous molds often require surgical debridement.

TABLE 12A – TREATMENT OF MYCOBACTERIAL INFECTIONS*

Tuberculin skin test (TST). Same as PPD [Chest 138:1456, 2010].

Criteria for positive TST after 5 tuberculin units (intermediate PPD) read at 48–72 hours:

- ≥5 mm induration: + HIV, immunosuppressed, ≥15 mg prednisone per day, healed TBc on chest x-ray, recent close contact
- ≥10 mm induration: foreign-born, countries with high prevalence; IVD Users; low income; NH residents; chronic illness; silicosis
- ≥15 mm induration: otherwise healthy

Two-stage to detect sluggish positivity: If 1st PPD + but <10 mm, repeat intermediate PPD in 1 wk. Response to 2nd PPD can also happen in 1 wk. Prior BCG may result in booster effect in 2-stage TST.

BCG vaccine as child: if ≥10 mm induration, & from country with TBc, should be attributed to MTB.

Routine anergy testing not recommended.

Interferon Gamma Release Assays (IGRAs): IGRAs detect sensitivities to MTB by measuring IFN-γ release in response to MTB antigens. May be used in place of TST in all situations in which TST may be used (MMWR 59 (RR–5), 2010). FDA approved tests available in the U.S.:

- QuantiFERON-TB Gold (QFT-G) (approved 2005)
- QuantiFERON-TB Gold In-Tube Test (QFT-GIT) (approved 2007)
- T-Spot (approved 2008)

IGRAs are relatively specific for MTB and do not cross-react with BCG or most nontuberculous mycobacteria. CDC recommends IGRA over TST for persons unlikely to return to TST & for follow-up testing since IGRAs do not produce "booster effect". May also be used without preference over TBc for occupational exposure. As with TST, testing with IGRAs in low prevalence populations will persons who have received BCG. TST is preferred in children age < 5 yrs (but IGRA is acceptable). IGRA or TST may be used without preference for recent contacts of TB with special utility for follow-up testing since IGRAs do not produce "booster effect". May also be used without preference over TBc for occupational exposure. As with TST, testing with IGRAs in low prevalence settings, inflating positivity and conversion rates, and result in false-positive results (CID 53:234, 2011). Manufacturer's IFN-gamma cutoff ≥0.35 IU/ml for QFT-GIT may be too low for low prevalence settings. A higher cut-off may be more appropriate (Am J Respir Crit Care Med 188:1005, 2013). For detailed discussion of IGRAs, see MMWR 59 (RR–5), 2010 and JAMA 308:241, 2012.

Rapid (24-hr or less) diagnostic tests for MTB: (1) the AMPLICOR Mycobacterium tuberculosis Test amplifies and detects MTB ribosomal RNA; (2) the AMPLIFIED Mycobacterium tuberculosis Direct Test amplifies and detects MTB DNA. Both tests have sensitivities & specificities >95% in sputum samples that are AFB-positive. In negative smears, specificity remains >95% but sensitivity is 40–77% (MMWR 58:7, 2009; CID 49:46, 2009) to 60–90% (see: http://www.cdc.gov/tb/publications/guidelines/amplification_tests/default.htm) (3) COBAS TaqMan MTB Test: real-time PCR test for detection of M. tuberculosis in respiratory specimens (not available in the U.S.) with performance characteristics similar to other rapid tests (J Clin Microbiol 51:3225, 2013).

Xpert MTB/RIF is a rapid test (2 hrs) for MTB in sputum samples which also detects RIF resistance with specificity of 99.2% and sensitivity of 72.5% in smear negative patients (NEJM 363:1005, 2011).
Current antibody-based and ELISA-based rapid tests for TBc not recommended by WHO because they are less accurate than microscopy ± culture (Lancet ID 11:736, 2011).

CAUSATIVE AGENT/DISEASE	MODIFYING CIRCUMSTANCES	SUGGESTED REGIMENS		
		INITIAL THERAPY	CONTINUATION PHASE OF THERAPY	
I. Mycobacterium tuberculosis exposure baseline TST/IGRA negative (household members & other close contacts of potentially infectious cases)	Neonate– Rx essential NOTE: If fever, abnormal CXR (pleural effusion, hilar adenopathy), infiltrate at baseline, treat for active TBc and rx with INH above.	INH (10 mg/kg/ day for 8–10 wks)	Repeat tuberculin skin test (TST) in 8–12 wks: If TST neg & infant age at exposure > 6 mos., stop INH, if TST (≥ 5 mm) or age ≤ 6 mos., treat with INH for total of 9 mos. If follow-up CXR abnormal, treat for active TBc.	
	As for neonate for 1st # (see below)		If repeat TST at 8–10 wks is negative, stop. If repeat TST ≥ 5 mm, continue INH for total of 9 mos. If INH not given initially, repeat TST at 3 mos., **If + Rx** with INH for 9 mos. (see Category 6 below).	
	Children <5 years of age—Rx indicated			
	Older children & adults— Risk 2–4%/¹yr		Pts at high risk of progression (e.g., HIV+, immunosuppressed or on immunosuppressive therapy) and no evidence of active infection should be treated for LTBI (see below). For others repeat TST/IGRA at 8–10 wks: no rx if repeat TST/IGRA neg.	

See page 2 for abbreviations   * Dosages are for adults (unless otherwise indicated) and assume normal renal function   † **DOT** = directly observed therapy

TABLE 12A (2)

CAUSATIVE AGENT/DISEASE	MODIFYING CIRCUMSTANCES	SUGGESTED REGIMENS	
		INITIAL THERAPY	ALTERNATIVE
II. Latent tuberculosis), infection (LTBI), positive TST or IGRA as above, active TB ruled out See FIGURE 1 for treatment algorithm for pt with abnormal baseline CXR (e.g., upper lobe fibronodular disease suspected active Tbc.) Review: NEJM 364:1414, 2011.	Age no longer an exclusion, all persons with LTBI should be offered therapy. If pre-anti-TNF therapy, recommend at least one month of treatment for LBTI prior to start of anti-TNF therapy (Arth Care & Res 64:625, 2012). Overall, regimens containing a rifamycin (RIF, RFB or RFP) are most effective at preventing active tuberculosis (AnnIM 161:419 & 449, 2014).	**INH** po once daily (adult: 5 mg/kg, max 300 mg/day; child: 10-15 mg/kg/day not to exceed 300 mg/day) x 9 mos. For current recommendations for monitoring hepatotoxicity on INH see MMWR 59:227, 2010. Supplemental pyridoxine 50 mg/day for HIV+ patients. A 12 dose once weekly DOT **INH + Rifapentine (RFP)**: **INH** po 15 mg/kg (max dose 900 mg); **RFP** po (wt-based dose): 10-14 kg: 300 mg; 14.1-25 kg: 450 mg; 25.1-32 kg: 600 mg; 32.1-49.9 kg: 750 mg; ≥50 kg: 900 mg. Not recommended for children age < 2 yrs; pts with HIV/AIDS on ART; pregnant women; or pts presumed infected with INH- or RIF-resistant MTB (MMWR 60:1650, 2011, NEJM 365:2155, 2011).	**INH** 300 mg once daily for 6 mo (but slightly less effective than 9 mos.; not recommended in children, HIV+ persons, or those with fibrotic lesions on chest film). **INH** 2x/wk (adult: 15 mg/kg, max 900 mg; child: 20-30 mg/kg, max dose 900 mg) x 9 mo. **RIF** once daily po (adult: 10 mg/kg/day, max dose 600 mg/day; child: 10-20 mg/kg/day, max dose 600 mg/day) for 4 mos. **INH + RIF** once daily x 3 mos.
	Pregnancy	Regimens as above. Once active disease is excluded may delay initiation of therapy until after delivery unless patient is recent contact to an active case, HIV+. Supplemental pyridoxine 10-25 mg/d recommended	
LTBI, suspected INH-resistant organism		**RIF** once daily po (adult: 10 mg/kg/day, max dose 600 mg/day; child: 10-20 mg/kg/day, max dose 600 mg/day) for 4 mos.	**RFB** 300 mg once daily po may be substituted for RIF (in HIV+ patient on anti-retrovirals, dose may need to be adjusted for drug interactions).
LTBI, suspected INH and RIF resistant organism		**Moxi:** 400 mg ± **EMB** 15 mg/kg once daily x 12 months	**Levo**: 500 mg once daily + (**EMB** 15 mg/kg or **PZA** 25 mg/kg) once daily x 12 months.

* Dosages are for adults (unless otherwise indicated) and assume normal renal function

See page 2 for abbreviations

¹ **DOT** = directly observed therapy

131

TABLE 12A (3)

CAUSATIVE AGENT/DISEASE

III. Mycobacterium tuberculosis
A. Pulmonary TB
General reference on rx in adults & children: MMWR 52 (RR-11):1, 2003. In pts with newly diagnosed HIV and TB, Rx for both should be started as soon as possible (NEJM 362:697, 2010).

Isolation essential! Hospitalized pts with suspected or documented active TB should be isolated in single rooms using airborne precautions until deemed non-infectious. DC isolation if 3 negative AFB smears at 8–12 hr intervals (NEJM 312:1353 & 1361, 2014).

USE DOT REGIMENS IF POSSIBLE
(continued on next page)

MODIFYING CIRCUMSTANCES: Rate of INH resistance known to be <4% (drug-susceptible organisms).

SUGGESTED REGIMENS — SEE COMMENTS FOR DOSAGE

INITIAL THERAPY

Regimen (in order of preference)	Drugs	Interval/Doses (min. duration)
1 (See Figure 2 page 135)	INH RIF PZA EMB	7 days per wk times 56 doses (8 wks) or 5 days per wk (DOT) times 40 doses (8 wks). If cavitary disease, treat for 9 mos. Fixed dose combination of INH, RIF, PZA & EMB currently being evaluated (JAMA 305:1415, 2011)
2 (See Figure 2 page 135)	INH RIF PZA EMB	7 days per wk times 14 doses (2 wks), then 2 times per wk times 12 doses (6 wks) or 5 days per wk (DOT) times 10 doses (2 wks) then 2 times per wk times 12 doses (6 wks)
3 (See Figure 2 page 135)	INH RIF PZA EMB	3 times per wk times 24 doses (8 wks)
4 (See Figure 2 page 135)	INH RIF EMB	7 days per wk times 56 doses (8 wks) or 5 days per wk (DOT) times 40 doses (8 wks)

CONTINUATION PHASE OF THERAPY AND DIRECTLY OBSERVED THERAPY (DOT) REGIMENS (in vitro susceptibility known)

Regimen	Drugs	Interval/Doses (min. duration)	Range of Total Doses (min. duration)
1a	INH/RIF	7 days per wk times 126 doses (18 wks) or 5 days per wk (DOT) times 90 doses (18 wks)	182–130 (26 wks)
1b	INH/RIF	2 times per wk times 36 doses (18 wks)	92–76 (26 wks) (Not AIDS pts)
1c	INH/RFP	1 time per wk times 18 doses (18 wks) (only if HIV-neg)	74–58 (26 wks)
2a	INH/RIF	2 times per wk times 36 doses (18 wks)	62–58 (26 wks) (Not AIDS pts)
2b	INH/RFP	1 time per wk times 18 doses (18 wks) (only if HIV-neg)	44–40 (26 wks)
3a	INH/RIF	3 times per wk times 54 doses (18 wks)	~78 (26 wks)
4a	INH/RIF	7 days per wk times 217 doses (31 wks) or 5 days per wk (DOT) times 155 doses (31 wks)	273–195 (39 wks)
4b	INH/RIF	2 times per wk times 62 doses (31 wks)	118–102 (39 wks)

COMMENTS

Dose in mg per kg (max. q24h dose)

Regimen* Q24h	INH	RIF	PZA	EMB	SM	RFB
Child	10–20 (300)	10–20 (600)	15–30 (2000)	15–25	20–40 (1000)	10–20
Adult	5 (300)	10 (600)	15–30 (2000)	15–25	15–25 (1000)	5 (300)
2 times per wk (DOT):						
Child	20–40 (900)	10–20 (600)	50–70 (4000)	50	25–30 (1500)	10–20 (300)
Adult	15 (900)	10 (600)	50–70 (4000)	50	25–30 (1500)	5 (300)
3 times per wk (DOT):						
Child	20–40 (900)	10–20 (600)	50–70 (3000)	25–30	25–30 (1500)	NA
Adult	15 (900)	10 (600)	50–70 (3000)	25–30	25–30 (1500)	NA

Second-line anti-TB agents can be dosed as follows to facilitate DOT: (5 times per wk)
Cycloserine 500–750 mg po q24h (5 times per wk)
Ethionamide 500–750 mg po q24h (5 times per wk)
Kanamycin or capreomycin 15 mg per kg IM/IV q24h (3–5 times per wk)
Ciprofloxacin 750 mg po q24h (5 times per wk)
Moxifloxacin 600–800 mg po q24h (5 times per wk)
Levofloxacin 750 mg po q24h (5 times per wk) (CID 21:1245, 1995)

Risk factors for drug-resistant (MDR) TB: Recent immigration from Latin America or Asia (esp. if living in area of ↑ resistance ≥4%) or previous rx, with exposure to known MDR TB. Incidence of MDR TB in US steady at 0.7%. Incidence of primary drug resistance is particularly high (>25%) in parts of China, Thailand, Russia, Estonia & Latvia, ~80% of US MDR cases in foreign born.

(continued on next page)

See page 2 for abbreviations   * Dosages are for adults (unless otherwise indicated) and assume normal renal function   † DOT = directly observed therapy

TABLE 12A (4)

CAUSATIVE AGENT/DISEASE	MODIFYING CIRCUM-STANCES	SUGGESTED REGIMEN[a]	DURATION OF TREATMENT (mos.)[b]	SPECIFIC COMMENTS[a]	COMMENTS
III. Mycobacterium tuberculosis **A. Pulmonary TB** *(continued from previous page)*	INH (±) RIF resistance	RIF, PZA, EMB (a FQ may strengthen the regimen for pts with extensive disease)	6	INH should be stopped in cases of INH resistance. Outcome similar for drug susceptible and INH-mono-resistant strains *(CID 48:179, 2009)*.	*(continued from previous page)* **Alternatives for resistant strains: Moxi** and **levo** are **FQs of choice**, not CIP. FQ resistance may be seen in pts previously treated with FQ. WHO recommends using moxi (if MIC ≤ 2) if resistant to earlier generation FQs *(AAC 54:4765, 2010)*. **Linezolid** 600 mg once daily has excellent in vitro activity, including MDR strains and effective in selected cases of MDR-TB and XDR TB but watch for toxicity *(NEJM 367:1508, 2012)*. **Bedaquiline** recently FDA approved for treatment of MDR TB based on efficacy in Phase 2 trials *(NEJM 360:2397, 2009; AAC 56:3271, 2012; NEJM 371:689, 723, 2014)*. Dose is 400 mg once daily for 2 weeks then 200 mg tiw for 22 weeks administered as directly observed therapy (DOT), taken with food, and always in combination with other anti-TB meds. **Consultation with an expert in MDR-TB management** strongly advised before use of this agent. For MDR-TB and XDR-TB, do drug susceptibility testing for ethambutol, PZA & other 2nd line drugs if possible *(CID 59:1364, 2014)*.
	Resistance to INH & RIF (± SM)	FQ, PZA, EMB, AMK or capreomycin (SM only if confirmed susceptible), see Comment	18–24	Extended rx is needed to ↓ the risk of relapse. In cases with extensive disease, the use of an additional agent (alternative agents) may be prudent to ↓ the risk of failure & additional acquired drug resistance. Resectional surgery may be appropriate.	
	Resistance to INH, RIF (± SM), & PZA	FQ (EMB or PZA if active), AMK or capreomycin (SM only if confirmed susceptible), see Comment	24	Use the first-line agents to which there is susceptibility. Add 2 or more alternative agents in case of extensive disease. Surgery should be considered. Survival ↑ in pts receiving active FQ & surgical intervention *(AJRCCM 169:1103, 2004)*.	
	Resistance to RIF	INH, EMB, FQ, supplemented with PZA for the first 2 mos (an IA may be included for the first 2–3 mos. for pts with extensive disease)	12–18	Extended use of an IA may not be feasible. An all-oral regimen times 12–18 mos. should be effective but for more extensive disease &/or to shorten duration (e.g. to 12 mos.), an IA may be added in the initial 2 mos. of rx.	
Multidrug-Resistant Tuberculosis (MDR TB): Defined as resistant to at least 2 drugs including INH & RIF. Pt clusters with high mortality *(NEJM 363:1050, 2010)*. **Extensively Drug-Resistant TB** (XDR-TB): Defined as resistant to INH & RIF plus any FQ and at least 1 of the 3 second-line drugs: capreomycin, kanamycin or amikacin *(MMWR 56:250, 2007; CID 51:379, 2010)*.					
	XDR-TB	Expert consultation strongly advised. See Comments	18–24	Therapy requires administration of 4–6 drugs to which infecting organism is susceptible, including second-line drugs *(MMWR 56:250, 2007)*. Increased mortality, seen primarily in HIV+ patients. Cure with outpatient therapy likely in non-HIV+ patients when regimens of 4 or 5 or more drugs to which organism is susceptible are employed *(NEJM 359:563, 2008; CID 47:496, 2008)*. Successful sputum culture conversion correlates to initial susceptibility to FQs and kanamycin *(CID 46:42, 2008)*. Bedaquiline and Linezolide are options.	
Reviews of therapy for MDR TB: *JAC 54:593, 2004; Med Lett 7:75, 2009. For XDR-TB see MMWR 56:250, 2007; NEJM 359:563, 2008*					

See page 2 for abbreviations *Dosages are for adults (unless otherwise indicated) and assume normal renal function **DOT** = directly observed therapy

TABLE 12A (5)

CAUSATIVE AGENT/DISEASE; MODIFYING CIRCUMSTANCES	SUGGESTED REGIMENS		COMMENTS
	INITIAL THERAPY	CONTINUATION PHASE OF THERAPY (in vitro susceptibility known)	
III. Mycobacterium tuberculosis (continued)			
B. Extrapulmonary TB Steroids: see Comment	INH + **RIF** (or **RFB**) + **PZA** + **EMB** q24h times 2 months. Some add pyridoxine 25–50 mg po q24h	INH + **RIF** (or **RFB**)	IDSA recommends 6 mos for lymph node, pleural, pericarditis, disseminated disease, genitourinary & peritoneal TBc; 6–9 mos for bone & joint; 9-12 mos for CNS (including meningeal) TBc. **Corticosteroids** "strongly rec" only for meningeal TBc (MMWR 52(RR-11):1, 2003). Steroids not recommended for pericarditis (NEJM 371:1121 & 1155, 2014).
C. Tuberculous meningitis Excellent summary of clinical aspects and therapy (including steroids) CMR 21:243, 2008. Also J Infect 59:167, 2009.	INH + **RIF** + **PZA** + prednisone 60 mg/day x 4 wks, then 30 mg/day x 4 wks, then 15 mg/day x 2 wks, then 5 mg/day x 1 wk	May add **EMB** when susceptibility to INH and RIF established. Can D/C PZA after 2 months. Treat for total of 12 months. See Table 9, page 87 for CSF drug penetration. Initial reg of INH + **RIF** + **SM** + **PZA** also effective, even in patients with INH resistant organisms.	3 drugs often rec for initial rx; we prefer 4 (J Infect 59:167, 2009). Infection with MDR TB ↑ mortality & morbidity. **Dexamethasone** (for 1st mo) shown to ↓ complications & ↑ survival (NEJM 351:1741, 2004). FQs (Levo, Gati, CIP) may be useful if started early (AAC 55:3244, 2011).
D. Tuberculosis during pregnancy	INH + **RIF** + **EMB** for 9 mos	SM should not be substituted for EMB due to toxicity. AMK, capreomycin, kanamycin, FQs also contraindicated. PZA is recommended for use by the WHO due to lack of safety data, although PZA has not been recommended for general use in U.S. due to lack of safety data. If PZA is not included in the initial treatment regimen, the minimum duration of therapy is 9 months. Pyridoxine, 25 mg/day, should be administered.
E. Treatment failure or relapse: Usually due to non-compliance or resistant organisms, or subtherapeutic drug levels (CID 55:169, 2012)	Directly observed therapy (DOT). Check susceptibilities. (See section III: A, page 131 & above)	INH + **RIF** (or **RFB**), q24h times 4 months (total 6 mos). Treat up to 9 mos. in pts with delayed response, cavitary disease	Pts whose sputum is culture-positive after 5–6 mos. = treatment failures. Failures may be due to non-compliance or resistant organisms, therefore obtain susceptibility to first and second line agents on current isolates. Non-compliance common, ones that the patient has not previously received if at all possible. Patients with MDR-TB usually convert sputum within 12 weeks of successful therapy.
F. HIV infection or AIDS— pulmonary or extrapulmonary	INH + **RIF** (or **RFB**) + **PZA** q24h x 2 mos. Add pyridoxine 50 mg q24h	INH + **RIF** (or **RFB**), q24h to regimens that include INH 50 mg po q24h to regimens that include INH	1. Co-administration of RIF not recommended for these anti-retroviral drugs: nevirapine, etravirine, rilpivirine, maraviroc, elvitegravir (integrase inhibitor in four drug combination Stribild®). (All HIV protease inhibitors. Use RFB instead). 2. Co-administration of RIF with raltegravir best avoided (use RFB instead) but if necessary increase raltegravir dose to 800 mg bid of latter. 3. Because of possibility of developing resistance to RIF or RFB in pts with low CD4 cell counts who receive weekly or biwkly therapy, daily dosing (preferred), or at a min 3x/wk dosing (failure rate likely higher) recommended for initial or continuation phase of rx. 4. Clinical & microbiologic response similar to that of HIV-neg patient 5. Post-treatment suppression not necessary for drug-susceptible strains.
Concomitant protease inhibitor (PI) therapy	INH 300 mg q24h + **RFB** (150 mg q24h or 300 mg tiw) + **EMB** 15 mg/kg q24h + **PZA** 25 mg/kg q24h x 2 mos; then **INH** + RFB times 4 mos. (up to 7 mos.) Alternative: **INH** + **FQ** + **PZA** + **EMB** x2 mos.	INH + **RFB** x 4 mos. (7 mos. in slow responders, cavitary disease) INH + **FQ** + **PZA** for additional 10 mos (up to 16 months if delayed response)	Rifamycins induce cytochrome CYP450 enzymes (RIF > RFB) & reduce serum levels of concomitantly administered PIs. Conversely, PIs inhibit CYP450 & cause ↑ serum levels of RFP & RFB. If dose of RFB is reduced, toxicity ↑. FQ either **levo** 500 mg q24h or **moxi** 400 mg q24h. May be used with any PI regimen.

See page 2 for abbreviations   * Dosages are for adults (unless otherwise indicated) and assume normal renal function   † **DOT** = directly observed therapy

134

TABLE 12A (6)
FIGURE 1 ALGORITHM FOR MANAGEMENT OF AT-RISK PATIENT WITH LOW OR HIGH SUSPICION OF ACTIVE TUBERCULOSIS WHILE CULTURES ARE PENDING (modified from MMWR 52(RR-11):1, 2003).

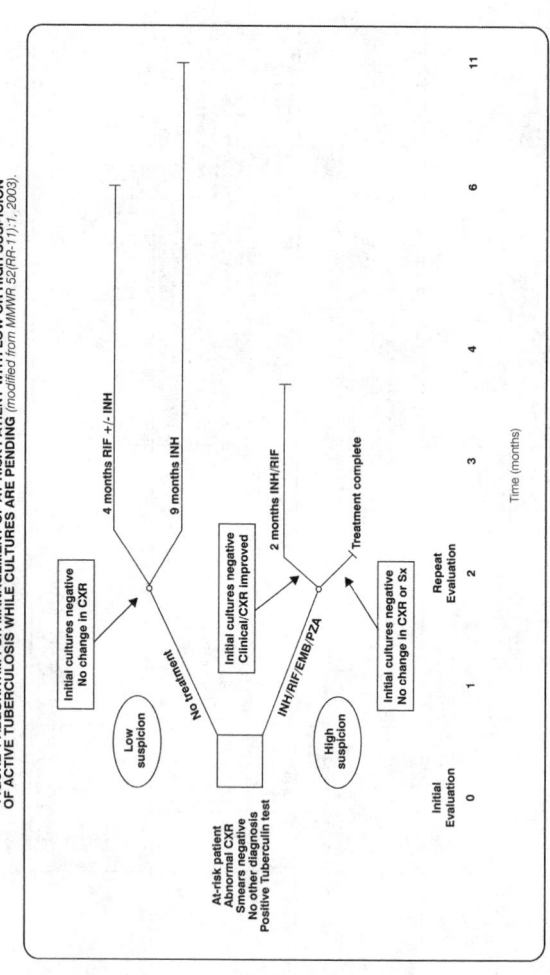

Patients at high clinical suspicion of active TB should be started on 4-drug therapy, pending results of cultures. If cultures are negative and there is no change in symptoms or CXR, the 4-drug regimen can be stopped and no further therapy is required. If cultures are negative and there is clinical or CXR improvement, continue INH/RIF for 2 additional months. For patients at low suspicion for active TB, treat for LTBI once cultures are negative.

See page 2 for abbreviations   * Dosages are for adults (unless otherwise indicated) and assume normal renal function   † **DOT** = directly observed therapy

TABLE 12A (7)

FIGURE 2 [Modified from MMWR 52(RR-11):1, 2003]

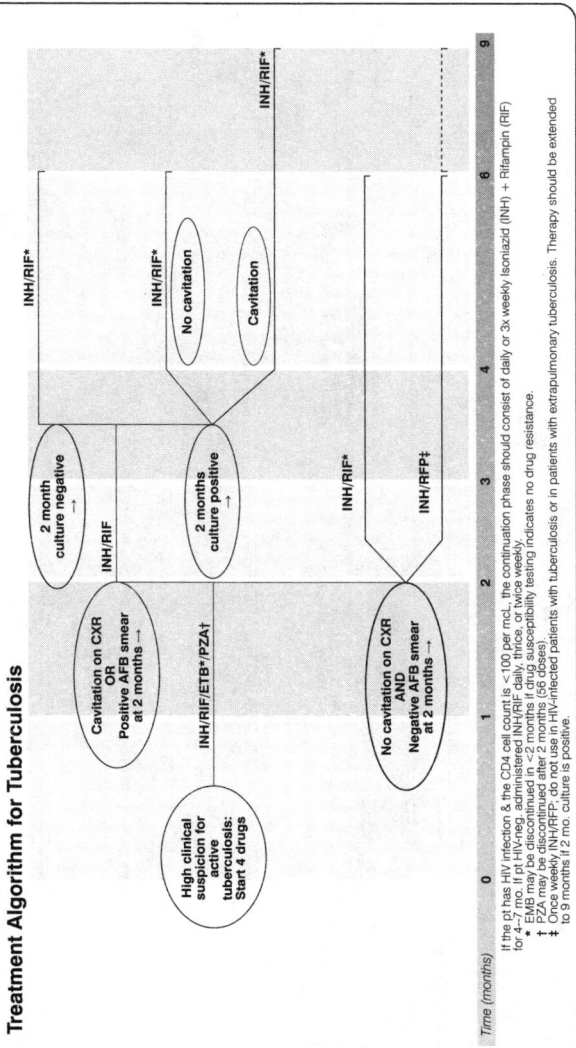

Treatment Algorithm for Tuberculosis

If the pt has HIV infection & the CD4 cell count is <100 per mcL, the continuation phase should consist of daily or 3x weekly Isoniazid (INH) + Rifampin (RIF) for 4–7 mo. If pt HIV-neg, administered INH/RIF daily, thrice, or twice weekly.

* EMB may be discontinued in <2 months if drug susceptibility testing indicates no drug resistance.
† PZA may be discontinued after 2 months (56 doses).
‡ Once weekly INH/RFP; do not use in HIV-infected patients with tuberculosis or in patients with extrapulmonary tuberculosis. Therapy should be extended to 9 months if 2 mo. culture is positive.

See page 2 for abbreviations.

TABLE 12A (8)

CAUSATIVE AGENT/DISEASE	MODIFYING CIRCUMSTANCES	SUGGESTED REGIMENS PRIMARY/ALTERNATIVE		COMMENTS
IV. Nontuberculous Mycobacteria (NTM) *A. M. bovis*		*AJRCCM 175:367, 2007; EID 17:506, 2011)*		The M. tuberculosis complex includes M. bovis and regimens effective for MTB (except PZA based) also likely to be effective for M. bovis. **All isolates resistant to PZA.** Isolation not required. Increased prevalence of extrapulmonary disease in U.S. born Hispanic populations and elsewhere *(CID 47:168, 2008; EID 14:909, 2008; EID 17:457, 2011).*
	Only fever (>38.5°C) for 12–24 hrs. Systemic illness or sepsis	**INH + RIF + EMB** for 2 months then INH + RIF for 7 months		
B. Bacillus Calmette-Guerin (BCG) (derived from M. bovis)		INH 300 mg q24h times 3 months. Same as for M. bovis.		Intravesical BCG effective in superficial bladder tumors and carcinoma in situ. With sepsis, consider initial adjunctive prednisolone. Also susceptible to RFB, CIP, ofibx, levo, moxi, streptomycin, amikacin, capreomycin *(AAC 53:316, 2009).* BCG may cause regional adenitis or pulmonary disease in HIV-infected children *(CID 37:1226, 2003).* **Resistant to PZA.**
C. M. avium-intracellulare complex (MAC, MAI, or Battey bacillus). *ATS/IDSA Consensus Statement: AJRCCM 175:367, 2007; See http://aidsinfo.nih.gov/ guidelines/html/4/adult-and-adolescent-oi-prevention-and-treatment-guidelines/o for updated CDC recommendations for AIDS patients.*	**Immunocompetent patients**			See *AJRCCM 175:367, 2007* for details of dosing and duration of therapy. Intermittent (tiw) therapy not recommended for patients with cavitary disease, patients who have been previously treated or patients with moderate or severe disease. The primary microbiologic goal of therapy is 12 months of negative sputum cultures on therapy.
	Nodular/Bronchiectatic disease	**[Clarithro** 1000 mg **or azithro** 500 mg], tiw + **EMB** 25 mg/kg tiw + [**RIF** 600 mg or **RFB** 300 mg] tiw		"Classic" **pulmonary MAC:** Men 50–75, smokers, COPD. May be associated with hot tub use *(Clin Chest Med 23:675, 2002).*
	Cavitary disease or severe nodular/bronchiectatic disease [**Clarithro** 500-1000 mg/day (lower	[**Clarithro** 500-1000 mg or **azithro** 250 mg/day] + **EMB** 15 mg/kg/day + [**RIF** 600 mg/day or **RFB** 150-300 mg/day] ± [**strep** or **AMK**]		"New" **pulmonary MAC:** Women 30–70, scoliosis, mitral valve prolapse, (bronchiectasis), pectus excavatum ("Lady Windermere syndrome") and fibronodular disease in elderly women *(EID 16:1576, 2010).* May also be associated with interferon gamma deficiency *(AJM 113:756, 2002).* For cervicofacial lymphadenitis (localized) in immunocompetent children, surgical excision is as effective as chemotherapy *(CID 44:1057, 2007).*
	HIV infection: **Primary prophylaxis**—Pt's CD4 count <50–100 per mm³. Discontinue when CD4 count >100 per mm³ in response to ART	**Azithro** 1200 mg po weekly OR **Clarithro** 500 mg po bid	**RFB** 300 mg q24h OR **Azithro** 1200 mg po weekly + **RIF** 300 mg po q24h	Moxifloxacin and gatifloxacin, active in vitro & in vivo *(AAC 51:4071, 2007).* **Many drug-drug interactions**, see Table 22, page 221. Drug-resistant MAI disease seen in 29–58% of pts in whom disease develops while taking clarithro prophylaxis & in 11% of those on azithro but has not been observed with RFB prophylaxis. Clarithro resistance more likely in pts with extremely low CD4 counts at initiation. Need to be sure no active MTB; RFB used for prophylaxis may promote selection of rifampicin-resistant MTB.
	Treatment Either presumptive dx or after + culture of blood, bone marrow, or usually, sterile body fluids, eg liver	**[Clarithro** 500 mg* po bid **or azithro** 500-600 mg/day) + **EMB** 15 mg/kg/day ± **RFB** 300 mg po q24h (adjust dose) * **Higher doses of clari (1000 mg bid) may be associated with ↑ mortality**	**Azithro** 500 mg po/day + **EMB** 15 mg/kg/day +/- **RFB** 300-450 mg po/day	Adjust RFB dose as needed for drug interactions.

(continued on next page) |

See page 2 for abbreviations   * Dosages are for adults (unless otherwise indicated) and assume normal renal function   † **DOT** = directly observed therapy

TABLE 12A (9)

CAUSATIVE AGENT/DISEASE	MODIFYING CIRCUMSTANCES	SUGGESTED REGIMENS		COMMENTS
		PRIMARY/ALTERNATIVE		
IV. Nontuberculous Mycobacteria (NTM) *(continued)*				
C. M. avium-intracellulare complex *(continued)*				*(continued from previous page)* Addition of a third or fourth drug should be considered for patients with advanced immunosuppression (CD4+ count <50 cells/μL), high mycobacterial loads (>2 log CFU/mL of blood), or in the absence of effective ART: AMK 10-15 mg/kg IV daily; Strep 1 gm IV or IM daily; CIP 500-750 mg PO bid; Levo 500 mg PO daily; Moxi 400 mg PO daily. Testing of susceptibility to clarithromycin and azithromycin is recommended. Short term (4-8 weeks) of systemic corticosteroid (equivalent to 20-40 mg of prednisone) can be used for IRIS.
	Chronic post-treatment suppression—secondary prophylaxis	**Always necessary.** [Clarithro or azithro] + EMB 15 mg/ kg/day (dosage above)	**Claritho or azithro** or RFB (dosage above)	Recurrences almost universal without chronic suppression. Can discontinue if no signs and symptoms of MAC disease and sustained (>6 months) CD4 count >100 cells/μL in response to ART.
D. Mycobacterium celatum	Treatment; optimal regimen not defined	May be susceptible to **claritho**. Treat as if MAC.		Isolated from pulmonary lesions and blood in AIDS patients . Easily confused with M. xenopi (and MAC).
E. Mycobacterium abscessus – – – – – – – – – – **Mycobacterium chelonae**	Treatment: Surgical excision may facilitate clarithro rx in subcutaneous abscess and is important adjunct to rx. For role of surgery in M. abscessus pulmonary disease, see *CID 52:565, 2011.*	Cutaneous: **Claritho** 500 mg po bid x 6 months. Pulmonary/disseminated: 2 or 3 IV drugs (check susceptibility (Amikacin, IMP, Cefoxitin, Tigecycline). Watch out for inducible resistance to Clarithro		M. abscessus susceptible in vitro to AMK (70%), clarithro (95%), cefoxitin (70%), CLO, cefmetazole, RFB, FQ, IMP, azithro, CIP, doxy, mino, tigecycline *(CID 42:1756, 2006; JIC 15:46, 2009).* Single isolates of M. abscessus often not associated with disease. Clarithro-resistant strains now described. Cefoxitin & Tigecycline active *(JID 209:905, 2014).* M. chelonae susceptible to AMK (80%), clarithro, azithro, tobramycin (100%), IMP (60%), moxifloxacin *(AAC 46:3283, 2002).* CIP, mino, doxy, linezolid (94%) *(CID 42:1756, 2006).* Resistant to cefoxitin, FQ. Tigecycline highly active in vitro and successfully used as salvage for M. chelonae infection in combination regimens *(J Antimicrob Chemother 69:1945, 2014).*
F. Mycobacterium fortuitum	Treatment; optimal regimen not defined. Surgical excision of infected areas.	**AMK + cefoxitin + probenecid** 2-6 wks, then po **TMP-SMX**, or **doxy** 2-6 mos. Usually responds to 6-12 mos of oral rx with 2 drugs to which it is susceptible.		**Resistant to all standard anti-TBc drugs.** Sensitive in vitro to doxycycline, minocycline, cefoxitin, IMP, AMK, TMP-SMX, CIP, oflox, azithro, clarithro, linezolid, tigecycline *(Clin Micro Rev 15:716, 2002),* but some strains resistant to azithromycin, rifabutin. For M. fortuitum pulmonary disease treat with at least 2 agents active in vitro until sputum cultures negative for 12 months *(AJRCCM 175:367, 2007).*
G. Mycobacterium haemophilum	Regimen(s) not defined in animal model, **clarithro + rifabutin** effective. Combination of **CIP + RFB + clarithro** reported effective but clinical experience limited *(CID 52:488, 2011).* Surgical debridement may be necessary.			Clinical: Ulcerating skin lesions, synovitis, osteomyelitis, cervicofacial lymphadenitis in children. Associated with permanent eyebrow makeup *(CID 52:488, 2011).* Lab: Requires supplemented media to isolate. Sensitive in vitro to: CIP, cycloserine, rifabutin, moxifloxacin. Over ⅓ resistant to: INH, RIF, EMB, PZA. For localized cervicofacial lymphadenitis in immunocompetent children, surgical excision as effective as chemotherapy *(CID 44:1057, 2007),* or "watchful waiting" *(CID 52:180, 2011).*

See page 2 for abbreviations   * Dosages are for adults (unless otherwise indicated) and assume normal renal function   † **DOT** = directly observed therapy

TABLE 12A (10)

CAUSATIVE AGENT/DISEASE	MODIFYING CIRCUMSTANCES	SUGGESTED REGIMENS PRIMARY/ALTERNATIVE	COMMENTS
IV. Nontuberculous Mycobacteria (NTM) (continued)			
H. Mycobacterium genavense	2 or more drugs: **Clarithro, EMB, RFB, CLO, Amikacin.** Moxifloxacin as alternatives.		Seen in AIDS patients with CD4 < 50 and in non-HIV severely immunocompromised hosts. For review see Clin Microbiol Infect 19:432, 2013.
I. Mycobacterium gordonae	Regimen(s) not defined, but consider **RIF + EMB + KM** or **CIP** (or **linezolid**)		Frequent colonizer, not associated with disease. In vitro: sensitive to EMB, RIF, AMK, CIP, clarithro, linezolid. Resistant to INH.
J. Mycobacterium kansasii	Q24h po: **INH** (300 mg) + **RIF** (600 mg) + **EMB** (25 mg per kg times 2 mos, then 15 mg per kg). Rx for 18 mos. (until culture-neg. sputum times 12 mos; 15 mos. If HIV+ pt.) (See Comment)	For **RIF** resistant organism: [**INH** 900 mg + **pyridoxine** 50 mg + **EMB** 25 mg/kg) po q24h + **Sulfamethoxazole** 1000 mg tid (if sulfamethoxazole is unavailable options include **TMP-SMX** two double strength tablets (320 mg TMP and 1600 mg SMX) bid OR **Clarithromycin** 500 mg po bid OR **Moxifloxacin** 400 mg po once daily. Treat for 12-15 mos or until 12-15 mos of culture-negative sputum.	**All isolates are resistant to PZA.** Highly susceptible to linezolid in vitro (AAC 47:1736, 2003) and to clarithro and moxifloxacin (AAC 55:950, 2005). If HIV+ pt taking protease inhibitor, substitute either clarithro (500 mg bid) or RFB (150 mg per day) for RIF. Because of variable susceptibility to INH, some substitute clarithro for INH. Resistance to clarithro reported.
K. Mycobacterium marinum	Two active agents for 1-2 months after surgical incision: **Clarithro** 500 mg bid + **EMB** 25 mg/kg q24h or **RIF** 600 mg q24h + **EMB** 25 mg/kg q24h Surgical excision.		For deep tissue involvement a three drug combination therapy with Rifampin 600 mg q24h + Minocycline 100-200 mg q24h or Doxycycline 100-200 mg q24h) + Clarithromycin 500 mg bid. Monotherapy may be considered for minimal disease: Minocycline 100-200 mg q24h or Doxycycline 100-200 mg q24h or TMP-SMX 160/800 mg po bid.
L. Mycobacterium scrofulaceum	Surgical excision. Chemotherapy seldom indicated. Although regimens not defined, **clarithro + CLO** with or **without EMB, INH, RIF, strep + cycloserine** have also been used.		In vitro resistant to INH, RIF, EMB, PZA, AMK, CIP. Susceptible to clarithro, strep, erythromycin.
M. Mycobacterium simiae	Regimen(s) not defined. Start 4 drugs as for disseminated MAC		Most isolates resistant to all 1st-line anti-tbc drugs. Isolates often not clinically significant.
N. Mycobacterium ulcerans (Buruli ulcer)	WHO recommends **RIF + SM** for 8 weeks. **RIF + CIP** recommended as alternatives by WHO (CMN 31:119, 2009).		Susceptible in vitro to RIF, strep, CLO, clarithro, CIP, oflox, amikacin, moxi, linezolid. Australian guidelines (MJA 200:267, 2014) recommend oral combination of RIF + Clarithro or RIF + a FQ (moxifloxacin or CIP). Surgery not required for those declining or intolerant of antibiotic, debridement of necrotic tissue, large defects.
O. Mycobacterium xenopi	Regimen(s) not defined. **Clarithro** 500 mg bid + **RIF** 600 mg q24h + **Rifabutin** 300 mg q24h or **EMB** 15 mg/kg once daily + **INH** 300 mg daily.		In vitro: sensitive to clarithro and many standard antimycobacterial drugs. MOXI active in vitro and may be an alternative.
V. Mycobacterium leprae (leprosy) Classification: CID 44:1096, 2007. Overview: Lancet ID 11:464, 2011.	There are 2 sets of therapeutic recommendations here, one from USA (National Hansen's Disease Programs [NHDP], Baton Rouge, LA) and one from WHO. Both are based on expert recommendations and neither has been subjected to controlled clinical trial.		

See page 2 for abbreviations   * Dosages are for adults (unless otherwise indicated) and assume normal renal function   † **DOT** = directly observed therapy

TABLE 12A (11)

Type of Disease	NHDP Regimen	WHO Regimen	COMMENTS
Paucibacillary Forms: (Intermediate, Tuberculoid, Borderline tuberculoid)	(**Dapsone** 100 mg/day + **RIF** 600 mg po/day) for 12 months	(**Dapsone** 100 mg/day (unsupervised)) + **RIF** 600 mg 1x/mo (supervised)) for 6 mos	Side-effects overall 0.4%
Single lesion paucibacillary	Treat as paucibacillary leprosy for 12 months.	Single dose ROM therapy: (RIF 600 mg + Oflox 400 mg + Mino 100 mg) (Ln 353:655, 1999).	
Multibacillary forms: **Borderline** **Borderline-lepromatous** **Lepromatous** See Comment for erythema nodosum leprosum Rev.: Lancet 363:1209, 2004	(**Dapsone** 100 mg/day + **CLO** 50 mg/day + **RIF** 600 mg/day) for 24 mos. **Alternative regimen:** (**Dapsone** 100 mg/day + **RIF** 600 mg/day + **Minocycline** 100 mg/day) for 24 mos if **CLO** is refused or unavailable.	(**Dapsone** 100 mg/day + **CLO** 50 mg/day (both unsupervised) + **RIF** 600 mg + **CLO** 300 mg once monthly (supervised)). Continue regimen for 12 months.	Side-effects overall 5.1%. For **erythema nodosum leprosum**: prednisone 60–80 mg/day or thalidomide 100–400 mg/day. Thalidomide available in US at 1-800-4-CELGENE. Altho thalidomide effective, WHO no longer rec because of potential toxicity however the majority of leprosy experts feel thalidomide remains drug of choice for ENL under strict supervision. **CLO (Clofazimine)** available from NHDP under IND protocol; contact at 1-800-642-2477. **Ethionamide** (250 mg q24h) or prothionamide (375 mg q24h) may be subbed for CLO. Etanercept effective in one case refractory to above standard therapy (CID 52:e133, 2011). Regimens incorporating clarithro, minocycline, dapsone monotherapy have been abandoned due to emergence of resistance (CID 52:e127, 2011), but older patients previously treated with dapsone monotherapy may remain on lifelong maintenance therapy. Moxi highly active in vitro and produces rapid clinical response (AAC 52:3113, 2008).

See page 2 for abbreviations   * Dosages are for adults (unless otherwise indicated) and assume normal renal function   † **DOT** = directly observed therapy

TABLE 12B – DOSAGE AND ADVERSE EFFECTS OF ANTIMYCOBACTERIAL DRUGS

AGENT (TRADE NAME)[1]	ROUTE/[a] DRUG RESISTANCE (RES) US[2],[§]	USUAL DOSAGE*	SIDE-EFFECTS, TOXICITY AND PRECAUTIONS	SURVEILLANCE
FIRST LINE DRUGS				
Ethambutol (Myambutol) (100, 400 mg tab)	RES: 0.3% (0-0.7%) po 400 mg tab	25 mg/kg/day for 2 mos then 15 mg/kg/day q24h or 15 mg/kg/day q24h as 1 dose 2x/wk (<10% protein binding) [Bacteriostatic to both extracellular & intracellular organisms]	**Optic neuritis** with decreased visual acuity, central scotomata, and loss of green and red perception, peripheral neuropathy and headache (−%), rashes (rare), arthralgia (rare), hyperuricemia (rare). Anaphylactoid reaction (rare). *Comment:* Primarily used to inhibit resistance. Disrupts outer cell membrane w/M. avium with 1 activity to other drugs.	Monthly visual acuity & red/green test. red/green with dose >15 mg/kg/day; ≥10% loss considered significant. Usually reversible if drug discontinued.
Isoniazid (INH) (Nydrazid, Laniazid, Teebaconin) (50, 100, 300 mg tab)	RES: 4.1% (2.6-8.5%) po 300 mg tab IM 100 mg/mL in 10 mL (IV route not FDA-approved but has been used, esp. in AIDS)	Q24h dose 5–10 mg/kg/day up to 300 mg/day as 1 dose. 2x/wk dose: 15 mg/kg (900 mg max dose) (< 10% protein binding) [Bactericidal to both extracellular and intracellular organisms] Add pyridoxine in alcoholic, pregnant, or malnourished pts.	Overall −1%. Liver. **Hep** (children 10%, mild ↑ SGOT, normalizes with continued rx, age <20 yrs rare, 20–34 yrs 1.2%, 250 yrs 2.3%) [also ↑ with ↓24h alcohol & previous exposure to Hep C (usually asymptomatic—*CID 36:293, 2003*]). May be fatal. With prodromal sx dark urine (less on LFTs; discontinue if SGOT >3–5x normal. **Peripheral neuropathy** (17% on 6 mg/kg per day, less on 300 mg, incidence ↑ in slow acetylators); **pyridoxine 10 mg q24h will decrease incidence**; other neurologic sequelae, convulsions, optic neuritis, toxic encephalopathy, psychosis, muscle twitching, dizziness, coma (all rare); allergic skin rashes, fever, minor disulfiram-like reaction, flushing after Swiss cheese; blood dyscrasias (rare); + antinuclear (20%). **Drug-drug interactions** common, see Table 22.	Pre-rx liver functions. Repeat if symptoms (fatigue, weakness, malaise, anorexia, nausea or vomiting) >3 days (*AJRCCM 152: 1705, 1995*). Some recommend SGOT at 2, 4, 6 mos esp. if age >50 yrs. Clinical evaluation every mo.
Pyrazinamide (500 mg tab)	po 500 mg tab	25 mg per kg per day (maximum 2.5 gm per day) q24h as 1 dose [Bactericidal for intracellular organisms]	**Arthralgia; hyperuricemia;** hepatitis (not over 2% if recommended dose not exceeded); gastric irritation; photosensitivity (rare).	Pre-rx liver functions. Monthly SGOT, uric acid. Measure serum uric acid if symptomatic gouty attack occurs.
Rifamate®— combination tablet	po (1 hr before meal)	2 tablets single dose q24h	1 tablet contains 150 mg INH, 300 mg RIF	As with individual drugs
Rifampin (Rifadin, Rimactane, Rifocin) (100, 300, 450, 600 mg cap)	RES: 0.2% (0–0.3%) po 300 mg cap (IV available, Merrell-Dow)	10.0 mg per kg per day up to 600 mg (one dose) as 1 dose (60–90% protein binding) [Bactericidal to all populations of organisms]	INH/RIF dc'd in −3% for toxicity, gastrointestinal irritation, antibiotic-associated colitis, drug fever (1%), pruritus with or without skin rash (1%), anaphylactoid reactions in HIV + pts, mental confusion, thrombocytopenia (1%), leukopenia (1%), hemolytic anemia, transient **abnormalities in liver function. "Flu syndrome"** (fever, chills, headache, bone pain, shortness of breath) seen if RIF taken irregularly or if q24h dose restarted after an interval of no rx. **Discolors urine, tears, sweat, contact lens an orange-brownish color.** May cause drug-induced lupus erythematosus (*Ln 349: 1521, 1977*).	Pre-rx liver function. Repeat if symptoms. **Multiple significant drug-drug interactions,** see Table 22.
Rifater®— combination tablet (See Side-Effects)	po (1 hr before meal)	Wt ≥65 kg, 6 tablets single dose q24h	1 tablet contains 50 mg INH, 120 mg RIF, 300 mg PZA. 4 tabs if <65 kg (PZA 25 mg per kg per day). Purpose is convenience in dosing, ↑ compliance (*AnIM 122: 951, 1995*) but cost 1.58 more. Side-effects = individual drugs.	As with individual drugs. PZA 25 mg per kg
Streptomycin (IV/IM soln)	RES: 3.9% (2.7–7.6%) IM (or IV)	15 mg per kg IM q24h, 0.75–1.0 gm per day initially for 60–90 days, then 1.0 gm 2–3 times per week (15 mg per kg per day) q24h as 1 dose	Overall 8%. **Ototoxicity:** vestibular dysfunction (vertigo); paresthesias; dizziness & nausea (all less in pts receiving 2–3 doses per week); tinnitus and high frequency loss (1%); nephrotoxicity; peripheral neuropathy (rare); allergic skin rashes (4–5%); drug fever. Available from X-Gen Pharmaceuticals, 607-732-4411. Ref. re. *IV—CID 19:1150, 1994.* Toxicity similar with qd vs tid dosing (*CID 38:1538, 2004*).	Monthly audiogram. In older pts, serum creatinine or BUN at start of rx and weekly if pt stable

[1] Note: Malabsorption of antimycobacterial drugs may occur in patients with AIDS enteropathy. For review of adverse effects, see *AJRCCM 167:1472, 2003.*

[2] **RES** = % resistance of M. tuberculosis

See page 2 for abbreviations.

* Dosages are for adults (unless otherwise indicated) and assume normal renal function

§ Mean (range) (higher in Hispanics, Asians, and patients <10 years old)

[a] Route of administration

[†] **DOT** = directly observed therapy

TABLE 12B (2)

AGENT (TRADE NAME)[1]	USUAL DOSAGE*	ROUTE/[1] DRUG RESISTANCE (RES) US[2],§	SIDE-EFFECTS, TOXICITY AND PRECAUTIONS	SURVEILLANCE
SECOND LINE DRUGS (more difficult to use and/or less effective than first line drugs)				
Amikacin (Amikin (IV soln)	7.5-10.0 mg per kg q24h [Bactericidal for extracellular organisms]	RES: (est. 0.1%) IM/IV 500 mg vial	See Table 10B, pages 107 & 110 Toxicity similar with qd vs tid dosing (CID 38:1538, 2004).	Monthly audiogram. Serum creatinine or BUN weekly if pt stable
Bedaquiline (Sirturo) (100 mg tab) Ref: JAC 69:2310, 2014; NEJM 371:723, 2014	Directly observed therapy (DOT): 400 mg once daily for 2 weeks, then 200 mg 3 times weekly for 22 weeks, taken with food and always used in combination with other anti-TB medications.	Does not exhibit cross-resistance to other TB drugs; always use in combination with other TB drugs to prevent selection of resistant mutants	Most common: nausea, vomiting, arthralgia, headache, hyperuricemia. Elevated transaminases. Bedaquiline in clinical trials was administered as one component of a multiple drug regimen, so side-effects were common, yet difficult to assign to a particular drug.	Moderate QTc increases (average of 10-16 ms over the 24 weeks of therapy. Potential risks of pancreatitis, myopathy, myocardial injury, severe hepatotoxicity.
Capreomycin sulfate (Capastat sulfate)	1 gm per day (15 mg per kg per day) q24h as 1 dose	RES: 0.1% (0-0.9%) IM/IV	Nephrotoxicity (36%), ototoxicity (auditory 11%), eosinophilia, leukopenia, skin rash, fever, hypokalemia, neuromuscular blockade.	Monthly audiogram, biweekly serum creatinine or BUN
Ciprofloxacin (Cipro) (250, 500, 750 mg tab)	750 mg bid	500 mg or 750 mg po IV 200-400 mg vial	TB not a FDA-approved indication for CIP. Desired CIP serum levels 4-6 mcg per mL. See Table 10A, page 103 & Table 10B, page 108 for adverse effects.	None
Clofazimine (Lamprene) (50, 100 mg cap)	50 mg per day (unsupervised) + 300 mg 1 time per month supervised or 100 mg per day	50 mg (with meals)	Skin: **pigmentation (pink-brownish black)** 75-100%; dryness 20%; pruritus 5%; GI: abdominal pain 50% (rarely severe leading to exploratory laparoscopy), splenic infarction (VR), bowel obstruction (VR), GI bleeding (VR). Eye: conjunctival irritation, retinal crystal deposits.	None
Cycloserine (Seromycin) (250 mg tab)	750–1000 mg per day (15 mg per kg per day) 2-4 doses per day [Bacteriostatic for both extra-cellular & intracellular organisms]	RES: 0.1% (0-0.3%) 250 mg cap	Convulsions, **psychoses** (5-10% of those receiving 1.0 gm per day); headache; somno-lence; hyperreflexia; increased CSF protein and pressure; **peripheral neuropathy.** 100 mg pyridoxine (or more) q24h should be given concomitantly. Contraindicated in epileptics.	None
Dapsone (25, 100 mg tab)	100 mg per day	100 mg tab	Blood: ↓ hemoglobin (1-2 gm) & ↑ retics (2-12%), in most pts. Hemolysis in G6PD deficiency. ↑ hemolysis due to concomitant atazanavir (AAC 56:1081, 2012). CNS: peripheral neuropathy (rare). GI: nausea, vomiting. Renal: albuminuria, nephrotic syndrome. Erythema nodosum leprosum in pts in rx for leprosy (½ pts 1st year). Hypersensitivity syndrome in 0.5-3.6% (See Surveillance). **Methemoglobinemia.**	Hypersensitivity syndrome: fever, rash, eosinophilia, lymphadenopathy, hepatitis, pneumonitis. Genetic marker identified (NEJM 369:1620, 2013).
Ethionamide (Trecator-SC) (120, 250 mg tab)	500–1000 mg per day (15-20 mg per kg per day) divided 1-3 doses per day [Bacteriostatic for extracellular organisms only]	RES: 0.8% (0-1.5%) 250 mg tab	**Gastrointestinal irritation** (up to 50% on large dose); goiter; peripheral neuropathy (rare); convulsions (rare); changes in affect (rare); difficulty in diabetes control; rashes; hepatitis; purpura; stomatitis; gynecomastia; menstrual irregularity. Give drug with meals or antacids; 50-100 mg pyridoxine per day concomitantly; SGOT monthly. Possibly teratogenic.	

See page 2 for abbreviations.   * Dosages are for adults (unless otherwise indicated) and assume normal renal function   [1] **DOT** = directly observed therapy
§ Mean (range) (higher in Hispanics, Asians, and patients <10 years old)

TABLE 12B (3)

AGENT (TRADE NAME)[1]	USUAL DOSAGE*	ROUTE/[1]° DRUG RESISTANCE (RES) US[2,§]	SIDE-EFFECTS, TOXICITY AND PRECAUTIONS	SURVEILLANCE
SECOND LINE DRUGS (continued)				
Linezolid (Zyvox) (600 mg tab, oral suspension 100 mg/mL)	600 mg once daily	PO or IV	Not FDA-approved indication. High rate of adverse events (>80% with 4 months or longer of therapy); myelosuppression, peripheral neuropathy, optic neuropathy. Avoid tyramine-containing foods, soy products, adrenergic agents (e.g., pseudoephedrine, phenylpropanolamine) MAO inhibitors, SSRIs; 600 mg > 300 mg dose for toxicity, consider reducing dose to 300 mg for toxicity or after 4 mos of therapy or culture-conversion to reduce toxicity.	Baseline and monthly complete blood count, monthly visual acuity checks, screen for symptoms of peripheral neuropathy, neurologic examination.
Moxifloxacin (Avelox) (400 mg tab)	400 mg qd	400 mg cap	Not FDA-approved indication. Concomitant administration of rifampin reduces serum levels of moxi (CID 45:1001, 2007).	None
Ofloxacin (Floxin) (200, 300, 400 mg tab)	400 mg bid	400 mg cap	Not FDA-approved indication. Overall adverse effects 11%, 4% discontinued due to side-effects. GI: nausea 3%, diarrhea 1%. **CNS:** insomnia 3%, headache 1%, dizziness 1%.	
Para-aminosalicylic acid (PAS, Paser) (Na+ or K+ salt) (4 gm cap)	4–6 gm bid (200 mg per kg per day) [Bacteriostatic for extracellular organisms only]	RES: 0.8% (0–1.5%) 450 mg tab (see Comment)	**Gastrointestinal irritation** (10–15%); goitrogenic action (rare); depressed prothrombin activity (rare); G6PD-mediated hemolytic anemia (rare), drug fever, rashes, hepatitis, myalgia, arthralgia. Retards hepatic enzyme induction, may ↓ INH hepatotoxicity. Available from CDC, (404) 639-3670, Jacobus Pharm. Co. (609) 921-7447.	None
Rifabutin (Mycobutin) (150 mg cap)	300 mg per day (prophylaxis or treatment)	150 mg tab	Polymyalgia, arthralgia, leukopenia, granulocytopenia. Anterior uveitis when given with concomitant clarithromycin; avoid 600 mg dose (NEJM 330:438, 1994). Uveitis reported with 300 mg per day (AnIM 12:510, 1994). Reddish urine, orange skin (pseudojaundice).	None
Rifapentine (Priftin) (150 mg tab)	600 mg twice weekly for 1st 2 mos., then 600 mg q week	150 mg tab	Similar to other rifabutins. (See RIF, RFB). Hyperuricemia seen in 21%. Causes red-orange discoloration of body fluids. Note ↑ prevalence of RIF resistance in pts on weekly rx. (Ln 353:1843, 1999).	None
Thalidomide (Thalomid) (50, 100, 200 mg cap)	100–300 mg po q24h (may use up to 400 mg po q24h for severe erythema nodosum leprosum)	50 mg tab	**Contraindicated in pregnancy. Causes severe life-threatening birth defects. Both male and female patients must take barrier contraceptive methods (Pregnancy Category X). Frequently causes drowsiness or somnolence. May cause peripheral neuropathy.** (AJM 108:487, 2000) For review, see Ln 363:1803, 2004.	In US: contact Celgene (800-4-CELGENE)

See page 2 for abbreviations.

* Dosages are for adults (unless otherwise indicated) and assume normal renal function
§ Mean (range) (higher in Hispanics, Asians, and patients <10 years old)

[1] **DOT** = directly observed therapy

TABLE 13A- TREATMENT OF PARASITIC INFECTIONS

- **See Table 13D for sources for antiparasitic drugs not otherwise commercially available.**
- The following resources are available through the Centers for Disease Control and Prevention (CDC) in Atlanta. Website is www.cdc.gov. General advice for parasitic diseases other than malaria: (+1) (404) 718-4745 (day), (+1) (770) 488-7100 (after hours). For CDC Drug Service 8:00 a.m. – 4:30 p.m. EST: (+1) (404) 639-3670; fax: (+1) (404) 639-3717. See www.cdc.gov/laboratory/drugservice/index.html For malaria: Prophylaxis advice (+1) (770) 488-7788; treatment (+1) (770) 488-7788; toll-free (US) 1-855-856-4713; website: www.cdc.gov/malaria
- **NOTE: All dosage regimens are for adults with normal renal function unless otherwise stated.** Many of the suggested regimens have not been FDA approved.
- For licensed drugs, suggest checking package inserts to verify dosage and side-effects. Occasionally, post-licensure data may alter dosage as compared to package inserts.

INFECTING ORGANISM	SUGGESTED REGIMENS — PRIMARY	SUGGESTED REGIMENS — ALTERNATIVE	COMMENTS
PROTOZOA—INTESTINAL (non-pathogenic): E. hartmanni, E. dispar, E. moshkovski, E. coli, Iodamoeba butschlii, Endolimax nana, Chilomastix mesnili)			
Balantidium coli	Tetracycline 500 mg po qid x 10 days	Metronidazole 750 mg po tid times 5 days	Another alternative: Iodoquinol 650 mg po tid x 20 days.
Blastocystis hominis Ref: *Trends Parasitol 28:305, 2012*	Metronidazole 1.5 gm po 1x/day x 10 days or 750 mg po tid x 10 days (need to treat is dubious)	Alternatives: **Iodoquinol** 650 mg po tid x 20 days OR **TMP-SMX-DS**, one bid x 7 days or **Nitazoxanide** 500 mg po bid x 3 days	Role as pathogen unclear: may serve as marker of exposure to contaminated food/water. Some genotypes may be more virulent.
Cryptosporidium parvum & hominis treatment is unsatisfactory Ref: *Curr Opin Infect Dis 23:494, 2010*	**Immunocompetent—No HIV: Nitazoxanide** 500 mg po bid x 3 days (expensive)	**HIV with immunodeficiency:** Effective antiretroviral therapy most important therapy. **Nitazoxanide** no clinical or parasite response compared to placebo.	**Nitazoxanide:** Approved in liquid formulation for rx of children & 500 mg tabs for adults who are immunocompetent. Ref.: *CID 40:1173, 2005.* **C. hominis** assoc. with ↑ in post-infection eye & joint pain, recurrent headache, & dizzy spells (*CID 39:504, 2004*).
Cyclospora cayetanensis; cyclosporiasis (*Clin Micro Rev 23:218, 2010*)	**Immunocompetent pts: TMP-SMX-DS** tab 1 po bid x 7-10 days. Other options: see *Comments.*	**AIDS pts: TMP-SMX-DS** tab 1 po qid for up to 3-4 wks (immunoincompetent pts: may require suppressive rx with **TMP-SMX-DS** 1 tab 3x/wk	If sulfa-allergic: **CIP** 500 mg po bid x 7 days but results inconsistent. Anecdotal success with Nitazoxanide. Biliary disease described in pts.
Dientamoeba fragilis See *AJTMH 82:614, 2010; Clin Micro Infect 14:601, 2008.*	**Iodoquinol** 650 mg po tid x 20 days or **Paromomycin** 25-35 mg/kg/day po in 3 div doses x 7 days or **Metronidazole** 750 mg tid x 10 days	For treatment failures: **Tetracycline** 500 mg po qid x 10 days + **Iodoquinol** 650 mg po tid x 10 days OR (**Iodoquinol** + **Paromomycin***)	Metronidazole in prospective random placebo-control DB study (*CID 58:1692, 2014*). In vitro tinidazole, metronidazole most active. *AAC 56:487, 2012*
Entamoeba histolytica; amebiasis. If available, use stool PCR for diagnosis. Asymptomatic cyst passer	**Paromomycin*** 25-35 mg/kg/day po in 3 divided doses x7 days OR **Iodoquinol*** 650 mg po tid x 20 days	**Diloxanide furoate*** (Furamide) 500 mg po tid x 10 days	Note: E. hartmanni and E. dispar are non-pathogenic.
Patient with diarrhea/dysentery; mild/moderate disease. Oral therapy possible	**Metronidazole** 500-750 mg po tid x 7-10 days or **tinidazole** 2 gm po daily x 3 days, followed by. Either [**paromomycin*** 25-35 mg/kg/day po divided in 3 doses x 7 days] or [**iodoquinol*** 650 mg po tid x 20 days] to clear intestinal cysts. See comment.		Colitis can mimic ulcerative colitis; ameboma can mimic adenocarcinoma of colon. **Nitazoxanide** 500 mg po bid x 3 days may be effective (*JID 184:381, 2001 & Tran R Soc Trop Med & Hyg 101:1025, 2007*).
Severe or extraintestinal infection, e.g. hepatic abscess	(**Metronidazole** 750 mg IV to PO tid x 10 days or **tinidazole** 2 gm 1x/day x 5 days) followed by **paromomycin*** 25-35 mg/kg/day po in 3 doses x 7 days or **iodoquinol*** 650 mg po tid x 20 days.		**Serology positive (antibody present) with extraintestinal disease.**
Giardia intestinalis also known as **Giardia lamblia, Giardia duodenalis.**	(**Tinidazole** 2 gm po x 1) OR (**nitazoxanide** 500 mg po bid x 3 days). **Metro & Paromomycin** are alternatives	**Metronidazole** 250 mg po tid x 5 days; Albendazole 400 mg po once daily with food x 5 days. Cochrane Database Syst Rev.2012 Dec 12:12:CD007787. **Pregnancy: Paromomycin*** 25-35 mg/kg/day po in 3 divided doses x 5-10 days.	**Refractory pts: (metro 750 mg po + quinacrine 100 mg po)** x 3 wks OR (**Paromomycin** 10 mg/kg/day 3x/day x 3 wks (*CID 33:22, 2001*) giardia genetically heterogeneous (*J Clin Invest 123:2346, 2013*)

* For source of drug, see Table 13D, page 157.

TABLE 13A (2)

INFECTING ORGANISM	SUGGESTED REGIMENS		COMMENTS
	PRIMARY	ALTERNATIVE	
PROTOZOA—INTESTINAL *(continued)*			
Cystoisospora belli (formerly **Isospora belli**) (AIDS ref: MMWR 58 (RR-4):1, 2009)	**Immunocompetent: TMP-SMX-DS** tab 1 po bid x 7–10 days. **Immunocompromised: TMP-SMX-DS** 1 po bid up to 4 wks. If CD4<200 may not respond, need ART.	**CIP** 500 mg po bid x 7 days is second-line alternative (AJM 132:885, 2000) OR **Pyrimethamine** 50–75 mg/day + **Folinic acid** (10–25 mg/day (po).	**Chronic suppression in AIDS pts:** either **TMP-SMX-DS** 1 tab 3x/wk OR tab 1 po daily OR **CIP** 500 mg po 3x/wk + **Pyrimethamine** 25 mg po + **folinic acid** 10 mg/day po OR as 2nd-line alternative: **CIP** 500 mg po 3x/wk.
Microsporidiosis			
Ocular: Encephalitozoon hellum or cuniculi, Vittaforma (Nosema) corneae, Nosema ocularum.	For HIV pts, antiretroviral therapy key. **Albendazole** 400 mg po bid x 3 wks plus fumagillin eye drops (see Comment).	In HIV+ pts, reports of response of E.hellum to **fumagillin** eyedrops (see Comment). For V. corneae, may need keratoplasty.	To obtain fumagillin: 800–292–6773 or www.leiters.com. Neutropenia & thrombocytopenia serious adverse events. Dx: Most labs use modified trichrome stain, electron micrographs for species identification. FA and PCR methods in development. Peds dose ref.: PIDJ 23:915, 2004
Intestinal (diarrhea): Enterocytozoon bieneusi, Encephalitozoon (Septata) intestinalis	**Albendazole** 400 mg po bid x 3 wks; peds dose: 15 mg/kg per day div. into 2 daily doses x7 days for E. intestinalis. Fumagillin equally effective.	Oral **fumagillin 20 mg po tid** reported effective for E. bieneusi (NEJM 346:1963, 2002) — see Comment	For Trachipleistophora sp., try itraconazole + albendazole (NEJM 351:42, 2004).
Disseminated: E. hellum, cuniculi or intestinalis; Pleistophora sp., others in 20 mg po tid (not available in US) Comment. Ref: JCM 52:3839, 2014.	**Albendazole** 400 mg po bid x 3 wks. Fumagillin	No established rx for Pleistophora sp.	Other pathogens: Brachiola vesicularum & algerae (NEJM 351:42, 2004).
PROTOZOA—EXTRAINTESTINAL			
Amebic meningoencephalitis (Clin Infect Dis 51:e7, 2010 (Balamuthia)) Mitefosine available from CDC for all species of free-living ameba, contact CDC Emergency Operations Center at 770-488-7100			
Acanthamoeba sp. — no proven rx Rev.: FEMS Immunol Med Micro 50:1, 2007	IV therapy: [Pentamidine + Albendazole ± (Fluconazole or Itraconazole) + Miltefosine 50 mg po tid. May and TMP-SMX, Metronidazole, and a Macrolide		For Acanthamoeba keratitis: miltefosine or voriconazole.
Balamuthia mandrillaris Naegleria fowleri: >95% mortality. Ref. MMWR 57:573, 2008.	[Pentamidine + Albendazole ± (Fluconazole or Itraconazole) + Miltefosine 50 mg po tid] Amphotericin B 1.5 mg/kg/day ± 1.5 mg/day intrathecal + Rifampin 10 mg/kg/day + Fluconazole 10 mg/kg/day IV/po + Miltefosine 50 mg po tid		
Babesia microti (US) and **Babesia divergens** (EU) (NEJM 366:2397, 2012)	For mild/moderate disease: **Atovaquone** 750 mg po bid + **Azithro** 500 mg po on day 1, then 250-1000 mg po daily for total of 7-10 days. If relapse, treat x 6 wks & until blood smear neg x 2 wks.	For severe babesiosis: (**Clindamycin** 600 mg po tid) + (**quinine** 650 mg po tid) x 7–10 days For adults, can give **clinda** IV as 1.2 gm bid.	Overwhelming infection in asplenic patients. In immunocompromised patients, treat for 6 or more weeks (CID 46:370, 2008). Transfusion related cases occur.
Leishmaniasis (Suggest consultation – CDC (+1) 404-718-4745) Note: Miltefosine approved for all forms of leishmania. Contact CDC for IND. Ref: Med Lett 56:89, 2014.			
Cutaneous: Mild Disease (< 4 lesions, none > 5 cm diameter, no lesions in cosmetically sensitive area, none over joints). Otherwise, consider Moderate Disease	Mild Disease (< 4 lesions, none > 5 cm): **Paromomycin** ointment 20 days (investigational), cryotherapy (freeze up to 3x with liquid nitrogen); intralesional Antimony 20 mg/kg into lesions weekly x 8-10 wks. CDC antimony IND does not cover intralesional use, common outside US.	**Moderate Disease:** **Sodium stibogluconate** (Pentostam) or **Meglumine antimonate** (Glucantime) 20 mg/kg/day IV/IM x 20 days. Dilute in 120 mL of D5W and infuse over 2 hrs. Alternatives: **Fluconazole** 200 mg po daily x 6 weeks (for L. mexicana, L. panamensis), **L. major**) or **ketoconazole** 600 mg po daily x 30 days (L. mexicana) or **Miltefosine** (dose as for mild disease	Oral therapy. Topical paromomycin* & other topical treatment (only when low potential for mucosal spread; never use for L. brasiliensis or L. guyanensis cutaneous lesions. Generic pentavalent antimony varies in quality and safety. Leishmania in travelers frequently responds to observation alone without therapy (CID 57:370, 2013). Miltefosine is preg cat D (do not use in pregnancy)
	Mild/moderate disease: Atovaquone 750 mg po daily x 20 days 50 mg/kg/day (divid) (wt <30-44 kg); 50 mg/kg (wt > 45 kg). Treat for 28 days. Response in about 70% of pts.		

* For source of drug, see Table 13D, page 157.

TABLE 13A (3)

INFECTING ORGANISM	SUGGESTED REGIMENS		COMMENTS
	PRIMARY	ALTERNATIVE	

PROTOZOA—EXTRAINTESTINAL *(continued)*

Leishmaniasis, Mucosal (Espundia).
All cutaneous lesions due to L. braziliensis. High cure rate with Lipo Ampho B *(Trans R Soc Trop Med Hyg* 108:176, 2014).

Primary: **Pentavalent antimony (Sb)*** 20 mg/kg/day IV or IM x 28 days for mucosal disease. 20 days for cutaneous disease **or liposomal amphotericin B** (regimens vary) with total cumulative dose of 20-60 mg/kg or **amphotericin B** 0.5-1 mg/kg IV daily or qod to total dose of 20-40 mg/kg. *See J Am Acad Dermatol 68:284, 2013.*

Alternative: **Miltefosine*** (w/food) 50 mg po bid (wt 30-44 kg); 50 mg po tid (wt ≥ 45 kg). Treat for 28 days. Complete resolution in 62% of pts.

Comments: Antimony available from CDC drug service; miltefosine FDA approved for leishmania in 2014 but not marketed in US at present. *See Table 13D for contact information.*

Visceral leishmaniasis – Kala-Azar –
New World & Old World
L. donovani: Old World India
L. infantum: Mediterranean
L. chagasi: New World

Primary (Immunocompetent): **Liposomal ampho B** 3 mg/kg once daily on days 1-5, 14, 21 **or Miltefosine*** (w/food) 50 mg po bid (wt 30-44 kg); 50 mg tid (wt ≥ 45 kg). Treat for 28 days. HIV/AIDS: **Liposomal Ampho B** 4 mg/kg qd on days 1-5, 10, 17, 24, 31, 38 (Curr Opin Infect Dis 26:1, 2013).

Alternative: **Standard Ampho B** 1 mg/kg IV daily x 15-20 days or every other day (total of 1-1.20 mg/kg) **or Miltefosine*** (w/food) 50 mg po bid (wt 30-44 kg); 50 mg tid (wt ≥ 45 kg). Treat for 28 days. HIV/AIDS: **Liposomal Ampho B** 4 mg/kg qd on days 1-5, 10, 17, 24, 31, 38 (Curr Opin Infect Dis 26:1, 2013), OR **pentavalent antimony*** 20 mg/kg/day IV/IM x 28 days.

Comments: In HIV patients, may need lifelong suppression with Amphotericin B q 2-4 wks.

Malaria (Plasmodia species) —NOTE: CDC Malaria info— prophylaxis/treatment (770) 488-7788. After hours: 770-488-7100. US toll-free 1-855-856-4713. CDC offers species confirmation and drug resistance testing. Refs: *JAMA* 297:2251, 2264 & 2285, 2007. Websites: www.cdc.gov/malaria; http://www.who.int/ith/ITH_chapter_7_pdf?ua= 1 Review of rapid diagnostic tests: *CID* 54:1637, 2012.

Prophylaxis—Drugs plus personal protection: screens, nets, 30-35% DEET skin repellent (avoid > 50% DEET) *(Med Lett* 54:75, 2012), permethrin spray on clothing and mosquito nets. Country risk in CDC Yellow Book.

For areas free of chloroquine (CQ)-resistant P. falciparum:
Central America (west of Panama Canal), Caribbean, Korea, Middle East (most)

Primary: **CQ** phosphate 500 mg po per wk starting 1-2 wks before travel, during travel, & 4 wks post-travel **or atovaquone-proguanil (AP)** 1 adult tablet per day (1 day prior to, during, & 7 days post-travel): **primaquine (PQ)** 30 mg base po daily in non-pregnant, G6PD-normal travelers; >92% effective vs P. vivax *(CID* 33:1990, 2001).

Alternative: **CQ Peds dose:** 8.3 mg/kg (5 mg/kg of base) po 1x/wk up to 300 mg (base) max. dose **or AP** (peds tabs): 11-20 kg, 1 tab; 21-30 kg, 2 tabs; 31-40 kg, 3 tabs; >40 kg, 1 adult tab per day. **Adults:** Doxy or MQ as below.

Comments: CQ safe during pregnancy. **The areas free of CQ-resistant falciparum malaria continue to shrink.** See CDC or WHO maps for most current information on CQ resistance.
Doxy AEs: photosensitivity, candida vaginitis, gastritis.

For areas with CQ-resistant P. falciparum

Primary: **Atovaquone 250 mg—proguanil 100 mg (Malarone)** comb. tablet, 1 adult tab po daily for adults & children > 8 yrs of age. Take 1-2 days prior to, during, & 7 days post-travel. Peds dose in footnote[1].
Note: **CQ** may exacerbate psoriasis.
Not in pregnancy. Malarone preferred for trips of a week or less; expense may preclude use for longer trips. Native population: intermittent pregnancy prophylaxis/treatment programs in a few countries. Fansidar 1 tab po 3 times during pregnancy *(Expert Rev Anti Infect Ther* 8:589, 2010).

Alternative: **Doxycycline** 100 mg po daily for adults & children > 8 yrs of age[1]. Take 1-2 days before, during, & 4 wks after travel. **OR**
Mefloquine (MQ) 250 mg (228 mg base) po once per wk, 1-2 wks before, during, & 4 wks after travel. Continue daily x 4 wks after leaving risk area.

Comments: **Pregnancy: MQ current best option.** Insufficient data with Malarone. Avoid doxycycline and primaquine.
Primaquine: Can cause hemolytic anemia if G6PD deficiency present.
MQ not recommended if cardiac conduction abnormalities, seizures, or psychiatric disorders, e.g. depression, psychosis.
MQ outside U.S.: 275 mg tab, contains 250 mg of base. If used, can start 3 wks before travel to assure tolerability.
Doxy AEs: photosensitivity, candida vaginitis, gastritis.

---

[1] Peds prophylaxis dosages: **Mefloquine** weekly dose by **weight**: <9 kg = 5 mg base = ⅛ adult tab weekly; 10-19 kg = ¼ adult tab weekly; 20-30 kg = ½ adult tab weekly; 31-45 kg = ¾ adult tab weekly; >45 kg = 1 tab weekly. **Atovaquone/proguanil** by **weight**: single daily dose using peds tab (62.5 mg atovaquone & 25 mg proguanil): 5-8 kg, 1/2 tab; 8-10 kg, 3/4 tab; 11-20 kg, 1 tab; 21-30 kg, 2 tabs; 31-40 kg, 3 tabs; ≥41 kg, one adult tab. **Doxycycline**, ages >8-12 yrs: 2 mg per kg per day up to 100 mg/day.

* For source of drug, see Table 13D, page 157.

TABLE 13A (4)

PROTOZOA—EXTRAINTESTINAL/Malaria (Plasmodia species) (continued)

Treatment of Malaria. Diagnosis is by microscopy. Alternative: rapid antigen detection test (Binax NOW): detects 96-100% of P. falciparum and 50% of other plasmodia (CID 49:908, 2009; CID 54:1637, 2012). Need microscopy to speciate. Can stay positive for over a month after successful treatment.

INFECTING ORGANISM	Region Acquired	SUGGESTED REGIMENS		COMMENTS
		PRIMARY	ALTERNATIVE	
Clinical Severity/ Plasmodia sp.		**Suggested Treatment Regimens (Drug)**		
		Adults	Peds	Comments
Uncomplicated / P. falciparum (or species not identified)	Cen. Amer., west of Panama Canal; Haiti; Dom. Repub., & most of Mid-East **CQ-sensitive**	**CQ** phosphate 1 gm salt (600 mg base) po, then 0.5 gm in 6 hrs, then 0.5 gm daily x 2 days. Total: 2500 mg salt	**Peds: CQ** 10 mg/kg of base po; then 5 mg/kg of base at 6, 24, & 48 hrs. Total: 25 mg/kg base	Other chloroquine salts available in some countries, total dose may differ. **Peds. dose should never exceed adult dose. CQ + MQ prolong QTc. Doses > 2x recommended may be fatal.**
	CQ-resistant or unknown resistance. Note: If >5% parasitemia or Hb <7, treat as severe malaria regardless of clinical findings or lack thereof.	**Adults: Atovaquone-proguanil** 1 gm-400 mg (4 adult tabs) po 1x/day x 3 days w/ food **OR [QS** 650 mg po tid x 3 days (7 days if SE Asia)] + **[(Doxy** 100 mg po bid) or **(tetra** 250 mg po qid) or **clinda** 20 mg/kg/d divided tid x 7 days] **Artemether-lumefantrine*** tabs 20/120 mg 4 tabs po (at 0, 8 hrs) then bid x 2 days (total 6 doses); take with food **OR** a less desirable adult alternative, **mefloquine** 750 mg po x 1 dose, then 500 mg x 1 dose 6-12 hr later. **MQ** is 2nd line alternative due to neuropsychiatric reaction and cannot use in SE Asia due to resistance. Clinda or tetracycline only if doxy not available.	**Peds: [QS** 10 mg/kg po tid x 3 days] + **[clinda** 20 mg/kg per day div. tid]—both x 7 days. Use doxy >8 yrs of age 2.2 mg/kg/ bid up to 100 mg per dose OR Atovaquone-proguanil (all once daily x 3 d) by weight: 5-8 kg: 2 peds tabs; 9-10 kg: 3 peds tabs; 11-20 kg: 1 adult tab; 21-30 kg: 2 adult tabs; 31-40 kg: 3 adult tabs; >40 kg: 4 adult tabs OR **MQ Salt:** 15 mg/kg x 1, then 10 mg/kg ALL po 6-12 hrs later. OR **Artemether-lumefantrine*** 5 kg to < 15 kg: 1 tablet (20 mg) as a single dose, then 1 tablet again after 8 hours, then 1 tablet every 12 hours for 2 days (40 mg). 15 kg to < 25 kg: 2 tablets (40 mg: 240 mg) as a single dose, then 2 tablets again after 8 hours, then 2 tablets every 12 hours for 2 days (360 mg). 25 kg to < 35 kg: 3 tablets (60 mg) as a single dose, then 3 tablets again after 8 hours, then 3 tablets every 12 hours for 2 days ≥ 35 kg: 4 tablets per dose x 6 doses as per adult dose	**Pregnancy:** • Artemether-lumefantrine 4 tablets (80 mg/480 mg) as a single dose, then 4 tablets again after 8 hours, then 4 tablets every 12 hours for 2 days (take with food). Drug of choice in 2nd/3rd trimester. Artemether-lumefantrine is safer than quinine in the first trimester of pregnancy. *Malar J. 13:197, 2014* OR • Quinine sulfate 10 mg/kg po tid x 3 days (7 days if SE Asia) + Clindamycin 20 mg/kg/day divided tid x 7 days • Do not initiate therapy if quinine available and artemether-lumefantrine is not in U.S. QS is only available as quinine 324 mg capsule, thus hard to treat children. **Note: Oral Artemether-lumefantrine tabs FDA-approved but not widely stocked. Call 1-800-COARTEM to obtain.**
Uncomplicated / P. malariae or P. knowlesi (JID 199: 1107 & 1143, 2009).	All regions – **CQ-sensitive**	**CQ** as above, adults & peds. In South Pacific, beware of P. knowlesi: looks like P. malariae, but behaves like P. falciparum (CID 46:165, 2007).	**Artemether-lumefantrine*** (20/120 mg tab): 4 tabs po x 1 dose, repeat in 8 hrs, then repeat q12h x 2 days (take with food) OR Atovaquone-proguanil (1000/400 mg) 4 adult tabs po daily x 3 days	

* For source of drug, see Table 13D, page 157.

TABLE 13A (5)

INFECTING ORGANISM	SUGGESTED REGIMENS		COMMENTS
	PRIMARY	ALTERNATIVE	

PROTOZOA—EXTRAINTESTINAL/Malaria (Plasmodia species)/Treatment of Malaria (continued)

Clinical Severity/ Plasmodia sp.	Region Acquired	Suggested Treatment Regimens (Drug)		Comments
		Adults	Peds	
Uncomplicated/ P. vivax or P. ovale	**CQ-sensitive** (except Papua New Guinea, Indonesia which are CQ-resistant–see below)	**CQ** as above + **PQ** base: 30 mg po once daily x 14 days Each primaquine phosphate tab is 26.3 mg of salt and 15 mg of base. 30 mg of base = 2 26.3 mg tabs prim. phos.	**Peds: CQ** as above + **PQ** base 0.5 mg po once daily x 14 days	PQ added to eradicate latent parasites in liver. **Screen for G6PD def. before starting PQ;** If G6PD deficient dose PQ as 45 mg po once weekly x 8 wks. **Note: rare severe reactions.** Avoid PQ in pregnancy. If P. vivax or P. ovale, after pregnancy check for G6PD deficiency & give PQ 30 mg po daily times 14 days.
Uncomplicated/ P. vivax	**CQ-resistant:** Papua, New Guinea & Indonesia	**QS** + (**doxy** or **tetra**) + **PQ** as above or **Artemether-Lumefantrine** (same dose as for P. falciparum)	**MQ** + **PQ** as above. **Peds** (<8 yrs old): **QS** alone x 7 days or **MQ** alone. If latter fail, add **doxy** or **tetra**	Rarely acute. Lung injury and other serious complications: LnID 8:449, 2008.

Clinical Severity/ Plasmodia sp.	Region Acquired	Suggested Treatment Regimens (Drug)		Comments
		Primary—Adults	Alternative & Peds	
Uncomplicated Malaria/Alternatives for Pregnancy Ref: LnID 7:118 & 136, 2007	CQ-sensitive areas	**CQ** as above	**CQ** as above	Doxy or tetra used if benefits outweigh risks.
	CQ-resistant P. falciparum	**QS** + **clinda** as above	If failing or intolerant: **QS** + **doxy**	No controlled studies of AP in pregnancy.
	CQ-resistant P. vivax	**QS** 650 mg po tid x 7 days		If P. vivax or P. ovale, after pregnancy check for G6PD deficiency & give PQ 30 mg po daily times 14 days.
	Intermittent pregnancy treatment (empiric)	Give treatment dose of [Sulfadoxine 500 mg + Pyrimethamine 25 mg (Fansidar) po] at 3 times during pregnancy to decrease maternal & fetal morbidity & mortality		
Severe malaria, i.e., impaired consciousness, severe anemia, renal failure, pulmonary edema, ARDS, DIC, jaundice, acidosis, seizures, parasitemia >5%. One or more of latter **Almost always P. falciparum.** Ref: NEJM 358:1829, 2008; Science 320:30, 2008.	All regions Note: •IV Artesunate is drug of choice but not FDA-approved. Available from CDC Drug Service under specific conditions, need to state quinidine not available or not tolerated. •IV quinidine uncommonly available. Possible emergency availability from Eli Lilly.	**Quinidine gluconate** in normal saline: 10 mg/kg (salt) IV over 1 hr then 0.02 mg/kg/min by constant infusion OR 24 mg/kg IV over 4 hrs & then 12 mg/kg over 4 hrs q8h. Continue until parasite density <1% & can take po. **PLUS** **QS** 650 mg po tid x 7 days (or Asia) **+ Doxy** 100 mg q12h (as tolerated), q8h x 7 days. **OR IV Artesunate[*]** 2.4 mg/kg IV x 7 days) OR Artesunate[*] 2.4 mg/kg IV at 0, 12, 24, 48 hrs, and Doxy 100 mg IV q12h x 7 days.)	**Peds: Quinidine gluconate IV**—same mg/kg dose as for adults **PLUS** (**Doxy:** if <45 kg, 4 mg per kg (V q12h; if ≥45 kg, dose as for adults) OR **Clinda, Clindamycin** 10 mg/kg IV (loading dose, then 5 mg/kg IV or po [as tolerated] q8h x 7 days) **Follow iV artesunate with a complete oral course of: Doxycycline, Atovaquone/proguanil, Artemether/lumefantrine or Dihydroartemisinin/piperaquine (not available in US)**	During quinidine IV, monitor BP, EKG (prolongation of QTc), & blood glucose (hypoglycemia). Exchange transfusion no longer recommended. Switch to QS po + (Doxy or Clinda) when patient able to take oral drugs. **Steroids not recommended for cerebral malaria.** IV artesunate from CDC (8 hr transport time post-approval), see Table 13D (Ref: CID 44:1067 & 1075, 2007).

* For source of drug, see Table 13D, page 157.

TABLE 13A (6)

INFECTING ORGANISM	SUGGESTED REGIMENS		COMMENTS
	PRIMARY	ALTERNATIVE	

PROTOZOA—EXTRAINTESTINAL/Malaria (Plasmodia species)/Treatment of Malaria (continued)

Malaria—self-initiated treatment: Only for people at high risk. Carry a reliable supply to recommended treatment (to counter local meds). Use only if malaria is lab-diagnosed and no available reliable meds.	Artemether-lumefantrine (20/120 mg tab) 4 tabs po x dose, repeat 8 hrs, then repeat q12h x 2 days (<35 kg, 1 tab. Peds dosing elsewhere) (AP)	Peds: Using adult AP tabs for 3 consecutive days: 5-20 kg, 1 tab; 21-30 kg, 2 tabs; 31-40 kg, 3 tabs; >40 kg, 4 tabs, see Uncomplicated/P. falciparum, page 146.	Do not use for renal insufficiency pts. Do not use if weight <11 kg, pregnant, or breast-feeding. Artemether-lumefantrine, sold as Riamet (EU) and Coartem (US & elsewhere).

Toxoplasma gondii (Reference: Ln 363:1965, 2004)

Immunologically normal patients (For pediatric doses, see reference)			
Acute illness w/ lymphadenopathy Acq. via transfusion (lab accident)	[No specific rx unless severe/persistent symptoms or evidence of vital organ damage		
Active chorioretinitis; meningitis; lowered resistance due to steroids or cytotoxic drugs	Treat as for active chorioretinitis.		For congenital toxo, toxo meningitis in adults, & chorioretinitis, add prednisone 1 mg/kg/day in 2 div. doses until CSF protein conc. falls or vision-threatening inflammation subsides.
	Pyrimethamine (pyri) 200 mg po once on "in" day, then 50-75 mg po q24h) + leucovorin (folinic acid) 5-20 mg 3x/wk)—see Comment. Treat 1-2 wks beyond signs/symptoms; continue leucovorin 1 wk after stopping pyri.	(Pyrimethamine (see footnote) [+] sulfadiazine (see Comment. 1-1.5 gm po qid) + leucovorin (folinic acid) 5-20 mg 3x/wk)—see Comment	Adjust folinic acid dose by following CBC results. Screen patients with IgG/IgM serology at commercial lab. IgG+ /IgM neg = remote past infection. IgG+/IgM+ = seroconversion. For Spiramycin, consult with Palo Alto Medical Foundation Toxoplasma Serology Lab: 650-853-4828 or toxlab@pamf.org.
Acute in pregnant women. Ref: CID 47:554, 2008.	If <18 wks gestation at diagnosis: Spiramycin* 1 gm po q8h until 16-18 wks; dc if amniotic fluid PCR is negative. Positive PCR: treat as below. If >18 wks gestation & documented fetal infection by positive amniotic fluid PCR: (Pyrimethamine 50 mg po q12h x 2 days, then 50 mg/day + sulfadiazine 75 mg/kg po x 1 dose, then 50 mg/kg q12h (max 4 gm/day) + folinic acid 10-20 mg po daily) for minimum of 4 wks or for duration of pregnancy.		Details in Ln 363:1965, 2004. Consultation advisable.
Fetal/congenital	Mgmt complex. Combo rx with pyrimethamine + sulfadiazine + leucovorin—see Comment		

AIDS

Cerebral toxoplasmosis Ref: MMWR 58/RR-4/ 1, 2009.	[Pyrimethamine (pyri) 200 mg x 1 po, then 75 mg/day po) + sulfadiazine (Wt based dose: 1 gm if <60 kg, po) or 1500 mg if ≥60 kg; q6h) + folinic acid (5-20 mg/day po) for minimum of 6 wks after resolution of signs/symptoms, and then suppressive rx (see below) OR TMP-SMX 10/50 mg/kg per day po or iv div. q12h	[Pyri + folinic acid (as in primary regimen)] + one of the following: (1) Clinda 600 mg po/IV q6h or (2) atovaquone 750 mg po q6h. Treat 4-6 wks after resolution of signs/symptoms, then suppression.	Use alternative regimen for pts with severe sulfa allergy. If multiple ring-enhancing brain lesions (CT or MRI), ~85% of pts respond to 7-10 days of empiric rx; if no response, suggest brain biopsy. Pyri penetrates brain even if no inflammation; folinic acid prevents pyrimethamine hematologic toxicity.
Primary prophylaxis. AIDS pts—IgG toxo antibody + CD4 count <100 per mcL	TMP-SMX 10/50 mg/kg per day po x 30 days (AAC 42:1346, 1998) TMP-SMX-DS, 1 tab po q24h or 3x/wk) or TMP-SMX-SS, 1 tab po q24h)	[(Dapsone 50 mg po q24h + (pyri 50 mg po q wk) + folinic acid 25 mg po q wk] OR atovaquone 1500 mg po q24h	Prophylaxis for pneumocystis also effective vs toxo. Ref: MMWR 58/RR-4/ 1, 2009. Another alternative: (Dapsone 200 mg po + pyrimethamine 75 mg po + folinic acid 25 mg po once weekly.
Suppression after rx of cerebral toxo	[Sulfadiazine 2-4 gm po divided in 2-4 doses/day) + (pyri 25-50 mg po q24h) + folinic acid 10-25 mg po q24h). DC if CD4 count >200 x3 mos	[(Clinda 600 mg po q8h) + (pyri 25-50 mg po q24h) + (folinic acid 10-25 mg po q24h)] OR atovaquone 750 mg po q6-12h	(pyri + sulfa) prevents PCP and toxo; (clinda + pyri) prevents toxo only. Additional drug needed to prevent PCP.

Trichomonas vaginalis	See Vaginitis, Table 1, page 26.		

---

[2] Sulfonamides for toxo. Sulfadiazine now commercially available. Sulfisoxazole much less effective.

* For source of drug, see Table 13D, page 157.

TABLE 13A (7)

INFECTING ORGANISM	SUGGESTED REGIMENS		COMMENTS
	PRIMARY	ALTERNATIVE	
PROTOZOA—EXTRAINTESTINAL/Toxoplasma gondii/AIDS (continued)			
Trypanosomiasis. Ref.: Ln 362:1469, 2003. **Note: Drugs for African trypanosomiasis may be obtained free from WHO or CDC. See Table 13D, page 157, for source information.**			
West African sleeping sickness (T. brucei gambiense)			
Early: Blood/lymphatic	**Pentamidine** 4 mg/kg IV/IM daily x 7-10 days	In US, free from CDC Drug service: **Suramin*** 100 mg IV (test dose), then 1 gm IV on days 1, 3, 7, 14, & 21 Peds: dose is 20 mg/kg.	Suramin effective but avoid if possible due to possible co-infection with O. volvulus in W. Africa.
Late: Encephalitis	Combination of IV **eflornithine** 400 mg/kg/day divided q12h x 7 days, plus **nifurtimox**, 15 mg/kg/day, divided q8h x 10 days (abbreviated NECT) now WHO standard of care (Lancet 374:56, 2009; CID 56:195 2013	Melarsoprol 2.2 mg/kg/day IV x 10 days; toxic arsenical now superseded by NECT†	
East African sleeping sickness (T. brucei rhodesiense)			
Early: Blood/lymphatic	**Suramin*** 100 mg IV (test dose), then 1 gm IV on days 1, 3, 7, 14, & 21	Peds: **Suramin*** 2 mg/kg test dose, then 20 mg/kg IV on days 1, 3, 7, 14, & 21	Suramin & Melarsoprol: CDC Drug Service or WHO (at no charge). (see Table 13D)
Late: Encephalitis (prednisolone may prevent encephalitis) Pre-treatment with Suramin advised by some.	**Melarsoprol***2.2 mg/kg/day IV x 10 days (PLoS NTD 6:e1695, 2012)	**Melarsoprol***From 2.2-3.6 mg/kg per day IV over 3 days; repeat 3.6 mg/kg after 7 days & for 3rd time at 3.6 mg/kg 7 days after 2nd course	Early illness: patient waiting for Suramin, use pentamidine 4 mg/kg/day IV/IM x 1-2 doses Does not enter CSF.
T. cruzi—**Chagas disease** or acute American trypanosomiasis For chronic disease: see Comment. Ref.: Ln 375:1388, 2010; LnID 10:556, 2010	Adult (Age ≥ 12) **Benznidazole*** 5-7 mg/kg/day po in 2 doses (q12h) x 60 days (Do not use in pregnancy) Pediatric (Age <12 years): **Benznidazole*** 10 mg/kg/day po in 2 doses (q12h) x 60 days	**Nifurtimox*** 8-10 mg/kg per day po div. 4x/day after meals x 120 days Age 11-16 yrs: 12.5-15.6 mg/kg per day div. qid po x 90 days Children <11yrs: 15-20 mg/kg per day div. qid po x 90 days.	Immunosuppression for heart transplant can reactivate chronic Chagas disease (J Card Failure 15:249, 2009). Can transmit by organ/transfusions (CID 48:1534, 2009).
NEMATODES—INTESTINAL (Roundworms). Eosinophilia? Think Strongyloides, toxocaria & filariasis: CID 34:407, 2005; 42:1781 & 1655, 2006-- See Table 13C.			
Anisakis simplex (anisakiasis) Anisakiasis differentiated from Anisakidosis (CID 51:806, 2010). Other--A. physistra, Pseudoterranova decipiens	Physical removal: endoscope or surgery IgE antibody test vs A. simplex may help diagnosis. No antimicrobial therapy.	Anecdotal reports of possible treatment benefit from albendazole (Ln 360:54, 2002; CID 41:1825, 2005)	Anisakiasis acquired by eating (raw) fish: herring, salmon, mackerel, cod, squid. Similar illness due to Pseudoterranova species acquired from cod, halibut, red snapper.
Ascaris lumbricoides (ascariasis) Ln 367:1521, 2006	**Albendazole** 400 mg po daily x 3 days or **mebendazole** 100 mg po x1 dose	**Ivermectin** 150-200 mcg/kg po x 1 dose	Review of efficacy of single dose: JAMA 299:1937, 2008.
Capillaria philippinensis (capillariasis)	**Mebendazole** 200 mg po bid x 20 days	**Albendazole** 200 mg po bid x 10 days	Albendazole preferred.
Enterobius vermicularis (pinworm)	**Mebendazole**US 100 mg po x 1, repeat in 2 wks OR **Pyrantel pamoate** 11 mg/kg base (to max. dose of 1 gm) po x1 dose, repeat in 2 wks	**Albendazole** 400 mg po x 1 dose, repeat in 2 wks.	Side-effects in Table 13B, page 156. Treat whole household.
Gongylonemiasis (adult worms in oral mucosa)	Surgical removal		Ref.: CID 32:1378, 2001; J Helminth 80:425, 2006.
Hookworm (Necator americanus and Ancylostoma duodenale)	**Albendazole** 400 mg po daily x 3 days	**Mebendazole**US 100 mg po bid x 3 days OR **Pyrantel pamoate** 11 mg/kg (to max. dose of 1 gm) po daily x 3 days	NOTE: Ivermectin not effective. Single dose therapy as used in public health programs has lower cure rates and 3-day albendazole superior to 3-day mebendazole. PLoS One 6:e25003, 2011
Strongyloides stercoralis (**strongyloidiasis**) (Hyperinfection, See Comment)	**Ivermectin** 200 mcg/kg per day po x 2 days	**Albendazole** 400 mg po bid x 7 days ; less effective	**For hyperinfection**, repeat at 15 days. For hyperinfection: veterinary ivermectin given subcutaneously or rectally (CID 49:1411, 2009).

† For source of drug, see Table 13D, page 157.

* For source of drug, see Table 13D, page 157.

TABLE 13A (8)

INFECTING ORGANISM	SUGGESTED REGIMENS		COMMENTS
	PRIMARY	ALTERNATIVE	
NEMATODES—INTESTINAL (Roundworms) *(continued)*			
Trichostrongylus orientalis, T. colubriformis	Pyrantel pamoate 11 mg/kg (max. 1 gm) po x 1	Albendazole 400 mg po x 1 dose	Mebendazole 100 mg po bid x 3 days
Trichuris trichiura (whipworm): *NEJM 370:610, 2014; PLoS One 6:e25003, 2011*	Mebendazole[NUS] 100 mg po bid x 3 days	Albendazole 400 mg po qd x 3 days **or Ivermectin** 200 mcg/kg po qd x 3 days	Mebendazole clearly superior for trichuris *(PLoS One 6:e25003, 2011; N Engl J Med 370:610, 2014)*
NEMATODES—EXTRAINTESTINAL (Roundworms)			
Ancylostoma braziliense & caninum: causes **cutaneous larva migrans**	Albendazole 400 mg po bid x 3-7 days *(Ln 17 8:302, 2008)*	Ivermectin 200 mcg/kg po x 1 dose/day x 1-2 days (not in children wt < 15 kg)	Also called "creeping eruption", dog and cat hookworm. Ivermectin cure rate 81-100% (1 dose) to 97% (2-3 doses) *(CID 31:493, 2000).*
Angiostrongylus cantonensis (Angiostrongyliasis) causes eosinophilic meningitis	Mild/moderate disease: Analgesics, serial LPs (if necessary). Adding **Albendazole** 15 mg/kg/day to prednisone 60 mg/day both for 14 days may reduce duration of headaches and need for LPs.	Adding **Albendazole** 15 mg/kg/day to prednisone 60 mg/day for 14 days may reduce duration of headaches and need for LPs.	**Do not use Albendazole without prednisone**, see *TRSMH 102:990, 2008.* Gnathostoma and Baylisascaris also cause eosinophilic meningitis.
Baylisascariasis (Raccoon roundworm); eosinophilic meningitis	No drug proven efficacious. Try po **albendazole**, Peds: 25–50 mg/day po; Adults: 400 mg po bid with corticosteroids. Treat for one month.		*Clin Microbiol Rev 18:703, 2005.* Other causes of eosinophilic meningitis: Gnathostoma & Angiostrongylus.
Dracunculus medinensis: **Guinea worm** *(Trans R Soc Trop Med Hyg 108:249, 2014)*	Slow extraction of pre-emergent worm over several days	No drugs effective. Oral analgesics, anti-inflammatory drugs, topical antiseptics/antibiotic ointments to alleviate symptoms and facilitate worm removal by gentle manual traction over several days.	
Filariasis: Determine if co-infection with either Loa loa or Onchocerca			
Lymphatic filariasis (**Elephantiasis**): Etiologies: Wuchereria bancrofti Brugia malayi, Brugia timori	*Mono-infection:* **Diethylcarbamazine[3](DEC)** * 6 mg/kg/day po in 3 divided doses x 12 days + **Doxy** 200 mg/day po x 6 wks	*Dual infection with Onchocerciasis:* Treat Onchocerciasis first: **Ivermectin** 150 mcg/kg po x 1 dose, wait 1 month, then start **DEC** as for *Dual infection with Loa Loa:* DEC drug of choice for both but can cause severe encephalopathy if >5000 Loa microfilaria/mL in blood. Refer to expert center for apheresis pre-DEC or prednisone + small doses of DEC. If <5000 microfilaria/mL, start regular dose of **DEC.**	Doxy x 6 wks may improve mild/moderate lymphedema independent of parasite infection *(CID 55:621, 2012).* **Note: DEC can cause irreversible eye damage if concomitant Onchocerciasis.**
Loiasis Loa loa: eye worm disease: **Look for dual infection with either Onchocerciasis or Lymphatic filariasis**	*Mono-infection with <5000 L. loa microfilaria/mL:* **DEC** 8-10 mg/kg/day po in 3 divided doses x 21 days *Mono-infection with >5000 L. loa microfilaria/mL:* Refer to expert center for apheresis prior to DEC therapy; alternatively: **Albendazole** 200 mg po bid x 21 days	*Dual infection with Lymphatic filariasis:* See Lymphatic filariasis, above *Dual infection with Onchocerciasis:* Treat Onchocerciasis first with **Ivermectin**, then treat L. loa with **DEC**	If >5000 L. loa microfilaria/mL in blood & given Ivermectin for Onchocerciasis, can facilitate entry of L. loa into CNS with severe encephalopathy.
Onchocerca volvulus (Onchocerciasis), river blindness: **Look for dual infection with either Loa loa or Lymphatic filariasis**	*Mono-infection:* **Ivermectin** 150 mcg/kg x 1 dose, then repeat every 3-6 months until asymptomatic + **Doxy** 200 mg/day x 6 wks. No accepted alternative therapy.	*Dual infection with Lymphatic filariasis:* See Lymphatic filariasis, above *Dual infection with Loa loa:* Treat Onchocerciasis first with **Ivermectin**, then treat L. loa with **DEC**. If >5000 L. Loa microfilaria/mL, refer to expert center for apheresis before starting DEC	Onchocerciasis and Loa loa are mildly co-endemic in West and Central Africa.

[3] May need antihistamine or corticosteroid for allergic reaction from disintegrating organisms

* For source of drug, see *Table 13D, page 157.*

TABLE 13A (9)

INFECTING ORGANISM	SUGGESTED REGIMENS		COMMENTS
	PRIMARY	ALTERNATIVE	
NEMATODES—EXTRAINTESTINAL (Roundworms)/Filariasis (continued)			
Body cavity Mansonella perstans	In randomized trial, doxy 200 mg once daily x 6 weeks cleared microfilaria from blood in 67 of 69 patients (NEJM 361:1448, 2009).	**Albendazole** in high dose x 3 weeks.	Efficacy of doxy believed to be due to inhibition of endosymbiont wolbachia. Ivermectin has no activity. Rev J Trop Med Hyg 100:458, 2006.
Mansonella streptocerca	**Ivermectin** 150 µg/kg x 1 dose.		May need antihistamine or corticosteroid for allergic reaction for pruritic hypopigmented lesions that may be confused with leprosy. Can be asymptomatic. Chronic pruritic, hypopigmented lesions that may be confused with leprosy.
Mansonella ozzardi	**Ivermectin** 200 µg/kg x 1 dose may be effective. Limited data but no other option. Am J Trop Med Hyg 90:1170, 2014		Usually asymptomatic. Articular pain, pruritus, lymphadenopathy reported. May have allergic reaction from dying organisms.
Dirofilariasis: **Heartworms** D. immitis, dog heartworm	No effective drugs; surgical removal only option		Can lodge in pulmonary artery → coin lesion. Eosinophilia rare.
D. tenuis (raccoon), D. ursi (bear), D. repens (dogs, cats)	No effective drugs		Worms migrate to conjunctive, subcutaneous tissue, scrotum, breasts, extremities. D. repens emerging throughout Europe Clin Microbiol Rev 25:507, 2012
Gnathostoma spinigerum Cutaneous larva migrans	**Albendazole** 400 mg q24h or bid times 21 days	**Ivermectin** 200 µg/kg/day x 2 days.	Other etiology of larva migrans: Ancylostoma sp. See page 150.
Eosinophilic meningitis	Supportive care; monitor for cerebral hemorrhage	Case reports of steroid use; both benefit and harm from Albendazole or ivermectin (EIN 17:1174, 2011).	Other causes of eosinophilic meningitis: **Angiostrongylus** (see page 150) & **Baylisascaris** (see page 150).
Toxocariasis (Ann Trop Med Parasit 103:3, 2010)	**Rx directed at relief of symptoms as infection self-limited, e.g., steroids & antihistamines; use of anthelmintics controversial.**		
Visceral larval migrans	**Albendazole** 400 mg bid x 5 days ± **Prednisone** 60 mg/day	**Mebendazole** 100–200 mg po bid times 5 days	Severe lung, heart or CNS disease may warrant steroids (Clin Micro Rev 16:265, 2003). Differential dx of larval migrans syndromes: Toxocara canis & catis, Ancylostoma spp., Gnathostoma spp., Spirometra spp.
Ocular larval migrans	First 4 wks of illness: (Oral) **prednisone** 30–60 mg po q24h + subtenon **triamcinolone** 40 mg/wk) x 2 wks (Surgery is sometimes necessary)		No added benefit of anthelmintic drugs; Rx of little effect after 4 wks. Some use steroids (Clin Microbiol Rev 16:265, 2003).
Trichinosis spiralis (**Trichinellosis**) — muscle infection (Review: Clin Micro Rev 22:127, 2009)	**Albendazole** 400 mg po bid x 8–14 days Concomitant **prednisone** 40–60 mg po q24h	**Mebendazole** 200–400 mg po tid x 3 days, then 400–500 mg po tid x 10 days	Use albendazole/mebendazole with caution during pregnancy. ↑ IgE, ↑ CPK, ESR 0, massive eosinophilia: >5000/µL.
TREMATODES (Flukes) – Liver, Lung, Intestinal. All flukes have snail intermediate hosts; transmitted by ingestion of metacercariae on plants, fish or crustaceans.			
Liver flukes: Clonorchis sinensis, Metorchis conjunctus, Opisthorchis viverrini	**Praziquantel** 25 mg/kg po tid x 2 days	**Albendazole** 10 mg/kg per day po x 7 days	Same dose in children
Fasciola hepatica (sheep liver fluke), Fasciola gigantica	**Triclabendazole** once, may repeat after 12–24 hrs. 10 mg/kg po x 1 dose. Single 20 mg/kg po dose effective in treatment failures.		
Intestinal flukes: Fasciola buski Heterophyes heterophyes, Metagonimus yokogawai, Nanophyetus salmincola	**Praziquantel** 25 mg/kg po tid x 1 days		Same dose in children

* For source of drug, see Table 13D, page 157.

TABLE 13A (10)

INFECTING ORGANISM	SUGGESTED REGIMENS		COMMENTS
	PRIMARY	**ALTERNATIVE**	
TREMATODES (Flukes) – Liver, Lung, Intestinal *(continued)*			
Lung fluke: Paragonimus sp.	**Praziquantel** 25 mg/kg po tid x 2 days	**Triclabendazole** 10 mg/kg po x two doses of 40 mg/kg or two doses of 20 mg/kg) 12-24 hrs.	Same dose in children
Schistosoma haematobium; GU bilharziasis,	**Praziquantel** 40 mg/kg po on the same day (one dose of 40 mg/kg or two doses of 20 mg/kg).		Same dose in children.
Schistosoma intercalatum	**Praziquantel** 20 mg/kg po on the same day in 1 or 2 doses		Same dose in children.
Schistosoma japonicum; Oriental schisto.	**Praziquantel** 60 mg/kg po on the same day (3 doses of 20 mg/kg).		Same dose in children. Cures 60-90% pts.
Schistosoma mansoni (intestinal bilharziasis)	**Praziquantel** 40 mg/kg po on the same day in (one dose of 40 mg/kg or two doses of 20 mg/kg).		Praziquantel: Same dose for children and adults. Cures 60-90% pts. No advantage to splitting dose in 2 Cochrane Database Syst Rev. 8:CD000053, 2014.
Schistosoma mekongi	**Praziquantel** 60 mg per kg po on the same day (3 doses of 20 mg/kg)		Same dose for children
Toxemic schisto; Katayama fever	**Praziquantel** 20 mg per kg po bid with short course of high dose prednisone. Repeat Praziquantel in 4-6 wks (*Clin Micro Rev 16:225, 2010*).		Reaction to onset of egg laying 4-6 wks after infection exposure in fresh water.
CESTODES (Tapeworms)			
Echinococcus granulosus (hydatid disease) (*LnID 12:871, 2012; Int Dis Clin No Amer 26:421, 2012*)	**Liver cysts:** Meta-analysis supports percutaneous aspiration-injection-reaspiration (**PAIR**) + albendazole for uncomplicated single liver cysts. Before & after drainage: **albendazole** ≥60 kg, 400 mg bid or < 60 kg, 15 mg/kg per day div. bid, with meals. After 1-2 days puncture (P) & needle aspirate (A) cyst content. Instill (I) hypertonic saline (15-30%) or absolute alcohol, wait 20-30 min, then re-aspirate (R) with final irrigation. **Continue albendazole for at least 30 days.**		
Echinococcus multilocularis (alveolar cyst disease) (*COID 11:415-437, 2003*)	Cure in 96% as comp. to 90% pts when cysts Albendazole efficacy not clearly demonstrated; can try in dosages used for hydatid disease. Wide surgical resection only reliable rx: technique evolving. Post-surgical prevention of recurrence (if inoperable). Albendazole for several years (*Acta Tropic 114:1, 2010*).		
Intestinal tapeworms			
Diphyllobothrium latum (fish), Diphylidium caninum (dog), T. saginata (beef), & Taenia solium (pork)	**Praziquantel** 5-10 mg/kg po x 1 dose for children and adults.	**Niclosamide** 2 gm po x 1 dose	Niclosamide from Expert Compounding Pharm, see *Table 13D*.
Hymenolepis diminuta (rats) and H. nana (humans)	**Praziquantel** 25 mg/kg po x 1 dose for children and adults.	**Niclosamide** 2 gm po daily x.7 days	
	NOTE: Treat concomitant T. solium intestinal tapeworms, if present, with **praziquantel** 5-10 mg/kg po x 1 dose after starting steroid.		
Neurocysticercosis (NCC): Larval form of *T. solium* Ref. *AJTMH 72:3, 2005*			
Parenchymal NCC 1-20 "Viable" or degenerating cysts by neuroimaging. Meta-analysis: Treatment assoc with cyst resolution, ↓ seizures, and ↓ seizure recurrence. Ref: *Neurology 80:1424, 2013.*	**Albendazole** 15 mg/kg/d po + **Praziquantel** 50 mg/kg/d po + **dexamethasone** 0.1 mg/kg/d po. Start steroid 1 day before anti-parasitics. Treat for 10 days. May need seizure meds for 1 yr.	**Albendazole** alone 800 mg po per day plus **Dexamethasone** 0.1 mg/kg per day ± Anti-seizure medication). See *Comment*	Ref: *LnID 14:687, 2014.* Steroids decrease serum levels of praziquantel so shouldn't use alone; can use w/high dose albendazole. NIH reports methotrexate at <20 mg/wk allows a reduction in steroid use (*CID 44:449, 2007*).
Dead calcified cysts	**No treatment indicated**		
Subarachnoid NCC	(**Albendazole** + **steroids** as above) + shunting for hydrocephalus prior to drug therapy. Ref: *Expert Rev Anti Infect Ther 9:123, 2011*		
Intraventricular NCC	**Neurocysticercosis (NCC):** removal is treatment of choice with or without obstruction of flow of CSF. **dexamethasone; observe closely for evidence of obstruction of flow of CSF.**		

---

* For source of drug, see *Table 13D, page 157.*

TABLE 13A (11)

INFECTING ORGANISM	INFECTING ORGANISM	SUGGESTED REGIMENS		COMMENTS
DISEASE	INFECTING ORGANISM	PRIMARY	ALTERNATIVE	COMMENTS

CESTODES (Tapeworms)/Neurocysticercosis (NCC) *(continued)*

Sparganosis (Spirometra mansonoides) Larval cysts; source—frogs/snakes		Surgical resection. No antiparasitic therapy. Can inject alcohol into subcutaneous masses.		

ECTOPARASITES. Ref.: *CID* 36:1355, 2003; *Ln* 363:889, 2004. **NOTE: Due to potential neurotoxicity and risk of aplastic anemia, lindane not recommended.**

Head lice *NEJM* 367:1687 & 1750, 2012; *Med Lett* 54:61, 2012.	Pediculus humanus, var. capitis	**Permethrin** 1% lotion. Apply to shampooed dried hair for 10 min., repeat in 9-10 days. **OR** **Malathion** 0.5% lotion (Ovide). Apply to dry hair for 8-12 hrs, then shampoo. 2 doses 7-9 days apart. **OR** **Spinosad** 0.9% suspension; wash off after 10 min (85% effective). Repeat in 7 days, if needed. Use nit comb initially & repeat in 7-10 days	**Ivermectin** 200-400 μg/kg po once, 3 doses at 7 day intervals effective in 95% (*IJID* 193:474, 2006). Topical ivermectin 0.5% lotion, 75% effective. **Malathion:** Report that 1-2 20-min. applications 98% effective (*Ped Derm* 21:670, 2004). In alcohol— potentially flammable. **Benzyl alcohol:** 76% effective	**Permethrin:** success in 78%. Resistance increasing. No advantage to 5% permethrin. **Spinosad** is effective, but expensive. Wash hats, scarves, coats & bedding in hot water, then dry in hot dryer for 20+ minutes.
Pubic lice (crabs)	Phthirus pubis	**Pubic hair: Permethrin OR malathion** as for head lice. Shave pubic hair.	**Eyelids: Petroleum jelly** applied qid x 10 days OR **yellow oxide of mercury** 1% qid x 14 days	**Do not use lindane.** Treat sex partners of the last 30 days.
Body lice	Pediculus humanus, var. corporis	No drugs for the patient. Organism lives in & deposits eggs in seams of clothing. Discard clothing; if not possible, treat clothing with 1% malathion powder or 0.5% permethrin powder. Success with ivermectin in homeless shelter: 12 mg po on days 0, 7, & 14 (*IJID* 193:474, 2006).		

Myiasis Due to larvae of flies

		Usually cutaneous/subcutaneous nodule with central punctum. Organism lives in & deposits eggs in seams of clothing. Treatment: Occlude punctum to prevent gas exchange with petrolatum, fingernail polish, makeup cream or bacon. When larva migrates, manually remove. Ref: *Clin Microbiol Rev* 25:79, 2012.		

Scabies Refs: *MMWR* 59(RR-12):89, 2010; *NEJM* 362:717, 2010.

Immunocompetent patients	Sarcoptes scabiei	**Permethrin** 5% cream (ELIMITE) under nails (finger and toe). Apply entire skin from chin down to and including under fingernails and toenails. Leave on 8-14 hrs. Repeat in 1-2 wks. Safe for children age >2 mos.	**Ivermectin** 250 μg/kg po with food x 1, then second dose in 1-2 wks. **Less effective: Crotamiton** 10% cream, apply x 24 hr, rinse off, then reapply x 24 hr.	Trim fingernails. Reapply cream to hands after handwashing. Treat close contacts; wash and heat dry linens. Pruritus may persist times 2 wks after mites are gone.
AIDS and HTLV-infected patients (CD4 <150 per mm³), debilitated or developmentally disabled patients (**Norwegian scabies**—see *Comments*)		For Norwegian crusted scabies: **Permethrin** 5% cream daily x 7 days, then twice weekly until cured. Add **ivermectin** po (dose in Alternative)	**Ivermectin** 250 mcg/kg po on days 1, 15 & 29 + **Permethrin** cream.	Norwegian scabies in AIDS pts: Extensive, crusted. Can mimic psoriasis. Not pruritic. Highly contagious—isolate!

* For source of drug, see *Table 13D, page 157.*

TABLE 13B – DOSAGE AND SELECTED ADVERSE EFFECTS OF ANTIPARASITIC DRUGS

Doses vary with indication. For convenience, drugs divided by type of parasite; some drugs used for multiple types of parasites, e.g., albendazole.

CLASS, AGENT, GENERIC NAME (TRADE NAME)	USUAL ADULT DOSAGE	ADVERSE REACTIONS/COMMENTS
Antiprotozoan Drugs		
Intestinal Parasites		
Diloxanide furoate[NUS] (Furamide)	500 mg po tid x 10 days	Source: See Table 13D, page 157. Flatulence, N/V, diarrhea.
Iodoquinol[NUS] (Yodoxin)	Adults: 650 mg po tid or 30-40 mg/kg/day div. tid; children: 40 mg/kg per day div. tid.	Rarely causes nausea, abdominal cramps, rash, acne. **Contraindicated if iodine intolerance** (contains 64% bound iodine). Can cause iododerma (papular or pustular rash) and/or thyroid enlargement.
Metronidazole	Side-effects similar for all. See metronidazole in Table 10B, page 108, & Table 10A, page 105	Source: See Table 13D, page 157.
Nitazoxanide (Alinia)	Adults: 500 mg po q12h. Children 4-11: 200 mg susp. po q12h. Take with food. Expensive.	Abdominal pain 7.8%, diarrhea 2.1%. Rev.: CID 40:1173, 2006; Expert Opin Pharmacother 7:953, 2006. Headaches, rarely yellow sclera (resolves after treatment).
Paromomycin (Humatin)	Up to 750 mg po qid (250 mg tabs). Source: See Table 13D	**Aminoglycoside similar to neomycin;** if absorbed due to concomitant inflammatory bowel disease can result in oto/nephrotoxicity. Doses >3 gm daily are associated with nausea, abdominal cramps, diarrhea.
Aminosidine IV in U.K.		
Quinacrine[NUS] (Atabrine, Mepacrine)	100 mg po tid. No longer available in U.S.; www.expertpharmacy.com; www.fagron.com	**Contraindicated for pts with history of psychosis or psoriasis. Yellow staining of skin.** Dizziness, headache, vomiting, toxic psychosis (1.5%), hemolytic anemia, leukopenia, thrombocytopenia, urticaria, rash, fever, minor disulfiram-like reactions.
Tinidazole (Tindamax)	250-500 mg tabs, with food. Regimen varies with indication.	**Chemical structure similar to metronidazole** but better tolerated. Seizures/peripheral neuropathy reported. **Adverse effects:** Metallic taste 4-6%, nausea 3-5%, anorexia 2-3%.
Antiprotozoan Drugs: Non-Intestinal Protozoa		
Extraintestinal Parasites		
Antimony compounds[NUS]	For IV use: vials with 100 mg antimony/mL. Dilute selected dose in 50 mL of D5W shortly before use. Infuse over at least 10 minutes.	**AEs in 1st 10 days:** headache, fatigue, elevated lipase/amylase, clinical pancreatitis. After 10 days: elevated AST/ALT/ALK/PHOS. **NOTE: Reversible T wave changes in 30-60%. Risk of QTc prolongation. Renal excretion; modify dose if renal insufficiency. Metabolized in liver; lower dose if hepatic insufficiency.** Generic drug may have increased toxicity due to antimony complex formation.
Stibogluconate sodium (Pentostam) from CDC or Meglumine antimoniate (Glucantime)—French trade name		
Artemether-Lumefantrine, po (Coartem, FDA-approved)	Tablets contain 20 mg Artemether and 120 mg Lumefantrine. Take with food. Can be crushed and mixed with a few teaspoons of water	**Can prolong QTc:** avoid in patients with congenital long QTc, family history of sudden death or long QTc, or need for drugs known to prolong QTc (see list under fluoroquinolones, Table 10A, page 107). Artemether and its active metabolite & Lumefantrine are metabolized by CYP3A4 (see drug-drug interactions, Table 22). Adverse effects experienced by >30% of adults: headache, anorexia, dizziness, arthralgia and myalgia.
Artesunate, IV Ref: NEJM 358:1829, 2008	Available from CDC Malaria Branch. 2.4 mg/kg IV at 0, 12, 24, & 48 hrs	**More effective & safer than quinidine.** Contact CDC at 770-488-7758 or 770-488-7100 after hours. No dosage adjustment for hepatic or renal insufficiency. No known drug interactions.
Atovaquone (Mepron) Ref.: AAC 46:1163, 2002	Suspension: 1 tsp (750 mg) po bid 750 mg/5 mL.	No. pts stopping rx due to side-effects was 9%.; rash 22%, GI 20%, headache 16%, insomnia 10%, fever 14%
Atovaquone and proguanil (Malarone) For prophylaxis of P. falciparum; little data on P. vivax. Generic available in US	**Prophylaxis:** 1 tab (250 mg + 100 mg) q24h with food **Treatment:** 4 tabs (1000 mg + 400 mg) once daily with food x 3 days Adult tab: 250/100 mg; Peds tab 62.5/25 mg Peds dosage: prophylaxis footnote 1 page 145; treatment see comment, page 146.	Adverse effects in rx trials: Adults—abd. pain 17%, N/V 12%, headache 10%, dizziness 5%. Rx stopped in 1%. Asymptomatic mild ↑ in ALT/AST. Children—cough, headache, anorexia, vomiting, abd. pain. See drug interactions, Table 22. Safe in G6PD-deficient pts. Can crush tabs for children and give with milk or other liquid nutrients. Renal insufficiency: contraindicated if CrCl <30 mL per min.

NOTE: Drugs available from CDC Drug Service indicated by "CDC." Call (+1) (404) 639-3670 (or -2888 (Fax)). **See Table 13D, page 157 for sources and contact information for hard-to-find antiparasitic drugs.**

TABLE 13B (2)

CLASS, AGENT, GENERIC NAME (TRADE NAME)	USUAL ADULT DOSAGE	ADVERSE REACTIONS/COMMENTS
Antiprotozoan Drugs: Non-intestinal Protozoa/Extraintestinal Parasites *(continued)*		
Benznidazole (CDC Drug Service)	7.5 mg/kg per day po. 100 mg tabs	**Photosensitivity in 50% of pts.** GI: abdominal pain, nausea/vomiting/anorexia. CNS: disorientation, insomnia, twitching/seizures, paresthesias, polyneuritis. **Contraindicated in pregnancy**
Chloroquine phosphate (Aralen)	Dose varies—see *Malaria Prophylaxis and rx, pages 145-146.*	Minor: anorexia/nausea/vomiting, headache, dizziness, blurred vision, pruritus in dark-skinned pts. Major: protracted rx in rheumatoid arthritis can lead to retinopathy. Can exacerbate psoriasis. Can block response to rabies vaccine. **Contraindicated in pts with epilepsy.**
Dapsone See *Comment re methemoglobinemia*	100 mg po q24h	Usually tolerated by pts with rash after TMP-SMX. **Dapsone is common etiology of acquired methemoglobinemia** (*NEJM 364:957, 2011*). Metabolite of dapsone converts heme iron to +3 charge (no O2 transport) from normal +2. Normal blood level 1%, cyanosis at 10%; headache, fatigue, tachycardia, dizziness at 30-40%; acidosis & coma at 60%, death at 70-80%. Low G6PD is a risk factor. Treatment: methylene blue 1-2 mg/kg IV over 5 min x 1 doses.
Eflornithine (Ornidyl) (WHO or CDC drug service)	200 mg/kg IV (slowly) q12h x 7 days for African trypanosomiasis	Diarrhea in ½ pts, vomiting, abdominal pain, anemia/leukopenia in ½ pts, seizures, alopecia, jaundice, ↓ hearing. Contraindicated in pregnancy.
Fumagillin	Eyedrops + po 20 mg po tid. Leiter's: 800-292-6772.	Adverse events: Neutropenia & thrombocytopenia
Mefloquine	One 250 mg tab/wk for **malaria prophylaxis**, for rx, 1250 mg x 1 or 750 mg & then 500 mg in 6-8 hrs. In U.S. 250 mg tab = 228 mg base; outside U.S. 275 mg tab = 250 mg base	Side-effects in roughly 3%. Minor: headache, irritability, insomnia, weakness, diarrhea. **Toxic psychosis, seizures can occur.** Do not use with quinine, quinidine, or halofantrine. Rare: Prolonged QT interval and toxic epidermal necrolysis (*Ln 349:101, 1997*). **Not used for self-rx due to neuropsychiatric side-effects.**
Melarsoprol (Mel B, Arsobal) (CDC)	See Trypanosomiasis for adult dose. Peds dose: 0.36 mg/kg IV, then gradual ↑ to 3.6 mg/kg q1-5 days for total of 9-10 doses.	**Post-rx encephalopathy (2-10%) with 50% mortality overall, risk of death 2° to rx 8-14%.** Prednisolone 1 mg per kg per day po may ↓ encephalopathy. Other: Heart damage, albuminuria, abdominal pain, vomiting, peripheral neuropathy, Herxheimer-like reaction, pruritus.
Miltefosine (Impavido) *Med Lett 56:69, 2014* FDA approved in 2014, but no commercialization in US at present	50 mg po bid (34-44 kg); 50 mg po tid (wt ≥45 kg). Treat for 28 days	Contact CDC for IND. **Pregnancy—No;** teratogenic. Side-effects vary, kala-azar pts, vomiting in up to 40%, diarrhea in 17%, "motion sickness", headache & increased creatinine. Metabolized by liver, virtually no urinary excretion.
Nifurtimox (Lampit) (CDC) Manufactured in Germany by Bayer	8-10 mg/kg per day po qid, 4 x per day for 90-120 days	**Side-effects in 40-70% of pts.** nausea/vomiting. CNS: polyneuritis (1/3), disorientation, insomnia, twitching, seizures. Skin rash. Hemolysis with G6PD deficiency.
Pentamidine (NebuPent)	300 mg via aerosol q month. Also used IM.	Hypotension, hypocalcemia, hypoglycemia followed by hyperglycemia, pancreatitis. Neutropenia (15%), thrombocytopenia. Nephrotoxicy. Others: nausea/vomiting, ↑ liver tests, rash.
Primaquine phosphate	26.3 mg (=15 mg base). Adult dose is 30 mg of base po daily.	**In G6PD def, pts, can cause hemolytic anemia with hemoglobinuria, esp. African, Asian peoples.** Methemoglobinemia. Nausea/abdominal pain if pt. fasting. **Pregnancy: No.**
Pyrimethamine (Daraprim, Malocide) Also combined with sulfadoxine as **Fansidar** (25-500 mg)	100 mg, then 25 mg/day. Cost of folinic acid (leucovorin)	**Major problem is hematologic:** megaloblastic anemia, ↓ WBC, ↓ platelets. Can give 5 mg folinic acid per day to ↓ bone marrow depression without interfering with antitoxoplasmosic effect. If sulfonamide used, add folinic acid to 10-50 mg/day. Pyrimethamine + sulfadiazine can cause mental changes due to carnitine deficiency (*AJM 95:112, 1993*). Other: Rash, vomiting, diarrhea, xerostomia.
Quinidine gluconate Cardiotoxicity ref: *LnID 7:549, 2007.*	Loading dose of 10 mg (equiv to 6.2 mg of quinidine base) / kg IV over 1-2 hr, then constant infusion of 0.02 mg of quinidine gluconate / kg per minute. May be available for compassionate use from Lilly.	**Adverse reactions of quinidine/quinine similar:** (1) IV bolus injection can cause rapid hypotension, (2) hyperinsulinemic hypoglycemia in pregnancy, (3) ↓ rate of infusion of IV quinidine if QT interval ↑ >25% of baseline, (4) reduce dose 30-50% after day 3 due to ↓ renal clearance and ↓ vol. of distribution. **See Table 13D, page 157 for**

NOTE: Drugs available from CDC Drug Service indicated by "CDC": Call (+1) (404) 639-3670 (or -2888 (Fax)). **See Table 13D, page 157 for sources and contact information for hard-to-find antiparasitic drugs.**

TABLE 13B (3)

CLASS, AGENT, GENERIC NAME (TRADE NAME)	USUAL ADULT DOSAGE	ADVERSE REACTIONS/COMMENTS
Antiprotozoan Drugs: Non-Intestinal Protozoa/Extraintestinal Parasites *(continued)*		
Quinine sulfate (Qualaquin)	324 mg tabs. No IV prep. In US. Oral rx of chloroquine-resistant falciparum malaria: 624 mg po tid x 3 days, then (tetracycline 250 mg po qid or doxy 100 mg bid) x 7 days	Cinchonism; tinnitus, headache, nausea, abdominal pain, blurred vision. Rarely: blood dyscrasias, drug fever, asthma, hypoglycemia. Transient blindness in <1% of 500 pts (*AnIM 136*:339, 2002). **Contraindicated if prolonged QTc, myasthenia gravis, optic neuritis or G6PD deficiency.**
Spiramycin (Rovamycin)	1 gm po q8h (see *Comment*).	GI and allergic reactions have occurred. Available at no cost after consultation with Palo Alto Medical Foundation Toxoplasma Serology Lab: 650-853-4828 or from U.S. FDA 301-796-1600.
Sulfadiazine	1–1.5 gm po q6h.	See *Table 10A, page 105, for sulfonamide side-effects*
Sulfadoxine & pyrimethamine combination (Fansidar)	Contains 500 mg sulfadoxine & 25 mg pyrimethamine	Long half-life of both drugs: Sulfadoxine 169 hrs, pyrimethamine 111 hrs allows weekly dosage. In African, used empirically in pregnancy for intermittent preventative treatment (ITPp) against malaria: dosing at 3 set times during pregnancy. Reduces material and fetal mortality if HIV+. See *Expert Rev Anti Infect Ther 8:589, 2010*. **Fatalities reported due to Stevens-Johnson syndrome and toxic epidermal necrolysis.** Renal excretion—caution if renal impairment.
DRUGS USED TO TREAT NEMATODES, TREMATODES, AND CESTODES		
Albendazole (Albenza)	Doses vary with indication. Take with food; fatty meal increases absorption.	**Pregnancy Cat. C;** give alert negative pregnancy test. Abdominal pain, nausea/vomiting, alopecia, ↑ serum transaminase. Rare leukopenia.
Diethylcarbamazine (CDC)	Used to treat filariasis.	Headache, dizziness, nausea, fever. Host may experience inflammatory reaction to death of adult worms: fever, urticaria, asthma, GI upset **(Mazzotti reaction). Pregnancy—No.**
Ivermectin (Stromectol, Mectizan) (3 mg tab & topical 0.5% lotion for head lice). Take on empty stomach.	Strongyloidiasis dose: 200 µg/kg/day po x 2 days Onchocerciasis: 150 µg/kg x 1 po Scabies: 200 µg/kg po x 1; if AIDS, wait 14 days & repeat	Mild side-effects: fever, pruritus, rash. In rx of onchocerciasis, can see tender lymphadenopathy, headache, bone/joint pain. Host may experience inflammatory reaction to death of adult worms: fever, urticaria, asthma, GI upset **(Mazzotti reaction).**
Mebendazole (Vermox) Not available in US, but widely available elsewhere.	Doses vary with indication.	Rarely causes abdominal pain, nausea, diarrhea. Contraindicated in pregnancy & children <2 yrs old.
Praziquantel (Biltricide)	Doses vary with parasite; see *Table 13A.*	Mild: dizziness/drowsiness, N/V, rash, fever. **Only contraindication is ocular cysticercosis.** Potential exacerbation of neurocysticercosis. Metab-induced by anticonvulsants and steroids; can negate effect with cimetidine 400 mg po tid. Reduce dose if advanced liver disease.
Pyrantel pamoate (over-the-counter)	Oral suspension. Dose for all ages: 11 mg/kg (to max. of 1 gm) x 1 dose	Rare GI upset, headache, dizziness, rash
Suramin (Germanin) *(CDC)*	Drug powder mixed to 10% solution with 5 mL water and used within 30 min. First give test dose of 0.1 gm IV. Try to avoid pregnancy.	Does not cross blood-brain barrier; no effect on CNS infection. Side-effects: vomiting, pruritus, urticaria, fever, paresthesias, albuminuria (discontinue drug if casts appear). Do not use if renal/liver disease present. Deaths from vascular collapse reported.
Triclabendazole (Egaten) (CDC)	Used for fasciola hepatica liver fluke infection: 10 mg/kg po x 1 dose. May repeat in 12-24 hrs. 250 mg tabs	AEs ≥10%: sweating and abdominal pain. AEs ≤10%: weakness, chest pain, fever, anorexia, nausea, vomiting. **Note: use with caution if G6PD def. or impaired liver function.**

NOTE: Drugs available from CDC Drug Service indicated by "CDC". Call (+1) (404) 639-3670 (or -2888 (Fax)). **See Table 13D, page 157 for sources and contact information for hard-to-find antiparasitic drugs.**

TABLE 13C – PARASITES THAT CAUSE EOSINOPHILIA (EOSINOPHILIA IN TRAVELERS)

Frequent and Intense (>5000 eos/mcL)	Moderate to Marked Early Infections	During Larval Migration; Absent or Mild During Chronic Infections	Other
Strongyloides (absent in compromised hosts); Lymphatic Filariasis; Toxocaria (cutaneous larva migrans)	Ascaris; Hookworm; Clonorchis; Paragonimis	Opisthorchis	Schistosomiasis; Cysticercosis; Trichuris; Angiostrongylus; Non-lymphatic filariasis; Gnathostoma; Capillaria; Trichostrongylus

TABLE 13D – SOURCES FOR HARD-TO-FIND ANTIPARASITIC DRUGS

Source	Drugs Available	Contact Information
CDC Drug Service	Artesunate, Benznidazole, Diethylcarbamazine (DEC), Eflornithine, Melarsoprol, Nifurtimox, Sodium stibogluconate, Suramin, Triclabendazole	www.cdc.gov/laboratory/drugservice/index.html (+1) 404-639-3670
WHO	Drugs for treatment of African trypanosomiasis	simarop@who.int; (+41) 794-682-726; (+41) 227-911-345 francoj@who.int; (+41) 796-198-535; (+41) 227-913-313
Compounding Pharmacies, Specialty Labs, Others		
Expert Compounding Pharmacy	Quinacrine, Iodoquinol, niclosamide	www.expertpharmacy.org 1-800-247-9767; (+1) 818-988-7979
Fagron Compounding Pharmacy (formerly Gallipot)	Quinacrine, Iodoquinol, Paromomycin, Diloxanide	www.fagron.com 1-800-423-6967; (+1) 651-681-9517
Leiter's Pharmacy	Fumagillin	www.leiterrx.com 1-800-292-6772, +1-408-292-6772
Victoria Apotheke Zurich will ship worldwide if sent physicians prescription.	Paromomycin (oral and topical). Triclabendazole. Other hard to find anti-parasitic drugs	www.pharmaworld.com (+41) 43-344-6060
Palo Alto Medical Foundation, Toxoplasma Serology Lab	Spiramycin (consultation required for release)	(+1) 650-853-4828; toxlab@pamf.org

TABLE 14A – ANTIVIRAL THERAPY*

For HIV, see Table 14D; For Hepatitis, see Table 14F and Table 14G

VIRUS/DISEASE	DRUG/DOSAGE	SIDE EFFECTS/COMMENTS
Adenovirus: Cause of RTIs including fatal pneumonia in children & young adults and 60% mortality in transplant pts (CID 43:331, 2006). Frequent cause of cystitis in immunosuppressed patients. Adenovirus 14 associated with severe pneumonia in otherwise healthy young adults (MMWR 56(45):1181, 2007). **Findings include:** fever, ↑ liver enzymes, leukopenia, thrombocytopenia, diarrhea, pneumonia, or hemorrhagic cystitis.	In severe cases of pneumonia or post HSCT[1]: **Cidofovir** • 5 mg/kg/wk x 2 wks, then q 2 wks + **probenecid** 1.25 gm/M² given 3 hrs before cidofovir and 3 & 9 hrs after each infusion. • 1 mg/kg 3x/wk. For adenovirus hemorrhagic cystitis (CID 40:199, 2005; Transplantation. 2006; 81:1398): Intravesical **cidofovir** (5 mg/kg in 100 mL saline instilled into bladder)	Cidofovir successful in 3/8 immunosuppressed children (CID 41: 1812, 2005) & 8 of 10 children with HSCT (CID 41; 1812, 2005). ↓ in virus load predicted response to cidofovir. Ribavirin has had mixed activity, appears restricted to group C serotypes. Vidarabine and Gancliclovir have in vitro activity against adenovirus; little to no clinical data. **Brincidofovir** (CMX001-Chimerix) oral cidofovir prodrug in Phase III.
Coronavirus—SARS-CoV Severe acute respiratory syndrome (NEJM 348:1953, 1967, 2003) **MERS-CoV:** Middle East respiratory syndrome (LnID 14:1090, 2014)	SARS: • Ribavirin—ineffective. • Interferon alfa ± steroids—small case series. • Pegylated alfa ± steroids: 1 serious fungal infections. • Low dose steroids alone successful in one Beijing hospital. High dose steroids + serious fungal infections. • Inhaled nitric oxide improved oxygenation & improved chest x-ray (CID 39:1531, 2004). **MERS:** Increased 14 day survival with Ribavirin po + PEG-IFN 180 mcg/kg sc x 2 wks (LnID 14:1090, 2014). Other therapies LnID 14:1136, 2014.	**SARS: Transmission by close contact:** effective infection control practices (**mask [changed frequently], eye protection, gown, gloves**) key to stopping transmission. **MERS:** Suspected reservoirs are camels and perhaps other animals. Review: Mayo Clinic Proc. 89: 1153, 2014.
Enterovirus—Meningitis: most common cause of aseptic meningitis. Rapid CSF PCR test is accurate, reduces costs and hospital length of stay (Peds 120:489, 2007)	No rx currently recommended; however, **pleconaril** still under investigation.	No clinical benefit from Pleconaril in double-blind placebo-controlled study in 21 infants with enteroviral aseptic meningitis (PID) 22:335, 2003). Some improvement among those with severe respiratory disease (AAC 2006 50:2409-14). Severe respiratory illness with enterovirus D68 (MMWR 63:798 & 901, 2014).
Hemorrhagic Fever Virus Infections: Review: LnID 6:203, 2006. **Congo-Crimean Hemorrhagic Fever** (HF) Tick-borne; symptoms include N/V, fever, headache, myalgias, & stupor (1/3). Signs: conjunctival injection, hepatomegaly, petechiae (1/3). Lab: ↓ platelets, ↑WBC, ↑ ALT, AST, LDH & CPK (100%)	Oral **ribavirin, 30 mg/kg** as initial loading dose & 15 mg/kg q6h x 4 days & then 7.5 mg/kg q8h x 6 days (WHO recommendation) (see Comment). Reviewed Antiviral Res 78:125, 2008.	3/3 healthcare workers in Pakistan had complete recovery (Ln 346:472, 1995) & 61/69 (88%) with confirmed CCHF rx with ribavirin survived in Iran (CID 36:1613, 2003). Shorter time of hospitalization among ribavirin treated pts (7.5 vs. 10.3 days), but no difference in mortality or transfusion needs in study done in Turkey (J Infection 52: 207-215, 2006). Suggested benefit from ribavirin & dexamethasone (281 pts) (CID 57:1270, 2013).
Ebola/Marburg HF (Central Africa) Largest ever documented outbreak of Ebola virus (EVD), West Africa, 2014. Diagnostic testing at U.S. CDC. Within a few days of symptom onset, diagnosis is most commonly made by antigen-capture enzyme linked immunosorbent assay (ELISA), IgM antibody ELISA, NAAT or viral culture. Updated in http://emergency.cdc.gov/han/han00365.asp. See also: http://www.bt.cdc.gov/han/han00364.asp	No effective antiviral rx (J Virol 77, 9733, 2003). **Brincidofovir** (Chimerix) (experimental prodrug of cidofovir) used in several US cases. Investigational antibody treatment 'ZMapp' used as compassionate use in a few selected patients (Mapp Biopharmaceutical; http://mappbio.com/). ZMapp is a 3 monoclonal antibody preparation derived from mice exposed to small fragments of Ebola virus.	**Abrupt onset of symptoms: typically, 8–10 days after exposure (range 2–21 days).** Nonspecific symptoms: fever, chills, malaise, and malaise. Fever, anorexia, asthenia / weakness are the most common signs and symptoms. Patients may develop a diffuse erythematous maculopapular rash (days 5–7) (usually involving the face, neck, trunk, and arms) that can desquamate. EVD can **often be confused with** other more common infectious diseases such as malaria, typhoid fever, meningococcemia, and other bacterial infections (e.g., pneumonia). Patients often have conjunctival injection. Hiccups reported. Patients may develop severe watery diarrhea, nausea, vomiting and abdominal pain. Patients may develop shortness of breath, headache or confusion, may also develop. Patients may develop. Seizures may occur, and cerebral edema reported. Bleeding is not universally present but can manifest later in the course as petechiae, ecchymosis/bruising, or oozing from venipuncture sites and mucosal hemorrhage. Frank hemorrhage is less common. Pregnant women may experience spontaneous miscarriages. **Gastrointestinal symptoms:** severe watery diarrhea, nausea, vomiting and abdominal pain. **Other:** chest pain, shortness of breath, headache or confusion, may also develop.

[1] HSCT = Hematopoietic stem cell transplant
* See page 2 for abbreviations. NOTE: All dosage recommendations are for adults (unless otherwise indicated) and assume normal renal function.

TABLE 14A (2)

VIRUS/DISEASE	DRUG/DOSAGE	SIDE EFFECTS/COMMENTS
Hemorrhagic Fever Virus Infections (*continued*)		
With pulmonary syndrome: Hantavirus pulmonary syndrome, "sin nombre virus"	**No benefit from ribavirin demonstrated** (*CID 39:1307, 2004*). Early recognition of disease and supportive (usually ICU) care is key to successful outcome.	Acute onset of fever, headache, myalgias, non-productive cough, thrombocytopenia, increased PT and capillary leak. Non-cardiogenic pulmonary edema with respiratory insufficiency following exposure to droppings of infected rodents.
With renal syndrome: Lassa, Venezuelan, Korean, HF, Sabia, Argentinian HF, Bolivian HF, Junin, Machupo	Oral **ribavirin, 30 mg/kg** as initial loading dose & 15 mg/kg q6h x 4 days & then 7.5 mg/kg x 6 days (WHO recommendation) (*see Comment*)	Toxicity low, hemolysis reported but recovery when treatment stopped. No significant changes in WBC, platelets, hepatic or renal function. *See CID 36:1254, 2003.*
Dengue and dengue hemorrhagic fever (DHF) www.cdc.gov/ncidod/dvbid/dengue/dengue-hcp.htm Think dengue in traveler to tropics or subtropics (incubation period usually 4-7 days) with fever, bleeding, thrombocytopenia, or hemoconcentration with shock. Dx by viral isolation or serology; serum to CDC (telephone 787-706-2399).	**No data on antiviral rx.** Fluid replacement with careful hemodynamic monitoring critical. Rx of **DHF** with colloids effective: 6% hydroxyethyl starch preferred in 1 study (*NEJM 353:9, 2005*). Review in *Semin Ped Infect Dis 16: 60-65, 2005.*	Of 77 cases dx at CDC (2001–2004), recent (2-wks) travel to Caribbean island 30%, Asia 17%, Central America 15%, S. America 15% (*MMWR 54:556, June 10, 2005*). 5 pts with severe **DHF** rx with dengue antibody-rx, gamma globulin 500 mg per kg q24h IV for 3-5 days; rapid ↑ in platelet counts (*CID 36:1623, 2003*). Diagnosis: ELISA detects IgM antibody. Has some cross-reactivity with West Nile Virus infection. Should only be used in pts with symptoms c/w Dengue Fever.
West Nile virus (*JAMA 310:308, 2013*) A flavivirus transmitted by mosquitoes, blood transfusions, transplanted organs & breast-feeding. Birds (>200 species) are main host with humans & horses incidental hosts. The US epidemic continues.	**No proven rx to date.** Reviewed in *Lancet Neurology 6: 171-181, 2007.*	Usually nonspecific febrile disease but 1/150 cases develops meningoencephalitis, aseptic meningitis or polio-like paralysis (*AnM 104:545, 2004; JC 113:1102, 2004*). Long-term sequelae (neuromuscular weakness & psychiatric) common (*CID 43:723, 2006*). Diagnosis: increased IgM antibody in serum & CSF or CSF PCR (contact State Health Dept./CDC). Blood supply now tested in 11/17 cases in U.S. Increased serum lipase in 11/17 cases (*NEJM 352:420, 2005*).
Yellow fever	**No data on antiviral rx. Guidelines for use of preventative vaccine:** (*MMWR 51: RR17, 2002*)	Reemergence in Africa & S. Amer. due to urbanization of susceptible population (*Lancet Inf 5:604, 2005*). Vaccination Diagnosis: increased IgM antibody safe and effective in HIV patients, especially in those with suppressed VL and higher CD4 counts (*XRX-001*) using the 17D strain proven safe and resulted in neutralizing antibodies after 2 doses in a de-escalation, phase I study. (*N Engl J Med 2011 Apr 7; 364:1326*)
Chikungunya fever: brake bone fever A self-limiting arbovirus illness spread by Aedes mosquito. High epidemic potential (Caribbean).	**No antiviral therapy.** Fluids, analgesics, anti-pyretics (*NEJM 371:885, 2014*).	Clinical presentation: high fever, severe myalgias & headache, macular papular rash with occ. thrombocytopenia. Rarely hemorrhagic complications. Dx by increase in IgM antibody or serum NAAT (CDC, Focus Diagnostics).
SFTSV (Severe fever with thrombocytopenia syndrome virus)	**No known therapy.**	New virus in the Bunyaviridae family described in China. Initially thought to be anaplasma infection; serology showed new virus. Possibly transmitted by *Haemaphysalis longicornis* ticks. (*N Engl J Med 2011; 364:1523-32*)
Hepatitis Viral Infections	*See Table 14F (Hepatitis A & B), Table 14G (Hepatitis C)*	

* See page 2 for abbreviations. NOTE: All dosage recommendations are for adults (unless otherwise indicated) and assume normal renal function.

TABLE 14A (3)

VIRUS/DISEASE	DRUG/DOSAGE	SIDE EFFECTS/COMMENTS
Herpesvirus Infections		
Cytomegalovirus (CMV)		
At risk pts: HIV/AIDS, cancer chemotherapy, post-transplant	**Primary prophylaxis** not generally recommended except in certain transplant populations (see Table 16). Preemptive therapy in pts with ↑ CMV DNA plasma VL & CD4 <100/mm³. If used: **valganciclovir** 900 mg po q12h (CID 32:783, 2001). Authors rec. primary prophylaxis be dc if response to ART with ↑ CD4 >100 for 6 mos.	Risk for developing CMV disease correlates with quantity of CMV DNA in plasma; each log₁₀ ↑ associated with 3.1-fold ↑ in disease (CID 28:758, 1999). Resistance demonstrated in 5% of transplant recipients receiving primary prophylaxis (J Antimicrob Chemother 65:2628, 2010). Consensus guidelines. Transplantation 96:333, 2013.
Ref: Transplantation 96:333, 2013; Am J Transplant 13(Suppl 4):93, 2013		
CMV :Colitis, Esophagitis, Gastritis	**Mild: Valganciclovir** 900 mg po with food x 14-21 days.	Diagnosis: Elevated whole blood quantitative PCR & histopathology
Symptoms relate to site of disease	**Severe: Ganciclovir** 5 mg/kg IV q12h x 14-21 days OR **Foscarnet** (60 mg/kg IV q8h or 90 mg/kg q12h) x14-21 days	
	Post-treatment suppression: **Valganciclovir** 900 mg po once daily until CD4 > 100 x 6 mos	
	Treat as for colitis, esophagitis, gastritis above	
CMV: Neurologic disease, Encephalitis		Diagnosis: Elevated whole blood and/or CSF quantitative PCR
Myelitis, polyradiculopathy, peripheral neuropathy		Note: **Severe or fatal IRIS** has occurred in AIDS pts; suggest delay starting ART for 2 wks after initiation of CMV therapy.
Symptoms relate to site of disease		
CMV: Pneumonia	*Viremic but no/mild symptoms:* **Valganciclovir** 900 mg po bid (Am J Transplant 7:2106, 2007)	*Post-treatment suppression:* Valganciclovir 900 mg po once daily x 1-3 months if high risk of relapse.
At risk: 1st 6 months post-transplant & 3 months post-stopping prophylaxis	*Severe in lung transplant or AIDS pts:* **Ganciclovir** 5 mg/kg IV q12h (adjust for renal insufficiency). Some data support adding CMV immune globulin (CytoGam). Treat until clinical resolution & neg blood PCR; min duration: 2 wks	Suspect resistant CMV if treatment failure or relapse. Do genotype resistance testing (CID 56:1018, 2013).
Diagnosis: prefer whole blood quantitative PCR and/or positive lung biopsy histopathology	*Ganciclovir-resistant:* **Foscarnet** (60 mg/kg IV q8h or 90 mg/kg q12h) IV (adjust for renal insufficiency). Try to reduce immunosuppression.	
Ref: Transplantation 96:333, 2013; Am J Transplant 13(Suppl 4):93, 2013		
CMV: Retinitis	*Not sight-threatening:* **Valganciclovir** 900 mg po with food x 14-21 days, then 900 mg po once daily until CD4 >100 x 6 months	Sight-threatening: <1500 microns from fovea or next to head of optic nerve. If can't use Valganciclovir, Ganciclovir 5 mg/kg IV q12h x 14-21 days, then 5 mg/kg IV once daily x 14-21 days.
Most common ocular complication of HIV/AIDS. Rare in pts on ART with CD4 >200. If not on ART, wait to start until after 2 wks of CMV therapy.	*Sight-threatening* (see Comment): **Valganciclovir** + intravitreal **Ganciclovir** 2 mg (1-4 doses over 7-10 days).	If suspect Ganciclovir resistance: Foscarnet (60 gm/kg IV q8h or 90 mg/kg q12h) x 14-21 days. Ganciclovir ocular implants no longer available.
Ref: aidsinfo.nih.gov/guidelines		
CMV immune recovery retinitis: new retinitis after starting ART. Do not stop ART or Valganciclovir. No steroids.		

CMV in Transplant patients: See Table 16 for discussion of prophylaxis. CMV disease can manifest as: CMV syndrome with or without end-organ disease (Transplantation 2013;96(4):333; and Am J Transplant. 2013;13 Suppl 4:93. **Ganciclovir** 5 mg/kg IV q12h OR **Valganciclovir** 900 mg po q12h (Am J Transplant 7:2106, 2007) are effective treatment options. **Guidelines for CMV therapy** (Transplantation). Treatment duration should be individualized. Continue treatment until (1) PCR or antigenemia has become undetectable, and (2) clinical evidence of disease has resolved, and (3) at least 2-3 weeks of treatment (Am J Transplant 13(Suppl 4):93, 2013; Blood 113:5711, 2009). Secondary prophylaxis (**Valganciclovir** 900 mg daily) should be considered for 1-3 month course in patients recently treated with high-dose immunosuppression such as lymphocyte depleting antibodies, or those with severe CMV disease, or those with >1 episode of CMV disease. In HSCT recipients, secondary prophylaxis should be considered in certain cases balancing the risk of recurrent infection with drug toxicity.

CMV in pregnancy: Hyperimmune globulin 200 IU/kg maternal weight as single dose during pregnancy (early), administered IV reduced complications of CMV in infant at one year of life. (CID 55: 497, 2012)

* See page 2 for abbreviations. NOTE: All dosage recommendations are for adults (unless otherwise indicated) and assume normal renal function.

TABLE 14A (4)

VIRUS/DISEASE	DRUG/DOSAGE	SIDE EFFECTS/COMMENTS
Herpesvirus Infections *(continued)*		
Epstein Barr Virus (EBV) — Mononucleosis (*Ln J ID* 3:131, 2003)	**No treatment.** Corticosteroids for tonsillar obstruction, CNS complications, or threat of splenic rupture.	**Etiology of atypical lymphocytes:** EBV, CMV, Hap A, Hap B, toxo, measles, mumps, drugs (*Int Pediatr* 18:20, 2003)
HHV-6—Implicated as cause of roseola (exanthem subitum) & other febrile diseases of childhood (*NEJM* 352:768, 2005). Fever & rash documented in transplant pts (*JID* 179:311, 1999). Reactivation in 47% of 110 U.S. hematopoietic stem cell transplant pts assoc. with meningoencephalitis in immunocompetent adults. Diagnosis made by pos. PCR in CSF. ↓ viral copies in response to **ganciclovir rx** (*CID* 40:890 & 894, 2005). Cidofovir is second line therapy (*Bone Marrow Transplantation* 2008) 42, 227–240).		
HHV-7—ubiquitous virus (>90% of the population is infected by age 3 yrs). No relationship to human disease. Infects CD4 lymphocytes via CD4 receptor, transmitted via saliva.		
HHV-8—The agent of Kaposi's sarcoma, Castleman's disease, & body cavity lymphoma. Associated with diabetes in sub-Saharan Africa (*JAMA* 299:2770, 2008).	**No antiviral treatment.** Effective anti-HIV therapy may help.	Localized lesions: radiotherapy, laser surgery or intralesional chemotherapy. Systemic: chemotherapy, Castleman's disease responded to ganciclovir (*Blood* 103:1632, 2004) & valganciclovir (*JID* 2006).
Herpes simplex virus (HSV Types 1 & 2) Bell's palsy H. simplex most implicated etiology. Other etiologic considerations: VZV, HHV-6, Lyme disease.	As soon as possible after onset of palsy. **Prednisone** 1 mg/kg po divided bid x 5 days then taper to 5 mg bid over the next 5 days (total of 10 days) prednisone) Alternate **Prednisone** (dose as above) + **Valacyclovir** 500 mg bid x 5 days	Prospective randomized double blind placebo controlled trial compared prednisolone vs acyclovir vs. (prednisolone + acyclovir) vs placebo. Best results with prednisolone: 85% recovery with placebo, 96% recovery with prednisolone, 93% with combination of acyclovir & prednisolone (*NEJM* 357:1598 & 1653, 2007). **Large meta-analysis confirms: Steroids alone, effective; antiviral drugs alone, not effective. Steroids + antiviral rx no more effective than steroids alone** (*JAMA* 302:985, 2009).
Encephalitis (Excellent reviews: *CID* 35: 254, 2002; UK experience (*EID* 9:234, 2003; *Eur J Neurol* 12:331, 2005.; *Antiviral Res*: 71:141-148, 2006) HSV-1 the most common cause of sporadic encephalitis. Survival & recovery from encephalitis are related to mental status at time of initiation of rx. **Early dx and rx imperative.** *NEJM* 371:68, 2014.	**Acyclovir** IV 10 mg/kg IV (infuse over 1 hr) q8h x 14-21 days. 20 mg/kg q8h in children <12 yrs. Dose calculation in obese patients uncertain. To lessen risk of nephrotoxicity with larger doses seems reasonable to infuse each dose over more than 1 hour. In morbid obesity, use actual body weight.	Mortality rate reduced from >70% to 19% with acyclovir rx. PCR analysis of CSF for HSV-1 DNA is 100% specific & 75–98% sensitive. 8/33 (25%) CSF samples drawn before day 3 were neg. by PCR (neg. PCR result with <10 WBC per mm³ in CSF (*CID* 36:1335, 2003). All were + after 3 days. Relapse after successful rx reported in 7/27 (27%) children. Relapse was associated with a lower total dose of initial acyclovir rx (285 ± 82 mg per kg in relapse group vs. 462 ± 149 mg per kg, p <0.03) (*Neuropediatrics* 35:371, 2004).
Genital Herpes: *Sexually Transmitted Treatment Guidelines 2010: MMWR 59 (RR-12), 2010.* Primary (initial episode)	**Acyclovir** (Zovirax or generic): 400 mg po tid x 7-10 days OR **Valacyclovir** (Valtrex): 1000 mg po bid x 7-10 days OR **Famciclovir** (Famvir): 250 mg po tid x 7-10 days	↓ by 2 days time to resolution of signs & symptoms, ↓ by 4 days time to healing of lesions, ↓ by 7 days duration of viral shedding. Does not prevent recurrences. For severe cases only: ↓ 5 mg per kg IV q8h times 5-7 days.
Episodic recurrences	**Acyclovir** 800 mg po bid **x 2 days** or 400 mg po tid **x 5 days** or **Famciclovir** 1000 mg po **x 1 day** or 125 mg po bid x 5 days of **Valacyclovir** 500 mg po bid **x 3 days** or 1 gm po once daily **x 5 days** For HIV patients, see **Comment**	An ester of acyclovir, which is well absorbed, bioavailability 3-5 times greater than acyclovir. Metabolized to penciclovir, which is active component. Side effects and activity similar to acyclovir. **Famciclovir** 250 mg po bid x 7-10 days **equal to acyclovir** 200 mg 5 times per day. For episodic recurrences in HIV patients: **acyclovir** 400 mg po tid x 5-10 days or **famciclovir** 500 mg po bid x 5-10 days or **valacyclovir** 1 gm po bid x 5-10 days

* See page 2 for abbreviations. NOTE: All dosage recommendations are for adults (unless otherwise indicated) and assume normal renal function.

TABLE 14A (5)

VIRUS/DISEASE	DRUG/DOSAGE	SIDE EFFECTS/COMMENTS
Herpesvirus Infections/ Herpes simplex virus (HSV Types 1 & 2) *(continued)*		
Chronic daily suppression	**Suppressive therapy reduces the frequency of genital herpes recurrences by 70–80% among pts who have frequent recurrences (i.e., >6 recurrences per yr) & many report no symptomatic outbreaks.** **Acyclovir** 400 mg po bid **or famciclovir** 250 mg po bid, **or valacyclovir** 1 gm po q24h; pts with <9 recurrences per yr could use 500 mg po q24h and then use **Valacyclovir** 1 gm po q24h if breakthrough at 500 mg. For HIV patients, see Comment	For chronic suppression in HIV patients: **acyclovir** 400–800 mg po bid or tid or **famciclovir** 500 mg po bid or **valacyclovir** 500 mg po bid
Genital, Immunocompetent:		
Gingivostomatitis, primary (children)	**Acyclovir** 15 mg/kg po 5x/day x 7 days	Efficacy in randomized double-blind placebo-controlled trial (*BMJ 314:1800, 1997*).
Keratoconjunctivitis and recurrent epithelial keratitis	**Trifluridine** (Viroptic), 1 drop 1% solution q2h (max. 9 drops per day) for max. of 21 days (*see Table 1, page 13*)	In controlled trials, response % > idoxuridine. Suppressive rx with acyclovir (400 mg) reduced recurrences of ocular HSV from 32% to 19% (*NEJM 339:300, 1998*).
Mollaret's recurrent "aseptic" meningitis (usually HSV-2) (*Ln 363:1772, 2004*)	No controlled trials of antiviral rx & resolves spontaneously. If therapy is to be given, **acyclovir** (15–30 mg/kg/day IV) or **valacyclovir** 1–2 gm po qid should be used.	Pos. PCR for HSV in CSF confirms dx (*EJCMID 23:560, 2004*). Daily suppression rx might ↓ frequency of recurrence but no clinical trials. Oral Valacyclovir ref: *JAC 47:855, 2001.*

Mucocutaneous (for genital see previous page)
Oral labial, "fever blisters":
Normal host
  See Ann Pharmacotherapy 38:705, 2004;
  JAC 53:703, 2004
	Start rx with prodrome symptoms (tingling/burning) before lesions show.
	
			Dose	Sx Decrease

Oral: Valacyclovir	2 gm po q12h x 1 day	1 day
Famciclovir	500 mg po bid x 7 days	2 days
Acyclovir[FDA]	400 mg po 5 x per day (q4h while awake) x 5 days	1½ day | **Topical:** | Penciclovir 1% cream	q2h during day x 4 days	1 day
Acyclovir 5% cream[¹]	q2h (q3h) x 7 days	1 day
	6x/day x 7 days	1½ day	 See Table 1, page 27	Penciclovir (*AAC 46:2848, 2002*). Oral acyclovir 5% cream (*AAC 46:2238, 2002*). Oral acyclovir 5% cream (*AAC 46:2238, 2002*). Topical fluocinonide (0.05% Lidex gel) q8h times 5 days in combination with famciclovir ↓ lesion size and pain when compared to famciclovir alone (*JID 181:1906, 2000*). Acyclovir 5% cream + 1% hydrocortisone (Xerese) superior to acyclovir alone (*AAC 58:1273, 2014*).
Herpes Whitlow		

² FDA approved only for HIV pts
³ Approved for immunocompromised pts
* See page 2 for abbreviations. NOTE: All dosage recommendations are for adults (unless otherwise indicated) and assume normal renal function.

TABLE 14A (6)

VIRUS/DISEASE	DRUG/DOSAGE	SIDE EFFECTS/COMMENTS
Herpesvirus Infections/ Herpes simplex virus (HSV Types 1 & 2) Mucocutaneous (continued)		
Oral labial or genital: Immunocompromised (includes pts with AIDS) and critically ill pts in ICU setting/large necrotic ulcers in perineum or face. (See Comment) Primary HSV in pregnancy, increased risk of dissemination, including severe hepatitis. Risk greatest in 3rd trimester (NEJM 370:211, 2014).	**Acyclovir** 5 mg per kg IV (infused over 1 hr) q8h times 7 days (250 mg per M²) or 400 mg po 5 times per day times 14 days (see Comment if suspect acyclovir-resistant) **OR** **Famciclovir:** In HIV infected, 500 mg po bid for 7 days for recurrent episodes of genital herpes **OR** **Valacyclovir**ᴬᴷᴬ: In HIV-infected, 500 mg po bid for 5–10 days for recurrent episodes of genital herpes or 500 mg po bid for chronic suppressive rx.	**Acyclovir-resistant HSV: IV foscarnet** 90 mg/kg IV q12h x 7 days. Suppressive therapy with famciclovir (500 mg po bid), valacyclovir (500 mg po bid) or acyclovir (400-800 mg po bid) reduces viral shedding and clinical recurrences.
Pregnancy and genital H. simplex	Acyclovir safe even in first trimester. No proof that acyclovir at delivery reduces risk/severity of neonatal Herpes. In contrast, C-section in women with active lesions reduces risk of transmission. Ref: Obstet Gyn 106:845, 2006	
Herpes simiae (Herpes B virus): **Monkey bite** CID 35:1191, 2002	**Postexposure prophylaxis: Valacyclovir** 1 gm po q8h times 14 days or acyclovir 800 mg po 5 times per day times 14 days. **Treatment of disease:** (1) CNS symptoms absent: **Acyclovir** 12.5–15 mg per kg IV q8h or ganciclovir 5 mg per kg IV q12h (2) CNS symptoms present: **Ganciclovir** 5 mg per kg IV q12h	Fatal human cases of myelitis and hemorrhagic encephalitis have been reported following bites, scratches, or eye inoculation of saliva from monkeys. Initial sx include fever, headache, myalgias and diffuse adenopathy, incubation period of 2–14 days (EID 9:246, 2003). In vitro ACV and ganciclovir less active than other nucleosides (ganciclovir or 5-ethyldeoxyuridine may be more active, clinical data needed) (AAC 51:2028, 2007).
Varicella-Zoster Virus (VZV) **Varicella:** Vaccination has markedly ↓ incidence of varicella & morbidity (MMWR 61:609, 2012). Guidelines for VZV vaccine (MMWR 56(RR-4) 2007).		
Normal host (chickenpox) Child (2–12 years)	In general, treatment not recommended. Might use oral **acyclovir** for healthy persons at ↑ risk for moderate to severe varicella, i.e., >12 yrs of age; chronic cutaneous or pulmonary diseases; chronic salicylate rx. (↑ risk of Reye syndrome). **acyclovir** dose: 20 mg/kg po qid x 5 days (start within 24 hrs of rash) or **valacyclovir** 20 mg/kg tid x 5 days.	Acyclovir slowed development and ↓ duration of disease in children: 9 to 7.6 days (PIDJ 21:739, 2002). Oral dose of acyclovir in children should not exceed 80 mg per kg per day or 3200 mg per day.
Adolescents, young adults	Start within 24 hrs of rash. **Valacyclovir** 1000 mg po tid x 5–7 days or **Famciclovir** 500 mg po tid (probably effective, but data lacking)	↓ duration of fever, time to healing, and symptoms.
Pneumonia or chickenpox in 3rd trimester of pregnancy	**Acyclovir** 800 mg po 5 times per day or 10 mg per kg IV q8h times 5 days. Risks and benefits to tetus and mother unknown. Many experts recommend rx, especially in 3ʳᵈ trimester. Some would add VZIG (varicella-zoster immune globulin).	Varicella pneumonia associated with 41% mortality in pregnancy. Acyclovir ↓ incidence and severity (JID 185:422, 2002). If varicella-susceptible mother exposed and respiratory symptoms develop within 10 days after exposure, start acyclovir

---

* See page 2 for abbreviations. NOTE: All dosage recommendations are for adults (unless otherwise indicated) and assume normal renal function.

TABLE 14A (7)

VIRUS/DISEASE	DRUG/DOSAGE	SIDE EFFECTS/COMMENTS
Herpesvirus Infections/Varicella-Zoster Virus (VZV) (continued)		
Immunocompromised host	**Acyclovir** 10–12 mg per kg (500 per M²) IV (infused over 1 hr) q8h times 7 days	Disseminated 1° varicella infection reported during infliximab rx of rheumatoid arthritis (J Rheum 31:2517, 2004). Continuous infusion of high-dose acyclovir (2 mg per kg per hr) successful in 1 pt with severe hemorrhagic varicella (NEJM 336:732, 1997).
Prevention—Postexposure prophylaxis Varicella deaths still occur in unvaccinated persons (MMWR 56 (RR-4) 1-40, 2007)	**CDC Recommendations for Prevention:** Since <5% of varicella-related deaths occur in adults >20 yrs of age, the CDC recommends a more aggressive approach in this age group: **1st, varicella-zoster immune globulin** (VZIG) (125 units/10 kg (22 lbs) body weight IM up to a max. of 625 units; minimum dose is 125 units) is recommended for postexposure prophylaxis in susceptible persons at greater risk for complications (immunocompromised such as HIV, malignancies, pregnancy, and steroid therapy) as soon as possible after exposure (<96 hrs). If varicella develops, initiate treatment quickly (<24 hrs of rash) with **acyclovir** as below. Some would rx presumptively with acyclovir in high-risk pts. **2nd,** susceptible adults should be vaccinated. Check antibody in adults with negative or uncertain history of varicella (10–30% will be Ab-neg.) and vaccinate those who are Ab-neg. **3rd,** susceptible children should receive vaccination. Recommended routinely before age 12–18 mos. but OK at any age.	
Herpes zoster (shingles) (See NEJM 369:255, 2013)		
Normal host • Effective therapy most evident in pts >50 yrs. (For treatment of post-herpetic neuralgia, see CID 36: 877, 2003; Ln 374:1252, 2009) • Vaccination↓ herpes zoster & post-herpetic neuralgia (NEJM 352: 2271, 2005; JAMA 292:157, 2006). Reviewed in J Am Acad Derm 58:361, 2008. • Analgesics for acute pain associated with Herpes zoster (NEJM 369:255, 2013)	**[NOTE: Trials showing benefit of therapy: only in pts treated within 3 days of onset of rash]** **Valacyclovir** 1000 mg tid times 7 days (adjust dose for renal failure) (See Table 17A) **OR** **Famciclovir** 500 mg tid x 7 days. Adjust for renal failure (See Table 17A) **OR** **Acyclovir** 800 mg po 5 times per day times 7–10 days **Add Prednisone** in pts over 50 yrs old for discomfort during acute phase of zoster. Does not decrease incidence of post-herpetic neuralgia. Dose: 30 mg po bid days 1–7, 15 mg bid days 8–14 and 7.5 mg bid days 15–21.	Increasing recognition of risk of stroke during 6 mos after episode of Shingles. Oral antivirals during clinical H. zoster infection may have protective effect (CID 58:1497, 1504, 2014). Time to healing more rapid. Reduced incidence of post-herpetic neuralgia (PHN) vs placebo in pts >50 yrs of age. Famciclovir similar to acyclovir in reduction of acute pain and incidence of PHN (J Micro Immunol Inf 37:75, 2004). In a meta-analysis of 4 placebo-controlled trials (691 pts), acyclovir accelerated by approx. 2-fold pain resolution and reduced incidence of post-herpetic neuralgia at 3 & 6 mos (CID 22:341, 1996); med. time to resolution of pain 41 days vs 101 days in those >50 yrs. In post-herpetic neuralgia, controlled trials demonstrated effectiveness of **gabapentin**, the role of antiviral drugs in rx of PHN unproven (Neurol 64:21, 2005) but 8 of 15 pt improved with IV acyclovir 10 mg/kg q 8 hrs x 14 days followed by oral valacyclovir 1gm 3x a day for 1 month (Arch Neur 63:940, 2006). Review: NEJM 371:1526, 2014.
		Role & opioid analgesic in controlling pain (Drugs 64:937, 2004; J Clin Virol 29:248, 2004). **Nortriptyline & amitriptyline** are equally effective but nortriptyline is better tolerated (CID 36:877, 2003). **Lidocaine patch** (5%) & **opioid analgesic** in controlling pain (Drugs 64:937, 2004; J Clin Virol 29:248, 2004).
Immunocompromised host Not severe	**Acyclovir** 800 mg po 5 times per day times 7 days. (Or, **famciclovir** 750 mg po q24h or 500 mg bid or 250 mg 3 times per day times 7 days **OR valacyclovir** 1000 mg po tid times 7 days, though both are not FDA-approved for this indication)	If progression, switch to IV. RA pts on TNF-alpha inhibitors at high risk for VZV. Zoster more severe, but less post-herpetic neuralgia (JAMA 301:737, 2009).
Severe: >1 dermatome, trigeminal nerve or disseminated	**Acyclovir** 10–12 mg per kg IV (infusion over 1 hr) q8h times 7–10 days. In older pts, ↓ to 7.5 mg per kg. If nephrotoxicity and pt improving, ↓ to 5 mg per kg q8h.	A common manifestation of immune reconstitution following HAART in HIV-infected children (J All Clin Immun 113:742, 2004). Rx must be begun within 72 hrs. For Acyclovir-resistant VZV in HIV+ pts previously treated with acyclovir: **Foscarnet** (40 mg per kg IV q8h for 14–26 days).

*See page 2 for abbreviations. NOTE: All dosage recommendations are for adults (unless otherwise indicated) and assume normal renal function.

TABLE 14A (8)

Influenza A & B and novel influenza viruses Refs: *http://www.cdc.gov/flu/professionals/antivirals/index.htm http://www.cdc.gov/flu/weekly/; NEJM 370:789, 2014.*
Vaccine Info (*http://www.cdc.gov/flu/professionals/acip/index.htm*); *Med Lett 56:97, 2014; MMWR 63:691, 2014.*

- **Oseltamivir and zanamivir are recommended drugs.** Amantadine and rimantadine should not be used because of widespread resistance.
- Guidelines: ACIP: (*MMWR 60 (RR01);1-24 2011*) *IDSA (CID 48:1003-1032, 2009)*
- Novel H1N1 (referred to as pandemic H1N1, pH1N1, H1N1pdm and formerly swine flu) emerged in 2009 and now is the dominant H1N1 strain worldwide. Old distinction from seasonal H1N1 is still sometimes used but not relevant
- Rapid influenza tests can be falsely negative in 20-50%
- Initiate therapy as close to the onset of symptoms as possible, and certainly within 48 hrs of onset of symptoms. Starting therapy after 48 hours of onset of symptoms is associated with reduced therapeutic benefit. However, starting therapy up to 5 days after onset in patients who are hospitalized is associated with improved survival (*Clin Infect Dis 55:1198, 2012*).
- Empiric therapy should be started for all patients who are hospitalized, have severe or progressive influenza or are at higher risk of complications due to age or underlying medical conditions.
- Look for concomitant bacterial pneumonia.
- Other important influenza viruses causing human disease
  - **H3N2v influenza:** 159 cases of influenza A/H3N2v reported over the summer of 2012. Most of the cases of influenza A/H3N2v occurred in children under the age of 10 with direct contact with pigs. This variant is susceptible to the neuraminidase inhibitors, oseltamivir and zanamivir. See *MMWR 61:619, 2012.*
  - **Avian influenza H5N1:** Re-emerged in Asia in 2003 and human cases detected in 15 countries mostly in Asia as well as Egypt, Nigeria and Djibouti. Circulation associated with massive poultry die diff. Imported cases rare – one in Canada. As of January 2014. 648 confirmed cases and 384 deaths (59%). Human infection associated with close contact with poultry; very limited human to human transmission. Mortality associated with high viral load, disseminated virus and high cytokine activity (*Nature Medicine 12:1203-1207 2006*). Sensitive to oseltamivir but oseltamivir resistance has emerged on therapy (*NEJM 353:267-272 2005*). Use oseltamivir and consider IV zanamivir
  - **Avian influenza H7N9:** Emerged in Eastern China in March 2013 and 132 cases documented during Spring 2013 with 44 deaths (33%). Cases appeared again in early winter 2013-2014 and continue to increase. Infection associated with close contact with live bird markets; extremely limited human to human transmission to date. Mortality highest among older persons and those with medical conditions. Oseltamivir active against most but not all strains. No zanamivir resistance documented to date.

Virus/Disease	Susceptible to (Recommended Drug/Dosage):	Resistant to:	Alternatives/Side Effects/Comments
A/H1N1 (current seasonal resembles pandemic H1N1) • Influenza B • Influenza A (A/H3N2, A/H3N2v*, A/H5N1, A/H7N9**)	**Oseltamivir** Adult: Oseltamivir 75 mg po bid × 5 days Pediatric (child age 1-12 years): Infant 2 wks-11 months: 3 mg/kg bid × 5 days ≤15 kg: 30 mg bid × 5 days >15 kg to 23 kg: 45 mg bid × 5 days >23 kg to 40 kg: 60 mg bid × 5 days >40 kg: 75 mg bid × 5 days or **Zanamivir** 2 inhalations (5 mg each) bid × 5 days or Peramivir 600 mg IV once daily × 5-10 days For IV Zanamivir, see **Comment**	Amantadine and rimantadine (100%) * A/H3N2v strain are susceptible ** A/H7N9 resistant to oseltamivir (rarely)	• **A/H1N1:** Higher dose (150 mg bid) **not** more effective for H1N1 • **Zanamivir** not recommended for children < 7 years or those with reactive airway disease • IV zanamivir is available under compassionate use IND and clinical trials for hospitalized influenza patients with suspected or known gastric stasis, gastric malabsorption, gastrointestinal bleeding, or for patients suspected or confirmed with oseltamivir-resistant influenza virus infection. For compassionate use, contact GlaxoSmithKline at (+1) 919-315-5215 or email: gsklinicalsupportHD@GSK.com. • **Influenza B:** One study suggested virologic benefit to higher dose oseltamivir for critically ill patients with influenza B • **A/H5N1:** Given high mortality, consider obtaining investigational drug. Zanamivir retains activity against most oseltamivir resistant H5N1

* See page 2 for abbreviations. NOTE: All dosage recommendations are for adults (unless otherwise indicated) and assume normal renal function.

TABLE 14A (9)

VIRUS/DISEASE	DRUG/DOSAGE	SIDE EFFECTS/COMMENTS
Measles Increasing reports of measles in unvaccinated children and adults *(MMWR 63:781, 2014; NEJM 371:358, 2014).*		
Children	No therapy or **vitamin A** 200,000 units po daily times 2 days	Vitamin A may ↓ severity of measles.
Adults	No rx or **ribavirin** IV: 20-35 mg per kg per day times 7 days	↓ severity of illness in adults *(CID 20:454, 1994).*
Metapneumovirus (HMPV) A paramyxovirus isolated from pts of all ages, with mild bronchiolitis/bronchospasm to pneumonia. Review: *Sem Resp Care Med 32:447, 2011.*	**No proven antiviral therapy** (intravenous ribavirin used anecdotally with variable results)	Human metapneumovirus isolated from 6-21% of children with RTIs *(NEJM 350:443, 2004).* Dual infection with RSV assoc. with severe bronchiolitis *(JID 191:382, 2005).*
Monkey pox (orthopox virus) *(see LnID 4:17, 2004).* Outbreak from contact with ill prairie dogs. Source likely imported Gambian giant rats *(CID 58:260, 2014).*	**No proven antiviral therapy.** Cidofovir is active in vitro & in mouse model	Incubation period of 12 days, then fever, headache, cough, adenopathy, & a vesicular papular rash that pustulates, umbilicates, & crusts on the head, trunk, & extremities. Transmission in healthcare setting rare.
Norovirus (Norwalk-like virus, or NLV) Vast majority of outbreaks of non-bacterial gastroenteritis *(NEJM 366:1121, 2013).*	**No antiviral therapy.** Replete volume. Transmission by contaminated food, fecal-oral contact with contaminated surfaces, or fomites.	Sudden onset of nausea, vomiting, and/or watery diarrhea lasting 12-60 hours. Ethanol-based hand rubs effective *(J Hosp Inf 60:144, 2005).*
Papillomaviruses: Warts External Genital Warts	**Patient applied:** **Podofilox** (0.5% solution or gel): apply 2x/day x 3 days, 4th day no therapy, repeat cycle 4x; OR **Imiquimod** 5% cream: apply once daily hs 3x/wk for up to 16 wks. **Sinecatechins:** Apply to external genital warts only 3x/day until effect or adverse effect **Provider administered:** Cryotherapy with liquid nitrogen; repeat q1-2 wks; OR **Podophyllin resin** 10-25% in tincture of benzoin. Repeat weekly as needed; OR **Trichloroacetic acid** (TCA): repeat weekly as needed; OR surgical removal.	**Podofilox:** Inexpensive and safe (pregnancy safety not established). Mild irritation after treatment. **Imiquimod:** Mild to moderate redness & irritation. Topical imiquimod effective for treatment of vulvar intraepithelial neoplasms *(NEJM 358:1465, 2008).* Safety in pregnancy not established. **Sinecatechins:** Local irritation, redness, pain, and itching **Cryotherapy:** Blistering and skin necrosis common. **Podophyllin resin:** Must air dry before treated area contacts clothing. Can irritate adjacent skin. **TCA:** Caustic. Can cause severe pain on adjacent normal skin. Neutralize with soap or sodium bicarbonate.
Warts on cervix	Need evaluation for evolving neoplasia	Gynecological consult advised.
Vaginal warts	Cryotherapy with liquid nitrogen or **TCA**	
Urethral warts	Cryotherapy with liquid nitrogen or **Podophyllin resin** 10-25% in tincture of benzoin	
Anal warts	Cryotherapy with liquid nitrogen or **TCA** or surgical removal	Advise anoscopy to look for rectal warts.
Skin papillomas	**Topical α-lactalbumin. Oleic acid** (from human milk) applied 1x/day for 3 wks	↓ lesion size & recurrence vs placebo (p <0.001) *(NEJM 350:2663, 2004).* Further studies warranted.

* See page 2 for abbreviations. NOTE: All dosage recommendations are for adults (unless otherwise indicated) and assume normal renal function.

TABLE 14A (10)

VIRUS/DISEASE	DRUG/DOSAGE	SIDE EFFECTS/COMMENTS
Parvo B19 Virus (Erythrovirus B19). *Review: NEJM 350:586, 2004. Wide range of manifestation.* **Treatment options for common symptomatic infections:**		
Erythema infectiosum	Symptomatic treatment only	Diagnostic tools: IgM & Igb antibody titers. Perhaps better: blood parvovirus PCR.
Arthritis/arthralgia	Nonsteroidal anti-inflammatory drugs (NSAID)	Dose of IVIG not standardized; suggest 400 mg/kg IV of commercial IVIG for 5 or 10 days of 1000 mg/kg IV for 3 days.
Transient aplastic crisis	Transfusions and oxygen	Most dramatic anemias in pts with pre-existing hemolytic anemia.
Fetal hydrops	Intrauterine blood transfusion	Bone marrow shows erythrocyte maturation arrest with giant pronormoblasts.
Chronic infection with anemia	**IVIG** and transfusion *(CID 56:968, 2013).* For dose, see *Comment*	
Chronic infection without anemia	Perhaps **IVIG**	
Papovavirus/Polyomavirus		
Progressive multifocal leukoencephalopathy (PML)	No specific therapy for JC virus. Two general approaches:	Failure of treatment with interferon alfa-2b, cytarabine and topotecan. Immunosuppressive **natalizumab** temporarily removed from market due to reported associations with PML. Mixed reports on **cidofovir.** Most likely effective for ART-experienced pts.
Serious demyelinating disease due to JC virus in immunocompromised pts.	1. In HIV pts: HAART. Cidofovir may be effective. 2. Stop or decrease immunosuppressive therapy.	
BK virus induced nephropathy in immunocompromised pts and hemorrhagic cystitis	Decrease immunosuppression if possible. Suggested antiviral therapy based on anecdotal data. If progressive renal dysfunction: 1. **Fluoroquinolone** first; 2. **IVIG** 500 mg/kg IV; 3. **Leflunomide** 100 mg po daily x 3 days, then 10-20 mg po daily; 4. **Cidofovir** only if refractory to all of the above (see *Table 14B for dose*).	Use PCR to monitor viral "load" in urine and/or plasma. Report of cidofovir as potentially effective for BK hemorrhagic cystitis *(CID 49:233, 2009).*
Rabies *(see Table 20B, page 216; diagnosis and management: www.cdc.gov/rabies)*		
Rabid dogs account for 50,000 cases per yr worldwide. Most cases in the U.S. are cryptic, 70% assoc. with 2 rare bat species *(EID 9:151, 2003).* An organ donor with early rabies infected 4 recipients (2 kidneys, liver & artery) all died avg. 13 days after transplant *(NEJM 352:1103, 2005).*	**Mortality 100% with only survivors those who receive rabies vaccine before the onset of illness/symptoms** *(CID 36:61, 2003).* A 15-year-old female who developed rabies 1 month post-bat bite survived after drug induction of coma (+ other rx) for 7 days; did not receive immunoprophylaxis *(NEJM 352:2508, 2005).*	Corticosteroids ↑ mortality rate and ↓ incubation time in mice. Therapies that have failed when symptoms develop include rabies vaccine, rabies immuno-globulin, rabies virus neutralizing antibody, ribavirin, alfa interferon, & ketamine. For post-exposure prophylaxis, see *Table 20B, page 216.*
Respiratory Syncytial Virus (RSV)	All ages: Hydration, O2 as needed. If wheezing, trial of beta-agonist.	In adults, RSV accounted for 10.6% of hospitalizations for pneumonia, 11.4% of AECB, 7.2% for asthma & 5.4% for CHF in pts >65 yrs of age *NEJM 352:1749, 2005).* RSV caused 11% of clinically important respiratory illnesses in military recruits *(CID 41:311, 2005).*
Major cause of morbidity in neonates/infants. Diagnosis: airway swab for RSV PCR	Corticosteroids: children-no; adults-maybe Nebulized Ribavirin: for severe RSV in children, adults *(CID 57:1731, 2013);* Nebulized Ribavirin + RSV immune globulin: immunocompromised adults (HSCT)*(CID 56:258, 2013).*	
Prevention of RSV in:		
(1) Children <24 mos. old with chronic lung disease of prematurity (formerly broncho-pulmonary dysplasia) requiring supple-mental O2, or	**Palivizumab** (Synagis) 15 mg per kg IM q month Nov-Apr. See *Pediatrics 126:e16, 2010.*	Expense argues against its use. Guidance from the Academy of Pediatrics recommends use of Palivizumab only in newborn infants born at 29 weeks gestation (or earlier) and in special populations (e.g., those infants with significant heart disease). *(Pediatrics 2014;134:415–420)*
(2) Premature infants (<32 wks gestation) and <6 mos. old at start of RSV season or		
(3) Children with selected congenital heart diseases		

* See page 2 for abbreviations. NOTE: All dosage recommendations are for adults (unless otherwise indicated) and assume normal renal function.

TABLE 14A (11)

VIRUS/DISEASE	DRUG/DOSAGE	SIDE EFFECTS/COMMENTS
Rhinovirus (Colds) *See Ln 361:51, 2003* Found in 1/2 of children with community-acquired pneumonia, role in pathogenesis unclear *(CID 39:681, 2004)*. High rate of rhinovirus identified in children with significant lower resp tract infections *(Ped Inf Dis 28:337, 2009)*	No antiviral rx indicated *(Ped Ann 34:53, 2005)*. Symptomatic rx: • **Ipratropium bromide** nasal (2 sprays per nostril tid) • **Clemastine** 1.34 mg 1–2 tab po bid-tid (OTC). Avoid zinc products *(see Comment)*.	Sx relief: ipratropium nasal spray ↓ rhinorrhea and sneezing vs placebo *(AnIM 125:89, 1996)*. Clemastine (an antihistamine) ↓ sneezing, rhinorrhea but associated with dry nose, mouth & throat in 6–19% *(CID 22:656, 1996)*. **Echinacea** didn't work *(CID 38:1367, 2004 & 40:807, 2005)*—put it to rest! Public health advisory advising that three over-the-counter cold remedy products containing **zinc** (e.g., Zicam) should not be used because of multiple reports of permanent anosmia *(www.fda.gov/Safety/MedWatch/SafetyInformation/ SafetyAlertsforHumanMedicalProducts/ucm166996.htm)*.
Rotavirus: Leading recognized cause of diarrhea-related illness among infants and children world-wide and kills ½ million children annually.	**No antiviral rx available;** oral hydration life-saving. In one study, **Nitazoxanide** 7.5 mg/kg 2x/d x 3 days reduced duration of illness from 75 to 31 hrs in Egyptian children. Impact on rotavirus or other parameters not measured. *(Lancet 368:100 & 124, 2006)*. Too early to recommend routine use *(Lancet 368:100, 2006)*	**Two live-attenuated vaccines highly effective (85 and 98%)** and safe in preventing rotavirus diarrhea and hospitalization *(NEJM 354: 1 & 23, 2006)*. ACIP recommends either of the two vaccines, RV1 or RV5, for infants *(MMWR 58(RR02): 1, 2009)*.
SARS-CoV: *See page 158*		
Smallpox *(NEJM 346:1300, 2002)*	Smallpox vaccine (if within 4 days of exposure) + cidofovir (dosage uncertain but likely similar to CMV (5 mg/kg IV once weekly for 2 weeks followed by once weekly dosing. Must be used with hydration and Probenecid; contact CDC: 770-488-7100)	
Contact vaccinia *(JAMA 288:1901, 2002)*	From vaccination: Progressive vaccinia—vaccinia immune globulin may be of benefit. To obtain immune globulin, contact CDC: 770-488-7100. *(CID 39:759, 776 & 819, 2004)*	
West Nile virus: *See page 159*		

* See page 2 for abbreviations. NOTE: All dosage recommendations are for adults (unless otherwise indicated) and assume normal renal function.

TABLE 14B – ANTIVIRAL DRUGS (NON-HIV)

DRUG NAME(S) GENERIC (TRADE)	DOSAGE/ROUTE IN ADULTS*	COMMENTS/ADVERSE EFFECTS
CMV (See SANFORD GUIDE TO HIV/AIDS THERAPY)		
Cidofovir (Vistide)	5 mg per kg IV once weekly for 2 weeks, then once every other week. **Properly timed IV prehydration with normal saline & Probenecid must be used with each cidofovir infusion:** 2 gm po 3 hrs before each dose and further 1 gm doses 2 & 8 hrs after completion of the cidofovir infusion. Renal function (serum creatinine and urine protein) must be monitored prior to each dose (see pkg insert for details). Contraindicated if creatinine >1.5 mg/dL, CrCl ≤55 mL/min or urine protein ≥ 100 mg/dL.	**Adverse effects: Nephrotoxicity:** dose-dependent proximal tubular injury (Fanconi-like syndrome): proteinuria, glycosuria, bicarbonaturia, phosphaturia, polyuria (nephrogenic diabetic insipidus). Concomitant saline prehydration, probenecid, extended dosing intervals allow use but still highly nephrotoxic. Other major toxicities: neutropenia (give G-CSF as needed); eye: monthly intra-ocular pressure. Dc cidofovir if pressure decreases 50% or uveitis occurs. **Black Box warning.** Renal impairment can occur after ≤2 doses. Contraindicated w/ concomitant nephrotoxic agents. Monitor for ↓ WBC. In animals, carcinogenic, teratogenic; causes ↓ sperm and ↓ fertility. FDA indication only CMV retinitis in HIV pts. **Comment:** Dose must be reduced or discontinued if changes in renal function occur during rx. For ↑ of 0.3-0.4 mg per dL in serum creatinine, cidofovir dose must be ↓ from 5 to 3 mg per kg; discontinue cidofovir if ↑ of 0.5 mg/dL above baseline or 3+ proteinuria develops (for 2+ proteinuria, observe pts carefully and consider discontinuation)
Foscarnet (Foscavir)	**Induction:** 90 mg per kg IV, over 1.5-2 hours, q12h **OR** 60 mg per kg, over 1 hour, q8h **Maintenance:** 90–120 mg per kg IV, over 2 hours, q24h Dosage adjustment with renal dysfunction (see Table 17A).	Use infusion pump to control rate of administration. **Adverse effects: Major toxicity is renal impairment (1/3 of patients).** Can cause ↓ Ca++ and/or ↓ Mg++, hence hypocalcemia manifests as arrhythmia, tetany, paresthesia, changes in mental status. Slow infusion rate and avoid drugs that lower Ca++, e.g., pentamidine. ↑↓ creatinine, proteinuria, mild (100%): diabetes insipidus, ↓K+, ↓Ca++, ↓ Mg++. Adequate hydration may ↓ toxicity. Other: headache, mild (100%); fatigue (100%), nausea (80%), fever (25%). CNS: seizures. Hematol: ↓ WBC, ↓ Hgb. Hepatic: liver function tests.† Neuropathy. Penile and oral ulcers.
Ganciclovir (Cytovene)	IV: 5 mg per kg q12h times 14 days (induction) 5 mg per kg IV q24h or 6 mg per kg 5 times per wk (maintenance) Dosage adjust. with renal dysfunction (see Table 17A)	**Adverse effects: Black Box warnings:** cytopenias, carcinogenicity/teratogenicity & aspermia in animals. Absolute neutrophil count dropped below 500 per mm³ in 15%, thrombocytopenia 21%, anemia 6%. Fever 48%, GI 50%: nausea, vomiting, diarrhea, abdominal pain 19%, rash 10%. Confusion, headache, psychiatric disturbances and seizures. Neutropenia may respond to granulocyte colony stimulating factor (G-CSF or GM-CSF). Severe myelosuppression may be ↑ with coadministration of zidovudine or azathioprine. 32% dc'd/interrupted rx, principally for neutropenia. Avoid pregnancy. A prodrug of ganciclovir with better bioavailability than oral ganciclovir: 60% with food.° Preg cat: C (may be teratogenic). Contraception recommended (♀ and ♂).
Valganciclovir (Valcyte)	450 mg tablets: take with food. Oral solution: 50 mg/mL. Adult dose: 900 mg. Treatment (induction): 900 mg po q12h with food. Prophylaxis (maintenance): 900 mg po q24h. Dosage adjustment for renal dysfunction (See Table 17A)	Adverse effects: Similar to ganciclovir. May cause dose limiting neutropenia, anemia, thrombocytopenia. Acute renal failure may occur. Diarrhea (16-41%), nausea (8-30%), vomiting (3-21%). **CMV retinitis** (sight-threatening lesions): 900 mg po q12h + intravenal Ganciclovir: 900 mg po q12h x 14-21 days, then 900 mg po q24h for maintenance
Herpesvirus		
Acyclovir (Zovirax or generic)	Doses: see Table 14A for various indications 400 mg or 800 mg tab 200 mg cap Suspension 200 mg per 5 mL Ointment or cream 5% IV injection Dosage adjustment for renal dysfunction (See Table 17A).	**po:** Generally well-tolerated with occ. diarrhea, vertigo, arthralgia. Less frequent rash, fatigue, insomnia, fever, menstrual abnormalities, acne, sore throat, muscle cramps, lymphadenopathy. **IV:** Phlebitis, caustic with vesicular lesions → obstructive uropathy (rapid infusion, dehydration, renal insufficiency and ↑ dose ↑ risk). Adequate pre-hydration may prevent such nephrotoxicity. Hepatic: ↑ ALT, AST.† Uncommon: neutropenia, rash, diaphoresis, hypotension, headache, nausea

---

* See page 2 for abbreviations. NOTE: All dosage recommendations are for adults (unless otherwise indicated) and assume normal renal function.

TABLE 14B (2)

DRUG NAME(S) GENERIC (TRADE)	DOSAGE/ROUTE IN ADULTS*	COMMENTS/ADVERSE EFFECTS
Herpesvirus (continued)		
Famciclovir (Famvir)	125 mg, 250 mg, 500 mg tabs. Dosage depends on indication: (see label and Table 14A).	Metabolized to penciclovir. **Adverse effects:** similar to acyclovir, included headache, nausea, diarrhea, and dizziness but incidence does not differ from placebo. May be taken without regard to meals. Dose should be reduced if CrCl <60 mL per min (see package insert & Table 14A, page 161 & Table 17A, page 211). May be taken with or without food.
Penciclovir (Denavir)	Topical 1% cream	Apply to area of recurrence of herpes labialis with start of sx, then q2h while awake times 4 days. Well tolerated.
Trifluridine (Viroptic)	Topical 1% solution: 1 drop q2h (max. 9 drops/day) until corneal re-epithelialization, then dose is ↓ for 7 more days (one drop q4h for at least 5 drops/day), not to exceed 21 days total rx.	Mild burning (5%), palpebral edema (3%), punctate keratopathy, stromal edema. For HSV keratoconjunctivitis or recurrent epithelial keratitis.
Valacyclovir (Valtrex)	500 mg, 1 gm tabs. Dosage depends on indication and renal function (see label, Table 14A & Table 17A)	An ester pro-drug of acyclovir that is well-absorbed, bioavailability 3-5 times greater than acyclovir. **Adverse effects** similar to acyclovir (see JID 186:S40, 2002). Thrombotic thrombocytopenic purpura/hemolytic uremic syndrome reported in pts with advanced HIV disease and transplant recipients participating in clinical trials at doses of 8 gm per day.
Valganciclovir (Valcyte)	450 mg tablets; take with food. Oral solution: 50 mg/mL. Adult does 900 mg, Treatment (induction): 900 mg po q12h with food; Prophylaxis (maintenance): 900 mg po q24h. Dosage adjustment for renal dysfunction (See Table 17A)	A prodrug of ganciclovir with better bioavailability than oral ganciclovir: 60% with food. Preg cat: C (may be teratogenic, contraceptive precaution for females). **Adverse effects:** Similar to ganciclovir. May cause dose limiting neutropenia, anemia, thrombocytopenia. Acute renal failure may occur. Diarrhea (16-41%), nausea (8-30%), vomiting (3-21%). **CMV retinitis** (sight-threatening lesions): 900 mg po q12h x 14-21 days, then 900 mg po q24h for maintenance
Hepatitis		
Adefovir dipivoxil (Hepsera)	10 mg po q24h (with normal CrCl); see Table 17A if renal impairment. 10 mg tab	It is an acyclic nucleotide analog with activity against hepatitis B (HBV) at 0.2-2.5 mM (IC₅₀). See Table 9 for Cmax & T½. Active against lamivudine-resistant HBV strains and in vitro vs. entecavir- resistant strains. To minimize resistance, use in combination with lamivudine for lamivudine-resistant virus: consider alternative therapy if viral load remains > 1,000 copies/mL with treatment. Primarily renal excretion—adjust dose. No food interactions. Generally few side effects, but **Black Box warning** regarding lactic acidosis/hepatic steatosis with nucleoside analogs. At 10 mg per day potential for delayed nephrotoxicity. Monitor renal function, esp. with pts with pre-existing or other risks for renal impairment. Pregnancy Category C. **Hepatitis may exacerbate when treatment discontinued;** Up to 25% of pts developed ALT ↑ 10 times normal within 12 wks, usually responds to re-treatment or self-limited, but hepatic decompensation has occurred. **Do not use adefovir in HIV infected patients**
Entecavir (Baraclude)	0.5 mg q24h. If refractory or resistant to lamivudine or telbivudine: 1 mg per day Tabs: 0.5 & 1 mg. Oral solution: 0.05 mg/mL. Administer on an empty stomach.	A nucleoside analog active against HBV including lamivudine-resistant mutants. Minimal adverse effects reported; headache, fatigue, dizziness, & nausea reported in 22% of pts. Alopecia, anaphylactoid reactions reported. Potential for lactic acidosis and exacerbation of hepB at discontinuation (**Black Box warning**). Do not use as single anti-retroviral agent in HIV co-infected pts; M184 mutation can emerge (NEJM 356:2614, 2007). Adjust dosage in renal impairment (see Table 17A, page 211).

* See page 2 for abbreviations. NOTE: All dosage recommendations are for adults (unless otherwise indicated) and assume normal renal function.

TABLE 14B (3)

DRUG NAME(S) GENERIC (TRADE)	DOSAGE/ROUTE IN ADULTS*	COMMENTS/ADVERSE EFFECTS
Hepatitis (continued)		
Interferon alfa is available as alfa-2a (Roferon-A) **alfa-2b** (Intron-A)	For HCV combination therapy, usual Roferon-A and Intron-A doses are 3 million international units 3x weekly subQ	Depending on agent, available in pre-filled syringes, vials of solution, or powder. **Black Box warnings:** can cause/aggravate psychiatric illness, ischemic events, infection. Withdraw therapy if symptoms worsen, esp. if depression or ideation of suicide.
PEG interferon alfa-2b (PEG-Intron)	0.5–1.5 mcg/kg subQ q wk	**Adverse effects: Flu-like syndrome** is common, esp. during 1st wk of rx: fever 98%, fatigue 89%, myalgia 73%, headache 71%, ↓ anorexia 46%, diarrhea 29%. CNS: dizziness 21%. Hemorrhage or ischemic stroke. Rash 18%, may progress to Stevens Johnson or exfoliative dermatitis. Alopecia. ↑ TSH: autoimmune thyroid disorders with ↓ or ↑ thyroidism. **Hemato:** ↓ WBC 49%, ↓
Peginterferon-40k interferon alfa-2a (Pegasys)	180 mcg subQ q wk	Hgb 27%, ↓ platelets 35%. Post-marketing reports of antibody-mediated pure red cell aplasia in pts receiving interferon/ribavirin with erythropoiesis-stimulating agents. Acute reversible hearing loss &/or tinnitus in up to 1/3 (Ln 343:1134, 1994). Optic neuropathy (retinal hemorrhage, cotton wool spots, ↓ in color vision) reported (AIDS 18:1805, 2004). Doses may require adjustment (or dc) based on individual response or adverse events, and can vary by product, indication (eg, HCV or HBV) and mode of use (mono- or combination+ of use). (Refer to labels of individual products and to ribavirin if used in combination for details of use.)
Lamivudine (3TC) (Epivir-HBV)	**HBV dose:** 100 mg po q24h Dosage adjustment with renal dysfunction (see Table 14D) Tabs 100 mg and oral solution 5 mg/mL	**Black Box warnings:** caution, dose is lower than HIV dose, so must exclude co-infection with HIV before using this formulation; lactic acidosis/hepatic steatosis; severe exacerbation of liver disease can occur on dc; YMDD-mutants resistant to lamivudine may emerge on treatment.
Ledipasvir + Sofosbuvir (Harvoni)	Combination formulation (Ledipasvir 90 mg + Sofosbuvir 400 mg) 1 tab po once daily	**Adverse effects:** See Table 14D. NS5A/NS5B inhibitor combination for Genotype 1 HCV. First agent for HCV treatment without Ribavirin or Interferon. No adjustment for mild/moderate renal or hepatic impairment. Most common AEs: fatigue (16%), headache (14%), nausea (7%), diarrhea (3%), insomnia (5%). Antacids and H2 blockers interfere with absorption of ledipasvir. The drug solubility decreases as pH increases. Recommended to separate administration of ledipasvir and antacid Rx by at least 4 hours.
Ribavirin (Rebetol, Copegus)	For use with an interferon for hepatitis C. Available as 200 mg caps and 40 mg/mL oral solution (Rebetol) or 200 mg and 400 mg tabs (Copegus) (See Comments regarding dosage)	**Black Box warnings (Preg Category X).** Drug may persist for 6 mos, avoid pregnancy for at least 6 mos in women or their partners. Only approved for pts with Ccr > 50 mL/min. Do not use in pts with severe heart disease or hemoglobinopathies. ARDS reported (Chest 124:406, 2003). **Adverse effects:** hemolytic anemia (may require dose reduction or dc), and all adverse effects of concomitant interferon used (see above). Postmarketing: retinal detachment, ↓ hearing, hypersensitivity reactions. See Table 14A for specific regimens, with different criteria in those with/without cardiac disease. **Initial Rebetol dose with Intron A (interferon alfa-2b) is wt-based:** 400 mg po for ≤ 75 kg, and 600 mg po am & 600 mg pm dose (≥ 75 kg), and with maximum prolonged doses of 1000 mg (≤ 75 kg) or 1200 mg (≥ 75 kg). **Copegus dose with PEG-Intron alfa-2a** are based in pts with genotype 1 or 4 (1000 mg for < 75 kg and 1200 mg for > 75 kg) divided into 2 doses (for 24 wks) than with genotypes 1 or 4 (1000 mg per day divided into 2 doses for < 75 kg and 1200 mg per day divided into 2 doses for ≥ 75 kg for 48 wks); in HIV/HCV co-infected pts, dose is 800 mg per day regardless of genotype. (See individual labels for details, including initial dosing and criteria for dose modification in those with/without cardiac disease.)
Simeprevir (Olysio)	150 mg 1 cap po once daily with food + both Ribavirin and Interferon	NS3/4A inhibitor. Need to screen patients with HCV genotype 1a for the Q80K polymorphism; if present consider alternative therapy. Contraindicated in pregnancy and in men whose female partners are pregnant (risk category C); concern is combination with ribavirin (risk category X). No dose adjustment required in patients with mild, moderate or severe renal impairment; no dose adjustment for mild hepatic impairment. Most common AEs (in combination with Ribavirin, Interferon): rash, pruritus, nausea. CYP3A inhibitors affect plasma concentration of Simeprevir.
Sofosbuvir (Sovaldi)	400 mg 1 tab po once daily with food + both Pegylated Interferon and Ribavirin. For combination formulation, see Ledipasvir.	NS5B inhibitor for Genotypes 1, 2, 3, 4 HCV. Efficacy established in patients awaiting liver transplant and in patients with HIV-1/HCV co-infection. No adjustment needed for mild to moderate renal impairment. No dose adjustment for mild, moderate, or severe hepatic impairment. Most common AEs (in combination with interferon and ribavirin): fatigue, headache, nausea, insomnia, anemia. Rifampin and St. Johns wort may alter concentrations of Sofosbuvir.

* See page 2 for abbreviations. NOTE: All dosage recommendations are for adults (unless otherwise indicated) and assume normal renal function.

TABLE 14B (4)

DRUG NAME(S) GENERIC (TRADE)	DOSAGE/ROUTE IN ADULTS*	COMMENTS/ADVERSE EFFECTS
Hepatitis *(continued)*		
Telbivudine (Tyzeka)	**HBV:** 600 mg orally q24h, without regard to food. Dosage adjustment with renal dysfunction, Ccr < 50 mL/min *(see label)*. 600 mg tabs; 100 mg for 5 mL solution.	An oral nucleoside analog approved for Rx of Hep B. It has ↑ rates of response and superior viral suppression than lamivudine *(NEJM 357:2576, 2007)*. **Black Box warnings** regarding lactic acidosis/hepatic steatosis with nucleosides and potential for severe exacerbation of HepB on dc. Generally well-tolerated with ↓ mitochondrial toxicity vs other nucleosides and no dose limiting toxicity observed *(Medical Letter 49:11, 2007)*. Myalgias, myopathy and rhabdomyolysis reported. Genotypic resistance rate was 4.4% by 2 yrs of treatment in 1 pt. Selects for YMDD mutation like lamivudine. Combination with lamivudine was inferior to monotherapy *(Hepatology 45:507, 2007)*.
Influenza A		
Amantadine (Symmetrel) or Rimantadine (Flumadine) Influenza B intrinsically resistant.	**Amantadine** 100 mg caps; 50 mg/mL oral solution & syrup. Treatment or prophylaxis: 100 mg bid; or 100 mg daily if age ≥65 y, dose reductions with CrCl starting at ≤50 mL/min. **Rimantadine** 100 mg tabs, 50 mg/5 mL syrup. Treatment or prophylaxis: 100 mg bid, or 100 mg daily in elderly nursing home pts, or severe hepatic disease, or CrCl ≤10 mL/min. For children, rimantadine only approved for prophylaxis.	**Side-effects/toxicity: CNS** (can be mild: nervousness, anxiety, difficulty concentrating, and lightheadedness). Serious: delirium, hallucinations, and seizures—are associated with high plasma drug levels resulting from renal insufficiency, esp. in older pts, those with prior seizure disorders, or psychiatric disorders.
Influenza A and B—For both drugs, initiate within 48 hrs of symptom onset		
Zanamivir (Relenza) For pts ≥ 7 yrs of age (treatment) or ≥ 5 yrs (prophylaxis)	Powder is inhaled by specially designed inhalation device. Each blister contains 5 mg zanamivir. **Treatment:** oral inhalation of 2 blisters (10 mg) bid for 5 days. **Prophylaxis:** oral inhalation of 2 blisters (10 mg) once daily for 10 days (household outbreak) to 28 days (community outbreak).	Active by inhalation against neuraminidase of both influenza A and B and inhibits release of virus from epithelial cells of respiratory tract. Approx. 4–17% of inhaled dose absorbed into plasma. Excreted by kidney but with low absorption, dose reduction not necessary in renal impairment. Minimal side-effects: <3% cough, sinusitis, diarrhea, nausea and vomiting. **Reports of respiratory adverse events in pts with or without h/o airways disease, should be avoided in pts with underlying respiratory disease.** Allergic reactions and neuropsychiatric events have been reported. **Caution: Do not reconstitute zanamivir powder for use in nebulizers or mechanical ventilators** (MedWatch report of Contact GSK (919-315-5275) for forms, then contact FDA: (301-796-1500 or 301-796-9900).
Oseltamivir (Tamiflu) For pts ≥ 1 yr (treatment or prophylaxis)	For CrCl: **Treatment,** 75 mg po bid for 5 days; 150 mg bid has been used for morbidly obese patients but this dose is not FDA-approved. **Prophylaxis,** 75 mg po once daily for 10 days to 6 wks. See label for pediatric weight-based dosing. Adult doses for CrCl ≤30 mL/min / CrCl: 75 mg caps, powder for oral suspension.	Well absorbed (80% bioavailability) from GI tract as ethyl ester of active compound GS 4071. ½ is 6–10 hrs; excreted unchanged by kidney. Adverse effects include diarrhea, nausea, vomiting, headache. Rarely, severe skin reactions (toxic epidermal necrolysis, Stevens-Johnson syndrome, erythema multiforme). **Delirium** & abnormal behavior reported *(CID 57:1511, 2013)*.
Peramivir (Rapivab)	600 mg IV single dose (acute uncomplicated influenza)	FDA indication is for single dose use in acute uncomplicated influenza. No approved dose for hospitalized patients but 200-400 mg IV daily for 5 days used in trial. Flu with H275Y oseltamivir resistance has moderate resistance to peramivir
Respiratory Syncytial Virus (RSV) monoclonal antibody		
Palivizumab (Synagis) Used for prevention of RSV infection in high-risk children	15 mg per kg IM q month throughout RSV season Single dose 100 mg vial	A monoclonal antibody directed against the surface F glycoprotein; **AEs:** uncommon, occ. ↑ ALT. Anaphylaxis <1/10 pts, acute hypersensitivity reactions <1/1000. Postmarketing reports: URI, otitis media, fever, ↑ pts, injection site reactions. Preferred over polyclonal immune globulin in high risk infants & children.
Warts Regimens are from drug labels specific for external genital and/or perianal condylomata acuminata only (see drug labels for indications, regimens, age limits).		
Interferon alfa-2b (IntronA)	Injection of 1 million international units into base of lesion, thrice weekly on alternate days for up to 3 wks. Maximum 5 lesions per course.	Interferons may cause "flu-like" illness and other systemic effects. 88% had at least one adverse effect. **Black box warning:** alpha interferons may cause or aggravate neuropsychiatric, autoimmune, ischemic or neoplastic disorders.
Interferon alfa-N3 (Alferon N)	Injection of 0.05 mL into base of each wart, up to 0.5 mL total per session, twice weekly for up to 8 weeks.	Contraindicated with allergy to mouse IgG, egg proteins, or neomycin.
Imiquimod (Aldara)	5% cream. Thin layer applied at bedtime, washing off after 6-10 hr, thrice weekly to maximum of 16 wks.	Erythema, itching & burning, erosions. Flu-like syndrome, increased susceptibility to sunburn (avoid UV).
Podofilox (Condylox)	0.5% gel or solution twice daily for 3 days, no therapy for 4 days; can use up to 4 such cycles.	Local reactions—pain, burning, inflammation in 50%. Can ulcerate. Limit surface area treated as per label.
Sinecatechins (Veregen)	15% ointment. Apply 0.5 cm strand to each wart three times per day until healing but not more than 16 weeks.	Application site reactions, which may result in ulcerations, phimosis, meatal stenosis, superinfection.

* See page 2 for abbreviations. NOTE: All dosage recommendations are for adults (unless otherwise indicated) and assume normal renal function.

TABLE 14C - AT A GLANCE SUMMARY OF SUGGESTED ANTIVIRAL AGENTS AGAINST TREATABLE PATHOGENIC VIRUSES

ANTIVIRAL AGENT	Adenovirus	BK virus	Cytomegalovirus	Hepatitis B	Hepatitis C	Herpes simplex virus	Influenza A / Influenza B	JC Virus	Respiratory Syncytial Virus	Varicella-zoster virus
Zanamivir	-	-	-	-	-	-	+++ / ++	-	-	-
Valganciclovir	±	-	+++	-	-	+	-	-	-	+
Valacyclovir	-	-	±	-	-	+++	-	-	-	+++
Rimantadine	-	-	-	-	-	-	±*** / -	-	-	-
Ribavirin	-	-	-	±	+++*	-	-	-	+	-
Oseltamivir	-	-	-	-	-	-	+++*** / ++	-	-	-
αInterferon Or PEG INF	-	-	-	+++	+++*	-	-	-	-	-
Ganciclovir/Valganciclovir	±	-	+++	-	-	+	-	-	-	+
Foscarnet	-	-	+++	-	-	++	-	-	-	-
Famciclovir	-	-	±	-	-	+++	-	-	-	+++
Cidofovir	+	+	+++	-	-	+	-	+	-	+
Sofosbuvir Simeprevir	-	-	-	-	+++	-	-	-	-	-
Adefovir Entecavir Lamivudine Tenofovir	-	-	-	+++	-	-	-	-	-	-
Amantadine	-	-	-	-	-	-	±*** / -	-	-	-
Acyclovir	-	-	±	-	-	+++	-	-	-	+

* 1st line rx = see Table 14G   **Influenza B is intrinsically resistant   *** High level resistance H1N1 (non-swine) in 2008; Swine H1N1 susceptible.

- = no activity; ± = possible activity; + = active, 3rd line therapy (least active)
++ = Active, 2nd line therapy (less active clinically); +++ = Active, 1st line therapy (usually active clinically)

TABLE 14D – ANTIRETROVIRAL THERAPY (ART) IN TREATMENT-NAÏVE ADULTS (HIV/AIDS)

A. Overview

- Antiretroviral therapy (ART) in treatment-naïve adult patients.
- Guidelines: www.aidsinfo.nih.gov and IAS-USA in *JAMA* 312:410, 2014.
- Design a regimen consisting of:
  - **Dual-nucleoside/-nucleotide reverse transcriptase inhibitor (NRTI component) PLUS either a:**
    - **Non-nucleoside reverse transcriptase inhibitor (NNRTI) OR**
    - **Protease Inhibitor (PI) OR**
    - **Strand-Transfer Integrase Inhibitor (STII)**
- Selection of components is influenced by many factors, including:
  - Results of viral resistance testing
  - Pregnancy (e.g., avoid Efavirenz—pregnancy risk category D)
  - HIV status (e.g., Nevirapine CONTRAINDICATED in women with CD4 >250 cells/μL and men with CD4 >400 cells/μL)
  - Potential drug interactions or adverse drug effects; special focus on tolerability (even low grade side effects can profoundly affect adherence)
  - Co-morbidities (e.g., lipid effects of PIs, liver or renal disease, cardiovascular disease risk, chemical dependency, psychiatric disease)
  - Convenience of dosing. Co-formulations increase convenience, but sometimes prescribing the two constituents individually is preferred, as when dose-adjustments are needed for renal disease.
  - HLA-B5701 testing required prior to using Abacavir (ABC)
  - Co-receptor tropism assay if considering Maraviroc (MVC)

B. Preferred Regimens (Non-pregnancy)

Single tablet Combinations	**Atripla** (Tenofovir/Emtricitabine/Efavirenz) 1 tablet once daily qhs OR **Stribild** (Elvitegravir/Cobicistat/Emtricitabine/Tenofovir) 1 tablet once daily OR **Complera/Eviplera** (Emtricitabine/Tenofovir/Rilpivirine) 1 tablet once daily with food (avoid when VL > 100,000 cells/mL) OR **Triumeq** (Abacavir/3TC/Dolutegravir) 1 tablet each once daily (see *Warnings below*)
NNRTI Multi-tablet regimens (Select one)	**Truvada** (Tenofovir/Emtricitabine) + **Efavirenz** 1 tablet each once daily qhs OR **Epzicom/Kivexa** (Abacavir/3TC) + **Efavirenz** 1 tablet each once daily qhs (see *Warnings below*)
Ritonavir-boosted PI Multi-tablet regimens (Select one)	**Truvada** (Tenofovir/Emtricitabine) + **Atazanavir/r** 1 tablet each once daily OR **Epzicom/Kivexa** (Abacavir/3TC) + **Atazanavir/r** 1 tablet each once daily (see *Warnings below*) OR **Truvada** (Tenofovir/Emtricitabine) + **Darunavir/r** 1 tablet each once daily OR
INSTI Multi-tablet regimens	**Truvada** (Tenofovir/Emtricitabine) + **Raltegravir** 1 tablet each once daily OR **Truvada** (Tenofovir/Emtricitabine) + **Dolutegravir** 1 tablet each once daily (see *Warnings below*) OR **Epzicom/Kivexa** (Abacavir/3TC) + **Dolutegravir** 1 tablet each once daily (see *Warnings below*) OR

NNRTI = non-nucleoside reverse transcriptase inhibitor, PI = protease inhibitor, INSTI = Strand transfer integrase inhibitor, /r = ritonavir boosted

- **Warnings:**
  - Epzicom/Kivexa (Abacavir/3TC) containing regimens: Use only in patients who are HLA-B5701 negative. Use Abacavir with caution in those with HIV RNA < 100,000 c/mL at baseline (this does not apply when Dolutegravir is the anchor drug of the regimen)
  - DO NOT USE Nevirapine if CD4 count > 250 cells/μL for women or > 400 cells/μL for men. Can result in life-threatening hypersensitivity reaction
- Co-formulations increase convenience, but sometimes prescribing the two components individually is preferred, as when dose adjustments are needed for renal disease.
- Rilpivirine is best used for patients with viral load < 100,000.
- Raltegravir 800 mg once daily is not quite as effective as 400 mg bid.

TABLE 14D (2)

C. Alternative Regimens (Non-pregnancy)

NNRTI Multi-tablet regimens (Select one)	• **Epzicom/Kivexa** (Abacavir/3TC) + **Rilpivirine** 1 tablet each once daily (see Warnings) OR • **Epzicom/Kivexa** (Abacavir/3TC) + **Nevirapine** 1 tablet each once daily (see Warnings) OR • **Truvada** (Tenofovir/Emtricitabine) + **Nevirapine** 1 tablet each once daily (see Warnings)
Boosted PI Multi-tablet regimens (Select one) **/c = cobicistat** **/r = ritonavir**	• **Epzicom/Kivexa** (Abacavir/3TC) + **Atazanavir/c** 1 tablet each once daily (see Warnings) OR • **Truvada** (Tenofovir/Emtricitabine) + **Atazanavir/c** 1 tablet each once daily OR • **Epzicom/Kivexa** (Abacavir/3TC) + **Darunavir/c** 1 tablet each once daily OR • **Truvada** (Tenofovir/Emtricitabine) + **Darunavir/c** 1 tablet each once daily OR • **Epzicom/Kivexa** (Abacavir/3TC) + **Darunavir/r** 1 tablet each once daily (see Warnings) OR • **Epzicom/Kivexa** (Abacavir/3TC) + **Kaletra** (Lopinavir/r) 1 tablet each once daily (see Warnings) OR • **Truvada** (Tenofovir/Emtricitabine) + **Kaletra** (Lopinavir/r) 1 tablet once daily
Nucleoside sparing (or limited) regimens	• **Darunavir/r** 1 tablet once daily with food + Raltegravir 400 mg bid OR • **Kaletra** (Lopinavir/r) 1 tablet once daily + Raltegravir 400 mg bid OR • **Kaletra** (Lopinavir/r) + Lamivudine 1 tablet each once daily

- Nevirapine 400 mg (Viramune XR) is the preferred formulation.
- Nevirapine should be used with caution with Abacavir owing to possible overlap of idiosyncratic hypersensitivity.
- Etravirine and Rilpivirine are options for some patients who have NNRTI resistance mutations, e.g., K103N, at baseline. Expert consultation is recommended.
- Boosted PIs can be administered once or twice daily.
- Cobicistat is now available as a PI-boosting agent
- Non-boosted PIs are no longer recommended
- Maraviroc is no longer recommended for initial treatment but may be used in cases of resistant viruses and as second line therapy (or beyond)

D. Pregnancy Regimens

• Timing of initiation of therapy and drug choice must be individualized • Viral resistance testing should be performed • Long-term effects of agents is unknown • Certain drugs are hazardous or contraindicated (Didanosine, Stavudine, Efavirenz)	• **Combivir** (Zidovudine/Lamivudine) 1 tablet bid + **Nevirapine** 1 tablet bid (fed or fasting)] after 14-day lead-in period or 1 tablet each once daily OR • **Combivir** (Zidovudine/Lamivudine) 1 tablet bid + **Kaletra** 2 tablets bid (without regard to food)

E. Selected Characteristics of Antiretroviral Drugs (*CPE = CSF penetration effectiveness: 1-4)

TABLE 14D (3)

1. **Selected Characteristics of Nucleoside or Nucleotide Reverse Transcriptase Inhibitors (NRTIs)**
All agents have Black Box warning: Risk of lactic acidosis/hepatic steatosis. Also, risk of fat redistribution/accumulation. For combinations, see warnings for component agents.

* CPE (CNS Penetration Effectiveness) value: 1 = Low Penetration; 2 - 3 = Intermediate Penetration; 4 = Highest Penetration into CNS (AIDS 25:357, 2011)

Generic/ Trade Name	Pharmaceutical Prep.	Usual Adult Dosage & Food Effect	% Absorbed, po	Serum T½, hrs	Intracellular T½, hrs	CPE*	Elimination	Major Adverse Events/Comments (See Table 14E)
Abacavir (ABC; Ziagen)	300 mg tabs or 20 mg/mL oral solution	300 mg po bid or 600 mg po q24h. Food OK	83	1.5	20	1	Live: metab, renal excretion of metabolites, 82%	**Hypersensitivity reaction:** fever, rash, N/V, malaise, diarrhea, abdominal pain, respiratory symptoms. (Severe reactions may be ↑ with 600 mg dose.) **Do not rechallenge!** Report to 800-270-0425. **Test HLA-B*5701 before use.** **See Comment Table 14E.** Studies raise concerns re ABC/3TC regimens in pts with VL ≥ 100,000 (www.niaid.nih.gov/news/newsreleases/2008/acIg52 02bulletin.htm). Controversy re increased CV events with use of ABC. Large meta-analysis shows no increased risk (AIDS 61. 441. 2012)
Abacavir (ABC)/lamivudine (Epzicom or Kivexa)	Film coated tabs ABC 600 mg + 3TC 300 mg	1 tab once daily (not recommended)						(See for individual components)
Abacavir (3TC)/dolutegravir (DTV)(Triumeq)	Film coated tabs: ABC 600 mg + 3TC 300 mg + DTV 50 mg	1 tab po once daily						**Black Box warning**— limited data for VL >100,000 copies/mL. Not recommended as initial therapy because of inferior virologic efficacy.
Abacavir (ABC)/ lamivudine (3TC)/ zidovudine (AZT) (Trizivir)	Film-coated tabs: ABC 300 mg + 3TC 150 mg + ZDV 300 mg	1 tab po bid (not recommended for wt <40 kg or CrCl <50 mL/min or impaired hepatic function)		(See individual components)				
Didanosine (ddI; Videx or Videx EC)	125, 200, 250, 400 enteric-coated caps; 100, 167, 250 mg powder for oral solution;	≥60 kg: Usually 400 mg enteric-coated po q24h 0.5 hr before or 2 hrs after meal. Do not crush. <60 kg: 250 mg EC po q24h. Food ↓ levels. See Comment	30-40	1.6	25-40	2	Renal excretion, 50%	**Pancreatitis,** peripheral neuropathy, lactic acidosis & hepatic steatosis (rare but life-threatening, esp. combined with stavudine in pregnancy). Retinal, optic nerve changes. **The combination ddI + TDF is generally avoided, but if used,** reduce dose of ddI-EC from 400 mg to 250 mg EC q24h (or from 400 mg to 200 mg EC for adults <60 kg). **Monitor for ↑ toxicity & possible ↓ in efficacy of this combination; may result in ↓ CD4.**

TABLE 14D (4)

E. Selected Characteristics of Antiretroviral Drugs (*CPE = CSF penetration effectiveness: 1-4)

1. Selected Characteristics of Nucleoside or Nucleotide Reverse Transcriptase Inhibitors (NRTIs) *(contd)*

Generic/ Trade Name	Pharmaceutical Prep.	Usual Adult Dosage & Food Effect	% Absorbed, po	Serum T½, hrs	Intracellular T½, hrs	CPE*	Elimination	Major Adverse Events/Comments *(See Table 14E)*
Emtricitabine (FTC, Emtriva)	200 mg caps; 10 mg per mL oral solution.	200 mg po q24h. Food OK	93 (caps), 75 (oral soln)	Approx. 10	39	3	Renal excretion 86%	Well tolerated; headache, nausea, vomiting & diarrhea occasionally, skin rash rarely. Skin hyperpigmentation. Differs only slightly in structure from lamivudine (5-fluoro substitution). **Exacerbation of Hep. B reported in pts after stopping FTC.** Monitor at least several months after stopping FTC in Hep B pts; some may need anti-HBV therapy.
Emtricitabine/ tenofovir disoproxil fumarate (Truvada)	Film-coated tabs: FTC 200 mg + TDF 300 mg	1 tab po q24h for CrCl ≥50 mL/min. Food OK	92/25	10/17	—	*(See individual components)*	Primarily renal/renal	*See Comments for individual agents.* **Black Box warning—Exacerbation of HepB after stopping FTC,** but preferred therapy for those with Hep B/HIV co-infection.
Emtricitabine/ tenofovir/efavirenz (Atripla)	Film-coated tabs: FTC 200 mg + TDF 300 mg + efavirenz 600 mg	1 tab po q24h on an empty stomach, preferably at bedtime. Do not use if CrCl <50 mL/min	*(See individual components)*					Not recommended for pts <18 yrs. *(See warnings for individual components.* **Exacerbation of Hep B** reported in pts discontinuing component drugs; some need anti-HBV therapy (tenofovir preferred). **Pregnancy category D**– Efavirenz may cause fetal harm. Avoid in pregnancy or in women who may become pregnant.
Emtricitabine/ tenofovir/rilpivirine (Complera; Eviplera)	Film-coated tabs: FTC 200 mg + TDF 300 mg + RPL 25 mg	1 tab po q24h with food	*(See individual components)*					*See individual components.* Preferred use in pts with HIV RNA level < 100,000 c/mL. Should not be used with PPI agents.
Lamivudine (3TC; Epivir)	150, 300 mg tabs; 10 mg/mL oral solution	150 mg po bid or 300 mg po q24h. Food OK	86	5–7	18	2	Renal excretion, minimal metabolism	**Use HIV dose, not Hep B dose.** Usually well-tolerated. **Risk of exacerbation of Hep B after stopping 3TC.** Monitor at least several months after stopping 3TC in Hep B pts; some may need anti-HBV therapy.
Lamivudine/ abacavir (Epzicom)	Film-coated tabs: 3TC 300 mg + abacavir 600 mg	1 tab po q24h. Food OK Not recommended for CrCl <50 mL/min or impaired hepatic function	86/86	5–7/1.5	16/20	*(See individual components)*	Primarily renal/ metabolism	*See Comments for individual agents.* **Note abacavir hypersensitivity Black Box warnings** (severe reactions may be somewhat more frequent with 600 mg dose) and 3TC Hep B warnings. Test HLA-B*5701 before use.
Lamivudine/ zidovudine (Combivir)	Film-coated tabs: 3TC 150 mg + ZDV 300 mg	1 tab po bid. Food OK Not recommended for CrCl <50 mL/min or impaired hepatic function Food OK	86/64	5–7/ 0.5–3	—	*(See individual components)*	Primarily renal/ metabolism with renal excretion of glucuronide	*See Comments for individual agents.* **Black Box warning**—exacerbation of Hep B in pts stopping 3TC

TABLE 14D (5)

E. Selected Characteristics of Antiretroviral Drugs (*CPE = CSF penetration effectiveness: 1-4)

1. Selected Characteristics of Nucleoside or Nucleotide Reverse Transcriptase Inhibitors (NRTIs) (continued)

Generic/ Trade Name	Pharmaceutical Prep.	Usual Adult Dosage & Food Effect	% Absorbed, po	Serum T½, hrs	Intracellular T½, hrs	CPE*	Elimination	Major Adverse Events/Comments (See Table 14E)
Stavudine (d4T, Zerit)	15, 20, 30, 40 mg capsules; 1 mg per mL oral solution	≥60 kg: 40 mg po bid <60 kg: 30 mg po bid Food OK	86	1.2–1.6	3.5	2	Renal excretion, 40%	Not recommended by DHHS as initial therapy because of adverse reactions. **Highest incidence of lipoatrophy, hyperlipidemia, & lactic acidosis of all NRTIs.** Pancreatitis. Peripheral neuropathy. (See didanosine comments.)
Tenofovir disoproxil fumarate (TDF; Viread)— a nucleotide	300 mg tabs	CrCl ≥50 mL/min: 300 mg po q24h. Food OK: high-fat meal ↑ absorption	39 (with food) 25 (fasted)	17	>60	1	Renal excretion	Headache, N/V. **Cases of renal dysfunction reported:** check renal function before using (dose reductions necessary if CrCl <50 cc/min); avoid concomitant nephrotoxic agents. One study found ↑ renal function at 48-wk in pts receiving TDF with a PI (mostly lopinavir/ritonavir) than with a NNRTI (JID 197:102, 2008). Avoid concomitant ddI. Atazanavir & lopinavir/ritonavir ↑ tenofovir concentrations: monitor for adverse effects. **Black Box warning—exacerbations of Hep B reported after stopping tenofovir.** Monitor liver enzymes if TDF stopped on HBV pts.
Zidovudine (ZDV, AZT; Retrovir)	100 mg caps, 300 mg tabs; 10 mg per mL IV solution; 10 mg/mL oral syrup	300 mg po q12h. Food OK	64	1.1	11	4	Metabolized to glucuronide & excreted in urine	Bone marrow suppression, GI intolerance, headache, insomnia, malaise, myopathy.

2. Selected Characteristics of Non-Nucleoside Reverse Transcriptase Inhibitors (NNRTIs)

Generic/ Trade Name	Pharmaceutical Prep.	Usual Adult Dosage & Food Effect	% Absorbed, po	Serum T½, hrs	Intracellular T½, hrs	CPE*	Elimination	Major Adverse Events/Comments (See Table 14E)
Delavirdine (Rescriptor)	100, 200 mg tabs	400 mg po three times daily. Food OK	85	5.8	3	—	Cytochrome P450 (3A inhibitor). 51% excreted in urine (<5% unchanged)	Rash severe enough to stop drug in 4.3%. ↑ AST/ALT, headaches. **Use of this agent is not recommended.**

TABLE 14D (6)

E. **Selected Characteristics of Antiretroviral Drugs** *CPE = CSF penetration effectiveness: 1-4)
2. **Selected Characteristics of Non-Nucleoside Reverse Transcriptase Inhibitors (NNRTIs)** *(continued)*

Generic/ Trade Name	Pharmaceutical Prep.	Usual Adult Dosage & Food Effect	% Absorbed, po	Serum T½, hrs	Intracellular T½, hrs	CPE	Elimination	Major Adverse Events/Comments *(See Table 14E)*
Efavirenz (Sustiva) New Guidelines indicate is OK to use in pregnant women (WHO Guidelines) or continue EFV in women identified as pregnant (HHS Guidelines).	50, 100, 200 mg capsules; 600 mg tablet	600 mg po q24h at bedtime, without food. Food may ↑ serum conc. which can lead to ↑ in risk of adverse events.	42	40–55 See Comment	3		Cytochrome P450 2B6 (3A-mixed inducer/ inhibitor), 14–34% excreted in urine as glucuroni-dated metabolites, 16–61% in feces	Severe rash in 1.7%. High frequency of CNS AEs: somnolence, dreams, confusion, agitation. Serious psychiatric symptoms. Certain CYP2B6 polymorphisms may predict exceptionally high plasma levels with standard doses *(CID 45:1230, 2007)*. False-pos. cannabinoid screen. Very long tissue T½. **If rx to be discontinued, stop efavirenz 1–2 wks before stopping companion drugs.** Otherwise, risk of developing efavirenz resistance as after 1–2 days only efavirenz in blood &/or tissue. Some bridge this gap by adding a PI to the NRTI backbone after efavirenz is discontinued. *(CID 42:401, 2006)*
Etravirine (Intelence)	100 mg tabs; 200 mg tabs	200 mg twice daily after a meal. May also be given as 400 mg once daily	Unknown (↓ systemic exposure if taken fasting)	41	2		Metabolized by CYP 3A4 (inducer) & 2C9, 2C19 (inhibitor). Fecal extraction.	For pts with HIV-1 resistant to NNRTIs & others. Active in vitro against most such isolates. Rash common, but rarely can be severe. Potential for multiple drug interactions. Generally, multiple mutations are required for high-level resistance. See Table 14E, page 186 for specific mutations and effects. Because of interactions, do not use with boosted atazanavir, boosted tipranavir, unboosted PIs, or other NNRTIs.
Nevirapine (Viramune) Viramune XR	200 mg tabs; 50 mg per 5 mL oral suspension; XR 400 mg tabs	200 mg po q24h x 14 days & then 200 mg po bid (see comments & Black Box warning) Food OK. If using Viramune XR, Still need the lead in dosing of 200 mg q24h prior to using 400 mg/d	>90	25–30	4		Cytochrome P450 (3A4, 2B6) inducer; 80% excreted in urine as glucuronidat-ed metabolites, 10% in feces	**Black Box warning—fatal hepatotoxicity.** Women with CD4 >250 esp. vulnerable, inc. pregnant women. Avoid in this group unless benefits clearly > risks *(www.fda.gov/cderrdrug/advisory/nevirapine.htm)*. intensive monitoring for liver toxicity required. Men with CD4 >400 also at ↑ risk. Severe rash in 7%, **severe or life-threatening skin reactions** in 2%. Do not restart if any suspicion of skin reactions. 2 wk dose escalation period may ↓ skin reactions. Because of long T½, consider continuing companion agents for several days if nevirapine is discontinued

TABLE 14D (7)

Generic/ Trade Name	Pharmaceutical Prep.	Usual Adult Dosage & Food Effect	% Absorbed, po	Serum T½, hrs	Intracellular T½, hrs	CPE	Elimination	Major Adverse Events/Comments (See Table 14E)

E. Selected Characteristics of Antiretroviral Drugs ("CPE = CSF penetration effectiveness: 1-4)

2. Selected Characteristics of Non-Nucleoside Reverse Transcriptase Inhibitors (NNRTIs) (continued)

Generic/ Trade Name	Pharmaceutical Prep.	Usual Adult Dosage & Food Effect	% Absorbed, po	Serum T½, hrs	Intracellular T½, hrs	CPE	Elimination	Major Adverse Events/Comments (See Table 14E)
Rilpivirine (Edurant)	25 mg tabs	25 mg daily with food	absolute bio-availability unknown; 40% lower Cmax in fasted state	50	unknown		Metabolized by Cyp3A4, 25% excreted unchanged in feces.	QTc prolongation with doses higher than 50 mg per day. Common AEs: depression, insomnia, headache, and rash. Do not co-administer with carbamazepine, phenobarbital, phenytoin, rifabutin, rifampin, rifapentine, proton-pump inhibitors, or multiple doses of dexamethasone. A fixed dose combination of rilpivirine + TDF/FTC (Complera/Eviplera) is approved. **Needs stomach acid for absorption. Do not administer with PPI.**

3. Selected Characteristics of Protease Inhibitors (PIs)

All PIs: Glucose metabolism: new diabetes mellitus or deterioration of glucose control; fat redistribution; possible hemophilia bleeding; hypertriglyceridemia. Exercise caution re: potential drug interactions & contraindications. QTc prolongation has been reported in a few pts taking PIs; some PIs can block hERG channels in vitro (Lancet 365:682, 2005).

Generic/ Trade Name	Pharmaceutical Prep.	Usual Adult Dosage & Food Effect	% Absorbed, po	Serum T½, hrs	CPE*	Elimination	Major Adverse Events/Comments (See Table 14E)
Atazanavir (Reyataz)	100, 150, 200, 300 mg capsules	400 mg po q24h with food. Ritonavir-boosted dose (atazanavir 300 mg po q24h + ritonavir 100 mg po q24h), with food, is recommended for ART-experienced pts. Use boosted dose when combined with either efavirenz 600 mg po q24h or TDF 300 mg po q24h. If used with buffered ddI, take with food 2 hrs pre or 1 hr post ddI.	Good oral bioavailability; food enhances bioavailability & ↓ pharmacokinetic variability. Absorption ↓ by antacids, H₂-blockers, proton pump inhibitors. Avoid unboosted drug with PPIs/H2-blockers. Boosted drug can be used with either >10 hr after H2-blockers or >12 hr after a PPI, if limited doses of the acid agents are used.	Approx. 7	2	Cytochrome P450 (3A4, 1A2 & 2C9 inhibitor) & UGT1A1 inhibitor, 13% excreted in urine (7% unchanged), 79% excreted in feces (20% unchanged)	Lower potential for ↑ lipids. Asymptomatic unconjugated hyperbilirubinemia common, jaundice especially likely in Gilbert's syndrome (AID 192:1381, 2005). Headache, rash, GI symptoms. Prolongation of PR interval (1st degree AV block) reported. Caution in pre-existing conduction system disease. Efavirenz & tenofovir ↓ atazanavir exposure: use atazanavir/ritonavir regimen; also, atazanavir exposure ↑ with ritonavir. In rx-experienced pts taking TDF and needing H2 blockers, atazanavir 400 mg with ritonavir 100 mg can be given; do not use PPIs. Rare reports of renal stones.
Darunavir (Prezista)	400 mg, 600 mg, 800 mg tablets	[600 mg darunavir + 100 mg ritonavir] po bid, with food or [800 mg darunavir + 100 mg ritonavir (two 400 mg tabs or one 800 mg tab) + 100 mg ritonavir] po once daily with food (**Preferred regimen in ART naive pts**)	82% absorbed (taken with ritonavir). Food ↑ absorption.	Approx 15 hr (with ritonavir)	3	Metabolized by CYP3A and is a CYP3A inhibitor	Contains sulfa moiety. Rash, nausea, headaches seen. Coadmin of certain drugs cleared by CYP3A is contraindicated (see label). Use with caution in pts with hepatic dysfunction (FDA warning about occasional hepatic dysfunction early in the course of treatment). Monitor carefully, esp. first several months of treatment. May cause hormonal contraception failure. With pre-existing liver disease. May cause hormonal contraception failure.

TABLE 14D (8)

E   Selected Characteristics of Antiretroviral Drugs (*CPE = CSF penetration effectiveness: 1-4)
3.   Selected Characteristics of Protease Inhibitors (PIs)*(continued)*

Generic/ Trade Name	Pharmaceutical Prep.	Usual Adult Dosage & Food Effect	% Absorbed, po	Serum T½, hrs	CPE*	Elimination	Major Adverse Events/Comments (See Table 14E)
Fosamprenavir (Lexiva)	700 mg tablet; 50 mg/mL oral suspension	1400 mg (two 700 mg tabs) po bid **OR** with ritonavir: [1400 mg] + fosamprenavir (2 tabs) + ritonavir 100 mg or 200 mg] po q24h **OR** (700 mg) fosamprenavir (1 tab) + ritonavir 100 mg] po bid	Bioavailability not established. Food OK	7.7 Ampre- navir	3	Hydrolyzed to amprenavir, then metabolized via cytochrome P450 (3A4 sub- strate, inhibitor, inducer)	Amprenavir prodrug. Contains sulfa moiety. Potential for serious drug interactions (see label). Rash including Stevens-Johnson syndrome. Once daily regimens: (1) not recommended for PI-experienced pts, (2) additional ritonavir needed if given with efavirenz (see label). Boosted twice daily regimen is recommended for PI-experienced pts. Potential for PI cross-resistance with darunavir.
Indinavir (Crixivan)	100, 200, 400 mg capsules Store in original container with desiccant	Two 400 mg caps (800 mg) po q8h, without food or with light meal. Can take with enteric-coated Videx. *[If taken with ritonavir (e.g., 800 mg indinavir + 100 mg ritonavir po q12h), no food restrictions]*	65	1.2-2	4	Cytochrome P450 (3A4 inhibitor)	**Maintain hydration. Nephrolithiasis,** nausea, inconsequential ↑ of indirect bilirubin (jaundice in Gilbert syndrome), ↑ AST/ALT, headache, asthenia, blurred vision, metallic taste, hemolysis. ↑ urine WBC (>100/hpf) has been assoc. with nephritis/ medullary calcification, cortical atrophy.
Lopinavir + ritonavir (Kaletra)	(200 mg lopinavir + 50 mg ritonavir) and (100 mg lopinavir + 25 mg ritonavir) tablets. Tabs do not need refrigeration. Oral solution: (80) mg lopinavir + 20 mg ritonavir) per mL. Refrigerate, but can be kept at room temp. (≤77°F) x 2 mos.	(400 mg lopinavir + 100 mg ritonavir)—2 tabs po bid. Higher dose may be needed in non-x-naive pts when used with efavirenz, nevirapine, or unboosted fosamprenavir. [Dose adjustment in con- comitant drugs may be necessary, see *Table 22B*.	No food effect with tablets.	5-6	3	Cytochrome P450 (3A4 inhibitor)	Nausea/vomiting/diarrhea (worse when administered with zidovudine), ↑ AST/ ALT, pancreatitis. Oral solution 42% alcohol. Lopinavir + ritonavir can be taken as a single daily dose of 4 tabs (total 800 mg lopinavir + 200 mg ritonavir), except in treatment-experienced pts or those taking concomitant efavirenz, nevirapine, amprenavir, or nelfinavir. Possible PR and QT prolongation. Use with caution in those with cardiac conduction abnormalities or when used with drugs with similar effects.
Nelfinavir (Viracept)	625, 250 mg tabs; 50 mg/gm oral powder	Two 625 mg tabs (1250 mg) po bid, with food	20-80 Food ↑ exposure & ↓ variability	3.5-5	1	Cytochrome P450 (3A4 inhibitor)	Diarrhea. Coadministration of drugs with life-threatening toxicities & which are cleared by CYP3A4 is contraindicated. Not recommended in initial regimens because of inferior efficacy; **prior concerns about EMS now resolved. Acceptable choice in pregnant women although it has inferior virologic efficacy than most other ARV anchor drugs.**

TABLE 14D (9)

E. Selected Characteristics of Antiretroviral Drugs

3. Selected Characteristics of Protease Inhibitors (PIs). (continued)

Generic/ Trade Name	Pharmaceutical Prep.	Usual Adult Dosage & Food Effect	% Absorbed, po	Serum T½, hrs	CPE	Elimination	Major Adverse Events/Comments (See Table 14F)
Ritonavir (Norvir)	100 mg capsules; 600 mg per 7.5 mL solution. Refrigerate caps but not solution. Room temperature for 1 mo. is OK.	Full dose not recommended (see comments). **With rare exceptions, used exclusively to enhance pharmacokinetics of other PIs, using lower ritonavir doses.**	Food ↑ absorption	3–5	1	Cytochrome P450. Potent 3A4 & D6 inhibitor.	Nausea/vomiting/diarrhea, extremity & circumoral paresthesias, hepatitis, pancreatitis, taste perversion, ↑ CPK & uric acid. **Black Box warning**—potentially fatal drug interactions. Many drug interactions—see Table 22A–Table 22B.
Saquinavir (Invirase—hard gel caps or tabs) + ritonavir	Saquinavir 200 mg caps, 500 mg film-coated tabs; ritonavir 100 mg caps	[2 tabs saquinavir (1000 mg) + 1 cap ritonavir (100 mg)] po bid with food	Erratic, 4 (saquinavir alone). Much more reliably absorbed when boosted with ritonavir.	1–2	1	Cytochrome P450 (3A4 inhibitor).	Nausea, diarrhea, headache, ↑ AST/ALT. Avoid rifampin with saquinavir + ritonavir: ↑ hepatitis risk. **Black Box warning**—Invirase to be used only with ritonavir. Possible QT prolongation. Use with caution in those with cardiac conduction abnormalities or when used with drugs with similar effects.
Tipranavir (Aptivus)	250 mg caps. Refrigerate unopened bottles. Use opened bottles within 2 mo. 100 mg/mL solution	[500 mg (two 250 mg caps) + ritonavir 200 mg] po bid with food.	Absorption low. ↑ intake with high fat meal. ↓ with Al⁺⁺⁺ & Mg⁺⁺ antacids.	5.5–6	1	Cytochrome 3A4 but with ritonavir, most of drug is eliminated in feces.	Contains sulfa moiety. **Black Box warning— reports of fatal/nonfatal intracranial hemorrhage, hepatitis, fatal hepatic failure.** Use cautiously in liver disease, esp. hepB, hepC; contraindicated in Child-Pugh class B-C. Monitor LFTs. Coadministration of certain drugs contraindicated (see label). **For highly ART-experienced pts or for multiple-PI resistant virus.** Do not use tipranavir and etravirine together owing to 76% reduction in etravirine levels.

4. Selected Characteristics of Fusion Inhibitors

Generic/ Trade Name	Pharmaceutical Prep.	Usual Adult Dosage	% Absorbed	Serum T½, hrs	CPE*	Elimination	Major Adverse Events/Comments (See Table 14F)
Enfuvirtide (T20, Fuzeon)	Single-use vials of 90 mg/mL when reconstituted. Vials should be stored at room temperature. Reconstituted vials can be refrigerated for 24 hrs only.	90 mg (1 mL) subcut. bid. Rotate injection sites, avoiding those currently inflamed.	84	3.8	1	Catabolism to its constituent amino acids with subsequent recycling of the amino acids in the body pool. Elimination pathway(s) have not been performed in humans. Does not alter the metabolism of CYP3A4, CYP2D6, CYP1A2, CYP2C19 or CYP2E1 substrates.	Local reaction site reactions 98%, 4% discontinue; erythema/induration ~80-90%, nodules/cysts ~80%. **Hypersensitivity reactions reported** (fever, rash, chills, N/V, ↓ BP, &/or ↑ AST/ALT)—do not restart if occur. Including background regimens, peripheral neuropathy 8.9%, insomnia 11.3%, ↓ appetite 6.3%, myalgia 5%, lymphadeno-pathy 2.3%, eosinophilia ~10%. ↑ incidence of bacterial pneumonias.

TABLE 14D (10)

E. **Selected Characteristics of Antiretroviral Drugs** (*CPE = CSF penetration effectiveness: 1-4) (continued)

5. **Selected Characteristics of CCR-5 Co-receptor Antagonists**

Generic/ Trade Name	Pharmaceutical Prep.	Usual Adult Dosage & Food Effect	% Absorbed	Serum T½, hrs	CPE	Elimination	Major Adverse Events/Comments (See Table 14E)
Maraviroc (Selzentry)	150 mg - 300 mg film-coated tabs	Without regard to food: - 150 mg bid if concomitant meds include CYP3A inhibitors including PIs (except tipranavir/ritonavir) and delavirdine (with/without) - 300 mg bid without significantly interacting meds including NRTIs, tipranavir/ritonavir, neveirapine - 600 mg bid if concomitant meds include CYP3A inducers, including elavirenz (without strong CYP3A inhibitors)	Est 33% with 300 mg dosage	14-18	3	CYP3A and P-glycoprotein substrate. Metabolites (via CYP3A) excreted feces > urine	**Black Box Warning-Hepatotoxicity,** may be preceded by rash; ↑ eos or IgE. NB: no hepatotoxicity was noted in MVC trials. Black box inserted owing to concern about potential CCR5 class effect. Data lacking in hepatic/renal insufficiency; ↑ concern with either could ↑ risk of ↓BP. Currently for treatment-experienced patients with multi-resistant strains. **Document CCR-5-tropic virus before use, as treatment failures assoc. with appearance of CXCR-4 or mixed-tropic virus.**

6. **Selected Characteristics of Strand Transfer Integrase Inhibitors**

Generic/ Trade Name	Pharmaceutical Prep.	Usual Adult Dosage & Food Effect	% Absorbed	Serum T½, hrs	CPE	Elimination	Major Adverse Events/Comments
Raltegravir (Isentress)	400 mg film-coated tabs	400 mg bid, without regard to food	Unknown	~ 9	3	Glucuronidation via UGT1A1, with excretion into feces and urine. (Therefore does NOT require ritonavir boosting)	For naive patients and treatment experienced pts with multiply-resistant virus. Well-tolerated. Nausea, diarrhea, headache, fever similar to placebo. CK↑ & rhabdomyolysis reported; unclear relationship. Increased depression in those with a history of depression. Low genetic barrier to resistance. Increase in CPK, myositis, rhabdomyolysis have been reported. Rare Stevens Johnson Syndrome. Better oral absorption if chewed (CID 57:480, 2013)
Elvitegravir/ cobicistat (Stribild)	150 mg - 150 mg	150 mg-150 mg once daily with or without food	<10%	12.9 (Cobi) 3.5 (ELV)	Unknown	The majority of **elvitegravir** metabolism is mediated by CYP3A enzymes. Elvitegravir also undergoes glucuronidation via UGT1A1/3 enzymes. **Cobicistat** is metabolized by CYP3A and to a minor extent by CYP2D6	For both treatment naive patients and treatment experienced pts with multiply-resistant virus. Generally well-tolerated. Use of cobicistat increases serum creatinine by ~ 0.1 mg/d via inhibition of proximal tubular enzyme; this does not result in reduction in true GFR but will result in erroneous apparent reduction in eGFR by MDRD or Cockcroft Gault calculations. Usual AEs are similar to those observed with ritonavir (cobi) and tenofovir/FTC.

TABLE 14D (11)

Generic/ Trade Name	Pharmaceutical Prep.	Usual Adult Dosage & Food Effect	% Absorbed	Serum T½, hrs	CPE	Elimination	Major Adverse Events/Comments (See Table 14E)
6. Selected Characteristics of Strand Transfer Integrase Inhibitors (continued)							
Elvitegravir (Vitekta)(EVG)	85 mg, 150 mg tabs	• EVG85 mg once daily + ATV/r 300/100 mg po once daily • EVG85 mg once daily + LPV/r 400/100 mg po bid • EVG150 mg once daily + DRV/r 600/100 mg po bid • EVG150 mg once daily + FOS/r 700/100 mg po bid • EVG150 mg once daily + TPV/r 500/200 mg po bid	ND	8.7	No	Hepatobiliary, metabolized by CYP3A	Well tolerated, mild diarrhea
Dolutegravir (Tivicay)	50 mg	50 mg po once daily 50 mg po BID (if STI resistance present or if co-admin with EFV, FOS, TIP, or Rif	Unknown	14	4	Glucuronidation via UGT1A1 (therefore does not require ritonavir or cobicistat boosting)	Hypersensitivity (rare). Most common: insomnia (3%) headache (2%), N/V (1%), rash (<1%). Watch for IRIS; Watch for elevated LFTs in those with HCV

F. Other Considerations in Selection of Therapy

Caution: Initiation of ART may result in immune reconstitution syndrome with significant clinical consequences. See Table 11B, of Sanford Guide to HIV/AIDS Therapy (AIDS Reader 16:199, 2006).

1. Resistance testing: Given current rates of resistance, resistance testing is recommended in all patients prior to initiation of therapy, including those with acute infection syndrome (may initiate therapy while waiting for test results and adjusting Rx once results return), at time of change of therapy owing to antiretroviral failure, when suboptimal virologic response is observed, and in pregnant women. **Resistance testing NOT recommended if pt is off ART for > 4 weeks or if HIV RNA is < 1000 c/mL.** See Table 6F of SANFORD GUIDE TO HIV/AIDS THERAPY.

2. Drug-induced disturbances of glucose & lipid metabolism (see Table 14E).
3. Drug-induced lactic acidosis & other FDA "box warnings" (see Table 14E)
4. Drug-drug interactions (see Table 22B)
5. Risk in pregnancy (see Table 8)
6. Use in women & children (see Table 14D)
7. Dosing in patients with renal or hepatic dysfunction (see Table 17A & Table 17B)

* CPE (CNS Penetration Effectiveness) value: 1 = Low Penetration; 2 - 3 = Intermediate Penetration; 4 = Highest Penetration into CNS (AIDS 25:357, 2011)

TABLE 14E– ANTIRETROVIRAL DRUGS & ADVERSE EFFECTS
(www.aidsinfo.nih.gov)

DRUG NAME(S): GENERIC (TRADE)	MOST COMMON ADVERSE EFFECTS	MOST SIGNIFICANT ADVERSE EFFECTS
Nucleoside Reverse Transcriptase Inhibitors (NRTI) Black Box warning for all nucleoside/nucleotide RTIs: lactic acidosis/hepatic steatosis, potentially fatal. Also carry Warnings that fat redistribution and immune reconstitution syndromes (including autoimmune syndromes with delayed onset) have been observed		
Abacavir (Ziagen)	Headache 7–13%, nausea 7–19%, diarrhea 7%, malaise 7–12%	**Black Box warning—Hypersensitivity reaction (HR)** in 8% with malaise, fever, GI upset, rash, lethargy & respiratory symptoms most commonly reported; myalgia, arthralgia, edema, paresthesia less common. **Discontinue immediately if HR suspected. Rechallenge contraindicated; may be life-threatening.** Severe HR may be more common with once-daily dosing. **HLA-B*5701 allele** predicts ↑ risk of HR in Caucasian pop., excluding pts with B*5701 ↓ ↓ HR incidence (*NEJM 358:568, 2008; CID 46:1111–1118, 2008).* DHHS guidelines recommend testing for B*5701 and use of abacavir-containing regimens only if HLA-B*5701 negative. Vigilance essential in all groups. Possible increased risk of MI with use of abacavir had been suggested (*JID 201:318, 2010).* Other studies found no increased risk of MI (*CID 52: 929, 2011).* A meta-analysis of randomized trials by FDA also did not show increased risk of MI (www.fda.gov/drugs/drugsafety/ucm245164.htm). Nevertheless, care is advised to optimize potentially modifiable risk factors when abacavir is used.
Didanosine (ddI) (Videx)	Diarrhea 28%, nausea 6%, rash 9%, headache 7%, fever 12%, hyperuricemia 2%	**Pancreatitis 1–9%. Black Box warning—Cases of fatal & nonfatal pancreatitis** have occurred in pts receiving ddI, especially when used in combination with d4T or d4T + hydroxyurea. Fatal lactic acidosis in pregnancy with ddI + d4T. Peripheral neuropathy in 20%, 12% required dose reduction. ↑ toxicity if used with TDF generally avoided but would require dose reduction of ddI because of ↑ toxicity and possible ↑ efficacy; may result in ↓ CD4. Rarely, retinal changes or optic neuropathy. Diabetes mellitus and rhabdomyolysis reported in post-marketing surveillance. Possible increased risk of MI under study (www.fda.gov/CDER; JID 201:318, 2010). Non-cirrhotic portal hypertension with ascites, varices, splenomegaly reported in post-marketing surveillance. See also *Clin Infect Dis 49:626, 2009; Amer J Gastroenterol 104:1707, 2009.*
Emtricitabine (FTC) (Emtriva)	Well tolerated. Headache, diarrhea, nausea, rash, skin hyperpigmentation	Potential for lactic acidosis (as with other NRTIs). Also **in Black Box—severe exacerbation of hepatitis B on stopping drug reported—monitor clinical/labs for several months after stopping in pts with hepB.** Anti-HBV rx may be warranted if FTC stopped.
Lamivudine (3TC) (Epivir)	Well tolerated. Headache 35%, nausea 33%, diarrhea 18%, abdominal pain 9%, insomnia 11% (all in combination with ZDV). Pancreatitis more common in pediatrics.	**Black Box warning.** Make sure to use HIV dosage, not Hep B dosage. **Exacerbation of hepatitis B on stopping drug. Patients with hepB who stop lamivudine require close clinical/lab monitoring for several months.** Anti-HBV rx may be warranted if 3TC stopped.
Stavudine (d4T) (Zerit)	Diarrhea, nausea, vomiting, headache	**Peripheral neuropathy** 15–20%. Pancreatitis 1%. Appears to produce lactic acidosis, hepatic steatosis and lipoatrophy/lipodystrophy more commonly than other NRTIs. **Black Box warning—Fatal & nonfatal pancreatitis with d4T + ddI.** Use with TDF generally avoided (but because of ↑ toxicity and possible ↑ efficacy, may result in ↓ CD4. Rarely, retinal changes or optic neuropathy. Diabetes mellitus and rhabdomyolysis reported in post-marketing surveillance. **Fatal lactic acidosis/steatosis in pregnant women receiving d4T + ddI.** Fatal and non-fatal lactic acidosis and severe hepatic steatosis can occur in others receiving d4T. Use with particular caution in patients with risk factors for liver disease, but lactic acidosis can even occur in those without known risk factors. Possible ↑ toxicity if used with ribavirin. Motor weakness in the setting of lactic acidosis mimicking the clinical presentation of Guillain-Barré syndrome (including respiratory failure) (rare)
Zidovudine (ZDV, AZT) (Retrovir)	Nausea 50%, anorexia 20%, vomiting 17%, **headache 62%.** Also reported: asthenia, insomnia, myalgias, nail pigmentation. Macrocytosis expected with all dosage regimens.	**Black Box warning—hematologic toxicity, myopathy. Anemia** (<8 gm, 1%), **granulocytopenia** (<750, 1.8%). Anemia may respond to epogen if endogenous serum erythropoietin levels are <500 milliU/mL. Possible ↑ toxicity if used with ribavirin. Co-administration with Ribavirin not advised. Hepatic decompensation may occur in HIV/HCV co-infected patients receiving zidovudine with interferon alfa ± ribavirin.

TABLE 14E (2)

DRUG NAME(S): GENERIC (TRADE)	MOST COMMON ADVERSE EFFECTS	MOST SIGNIFICANT ADVERSE EFFECTS
Nucleotide Reverse Transcriptase Inhibitor (NRTI). Black Box warning for all nucleoside/nucleotide RTIs: lactic acidosis/hepatic steatosis, potentially fatal. Also carry Warnings that fat redistribution and immune reconstitution syndromes (including autoimmune syndromes with delayed onset) have been observed *(continued)*		
Tenofovir disoproxil fumarate (TDF) (Viread)	Diarrhea 11%, nausea 8%, vomiting 5%, flatulence 4% (generally well tolerated)	**Black Box Warning—Severe exacerbations of hepatitis B reported in pts who stop tenofovir.** Monitor carefully if drug is stopped; anti-HBV rx may be warranted if TDF stopped. Reports of renal injury from TDF including Fanconi syndrome *(CID 37:e174, 2003; J AIDS 35:269,204; CID 42:283, 2006)*. Fanconi syndrome and diabetes reported with TDF + ddI *(AIDS Reader 19:114, 2009)*. Modest decline in renal function appears greater with TDF than with NRTIs *(CID 51:296, 2010)* and may be greater in pts receiving TDF with a PI instead of an NNRTI *(JID 197:102, 2008; AIDS 26:567, 2012)*. In a VA study that followed ~10,000 HIV-infected individuals, TDF exposure was significantly associated with increased risk of proteinuria, a more rapid decline in renal function and chronic kidney disease *(AIDS 26:867, 2012)*. Monitor Ccr, serum phosphate and urinalysis, especially carefully in those with pre-existing renal dysfunction or nephrotoxic medications. TDF also appears to be associated with increased risk of bone loss. In a substudy of an ACTG comparative treatment trial, those randomized to TDF-FTC experienced greater decreases in spine and hip bone mineral density (BMD) at 96 weeks compared with those treated with ABC-3TC *(JID 203:1791, 2011)*. Consider monitoring BMD in those with history of pathologic fractures, or who have risks for osteoporosis or bone loss.
Non-Nucleoside Reverse Transcriptase Inhibitors (NNRTI). Labels caution that fat redistribution and immune reconstitution can occur with ART.		
Delavirdine (Rescriptor)	Nausea, diarrhea, vomiting, headache	Skin rash has occurred in 18%; can continue or restart drug in most cases. Stevens-Johnson syndrome & erythema multiforme have been reported rarely. ↑ in liver enzymes in <5% of patients.
Efavirenz (Sustiva)	**CNS side effects 52%;** symptoms include dizziness, insomnia, somnolence, impaired concentration, psychiatric sx. & abnormal dreams; symptoms are worse after 1st or 2nd dose & improve over 2–4 weeks; discontinuation rate 2.6%. Rash 26% (vs. 17% in comparators), often improves with oral antihistamines; discontinuation rate 1.7%. Can cause false-positive urine test results for cannabinoid with CEDIA DAU multi-level THC assay. Metabolite can cause false-positive urine screening test for benzodiazepines *(CID 48:1787, 2009)*.	**Caution:** CNS effects may impair driving and other hazardous activities. Serious neuropsychiatric symptoms reported, including severe depression (2.4%) & suicidal ideation (0.7%). Elevation in liver enzymes. Fulminant hepatic failure reported *(see FDA label)*. **Teratogenicity reported in primates; pregnancy category D—may cause fetal harm, avoid in pregnant women or those who might become pregnant.** NOTE: No single method of contraception is 100% reliable. Barrier + 2nd method of contraception advised, continued 12 weeks after stopping efavirenz. Contraindicated with certain drugs metabolized by CYP3A4. Slow metabolism in those homozygous for the CYP-2B6 G516T allele can result in exaggerated toxicity and intolerance. This allele more common in blacks and women *(CID 42:408, 2006)*. Stevens-Johnson syndrome and erythema multiforme reported in post-marketing surveillance.
Etravirine (Intelence)	Rash 9%, generally mild to moderate and spontaneously resolving; 2% dc clinical trials for rash. More common in women. Nausea 5%.	Severe rash (erythema multiforme, toxic epidermal necrolysis), Stevens-Johnson syndrome has been reported. Hypersensitivity reactions can occur with rash, constitutional symptoms and organ dysfunction, including hepatic failure *(see FDA label)*. Potential for CYP450-mediated drug interactions. Rhabdomyolysis has been reported in post-marketing surveillance.
Nevirapine (Viramune)	**Rash 37%** usually occurs during 1st 6 wks of therapy. Follow recommendations for 14-day lead-in dose to reduce risk of rash *(see Table 14D)*. Women experience 7-fold ↑ in risk of severe rash *(CID 32:124, 2001)*. 50% resolve within 2 wks of dc of drug & 80% by 1 month. 6.7% discontinuation rate.	Severe rash: Stevens-Johnson syndrome, toxic epidermal necrolysis (DRESS) & systemic symptoms (DRESS) *(AIM 161:2501, 2001)*. Rx rashes immediately; do not restart rx. In a clinical trial, the use of prednisone ↑ the risk of rash. **Black Box warning—Severe hepatotoxicity reported,** 2/3 during the first 12 wks of rx. Overall 1% develops hepatitis. Pts with pre-existing ↑ in ALT &/or history of chronic Hep B or C ↑ susceptible *(Hepatol 35:182, 2002)*. Women with CD4 >250, including pregnant women, at ↑ risk. Avoid in this group unless no other option. Men with CD4 >400 also at ↑ risk. Monitor pts intensively (clinical & LFTs), esp. during the first 12 wks of rx. If clinical hepatotoxicity, severe skin or hypersensitivity reactions occur, dc drug & never rechallenge.

TABLE 14E (3)

DRUG NAME(S): GENERIC (TRADE)	MOST COMMON ADVERSE EFFECTS	MOST SIGNIFICANT ADVERSE EFFECTS
Non-Nucleoside Reverse Transcriptase Inhibitors (NNRTI) *(continued)*		
Rilpivirine (Edurant)	Headache (3%), rash (3%; led to discontinuation in 0.1%), insomnia (3%), depressive disorders (4%), Psychiatric disorders led to discontinuation in 1%. Increased liver enzymes observed.	Drugs that induce CYP3A or increase gastric pH may decrease plasma concentration of rilpivirine and co-administration with rilpivirine should be avoided. Among these are potent anticonvulsants, rifamycins, PPIs, dexamethasone and St. John's wort. At supra-therapeutic doses, rilpivirine can increase QTc interval; use with caution with other drugs known to increase QTc. May cause depressive disorder, including suicide or suicidal ideation. Overall, appears to cause fewer neuropsychiatric side effects than efavirenz (*JAIDS 60:33, 2012*).
Protease Inhibitors (PI)		
Diarrhea is common AE (**crofelemer** 125 mg bid may help, but perhaps. Abnormalities in glucose metabolism, dyslipidemias, fat redistribution syndromes are potential problems. Pts taking PI may be at increased risk for developing osteopenia/osteomalacia. Spontaneous bleeding episodes have been reported in HIV+ pts with hemophilia being treated with PI. Rheumatoid complications have been reported (*An Rheum Dis 61:82, 2002*). Potential for QTc prolongation. **Caution for all PIs**—Coadministration with drugs dependent on CYP3A or other enzymes for elimination & for which ↑ levels can cause serious toxicity may be contraindicated. ART may result in immune reconstitution syndromes, which may include early or late presentations of autoimmune syndromes. Increased premature births among women receiving ritonavir-boosted PIs as compared with those receiving other antiretroviral therapy, even after accounting for other potential risk factors (*CID 54:1348, 2012*).		
Atazanavir (Reyataz)	Asymptomatic unconjugated hyperbilirubinemia in up to 60% of pts, jaundice in 7–9% [especially with Gilbert syndrome (*JID 192: 1381, 2005*)]. Moderate to severe events: Diarrhea 1–3%, nausea 6–14%, abdominal pain 4%, headache 6%, rash 20%.	Prolongation of PR interval (1st degree AV block (1st degree AV block in 5–6%) reported, rarely 2° AV block. QTc increase and torsades reported (*CID 44:e67, 2007*). Acute interstitial nephritis (*Am J Kid Dis 44:E31, 2004*) and urolithiasis (atazanavir stones) reported (*AIDS 20:2131, 2006; NEJM 355:2158, 2006*). Potential ↑ transaminases in pts co-infected with HBV or HCV. Severe skin eruptions (Stevens-Johnson syndrome, erythema multiforme, and toxic eruptions, or DRESS syndrome) have been reported.
Darunavir (Prezista)	With background regimens, headache 15%, nausea 18%, diarrhea 20%, ↑ amylase 17%. Rash in 10% of treated; 0.5% discontinuation.	Hepatitis in 0.5%, some with fatal outcome. Use caution in pts with HBV or HCV co-infections or other hepatic dysfunction. Monitor for clinical symptoms and LFTs. Stevens-Johnson syndrome, toxic epidermal necrolysis, erythema multiforme. Contains sulfa moiety. Potential for major drug interactions. May cause failure of hormonal contraceptives.
Fosamprenavir (Lexiva)	Skin rash ~ 20% (moderate or worse in 3–8%), nausea, headache, diarrhea.	Rarely Stevens-Johnson syndrome, hemolytic anemia. Pro-drug of amprenavir. Contains sulfa moiety. Angioedema, and nephrolithiasis reported in post-marketing experience. Potential increased risk of MI (see FDA label). Angioedema, oral paresthesias, myocardial infarction and nephrolithiasis reported in post-marketing experience. Elevated LFTs seen with higher than recommended doses; increased risk in those with pre-existing liver abnormalities. Acute hemolytic anemia reported with amprenavir.
Indinavir (Crixivan)	↑ in indirect bilirubin 10–15% (≥2.5 mg/dl, with overt jaundice especially likely in those with Gilbert syndrome (*JID 192: 1381, 2005*). Nausea 12%, vomiting 4%, diarrhea 5%. Metallic taste. Paronychia and ingrown toenails reported (*CID 32:140, 2001*).	**Kidney stones.** Due to indinavir crystals in collecting system. Nephrolithiasis in 12% of adults, higher in pediatrics. Minimize risk with good hydration (at least 48 oz. water/day) (*AAC 42:332, 1998*). Tubulointerstitial nephritis/renal cortical atrophy reported in association with asymptomatic ↑ urine WBC. Severe hepatitis reported in 3 cases (*Ln 349:924, 1997*). Hemolytic anemia reported.
Lopinavir/Ritonavir (Kaletra)	GI: **diarrhea** 14–24%, nausea 2–16%. More diarrhea with q24h dosing.	Lipid abnormalities in up to 20–40%. Possible increased risk of MI with cumulative exposure (*JID 201:318, 2010*). ↑ PR interval, 2° or 3° heart block described. Post-marketing reports of ↑ QTc and torsades: avoid use in congenital QTc prolongation or in other circumstances that prolong QTc or increase susceptibility to torsades. Hepatitis, with hepatic decompensation; caution especially in those with pre-existing liver disease. Pancreatitis. Inflammatory edema of legs (*AIDS 16:673, 2002*). Stevens-Johnson syndrome & erythema multiforme reported. Note high drug concentration in oral solution. Toxic potential of oral solution (contains ethanol and propylene glycol) in neonates.
Nelfinavir (Viracept)	Mild to moderate **diarrhea** 20%. Oat bran tabs, calcium, or oral anti-diarrheal agents (e.g., loperamide, diphenoxylate/atropine sulfate) can be used to manage diarrhea	Potential for drug interactions. Powder contains phenylalanine.

TABLE 14E (4)

DRUG NAME(S): GENERIC (TRADE)	MOST COMMON ADVERSE EFFECTS	MOST SIGNIFICANT ADVERSE EFFECTS
Protease Inhibitors (PI) *(continued)*		
Ritonavir (Norvir) (Currently, primary use is to enhance levels of other anti-retrovirals, because of ↑ toxicity/interactions with full-dose ritonavir)	GI: bitter aftertaste ↓ by taking with chocolate milk, Ensure, or Advera; nausea 23%, ↓ by initial dose esc (titration) regimen; vomiting 13%, diarrhea 15%. Circumoral paresthesias 5-6%. Dose >100 mg bid assoc. with ↑ GI side effects & ↑ in lipid abnormalities.	**Black Box** warning relates to many important drug-drug interactions—inhibits P450 CYP3A & CYP2 D6 system— may be life-threatening (see Table 22A). Several cases of iatrogenic Cushing's syndrome reported with concomitant use of ritonavir and corticosteroids, including dosing of the latter by inhalation, ocular injection or a single IM injection. Rarely Stevens-Johnson syndrome, toxic epidermal necrolysis anaphylaxis. Primary A-V block (and higher) injection. Rarely Stevens-Johnson syndrome, toxic epidermal necrolysis anaphylaxis. Primary A-V block (and higher) injection. Rarely Stevens-Johnson syndrome, toxic epidermal necrolysis anaphylaxis. Primary A-V block (and higher) injection. Rarely Stevens-Johnson syndrome, including fatalities. Monitor LFTs carefully during therapy, especially in those with pre-existing liver disease, including HBV and HCV.
Saquinavir (Invirase: hard cap, tablet)	**Diarrhea,** abdominal discomfort, nausea, headache	**Warning—Use Invirase only with ritonavir.** Avoid garlic capsules (may reduce SQV levels) and use cautiously with proton-pump inhibitors (increased SQV levels significant). Use of saquinavir/ritonavir can prolong QTc interval or may rarely cause 2° or 3° heart block; torsades reported. Contraindicated in patients with prolonged QTc or those taking drugs or who have other conditions (e.g., low K+ or Mg+ +) that pose a risk with prolonged QTc (http://www.fda.gov/drugs/DrugSafety/ucm230096.htm, accessed May 25, 2011). Contraindicated in patients with complete AV block, or those at risk, who do not have pacemaker. Hepatic toxicity encountered in patients with pre-existing liver disease or in individuals receiving concomitant rifampin. Rarely, Stevens Johnson syndrome
Tipranavir (Aptivus)	Nausea & vomiting, diarrhea, abdominal pain. Rash in 8-14%, more common in women, & 33% in women taking ethinyl estradiol. Major lipid effects.	**Black Box Warning—associated with hepatitis & fatal hepatic failure.** Risk of hepatotoxicity increased in hepB or hepC co-infection. Possible photosensitivity skin reactions. Contraindicated in Child-Pugh Class B or C hepatic impairment. **Associated with fatal/nonfatal intracranial hemorrhage (can inhibit platelet aggregation).** Caution in those with bleeding risks. Potential for major drug interactions. Contains sulfa moiety and vitamin E.
Fusion Inhibitor		
Enfuvirtide (T20, Fuzeon)	Local injection site reactions (98%; at least 1 local ISR, 4% dc because of ISR) (pain & discomfort, induration, erythema, nodules & cysts, pruritus, & ecchymosis). Diarrhea 32%, nausea 23%, fatigue 20%.	↑ Rate of bacterial pneumonia (3.2 pneumonia events/100 pt yrs), **hypersensitivity reactions** ≤1% (rash, fever, nausea & vomiting, chills, rigors, hypotension, & ↑ serum liver transaminases); can occur with reexposure. Cutaneous amyloid deposits containing enfuvirtide peptide reported in skin plaques persisting after discontinuation of drug (*J Cutan Pathol* 39:220, 2012).
CCR5 Co-receptor Antagonists		
Maraviroc (Selzentry)	With ARV background: Cough 13%; fever 12%, rash 10%, abdominal pain 8%. Also, dizziness, myalgia, arthralgias. ↑ Risk of URI, HSV infection.	**Black box warning-Hepatotoxicity.** May be preceded by allergic features (rash, ↑eosinophils or ↑IgE levels). Use with caution in pts with HepB or C. Cardiac ischemia/infarction in 1.3%. May cause ↓BP, orthostatic syncope, especially in patients with renal dysfunction. Significant interactions with CYP3A inducers/inhibitors. Long-term risk of malignancy unknown. Stevens-Johnson syndrome reported post-marketing. Generally favorable safety profile during trial of ART-naive individuals (*JID* 201: 803, 2010).
Integrase Inhibitors		
Raltegravir (Isentress)	Diarrhea, headache, insomnia, nausea. LFT ↑ may be more common in pts co-infected with HBV or HCV.	Hypersensitivity reactions can occur. Rash, Stevens-Johnson syndrome, toxic epidermal necrolysis reported. Hepatic failure reported in 4 pts; ↑CK, myopathy and rhabdomyolysis reported (*AIDS* 22:1382, 2008), ↑ of preexisting depression reported in 4 pts; all could continue raltegravir after adjustment of psych. meds (*AIDS* 22:1890, 2008).
Elvitegravir+ Cobicistat (Stribild), Elvitegravir (Vitekta)	Nausea and diarrhea are the two most common AEs. Increased serum creatinine 0.1-0.15 mg/dL due to inhibition of prox. tubular enzymes by cobicistat with no decrease in GFR.	**Same Black Box warnings as ritonavir and tenofovir.** Rare lactic acidosis syndrome. Owing to renal toxicity, should not initiate Rx when pre-Rx eGFR is < 70 cc/min. Follow serial serum creatinine and urinary protein and glucose. Discontinue drug if serum Cr rises > 0.4 mg/dl above baseline value. Chewable tablets contain phenylalanine.
Dolutegravir (Tivicay)	Insomnia and headache (2-4%)	Rash, liver injury reported. Increased ALT/AST in 203%. Competition with creatinine for tubular secretion increased serum creatinine by a mean of 0.1 mg/dl, with no change in GFR.

TABLE 14F– HEPATITIS A & HBV TREATMENT

Hepatitis A Virus (HAV)

1. **Drug/Dosage:** No therapy recommended. If within 2 wks of exposure, prophylactic IVIG 0.02 mL per kg IM times 1 protective. Hep A vaccine equally effective as IVIG in randomized trial and is emerging as preferred Rx *(NEJM 357:1685, 2007).*

2. **HAV Superinfection:** 40% of pts with chronic Hepatitis C virus (HCV) infection who developed superinfection with HAV developed fulminant hepatic failure *(NEJM 338:286, 1998).* Similar data in pts with chronic Hepatitis B virus (HBV) infection that suffer acute HAV *(Ann Trop Med Parasitol 93:745, 1999).* **Hence, need to vaccinate all HBV and HCV pts with HAV vaccine.**

HBV Treatment Review: screening and treatment *(AnIM 161:31, 58, 2014).*

				When to Treat HBV	
HBeAg status	**HBV DNA: "viral load"**	**ALT**	**Fibrosis***	**Treatment** IFN = interferon; NUC = nucleoside/ tide analogue	**Comments**
+	> 20,000	< 2xULN	F0 –F2	Observe	Low efficacy with current Rx; biopsy helpful in determining whether to Rx. Lean toward Rx if older age or + Family Hx HCC
+	> 20,000	< 2x ULN	F3-F4	Treat: IFN or NUC	**No IFN if decompensated cirrhosis**
+	>20,000	> 2x ULN	Any	Treat: IFN or NUC	INF has higher chance of seroconversion to HBeAg Negative and HBsAg Negative status.
-	< 2000	< 1xULN	Any	Observe	Might Treat if F4; **No IFN if decompensated cirrhosis**
-	2000-20,000	< 2x ULN	F0 – F2	Observe	
-	2000-20,000	< 2x ULN	F3 – F4	Treat: NUC or (IFN)	NUCs favored if HBeAg negative; Treatment duration ill-defined. Certainly > 1 year, likely chronic Rx (indefinitely)
-	> 20,000	> 2xULN	Any	Treat: NUC or IFN	NUCs favored if HBeAg negative; Treatment duration chronic / indefinite

Modified from *AASLD HBV Treatment Guidelines (www.aasld.org); Lok/ McMahon, Hepatology .2009; 50. p. 1-36*
* Liver Biopsy or fibrosure assay is helpful in determining when and how to treat
** Treatment options listed below

HBV Treatment Regimens. Single drug therapy is usually sufficient; combination therapy for HIV co-infection.

	Drug/Dose	**Comments**
Preferred Regimens	**Pegylated-Interferon-alpha 2a** 180 µg sc once weekly OR **Entecavir** 0.5 mg po once daily OR **Tenofovir** 300 mg po once daily	PEG-IFN: Treat for 48 weeks Entecavir: Do not use Entecavir if Lamivudine resistance present. Entecavir/Tenofovir: Treat for at least 24-48 weeks after seroconversion from HBeAg to anti-HBe. Indefinite chronic therapy for HBeAg negative patients. Renal impairment dose adjustments necessary.
Alternative Regimens	**Lamivudine** 100 mg po once daily OR **Telbivudine** 600 mg po once daily OR **Emtricitabine** 200 mg po once daily (investigational) OR **Adefovir** 10 mg po once daily	These alternative agents are rarely used except in combination. When used, restrict to short term therapy owing to high rates of development of resistance. Not recommended as first-line therapy. Use of Adefovir has mostly been replaced by Tenofovir.
Preferred Regimen for HIV-HBV Co-Infected Patient	**Truvada** (Tenofovir 300 mg + Emtricitabine 200 mg) po once daily + another anti-HIV drug	ALL patients if possible as part of a fully suppressive anti-HIV/anti-HBV regimen. Continue therapy indefinitely.

TABLE 14G– HCV TREATMENT REGIMENS AND RESPONSE

1. **Indications for Treatment.** Treatment is indicated for all patients with chronic HCV. Priority for Rx should be given to those with more advanced fibrosis (F3 / F4) and those with underlying co-morbid conditions due to HCV. Type and duration of Rx is based on genotype. Pegylated interferon (Peg-IFN) is no longer a recommended regimen; all DAA regimens with or without ribavirin are the preferred choice.

2. **Definitions of Response to Therapy.**

Null	Failure to decrease HCV VL by >2 log at week 12. (applies to PEG-IFN Rx)
End of Treatment Response (ETR)	Undetectable at end of treatment.
Relapse	Undetectable at end of therapy (ETR) but rebound (detectable) virus within 12 weeks after therapy stopped.
Sustained Virologic Response (SVR)	CURE! Still undetectable at end of therapy and beyond 12 weeks after therapy is stopped.

3. **HCV Treatment Regimens**

- Biopsy is a 'gold standard' for staging HCV infection and is helpful in some settings to determine the ideal timing of HCV treatment. When bx not obtained, "non-invasive" tests are often employed to assess the relative probability of advanced fibrosis or cirrhosis. Fibroscan (elastography) is now approved in the US and most of the world as a means of assessing liver fibrosis. Elastography values of > 10 kPa (Kilopascals) correlates with significant fibrosis (F3 or F4 disease).

- Resistance tests: Genotypic resistance assays are available that can determine polymorphisms associated with reduction in susceptibility to some DAAs (Direct Acting Agents, e.g., protease inhibitors). **However, resistance tests are not routinely recommended since response to therapy is typically still preserved even when resistance conferring mutations are identified for most DAAs.**

- **IMPORTANT NOTE REGARDING TREATMENT DECISION-MAKING:** Newer drugs are in development and options for Rx are changing rapidly (i.e., several times per year). Monitor updates at *webedition.sanfordguide.com* or *hcvguidelines.org.*

INITIAL TREATMENT FOR PATIENTS WITH CHRONIC HCV

For retreatment and special populations (e.g., decompensated cirrhotics) see *www.hcvguidelines.org.*

Drug	Abbreviation	Formulation/Dose
Boceprevir	BOC	No longer recommended
Dasabuvir	DBV	250 mg tablet po twice daily
Paritaprevir + Ritonavir + Ombitasvir	PTV/r/OBV	Fixed dose combination tablet (Paritaprevir 150 mg + Ritonavir 100 mg + Ombitasvir 25 mg) po once daily
Pegylated Interferon (alfa 2a)	PEG-IFN	180 mcg sc per week
Ribavirin	RBV	Weight based dosing: 1000 mg (< 75 kg) or 1200 mg (> 75 kg)) po twice daily
Simeprevir	SMV	150 mg tablet po once daily
Sofosbuvir	SOF	400 mg tablet po once daily
Sofosbuvir + Ledipasvir	SOF/LDV	Fixed dose combination tablet (Sofosbuvir 400 mg + Ledipasvir 90 mg) po once daily
Telaprevir	TVR	No longer recommended

TABLE 14G (2)

Genotype	Recommended	Alternative	Not Recommended
1a	• **SOF/LDV** x 12 weeks OR • **PTV/r/OBV + DBV + RBV X 12** weeks OR • **SOF/SMV ± RBV** x 12 weeks	None	• SOF + RBV x 24 weeks • SOF + PEG-IFN/RBV x 12 weeks • SMV + PEG-IFN/RBV X 24 or 48 weeks (RGT) TVR + PEG-IFN/RBV x 24 or 48 weeks (RGT)
1b	• **SOF/LDV** x 12 weeks * OR • **PTV/r/OBV + DBV ± RBV** (cirrhosis) X 12 weeks OR • **SOF + SMV** x 12 weeks	None	• BOC + PEG-IFN/RBV x 28 or 48 weeks (RGT) • PEG-IFN/RBV x 48 weeks • Monotherapy with PEG-IFN, RBV, or a DAA Do not treat with PEG-IFN or combination DAA regimens. See www.hcvguidelines.org
2	**SOF + RBV** x 12-16 weeks (if cirrhosis: extend course)	None	• PEG-IFN/RBV x 24 weeks • Monotherapy with PEG-IFN, RBV or a DAA • Any regimen with TVR, BOC or SMV
3	**SOF + RBV** x 24 weeks	**SOF + PEG-IFN/RBV** x 12 weeks	• PEG-IFN/RBV x 24 -48 weeks • Monotherapy with PEG-IFN, RBV or a DAA • Any regimen with TVR, BOC or SMV
4	• **PTV/r/OBV + DBV + RBV** x 12 weeks OR • **SOF + RBV** x 24 weeks OR • **SOF/LDV** x 12 weeks	• **SOF + PEG-IFN/RBV** x 12 weeks • **SOF/SMV +/- RBV** x 12 weeks	• SMV x 12 weeks + PEG-IFN/RBV x 24-48 weeks • SMV x 12 weeks + PEG-IFN/RBV x 24-48 weeks • Monotherapy with PEG-IFN, RBV, or a DAA • Any regimen with TVR or BOC
5	**SOF + PEG-IFN + RBV** x 12 weeks	**PEG-IFN + RBV** x 48 weeks	• Monotherapy with PEG-IFN, RBV, or a DAA • Any regimen with TVR or BOC
6	**SOF/LDV** x 12 weeks	**SOF + PEG-IFN + RBV** x 12 weeks	

* 8 weeks of therapy can be used in selected patients (see www.hcvguidelines.org)

The regimens will change. For updates go to: webedition.sanfordguide.com and www.hcvguidelines.org

TABLE 15A – ANTIMICROBIAL PROPHYLAXIS FOR SELECTED BACTERIAL INFECTIONS*

CLASS OF ETIOLOGIC AGENT/DISEASE/CONDITION	PROPHYLAXIS AGENT/DOSE/ROUTE/DURATION	COMMENTS
Group B streptococcal disease (GBS), neonatal: Approaches to management [CDC Guidelines, *MMWR 59 (RR-10):1, 2010*]:		
Pregnant women—intrapartum antimicrobial prophylaxis procedures:		**Regimens for prophylaxis against early-onset group B streptococcal disease in neonate used during labor:**
1. Screen all pregnant women with vaginal & rectal swab for GBS at 35–37 wks gestation (unless other indications for prophylaxis exist: GBS bacteriuria during this pregnancy or previously delivered infant with invasive GBS disease; even then cultures may be useful for susceptibility testing). Use transport medium; GBS survive at room temp. up to 96 hrs. **Rx during labor if swab culture positive.**		**Penicillin G** 5 million Units IV (initial dose) then 2.5 to 3 million Units IV q4h until delivery Alternative: **Ampicillin** 2 gm IV (initial dose) then 1 gm IV q4h until delivery Penicillin-allergic patients:
2. Rx during labor if previously delivered infant with invasive GBS infection, or if any GBS bacteriuria during this pregnancy.		• Patient not at high risk for anaphylaxis: **Cefazolin** 2 gm IV (initial dose) then 1 gm IV q8h until delivery
3. Rx if GBS status unknown but if any of the following are present: (a) delivery at <37 wks gestation [see *MMWR 59 (RR-10): 1, 2010* algorithms for preterm premature rupture of membranes]; or (b) duration of ruptured membranes ≥18 hrs; or (c) intrapartum temp. ≥100.4°F (≥38.0°C). If amnionitis suspected, broad-spectrum antibiotic coverage should include an agent active vs. group B streptococci.		• Patient at high risk for anaphylaxis from β-lactams. □ If organism is both clindamycin- and erythromycin-susceptible, **or** if erythromycin-resistant, but clindamycin-susceptible confirmed by D-zone test (or equivalent) showing lack of inducible resistance: **Clindamycin** 900 mg IV q8h until delivery
4. Rx if positive intra-partum NAAT for GBS.		□ If susceptibility of organism unknown, lack of inducible resistance to clindamycin has not been excluded, or patient is allergic to clindamycin: **Vancomycin** 1 gm IV q12h until delivery
5. Rx not indicated if: negative vaginal/rectal cultures at 35-37 wks gestation or C-section performed before onset of labor with intact amniotic membranes (use standard surgical prophylaxis).		
Neonate of mother given prophylaxis	*See detailed algorithm in MMWR 59 (RR-10):1, 2010.*	
Preterm, premature rupture of the membranes: Grp B strep-negative women Cochrane Database Rev 12:CD00:1058, 2013; Obstet&Gyn 124:515:2014; Am J Obstet-Gyn 207:475. 2012.	No Pen Allergy: (**AMP** 2 gm IV q6h x 48h, then **AM-CL** 875/125 po bid x 5d) + **Azithro** 1 gm po x 1 dose (**Azithro** for genital mycoplasma sp.) Mild non-IgE Pen Allergy, e.g., rash only: **Cefazolin** 1 g. IV q8h x 48h, then (**Cephalexin** 500 mg po q6h x 5d + **Azithro** 1 gmpo x 1 dose) Severe IgE-mediated Pen Allergy: (**Clinda** 900 mg IV q8h x 48h + **Gent** 7 mg/kg IV once daily x 2d), then (**Clinda** 300 mg po id x 5d + **Azithro** 1 gmpo x 1 dose)	
Post-splenectomy bacteremia. Usually encapsulated bacteria: pneumococci, meningococci, H. flu type B, bacteremia: Enterobacter, S. aureus, Capnocytophaga, P. aeruginosa. Also at risk for fatal malaria, severe babesiosis	Protein conjugate pneumococcal H. influenza type B and meningococcal vaccine (CID 58:309, 2014). Daily Prophylaxis. Asplenic Children(daily until age 5/min 1yr): **Amox** 125 mg po bid (age 2mo-3yr); **Amox** 250 mg po bid (age >3yr-5yr). If allergic, e.g. rash only: **Cephalexin** 250 mg po bid. If IgE-mediated reaction, no good choice. Fever in Children & Adults: **AM-CL** 875/125 po bid (adult); 90 mg/kg po div bid (child); Alternative: **Levo** 750 mg po or **Moxi** 400 mg once daily. Seek immediate medical care. Some recommend **Amox** 2 gmpo before sinus or airway procedures.	

TABLE 15A (2)

CLASS OF ETIOLOGIC AGENT/DISEASE/CONDITION	PROPHYLAXIS AGENT/DOSE/ROUTE/DURATION	COMMENTS
Sexual Exposure		
Sexual assault survivor [likely agents and risks, see *MMWR 59 (RR-12);1, 2010*] For review of overall care: *NEJM 365:834, 2011.*	[(**Ceftriaxone** 250 mg IM)] + (**Metronidazole** 2 gm po as single dose) + (**Azithromycin** 1 gm po once) or (**Doxycycline** 100 mg po bid for 7 days)]	• Obtain expert advice re: forensic exam & specimens, pregnancy, physical trauma, psychological trauma. Check wet mount for T. vaginalis (and culture), check specimen for bacterial vaginosis and Candida if appropriate. • Test for gonococci and chlamydia (NAAT) at appropriate sites. • Serologic evaluation for syphilis, HIV, HBV, HCV not easily transmitted from sexual activity, but consider test in high-risk circumstances (*MMWR 60:945, 2011*). • Initiate post-exposure protocols for HBV vaccine, HIV post-exposure prophylaxis as appropriate (see *Table 15D*). • Follow-up for STDs in 1-2 weeks; retest if prophylaxis not given initially or if symptomatic. • Follow-up serologies for syphilis, HIV, HBV (and HCV if done) at 6 wks, 3 mos and 6 mos. **Notes:** Ceftriaxone is preferred over cefixime for treatment of gonorrhoea; the latter is less effective for pharyngeal infection and strains with decreased susceptibility to cephalosporins are beginning to appear; those with decreased susceptibility to cefixime are more prevalent than those with decreased susceptibility to ceftriaxone (*MMWR 60:873, 2011*). Cefixime 400 mg po once can be used in place of ceftriaxone, if the latter is unavailable (*Derived from CDC STD treatment update MMWR 61:590, 2012*). Azithromycin is preferred to doxycycline because it also provides activity against some GC with reduced susceptibility to cephalosporins (*MMWR 60:873, 2011*). In patients highly allergic to cephalosporins, azithromycin 2 gm po once can be used in place of ceftriaxone.
Contact with specific sexually transmitted diseases	See comprehensive guidelines for specific pathogens in *MMWR 59 (RR-10);1, 2010.*	
Syphilis exposure		Presumptive rx for exposure within 3 mos., as tests may be negative. *See Table 1, page 24.* If exposure occurred > 90 days prior, establish dx or treat empirically (*MMWR 59 (RR-12): 1, 2010*).
Sickle-cell disease. Likely agent: S. pneumoniae (see post-splenectomy, above) Ref.: *2009 Red Book Online, Amer Acad Pediatrics*	Children <5 yrs: **Penicillin V** 125 mg po bid ≥5 yrs: **Penicillin V** 250 mg po bid. (Alternative in children: Amoxicillin 20 mg per kg per day)	Start prophylaxis by 2 mos. (*Pediatrics 106:367, 2000*); continue until at least age 5. When to stop must be individualized. Age-appropriate vaccines, including pneumococcal, Hib, influenza, meningococcal. Treating infections, consider possibility of penicillin non-susceptible pneumococci.

TABLE 15B – ANTIBIOTIC PROPHYLAXIS TO PREVENT SURGICAL INFECTIONS IN ADULTS*

2013 Guidelines: Am J Health Syst Pharm 70:195, 2013

General Comments:
- To be optimally effective, antibiotics must be started within 60 minutes of the surgical incision. Vancomycin and FQs may require 1-2 hr infusion time, so start dose 2 hrs before the surgical incision.
- Most applications employ a single preoperative dose of prophylactic agent, intraoperative supplementary dose(s) may be required.
- For procedures lasting > 2 half-lives of prophylactic agent, intraoperative supplementary dose(s) may be required.
- Dose adjustments may be desirable in pts with BMI >30.
- Prophylaxis does carry risk: e.g., C. difficile colitis, allergic reactions
- Active screening for S. aureus nasal colonization and application of chlorhexidine washes and intranasal mupirocin reported as a strategy that decreases surgical site infection
- In general, recommendations are consistent with those of the Surgical Care Improvement Project (SCIP)

Use of Vancomycin:
- For many common prophylaxis indications, vancomycin is considered an alternative to β-lactams in pts allergic to or intolerant of the latter.
- Vancomycin use may be justified in centers where rates of post-operative infection with methicillin-resistant staphylococci are high or in pts at high risk for these.
- Unlike β-lactams in common use, vancomycin has no activity against gram-negative organisms. **When gram-negative bacteria are a concern following specific procedures, it may be necessary or desirable to add a second agent with appropriate in vitro activity.** This can be done using cefazolin with vancomycin in the non-allergic pt, or in pts intolerant of β-lactams using vancomycin with another gram-negative agent (e.g., aminoglycoside, fluoroquinolone, possibly aztreonam, if pt not allergic; local resistance patterns and pt factors would influence choice).
- Infusion of vancomycin, especially too rapidly, may result in hypotension or other manifestations of histamine release (red person syndrome). Does not indicate an allergy to vancomycin.

TABLE 15B (2)

TYPE OF SURGERY	PROPHYLAXIS	COMMENTS
Cardiovascular Surgery Antibiotic prophylaxis in cardiovascular surgery has been proven beneficial in the following procedures: • Reconstruction of abdominal aorta • Procedures on the leg that involve a groin incision • Any vascular procedure that inserts prosthesis/foreign body • Lower extremity amputation for ischemia • Cardiac surgery • Permanent Pacemakers (*Circulation 121:458, 2010*) • Heart transplant	**Cefazolin** 1-2 gm (Wt <120 kg) or 3 gm (Wt >120 kg) IV as a single dose or q8h for 1-2 days **or cefuroxime** 1.5 gm IV as a single dose or q12h for total of 6 gm **or vancomycin** 1 gm IV as single dose for 1-2 days. For pts weighing >90 kg, use vanco 1.5 gm IV as a single dose or q12h for 1-2 days. Re-dose cefazolin q4h if CrCl >30 mL/min or q8h if CrCl ≤30 mL/min Consider **intranasal mupirocin** evening before, day of surgery & bid for 5 days post-op in pts with pos. nasal culture for S. aureus. Mupirocin resistance has been encountered.	**Timing & duration:** Single infusion just before surgery as effective as multiple doses. No prophylaxis needed for cardiac catheterization. For prosthetic heart valves, customary to stop prophylaxis either after removal of retrosternal drainage catheters or just a 2nd dose after coming off bypass. **Vancomycin** may be preferable in hospitals with ↑ freq of MRSA, in high-risk pts, those colonized with MRSA or for Pen-allergic pts. Clindamycin 900 mg IV is another alternative for Pen-allergic or Vanco-allergic pt.
Gastric, Biliary and Colonic Surgery **Gastroduodenal/Biliary** Gastroduodenal, includes percutaneous endoscopic gastrostomy (high risk only), pancreaticoduodenectomy (Whipple procedure)	**Cefazolin** (1-2 gm IV) or **cefoxitin** (1-2 gm IV) or **cefotetan** (1-2 gm IV) or **ceftriaxone** (2 gm IV) as a single dose (some give additional doses q12h for 2-3 days). See Comment	Gastroduodenal (PEG placement): High-risk pts: marked obesity, obstruction, ↓ gastric acid or ↓ motility. Re-dose cefazolin q4h and cefoxitin q2h if CrCl >30 mL/min; q6h and q4h, respectively, if CrCl ≤30 ml/min
Biliary, includes laparoscopic cholecystectomy	Low risk, laparoscopic: No prophylaxis Open cholecystectomy: **cefazolin, cefoxitin, cefotetan, ampicillin-sulbactam**	Biliary high-risk or open procedure: age >70, acute cholecystitis, non-functioning gallbladder, obstructive jaundice or common duct stones. With cholangitis, treat as infection, not prophylaxis.
Endoscopic retrograde cholangiopancreatography	No rx without obstruction. If obstruction: **Ciprofloxacin** 500-750 mg po or 400 mg IV 2 hrs prior to procedure or **PIP-TZ** 4.5 gm IV 1 hr prior to procedure	Most studies show that achieving adequate drainage will prevent post-procedural cholangitis or sepsis and no further benefit from prophylactic antibiotics: greatest benefit likely when complete drainage cannot be achieved. See *Gastroint Endosc 67:791, 2008; Gut 58:868, 2009.*
Colorectal Recommend combination of: • Mechanical bowel prep • PO antibiotic (See Comment) • IV antibiotic	**Parenteral regimens** (emergency or elective): **Cefazolin** 1-2 gm IV + **metronidazole** 0.5 gm IV) (see Comment) or **cefoxitin** or **cefotetan** 1-2 gm IV (if available) or **Ceftriaxone** 2 gm IV + **Metro** 0.5 gm IV or **ERTA** 1 gm IV Beta-lactam allergy: see Comment	**Oral regimens: Neomycin + erythromycin.** Pre-op day: (1) 10 am 4L polyethylene glycol electrolyte solution (Colyte, GoLYTELY) po over 2 hr. (2) Clear liquid diet only. (3) 1 pm, 2 pm & 11 pm, neomycin 1 gm + erythro base 1 gm po. (4) NPO after midnight. Alternative regimens have been less well studied: GoLYTELY 1-6 pm, then neomycin 2 gm po + metronidazole 2 gm po at 7 pm & 11 pm. Oral regimen as effective as parenteral; parenteral in addition to oral not required but often used (*Am J Surg 189:395, 2005*). Study found **Ertapenem** more effective than cefotetan, but associated with non-significant ↑ risk of C. difficile (*NEJM 355:2640, 2006*). Beta lactam allergy: **Clindamycin** 900 mg IV + (**Gentamicin** 5 mg/kg or **Aztreonam** 2 gm IV) or **Ciprofloxacin** 400 mg IV)
Ruptured viscus: See *Peritoneum/Peritonitis, Secondary, Table 1, page 47.*		

TABLE 15B (3)

TYPE OF SURGERY	PROPHYLAXIS	COMMENTS
Head and Neck Surgery	**Cefazolin** 2 gm IV (Single dose) (some add **metronidazole** 500 mg IV) **OR** **Clindamycin** 600-900 mg IV (single dose) ± **gentamicin** 5 mg/kg IV (single dose) (*See Table 10D for weight-based dose calculation*).	Antimicrobial prophylaxis appears efficacious only for procedures involving oral/pharyngeal mucosa (e.g., laryngeal or pharyngeal tumor) but even with prophylaxis, wound infection rate can be high. **Clean, uncontaminated head & neck surg does not require prophylaxis.** Re-dose cefazolin q4h if CrCl >30 mL/min or q8h if CrCl ≤30 mL/min
Neurosurgical Procedures Clean, non-implant; e.g., elective craniotomy	**Cefazolin** 1-2 gm IV once. Alternative: **vanco** 1 gm IV once; for pts weighing > 90 kg, use vanco 1.5 gm IV as single dose.	Clindamycin 900 mg IV is alternative for vanco-allergic or beta-lactam allergic pt. Re-dose cefazolin q4h if CrCl >30 mL/min or q8h if CrCl ≤30 mL/min
Clean, contaminated (cross sinuses, or naso/oropharynx)	**Clindamycin** 900 mg IV (single dose)	British recommend amoxicillin-clavulanate 1.2 gm IV[a,c] or (cefuroxime 1.5 gm IV + metronidazole 0.5 gm IV).
CSF shunt surgery, intrathecal pumps:	**Cefazolin** 1-2 gm (Wt <120 kg) or 3 gm (Wt > 120 kg) IV once. Alternative: **vanco** 1 gm IV once; for pts weighing > 90 kg, use vanco 1.5 gm IV as single dose OR **Clindamycin** 900 mg IV	Randomized study in a hospital with high prevalence of infection due to methicillin-resistant staphylococci showed vancomycin was more effective than cefazolin in preventing CSF shunt infections (*J Hosp Infect* 69:337, 2008). Re-dose cefazolin q4h if CrCl >30 mL/min or q8h if CrCl ≤30 mL/min
Obstetric/Gynecologic Surgery Vaginal or abdominal hysterectomy	**Cefazolin** 1-2 gm or **cefotetan** 1-2 gm or **cefoxitin** 1-2 gm or **ampicillin-sulbactam** 3 gm IV 30 min. before surgery.	Alternative: (**Clindamycin** 900 mg IV or **Vancomycin** 15 mg/kg x 1 dose and **Aztreonam** 2 gm IV) OR (**Metronidazole** 500 mg IV + **Ciprofloxacin** 400 mg IV)
Cesarean section for premature rupture of membranes or active labor	**Cefazolin** 1-2 gm IV (See Comments). Alternative: **Clindamycin** 900 mg IV + (**Gentamicin** 5 mg/kg IV or **Tobramycin** 5 mg/kg IV) x 1 dose	Prophylaxis decreases risk of endometritis and wound infection. Traditional approach had been to administer antibiotics after cord is clamped to avoid exposing infant to antibiotic. However, studies suggest that administering prophylaxis before the skin incision results in fewer surgical site infections (*Obstet Gynecol* 115:187, 2010; *Amer J Obstet Gynecol* 199:301.e1 and 310.e1, 2008) and endometritis (*Amer J Obstet Gynecol* 196:455.e1, 2007).
Surgical Abortion (1st trimester)	1st trimester **Doxycycline** 300 mg po. 100 mg 1 hr before procedure + 200 mg post-procedure.	Meta-analysis showed benefit of antibiotic prophylaxis in all risk groups.
Orthopedic Surgery Hip arthroplasty, spinal fusion	Same as cardiac surgery	Customarily stopped after "Hemovac" removed. 2013 Guidelines recommend stopping prophylaxis within 24 hrs of surgery (*Am J Health Syst Pharm* 70:195, 2013).
Total joint replacement (other than hip)	**Cefazolin** 1-2 gm IV pre-op (± 2nd dose) or **vancomycin** 1 gm IV. For pts weighing > 90 kg, use vanco 1.5 gm IV as single dose or **Clindamycin** 900 mg IV.	2013 Guidelines recommend stopping prophylaxis within 24 hrs of surgery (*Am J Health Syst Pharm* 70:195, 2013). Usual to administer before tourniquet inflation. Intranasal mupirocin if colonized with S. aureus.
Open reduction of closed fracture with internal fixation	**Ceftriaxone** 2 gm IV once	3.6% (ceftriaxone) vs 8.3% (for placebo) infection found in Dutch trauma trial (*Ln* 347:1133, 1996). Several alternative antimicrobials can ↓ risk of infection (*Cochrane Database Syst Rev* 2010; CD 000244).

TABLE 15B (4)

TYPE OF SURGERY	PROPHYLAXIS	COMMENTS
Orthopedic Surgery, (contd) Prophylaxis to protect prosthetic joints from hematogenous infection related to distant procedures (patients with plates, pins and screws only are not considered to be at risk)		• In 2003, the American Academy of Orthopedic Surgeons (AAOS), in conjunction with the American Dental Association and the American Urological Association, developed Advisory Statements on the use of antibiotic prophylaxis to prevent infection of implanted joint prostheses for procedures that may cause bacteremia. (*Am J Dent Assoc 134:895, 2003; J Urol 169:1796, 2003*). These documents stratified procedures for risk of bacteremia, identified patients at risk of infection (incl. all pts in first 2 years after insertion), and offered antibiotic options. (*See also Med Lett 47:59, 2005 and review in Infect Dis Clin N Amer 19:931, 2005*) • A February 2009 Information Statement from the AAOS listed patient factors that may ↑ risk of infection, but recommended that antibiotic prophylaxis be considered for any invasive procedure that may cause bacteremia in all patients with a joint replacement (http://aaos.org/about/papers/advistmt/1033.asp) • The editors believe that the latter approach is excessively broad and exposes many to the risks of antibiotics without definite evidence of benefit. As pointed out in guidelines for prevention of endocarditis, transient bacteremias occur with routine daily activities (*Circulation 2007; 116:1736*). • **A recent prospective, case-control study concluded that antibiotic prophylaxis for dental procedures *did not decrease the risk of hip or knee prosthesis infection* (Clin Infect Dis 50:8, 2010).** • For patients with prosthetic joints, infections involving tissue to be manipulated surgically should be treated before surgery whenever possible. Prophylaxis with an anti-staphylococcal β-lactam or vancomycin (according to susceptibility of the organism) for procedures involving tissues colonized by staphylococci would be appropriate, as these organisms are common causes of prosthetic joint infections. For now, the 2003 documents cited above appear to provide the best information on which to base such decisions.
Peritoneal Dialysis Catheter Placement	Vancomycin single 1 gm IV dose 12 hrs prior to procedure	Effectively reduced peritonitis during 14 days post-placement in 221 pts: vanco 1%, cefazolin 7%, placebo 12% (p=0.02) (*Am J Kidney Dis 36:1014, 2000*).
Urologic Surgery/Procedures	• See Best Practice Policy Statement of Amer. Urological Assoc. (AUA) (*J Urol 179:1379, 2008*) and 2013 Guidelines (*Am J Health Syst Pharm 70:195, 2013*) • Selection of agents targeting urinary pathogens may require modification based on local resistance patterns; ↑ TMP-SMX and/or fluoroquinolone (FQ) resistance among enteric gram-negative bacteria is a concern.	
Cystoscopy	*Prophylaxis generally not necessary if urine is sterile (however, AUA recommends FQ or TMP-SMX for those with several potentially adverse host factors (e.g., advanced age, immunocompromised state, anatomic abnormalities, etc.)* • Treat patients with UTI prior to procedure using an antimicrobial active against pathogen isolated	
Cystoscopy with manipulation	**Ciprofloxacin** 500 mg po or **TMP-SMX** 1 DS tablet po may be an alternative in populations with low rates of resistance)	Procedures mentioned include ureteroscopy, biopsy, fulguration, TURP, etc. Treat UTI with targeted therapy before procedure if possible.
Transrectal prostate biopsy	**Ciprofloxacin** 500 mg po 12 hrs prior to biopsy and repeated 12 hrs after 1st dose. *See Comment.*	Bacteremia 7% with CIP vs 37% with **gentamicin** (*JAC 39:115, 1997*). **Levofloxacin** 500 mg 30-60 min before procedure was effective in low risk pts; additional doses were given for ↑ risk (*J Urol 168:1021, 2002*). Serious bacteremias due to FQ-resistant organisms have been encountered in patients receiving FQ prophylaxis. Clinicians should advise patients to immediately report symptoms suggesting infection. Pre-operative prophylaxis should be determined on an institutional basis based on susceptibility profiles of prevailing organisms. Although 2nd or 3rd generation cephalosporins or addition of single-dose gentamicin has been suggested, infections due to ESBL-producing and genl-resistant organisms have been encountered (*Urol 74:332, 2009*).
Other		
Breast surgery, herniorrhaphy	**Cefazolin** 1-2 gm IV x 1 dose or **Ampicillin-sulbactam** 3 gm IV x 1 dose or **Clindamycin** 900 mg IV x 1 dose or **Vancomycin** 1 gm IV x 1 dose (1.5 gm if wt > 90 kg)	Benefits of prophylaxis for clean surgical procedures to reduce risk of surgical site infection in breast surgery (studies not examining immediate reconstruction), but great variability in regimens selected (*Cochrane Database Syst Rev 2006; (2): CD 005360*). For inguinal hernia repair, one analysis found prophylaxis to be beneficial in repairs with mesh (*J Hosp Infect 62: 427, 2006*), while another concluded that antibiotics may reduce risk of infection in pooled population or in those repaired with prosthetic material (mesh), but that the data were not sufficiently strong to make firm recommendations for or against their use universally (*Cochrane Database Syst Rev 2007; (3): CD 003769*).

TABLE 15C – ANTIMICROBIAL PROPHYLAXIS FOR THE PREVENTION OF BACTERIAL ENDOCARDITIS IN PATIENTS WITH UNDERLYING CARDIAC CONDITIONS*

In 2007, the American Heart Association guidelines for the prevention of bacterial endocarditis were updated. The resulting document (*Circulation 2007; 116:1736-1754 and http://circ.ahajournals.org/reprint/116/15/1736*), which was also endorsed by the Infectious Diseases Society of America, represents a significant departure from earlier recommendations.

- Antibiotic prophylaxis for dental procedures is now directed at individuals who are likely to suffer the most devastating consequences should they develop endocarditis.
- Prophylaxis to prevent endocarditis is no longer specified for gastrointestinal or genitourinary procedures. The following is adapted from and reflects the new AHA recommendations. *See original publication for explanation and precise details.*

SELECTION OF PATIENTS FOR ENDOCARDITIS PROPHYLAXIS

FOR PATIENTS WITH ANY OF THESE HIGH-RISK CARDIAC CONDITIONS ASSOCIATED WITH ENDOCARDITIS:	WHO UNDERGO DENTAL PROCEDURES INVOLVING:	WHO UNDERGO INVASIVE RESPIRATORY PROCEDURES INVOLVING:	WHO UNDERGO INVASIVE PROCEDURES OF THE GI OR GU TRACTS:	WHO UNDERGO PROCEDURES INVOLVING INFECTED SKIN AND SOFT TISSUES:
Prosthetic heart valves Previous infective endocarditis Congenital heart disease with any of the following: • Completely repaired cardiac defect using prosthetic material (Only for 1st 6 months) • Partially corrected but with residual defect near prosthetic material • Uncorrected cyanotic congenital heart disease • Surgically constructed shunts and conduits Valvulopathy following heart transplant	Any manipulation of gingival tissue, dental periapical regions, or perforating the oral mucosa. **PROPHYLAXIS RECOMMENDED‡** *(See Dental Procedures Regimens table below)* (Prophylaxis *is not* recommended for routine anesthetic injections (unless through infected area), dental x-rays, shedding of primary teeth, adjustment of orthodontic appliances or placement of orthodontic brackets or removable appliances).	Incision of respiratory tract mucosa **CONSIDER PROPHYLAXIS** *(see Dental Procedures Regimens table)* Or For treatment of established infection **PROPHYLAXIS RECOMMENDED** *(see Dental Procedures Regimens table for oral flora, but include anti-staphylococcal coverage when S. aureus is of concern)*	PROPHYLAXIS is no longer recommended solely to prevent endocarditis, **but the following approach is reasonable:** For patients with enterococcal UTIs • treat before elective GU procedures • include enterococcal coverage in perioperative regimen for non-elective procedures† For patients with existing GU or GI infections or those who receive perioperative antibiotics to prevent surgical site infections or sepsis • it is reasonable to include agents with anti-enterococcal activity in perioperative coverage†	Include coverage against staphylococci and β-hemolytic streptococci in treatment regimens

PROPHYLACTIC REGIMENS FOR DENTAL PROCEDURES

SITUATION	AGENT	REGIMEN†
Usual oral prophylaxis	Amoxicillin	Adults 2 gm, children 50 mg per kg, orally 1 hour before procedure.
Unable to take oral medications	Ampicillin² OR	Adults 2 gm, children 50 mg per kg; IV or IM, within 30 min before procedure.
	Cephalexin³ OR	Adults 2 gm, children 50 mg per kg, orally, 1 hour before procedure
	Clindamycin	Adults 600 mg, children 20 mg per kg; orally, 1 hour before procedure
Allergic to penicillins	Azithromycin or clarithromycin	Adults 500 mg, children 15 mg per kg; orally, 1 hour before procedure
	Clindamycin	Adults 1 gm, children 50 mg per kg; IV or IM, within 30 min before procedure
Allergic to penicillins and unable to take oral medications	Cefazolin³ OR	Adults 1 gm, children 50 mg per kg; IV or IM, within 30 min before procedure
	Clindamycin	Adults 600 mg, children 20 mg per kg; IV or IM, within 30 min before procedure

† Agents with anti-enterococcal activity include penicillin, ampicillin, amoxicillin, piperacillin, vancomycin and others. Check susceptibility if available. (See Table 5 for highly resistant organisms.)
‡ 2008 AHA/ACC focused update of guidelines on valvular heart disease use term "is reasonable" to reflect level of evidence (*Circulation 118:887, 2008*).

1 Children's dose should not exceed adult dose. AHA document lists all doses as 30-60 min before procedure.
2 AHA lists cefazolin or ceftriaxone (at appropriate doses) as alternatives to ampicillin.
3 Cephalosporins should not be used in individuals with immediate-type hypersensitivity reaction (urticaria, angioedema, or anaphylaxis) to penicillins or other β-lactams. AHA proposes ceftriaxone as potential alternative to cefazolin; and other 1st or 2nd generation cephalosporin in equivalent doses as potential alternatives to cephalexin.

TABLE 15D – MANAGEMENT OF EXPOSURE TO HIV-1 AND HEPATITIS B AND C*

OCCUPATIONAL EXPOSURE TO BLOOD, PENILE/VAGINAL SECRETIONS OR OTHER POTENTIALLY INFECTIOUS BODY FLUIDS OR TISSUES WITH RISK OF TRANSMISSION OF HEPATITIS B/C AND/OR HIV-1 (E.G., NEEDLESTICK INJURY)

Free consultation for occupational exposures, call (PEPline) 1-888-448-4911. *[Information also available at www.aidsinfo.nih.gov]*

General steps in management:

1. Wash clean wounds/flush mucous membranes immediately (use of caustic agents or squeezing the wound is discouraged; data lacking regarding antiseptics).
2. Assess risk by doing the following: (a) Characterize exposure; (b) Determine/evaluate source of exposure by medical history, risk behavior, & testing for hepatitis B/C, HIV; (c) Evaluate and test exposed individual for hepatitis B/C & HIV.

Hepatitis B Occupational Exposure Prophylaxis *(MMWR 62(No.10, Suppl):1, 2013)*

Exposed Person Vaccine Status	Exposure Source		
	HBs Ag+	HBs Ag–	Status Unknown or Unavailable for Testing†
Unvaccinated	Give HBIG 0.06 mL per kg IM & initiate HB vaccine	Initiate HB vaccine	Initiate HB vaccine
Vaccinated (antibody status unknown)	Do anti-HBs on exposed person: If titer ≥10 milli-International units per mL, no rx If titer <10 milli-International units per mL, give HBIG + 1 dose HB vaccine**	No rx necessary	Do anti-HBs on exposed person: If titer ≥10 milli-International units per mL, no rx § If titer <10 milli-International units per mL, give 1 dose of HB vaccine**

†Persons previously infected with HBV are immune to reinfection and do not require postexposure prophylaxis.

For known vaccine series responder (titer ≥10 milli-International units per mL), monitoring of levels or booster doses not currently recommended. Known non-responder (<10 milli-International units per mL) to 1° series HB vaccine & exposed to either HBsAG+ source or suspected high-risk source—rx with HBIG & re-initiate vaccine series **or** give 2 doses HBIG 1 month apart. For non-responders after a 2nd vaccine series, 2 doses HBIG 1 month apart is preferred approach to new exposure.

§ If known high risk source, treat as if source were HBsAG positive
** Follow-up to assess vaccine response or address completion of vaccine series.

Hepatitis B Non-Occupational Exposure & Reactivation of Latent Hepatitis B

Non-Occupational Exposure *(MMWR 59(RR-10):1, 2010)*

- Exposure to blood or sexual secretion of HBsAg-positive person
  - Percutaneous (bite, needlestick)
  - Sexual assault
- Initiate immunoprophylaxis within 24 hrs or sexual exposure & no more than 7 days after parenteral exposure
- Use Guidelines for occupational exposure for use of HBIG and HBV vaccine

TABLE 15D (2)

Hepatitis B Non-Occupational Exposure & Reactivation of Latent Hepatitis B *(continued)*

Reactivation of Latent HBV *(Eur J Cancer 49:3486, 2013; Semin/ar of Liver Dis 33:167, 2013; Crit Rev Oncol-Hematol 87:12, 2013)*

- Patients requiring administration of anti-CD 20 monoclonal antibodies as part of treatment selected malignancies, rheumatoid arthritis and vasculitis are at risk for reactivation of latent HBV
- Two FDA-approved anti-CD 20 drugs: ofatumumab (Azerra) & rituximab (Rituxan)
- Prior to starting anti-CD 20 drug, test for latent HBV with test for HBsAg and Anti IgG HB core antibody
- If pt has latent HBV & anti-CD 20 treatment is necessary, treatment should include an effective anti-HBV drug

Hepatitis C Exposure

Determine antibody to hepatitis C for both exposed person &, if possible, exposure source. If source + or unknown and exposed person negative, follow-up HCV testing for HCV RNA (detectable in blood in 1-3 weeks) and HCV antibody (90% will seroconvert will do so by 3 months) is advised. **No recommended prophylaxis;** immune serum globulin not effective. Monitor for early infection, as therapy may ↓ risk of progression to chronic hepatitis. Persons who remain viremic 8-12 weeks after exposure should be treated with a course of pegylated interferon *(Gastro 130:632, 2006 and Hpt 43:923, 2006). See Table 14G.* Case-control study suggested risk factors for occupational HCV transmission include percutaneous exposure to needle that had been in artery or vein, deep injury, male sex of HCW, & was more likely when source VL >6 log10 copies/mL.

HIV: Occupational exposure management *[Adapted from CDC recommendations, Infect Control Hosp Epi 34: 875, 2014]*

- The decision to initiate postexposure prophylaxis (PEP) for HIV is a clinical judgment that should be made in concert with the exposed healthcare worker (HCW). It is based on:
  1. Likelihood of the source patient having HIV infection: † with history of high-risk activity—injection drug use, sexual activity with known HIV+ person, unprotected sex with multiple partners (either hetero- or homosexual), receipt of blood products 1978-1985. † with clinical signs suggestive of advanced HIV (unexplained wasting, night sweats, thrush, seborrheic dermatitis, etc.).
  2. Type of exposure (approx. 1 in 300-400 needlesticks from infected source will transmit HIV).
  3. Limited data regarding efficacy of PEP drugs & potential for drug interactions.
  4. Significant adverse effects of PEP drugs & potential for drug interactions.
  - Substances considered potentially infectious include: blood, tissues, semen, vaginal secretions, CSF, synovial, pleural, peritoneal, pericardial and amniotic fluids; and other visibly bloody fluids.
  - Fluids normally considered low risk for transmission, unless visibly bloody, include: urine, vomitus, stool, sweat, saliva, nasal secretions, tears and sputum.
- If source person is **known positive for HIV or likely to be infected** and **status of exposure warrants PEP,** antiretroviral drugs should be started **immediately.** If source person is HIV antibody negative, drugs can be stopped **unless source is suspected of having acute HIV infection.** The HCW should be re-tested at **3-4 weeks, 3 & 6 months whether PEP is used or not** (the vast majority of seroconversions will occur by 3 months; delayed conversions after 6 months are exceedingly rare). Tests for HIV RNA should not be used for dx of HIV infection in HCW because of false-positives (esp. at low titers) & these tests are only approved for established HIV infection [a possible exception is if pt develops signs of acute HIV (mononucleosis-like) syndrome within the 1st 4-6 wks of exposure when antibody tests might still be negative.]
- PEP for HIV is usually given for **4 wks** and monitoring of adverse effects recommended; baseline **complete blood count, renal and hepatic panel** to be **repeated at 2 weeks.** 50-75% of HCW on PEP demonstrate mild side-effects (nausea, diarrhea, headache, etc.) but in up to ½ severe enough to discontinue PEP. Consultation with infectious diseases/ HIV specialist valuable when questions regarding PEP arise. **Seek expert help in special situations, such as pregnancy, renal impairment, treatment-experienced source.**

TABLE 15D (3)

3 Steps to HIV Postexposure Prophylaxis (PEP) After Occupational Exposure: *[Latest CDC recommendations available at www.aidsinfo.nih.gov]*

Step 1: Determine the exposure code (EC)

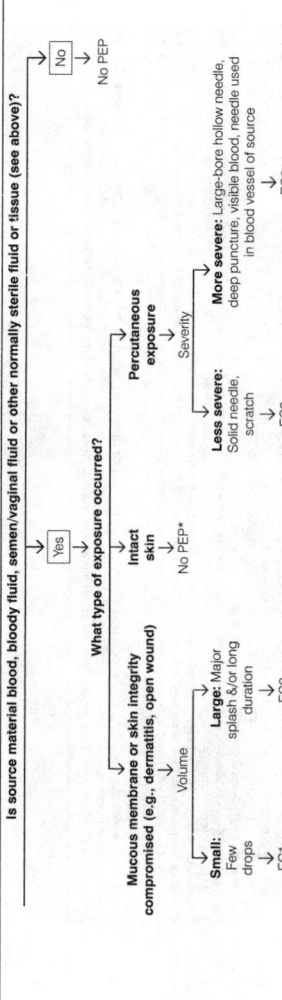

Is source material blood, bloody fluid, semen/vaginal fluid or other normally sterile fluid or tissue (see above)?

No → No PEP

Yes →

What type of exposure occurred?

→ **Intact skin** → No PEP*

→ **Mucous membrane or skin integrity compromised (e.g., dermatitis, open wound)**

Volume

→ **Small:** Few drops → EC1

→ **Large:** Major splash &/or long duration → EC2

→ **Percutaneous exposure**

Severity

→ **Less severe:** Solid needle, scratch → EC2

→ **More severe:** Large-bore hollow needle, deep puncture, visible blood, needle used in blood vessel of source → EC3

* *Exceptions can be considered when there has been prolonged, high-volume contact.*

Step 2: Determine the HIV Status Code (HIV SC)

What is the HIV status of the exposure source?

→ **HIV negative** → No PEP

→ **HIV positive**

→ **Low titer exposure:** asymptomatic & high CD4 count, low VL (<1500 copies per mL) → HIV SC 1

→ **High titer exposure:** advanced AIDS, primary HIV high viral load or low CD4 count → HIV SC 2

→ **Status unknown** → HIV SC unknown

→ **Source unknown** → HIV SC unknown

TABLE 15D (4)

3 Steps to HIV Postexposure Prophylaxis (PEP) After Occupational Exposure *(continued)*

Step 3: Determine Postexposure Prophylaxis (PEP) Recommendation

EC	HIV SC	PEP
1	1	Consider basic regimen[a]
1	2	Recommend basic regimen[a,b]
2	1	Recommend basic regimen[b]
2	2	Recommend expanded regimen
3	1 or 2	Recommend expanded regimen
1, 2, 3	Unknown	If exposure setting suggests risks of HIV exposure, consider basic regimen[c]

[a] Based on estimates of ↓ risk of infection after mucous membrane exposure in occupational setting compared with needlestick.

[b] Or, consider expanded regimen[c].

[c] In high risk circumstances, consider expanded regimen[c] on case-by-case basis.

Around the clock, urgent expert consultation available from: National Clinicians' Postexposure Prophylaxis Hotline (PEPline) at 1-888-448-4911 (1-888-HIV-4911) and on-line at http://www.ucsf.edu/hivcntr

Regimens: (Treat for 4 weeks; monitor for drug side-effects every 2 weeks)

Basic regimen: ZDV + 3TC, FTC + TDF, or as an alternative d4T + 3TC.

Expanded regimen: Basic regimen + one of the following: lopinavir/ritonavir *(preferred)*, or *(as alternatives)* atazanavir/ritonavir or fosamprenavir/ritonavir. Efavirenz can be considered (except in pregnancy or potential for pregnancy—**Pregnancy Category D**), but CNS symptoms might be problematic. [**Do not use nevirapine;** serious adverse reactions including hepatic necrosis reported in healthcare workers.]

Other regimens can be designed. If possible, use antiretroviral drugs for which resistance is unlikely based on susceptibility data or treatment history of source pt (if known). Seek expert consultation if ART-experienced source on pregnancy or potential for pregnancy.

NOTE: Some authorities feel that an expanded regimen should be employed whenever PEP is indicated. Expanded regimens are likely to be advantageous with ↑ numbers of ART-experienced source pts or when there is doubt about exact extent of exposures in decision algorithm. Mathematical model suggests that under some conditions, completion of full course basic regimen is better than prematurely discontinued expanded regimen. However, while expanded PEP regimens have ↑ adverse effects, there is not necessarily ↑ discontinuation.

POSTEXPOSURE PROPHYLAXIS FOR NON-OCCUPATIONAL EXPOSURES TO HIV-1
[Adapted from CDC recommendations, MMWR 54 (RR2), 2005, available at www.cdc.gov/mmwr/indrr 2005.html]

Because the risk of transmission of HIV via sexual contact or sharing needles by injection drug users may reach or exceed that of occupational needlestick exposure, it is reasonable to consider PEP in persons who have had a non-occupational exposure to blood or other potentially infected fluids (e.g., genital/rectal secretions, breast milk) from an HIV+ source. Risk of HIV acquisition per exposure varies with the act (for needle sharing and receptive anal intercourse, ≥0.5%; approximately 10-fold lower with insertive vaginal and anal intercourse, 0.05–0.07%). Overt or occult traumatic lesions may ↑ risk in survivors of sexual assault.

For pts at risk of HIV acquisition through non-occupational exposure to HIV+ source material having occurred ≤72 hours before evaluation, DHHS recommendation is to treat for 28 days with an antiretroviral **expanded regimen,** using preferred regimens [efavirenz *(not in pregnancy or pregnancy risk—Pregnancy Category D)* + (3TC or FTC) + (ZDV or TDF)] **or** lopinavir/ritonavir + (3TC or FTC) + ZDV] or one of several alternative regimens *[see Table 14D & MMWR 54(RR-2):1, 2005]*. Failures of prophylaxis have been reported, and may be associated with longer interval from exposure to start of PEP; this supports prompt initiation of PEP if it to be used.

Areas of uncertainty: (1) expanded regimens are not proven to be superior to 2-drug regimens, (2) while PEP not recommended for exposures >72 hours before evaluation, it may possibly be effective in some cases, (3) when HIV status of source patient is unknown, decision to treat and regimen selection must be individualized based on assessment of specific circumstances.

Evaluate for exposures to Hep B, Hep C *(see Occupational PEP above)* and bacterial sexually-transmitted diseases *(see Table 15A)* and treat as indicated. DHHS recommendations for sexual exposures to HepB and bacterial pathogens are available in *MMWR 55(RR-11), 2006.* Persons who are unvaccinated or who have not responded to full HepB vaccine series should receive hepB immune globulin preferably within 24-hours of percutaneous or mucosal exposure to blood or body fluids of an HBsAg-positive person, along with hepB vaccine, with follow-up to complete vaccine series. Unvaccinated or not-fully-vaccinated persons exposed to a source with unknown HepBsAg-status should receive vaccine and complete vaccine series. See *MMWR 55(RR-11), 2006* for details and recommendations in other circumstances.

TABLE 16 – PREVENTION OF SELECTED OPPORTUNISTIC INFECTIONS IN HUMAN HEMATOPOIETIC CELL TRANSPLANTATION (HCT) OR SOLID ORGAN TRANSPLANTATION (SOT) IN ADULTS WITH NORMAL RENAL FUNCTION.

General comments: Medical centers performing transplants will have detailed protocols for the prevention of opportunistic infections which are appropriate to the infections encountered, patients represented and resources available at those sites. Regimens continue to evolve and protocols adopted by an institution may differ from those at other centers. Care of transplant patients should be guided by physicians with expertise in this area.

References:

For HCT: Expert guidelines endorsed by the IDSA, updating earlier guidelines (*MMWR 49 (RR-10):1, 2000*) in: *Biol Blood Marrow Transpl 15:1143, 2009*. These guidelines provide recommendations for prevention of additional infections not discussed in this table and provide more detailed information on the infections included here.

For SOT: Recommendations of an expert panel of The Transplantation Society for management of CMV in solid organ transplant recipients in: *Transplantation 89:779, 2010*. Timeline of infections following SOT in: *Amer J Transpl 9 (suppl 4):S3, 2009.*

OPPORTUNISTIC INFECTION	TYPE OF TRANSPLANT	PROPHYLACTIC REGIMENS
CMV (Recipient + **or** Donor +/Recipient –) Ganciclovir resistance: risk, detection, management (*CID 56:1018, 2013*)	SOT	**Prophylaxis: Valganciclovir** 900 mg po q24h Alternatives include **Ganciclovir** 1000 mg po 3 x/day, **Valganciclovir** 2 gm po 4 x/day (*kidney only, see comment*), CMV IVIG or IVIG. **Also consider preemptive therapy** (monitor weekly for CMV viremia by PCR (or antigenemia) for 3-6 months post transplant. If viremia detected, start Valganciclovir 900 mg po bid or Ganciclovir 5 mg/kg IV q12h until clearance of viremia, but for not less than 2 weeks followed by secondary prophylaxis or preemptive approach. Prophylaxis vs pre-emptive rx compared: *CID 58:785, 2014*. CMV hyper IVIG is as adjunct to prophylaxis in high-risk lung, heart/lung, heart, or pancreas organ transplant recipients. Dosing: 150 mg/kg within 72 hrs of transplant and at 2, 4, 6 and 8 weeks; then 100 mg/kg at weeks 12 and 16.
	HCT	Preemptive Strategy: Monitor weekly for CMV viremia by PCR (or antigenemia) for 3-6 months post transplant with consideration for more prolonged monitoring in patients at risk for late-onset CMV disease (chronic GVHD, requiring systemic treatment, patients receiving high-dose steroids, T-cell depleted or cord blood transplant recipients, and CD4 < 100 cells/mL). Start treatment with identification of CMV viremia or antigenemia as above. Consider prophylaxis (beginning post-engraftment) with **Valganciclovir** 900 mg po q24h. *National Comprehensive Cancer Network Guidelines on Prevention and Treatment of Cancer-Related Infections, Version 1.2013, Blood 113:5711, 2009, and Biol Blood Marrow Transpl 15:1143, 2009.*
Hepatitis B	SOT	For anti-viral agents with activity against HBV, see Table 14B, page 170 to 172. For discussion of prevention of HBV re-infection after transplantation and prevention of donor-derived infection see *Am J Transplant 9: S116, 2013*
	HCT	Patients who are anti-HBc positive and anti-HBs positive, but without evidence of active viral replication, can be monitored for ↑LFTs and presence of +HBV-DNA, and given pre-emptive therapy at that time. Alternatively, prophylactic anti-viral therapy can be given, commencing before transplant. (*See guidelines for other specific situations: Biol Blood Marrow Transpl 15:1143, 2009.*) These guidelines recommend Lamivudine 100 mg po q24h as an anti-viral.
Herpes simplex	SOT	**Acyclovir** 400 mg po bid, starting early post-transplant (*Clin Microbiol Rev 10:86, 1997*).
	HCT	**Acyclovir** 250 mg per meter-squared iv q12h **or Acyclovir** 400 mg to 800 mg po bid, from conditioning to engraftment or resolution or mucositis. For those requiring prolonged suppression of HSV, the higher dose (Acyclovir 800 mg po bid) is recommended to minimize the risk of emerging resistance.

* See page 2 for abbreviations

TABLE 16 (2)

PROPHYLACTIC REGIMENS

OPPORTUNISTIC INFECTION	TYPE OF TRANSPLANT	PROPHYLACTIC REGIMENS
Aspergillus spp.	SOT	Lung and heart/lung transplant: Inhaled **Amphotericin B** and/or a mold active oral azole are commonly used, but optimal regimen not defined. Aerosolized **Amphotericin B** 6 mg qbh (or 25 mg/day) OR aerosolized **LAB** 25 mg/day OR **Voriconazole** 200 mg po bid OR **Itraconazole** 200 mg po bid. 59% centers employ universal prophylaxis for 6 months in lung transplant recipients with 97% targeting Aspergillus. Most use Voriconazole alone or in combination with inhaled Amphotericin B *(Am J Transplant 11:361, 2011)*. Consider restarting prophylaxis during periods of intensified immune suppression. Liver transplant: Consider only in high-risk, re-transplant and/or those requiring renal-replacement therapy. Recommendations on aspergillus prophylaxis in SOT can be found at *(Am J Transplant 13:228, 2013)*.
	HCT/Heme malignancy	Indications for prophylaxis against aspergillus include AML and MDS with neutropenia and HCT with GVHD. Posaconazole 200 mg po tid approved this indication *(NEJM 356:335, 2007 and NEJM 356:348,2007)* Posaconazole ER tablets, also approved for prophylaxis (300 mg po BID x 1 day, then 300 daily). Retrospective analysis suggests that Voriconazole would have efficacy in steroid-treated patients with GVHD *(Bone Marrow Transpl 45:662, 2010)*, but is not approved for this indication. Amphotericin B and echinocandins are alternatives as well.
Candida spp.	SOT	Consider in select, high risk patients (liver, small bowel, pancreas). Consider in select, high-risk patients (re-transplants, dialysis). **Fluconazole** 400 mg daily for 4 weeks post-transplant. *(Amer J Transpl 13:200, 2013)*
	HCT	**Fluconazole** 400 mg po or iv once daily from day 0 to engraftment or when ANC consistently >1000, or **Posaconazole** solution 200 mg po tid or Posa ER tablets (300 mg po BID x 1 day, then 300 daily). Approved for high-risk patients (e.g., with GVHD or prolonged neutropenia), or Micafungin 50 mg iv once daily.
Coccidioides immitis	Any	**Fluconazole** 200-400 mg po q24h *(Transpl Int Dis 5:3, 2003; Am J Transpl 6:340, 2006)*. See *COID 21:45, 2008* for approach at one center in endemic area; e.g., Fluconazole 400 mg q24h for first year post-transplant, then 200 mg q24h thereafter. Fluconazole 400 mg q24h for positive serology without evidence of active infection.
Pneumocystis jiroveci	SOT	**TMP-SMX:** 1 single-strength tab po q24h or 1 double-strength tab po once daily for 3 to 7 days per week. Duration: kidney: 6 mos to 1 year *(Amer J Transpl 9 (suppl 3): S59, 2009)*; heart, lung, liver: ≥ 1 year to life-long *(Amer J Transpl 4 (suppl 10): 135, 2004)*.
	HCT	**TMP-SMX:** 1 single-strength tab po q24h or 1 double-strength tab po once daily or once a day for 3 days per week, from engraftment to ≥ 6 mos post-transplant.
Toxoplasma gondii	SOT	**TMP-SMX** (1 SS tab po q24h or 1 DS tab po once daily) x 3-7 days/wk for 6 mos post-transplant. (See *Clin Micro Infect 14:1089, 2008*).
	HCT	**TMP-SMX:** 1 single-strength tab po q24h or 1 double-strength tab po once daily or once a day for 3 days per week, from engraftment to ≥ 6 mos post transplant for seropositive allogeneic transplant recipients.
Trypanosoma cruzi	Heart	May be transmitted from organs or transfusions *(CID 48:1534, 2009)*. Inspect peripheral blood of suspected cases for parasites *(MMWR 55:798, 2006)*. Risk of reactivation during immunosuppression is variable *(JAMA 298:2171, 2007; JAMA 299:1134, 2008; J Cardiac Fail 15:249, 2000)*. If known Chagas disease in donor or recipient, contact CDC for treatment options *(phone 770-488-7775 or in emergency 770-488-7100). Am J Transplant 11:672, 2011*

* See page 2 for abbreviations

TABLE 17A – DOSAGE OF ANTIMICROBIAL DRUGS IN ADULT PATIENTS WITH RENAL IMPAIRMENT

- For listing of drugs with NO need for adjustment for renal failure, see *Table 17B*.
- Adjustments for renal failure are based on an estimate of creatinine clearance (CrCl) which reflects the glomerular filtration rate.
- **Different methods for calculating estimated CrCl are suggested for non-obese and obese patients.**
  - Calculations for ideal body weight (IBW) in kg:
    - **Men:** 50 kg plus 2.3 kg/inch over 60 inches height.
    - **Women:** 45 kg plus 2.3 kg/inch over 60 inches height.
  - Obese is defined as 20% over ideal body weight or body mass index (BMI) >30

- Calculations of estimated CrCl (*References, see (NEJM 354:2473, 2006 (non-obese), AJM 84:1053, 1988 (obese))*
  - **Non-obese patient**—
    - Calculate ideal body weight (IBW) in kg (as above)
    - Use the following formula to determine estimated CrCl

$$\frac{(140 \text{ minus age})(\text{IBW in kg})}{72 \times \text{serum creatinine}} = \begin{array}{l} \text{CrCl in mL/min for men.} \\ \text{Multiply answer by 0.85} \\ \text{for women (estimated)} \end{array}$$

  - **Obese patient**—
    - Weight ≥20% over IBW or BMI >30
    - Use the following formulas to determine estimated CrCl

$$\frac{(137 \text{ minus age}) \times [(0.285 \times \text{wt in kg}) + (12.1 \times \text{ht in meters}^2)]}{51 \times \text{serum creatinine}} = \text{CrCl (obese male)}$$

$$\frac{(146 \text{ minus age}) \times [(0.287 \times \text{wt in kg}) + (9.74 \times \text{ht in meters}^2)]}{60 \times \text{serum creatinine}} = \text{CrCl (obese female)}$$

- If estimated CrCl ≥90 mL/min, see *Tables 10A and 10D* for dosing.
- What weight should be used to calculate dosage on a mg/kg basis?
  - If less than 20% over IBW, use the patient's actual weight for all drugs.
  - **For obese patients** (≥20% over IBW or BMI >30):
    - **Aminoglycosides:** (IBW plus 0.4(actual weight minus IBW) = adjusted weight.
    - **Vancomycin:** actual body weight whether non-obese or obese.
    - **All other drugs:** insufficient data (*Pharmacotherapy 27:1081, 2007*).

- For slow or sustained extended daily dialysis (**SLEDD**) over 6-12 hours, adjust does as for CRRT. For details, see *CID 49:433, 2009; CCM 39:560, 2011.*
- General reference: Drug Prescribing in Renal Failure, 5th ed. Aronoff, et al. (eds) (*Amer College Physicians, 2007 and drug package inserts*).

TABLE 17A (2)

ANTIMICROBIAL	HALF-LIFE (NORMAL/ESRD) hr	DOSE FOR NORMAL RENAL FUNCTION	METHOD (see footer)	ADJUSTMENT FOR RENAL FAILURE — Estimated creatinine clearance (CrCl), mL/min			HEMODIALYSIS, CAPD	COMMENTS & DOSAGE FOR CRRT
				>50–90	10–50	<10		
ANTIBACTERIAL ANTIBIOTICS **Aminoglycoside Antibiotics: Traditional multiple daily doses—adjustment for renal disease**								
Amikacin	1.4–2.3/17–150	7.5 mg per kg q12h or 15 mg/kg once daily (see below)	I	7.5 mg/kg q12h	30–50: 7.5 mg/kg q24h; 10–50: 7.5 mg/kg q48h	7.5 mg/kg q72h	HEMO: 7.5 mg/kg AD. CAPD: 15–20 mg lost per L dialysate per day (see Comment)	**High flux hemodialysis** membranes lead to unpredictable aminoglycoside clearance; measure post-dialysis drug levels for efficacy and toxicity. With **CAPD**, pharmacokinetics highly variable—**check serum levels.** Usual method for CAPD: 2 liters of dialysis fluid placed qid or 8 liters per day (give 8&20 mg lost per L = 160 mg of amikacin supplement IV per day)
Gentamicin, Tobramycin (Monitor levels)	2–3/20–60	1.7 mg per kg q8h. Once daily dosing below	I	5–7 mg/kg once daily or 1.7–2.3 mg/kg q8h	1.7 mg/kg q12-48h / 2.3 mg/kg q8h — **Same dose for CRRT** See Comment for SLEDD dose	1.7 mg/kg q48-72h	HEMO: 3 mg/kg AD. Monitor levels. CAPD: 3–4 mg lost per L dialysate per day	Adjust dosing weight for obesity: [ideal body weight + 0.4 (actual body weight – ideal body weight)] (CID 25:112, 1997).
Netilmicin[NUS]	2–3/35–72	2 mg per kg q8h. Once daily dosing below	I	2 mg/kg q8h or 6.5 mg/kg once daily	2 mg/kg q12-24h — **Same dose for CRRT**	2 mg/kg q48h	HEMO 3 mg/kg AD CAPD: 3–4 mg lost per L dialysate per day	**Gent SLEDD dose** in critically ill: 6 mg IV q48h starting 30 min before start of SLEDD (daily SLEDD; q48h Gent). (AAC 54:3635, 2010).
Streptomycin	2–3/30–80	15 mg per kg (max. of 1 gm) q24h. Once daily dosing below	I	15 mg/kg q24h	15 mg/kg q24-72h — **Same dose for CRRT**	15 mg/kg q72-96h	HEMO: 7.5 mg/kg AD CAPD: 20–40 mg lost per L dialysate per day	

ONCE-DAILY AMINOGLYCOSIDE THERAPY: ADJUSTMENT IN RENAL INSUFFICIENCY (see Table 10D for OD dosing/normal renal function)

Creatinine Clearance (mL per min.) Drug	>80	60–80	40–60	30–40	20–30	10–20	<10
		Dose q24h (mg per kg)			Dose q48h (mg per kg)		Dose q72h and AD
Gentamicin/Tobramycin	5.1	4	3.5	2.5	4	3	2
Amikacin/Kanamycin/streptomycin	15	12	7.5	4	8	7.5	3
Isepamicin[NUS]	8	8	4	2.5	8		2
Netilmicin[NUS]	6.5	5	4	2	2.5	2	2

ANTIMICROBIAL	HALF-LIFE (NORMAL/ESRD) hr	DOSE FOR NORMAL RENAL FUNCTION	METHOD	>50–90	10–50	<10	HEMODIALYSIS, CAPD	COMMENTS & DOSAGE FOR CRRT
Carbapenem Antibiotics								
Doripenem	1/18	500 mg IV q8h	D&I	500 mg IV q8h	≥30–≤50: 250 mg IV q8h; >10–<30: 250 mg q12h	No data	HEMO: CAPD: No data	CRRT: 500 mg q8h (JAC 69:2508, 2014)
Ertapenem	4/>4	1 gm q24h	D	1 gm q24h	0.5 gm q24h (CrCl <30) CRRT: 1 gm q24h (AAC 58:1320, 2014)	0.5 gm q24h	HEMO: Dose as for CrCl <10; if dosed <6 hrs prior to HD, give 150 mg supplement AD	↑ potential for seizures if recommended doses exceeded in pts with CrCl <20 mL per min. See pkg insert, esp. for pts <70 kg
Imipenem (see Comment)	1/4	0.5 gm q6-8h	D&I	250–500 mg q6-8h	250 mg q8-12h Dose for CRRT: 0.5–1 gm q12h (AAC 49:2421, 2005)	125–250 mg q12h	HEMO: Dose AD CAPD: Dose for CrCl <10	
Meropenem	1/6–8	1 gm q8h	D&I	1 gm q8h	1 gm q12h **Same dose for CRRT**	0.5 gm q24h	HEMO: Dose AD CAPD: Dose for CrCl <10	

Abbreviation Key: Adjustment Method: **D** = dose adjustment; **I** = interval adjustment; **CAPD** = continuous ambulatory peritoneal dialysis; **CRRT** = continuous renal replacement therapy; **HEMO** = hemodialysis; **AD** = after dialysis; "**Supplement**" or "**Extra**" is to replace drug lost during dialysis – additional drug beyond continuation of regimen for CrCl < 10 mL/min.

TABLE 17A (3)

ANTIMICROBIAL	HALF-LIFE (NORMAL/ ESRD) hr	DOSE FOR NORMAL RENAL FUNCTION	METHOD (see footer)	ADJUSTMENT FOR RENAL FAILURE Estimated creatinine clearance (CrCl), mL/min			HEMODIALYSIS, CAPD	COMMENTS & DOSAGE FOR CRRT
				>50-90	10-50	<10		
ANTIBACTERIAL ANTIBIOTICS (continued)								
Cephalosporin Antibiotics: DATA ON SELECTED **PARENTERAL** CEPHALOSPORINS								
Cefazolin	1.9/40-70	1-2 gm q8h	I	q8h	q12h **Same dose for CRRT**	q24-48h	HEMO: Extra 0.5-1 gm AD CAPD: 0.5 gm q12h	
Cefepime	2.2/18	2 gm q8h (max. dose)	D&I	2 gm q8h	2 gm q12-24h **Same dose for CRRT**	1 gm q24h	HEMO: Extra 1 gm AD CAPD: 1-2 gm q48h	
Cefotaxime, Ceftizoxime	1.7/15-35	2 gm q8h	I	q8-12h	q12-24h **Same dose for CRRT**	q24h	HEMO: Extra 1 gm AD CAPD: 0.5-1 gm q24h	Active metabolite of cefotaxime in ESRD. ↓ dose further for hepatic & renal failure.
Cefotetan	3.5/13-25	1-2 gm q12h	D	100%	1-2 gm q24h **Same dose for CRRT**	1-2 gm q48h	HEMO: Extra 1 gm AD CAPD: 1 gm q24h	CRRT dose: 750 mg q12h
Cefoxitin	0.8/13-23	2 gm q8h	I	q8h	q8-12h **Same dose for CRRT**	q24-48h	HEMO: Extra 1 gm AD CAPD: 1 gm q24h	May falsely increase serum creatinine by interference with assay.
Ceftaroline	1.6/–	600 mg q12h	D	600 mg IV q12h	30-50: 400 mg q12h 15-30: 300 mg q12h	< 15: 200 mg q12h	HEMO: 200 mg q12h	1-hr infusion for all doses
Ceftazidime	1.2/13-25	2 gm q8h	I	q8-12h	q12-24h **Same dose for CRRT**	q24-48h	HEMO: Extra 1 gm AD CAPD: 0.5 gm q24h	Since 1/2 dose is dialyzed, post-dialysis dose is max of 3 gm.
Ceftobiprole	2.9-3.3/21	500 mg IV q8-12h	I	500 mg IV q8-12h	≥30 & ≤50: 500 mg q12h over 2 hrs ≥10 & <30: 250 mg q12h over 2 hrs **Same dose for CRRT**	No data	No data	
Cefuroxime sodium	1.2/17	0.75-1.5 gm q8h	I	q8h	q8-12h **Same dose for CRRT**	q24h	HEMO: Dose AD CAPD: Dose for CrCl <10	
Fluoroquinolone Antibiotics								
Ciprofloxacin	3-6/6-9	500-750 mg po (or 400 mg IV) q12h	D	100%	50-75% CRRT 400 mg IV q24h	50%	HEMO: 250 mg po or 200 mg IV q12h CAPD: 250 mg po or 200 mg IV q8h	
Gatifloxacin[NUS]	7-14/11-40	400 mg po/IV q24h	D	400 mg q24h	400 mg, then 200 mg q24h Same dose for CRRT	400 mg, then 200 mg q24h	HEMO: 200 mg q24h AD CAPD: 200 mg q24h	
Gemifloxacin	7/>7	320 mg po q24h	D	320 mg q24h	160 mg q24h	160 mg q24h	HEMO: 160 mg q24h AD CAPD: 160 mg q24h	
Levofloxacin	6-8/76	750 mg q24h IV, PO	D&I	750 mg q48h	20-49: 750 mg q48h	<20: 750 mg once, then 500 mg q48h	HEMO/CAPD: Dose for CrCl <20	CRRT 750 mg once, then 500 mg q48h, although not FDA-approved.
Ofloxacin	7/28-37	200-400 mg q12h	D	200-400 mg q12h	200-400 mg q24h **Same dose for CRRT**	200 mg q24h	HEMO: Dose for CrCl <10, AD CAPD: 300 mg q24h	
Macrolide Antibiotics								
Clarithromycin	5-7/22	500-1000 mg q12h	D	500 mg q12h	500 mg q12-24h	500 mg q24h	HEMO: Dose AD CAPD: None	CRRT as for CrCl 10-50
Erythromycin	1.4/5-6	250-500 mg q6h	D	100%	100%	50-75%	HEMO/CAPD/CRRT: None	Ototoxicity with high doses in ESRD

Abbreviation Key: Adjustment Method: **D** = dose adjustment; **I** = interval adjustment; **CAPD** = continuous ambulatory peritoneal dialysis; **CRRT** = continuous renal replacement therapy; **"Supplement"** or **"Extra"** is to replace drug lost during dialysis – additional drug beyond continuation of regimen for CrCl < 10 mL/min.
HEMO = hemodialysis; **AD** = after dialysis.

TABLE 17A (4)

ANTIMICROBIAL	HALF-LIFE (NORMAL/ESRD) hr	DOSE FOR NORMAL RENAL FUNCTION	METHOD (see footer)	ADJUSTMENT FOR RENAL FAILURE — Estimated creatinine clearance (CrCl), mL/min			HEMODIALYSIS, CAPD	COMMENTS & DOSAGE FOR CRRT
				>50-90	10-50	<10		
ANTIBACTERIAL ANTIBIOTICS (continued)								
Miscellaneous Antibacterial Antibiotics								
Colistin (Polymyxin E) Based on 105 pts (AAC 55:3284, 2011). All doses refer to Colistin "base" in mg	<6/>48	See Table 10A, page 104 for loading dose and maintenance dose	D & I	$3.5 \times [(1.5 \times CrCln) + 30] \times$ (pt BSA in m2/1.73m³) = total daily dose of Colistin base. Divide and give q12h. CrCln = normalized CrCl based on body surface area (BSA): Pt BSA in m²/1.73m².			**Intermittent Hemodialysis:** • Calculation of dose: 3.5 (30) = 105 mg. (CrCl is zero). On days with no hemodialysis, give total daily dose of 105 mg divided bid. • On dialysis days, need to supplement the dose by 50 % due to colistimethate filtration by the dialysis membrane. • So, on dialysis days the total dose is 150 mg; divide and give half the dose during the last hour of hemodialysis and the second half 12 hours later.	**CAPD:** • 160 mg q24h (unable to locate modern CAPD data) **CRRT:** • For average serum steady state concentration of 3.5 μg/mL, the total daily dose is 672 mg; the dose is divided and given q12h. **The dose is necessarily high due to removal of drug by the dialysis membranes.** Rationale: 3.5 μg/mL as the targeted serum level X 192 mg for each 1 μg/mL of targeted serum level = total daily dose, i.e., 3.5 x 192 = 672. See AAC 55: 3284, 2011 for data.
Dalbavancin	150-260/-	1000 mg x 1, then 500 mg one wk later	D	No change	<30: 750 mg x 1, then 375 mg 1 wk later		Regularly scheduled HEMO: No adjustment	
Daptomycin	9.4/30	4-6 mg per kg per day	I	4-6 mg per kg per day	CrCl <30, 6 mg per kg q48h (CCM 39:19, 2011)	CRRT: 8 mg/kg q48h (AAC 39/19, 2011)	**HEMO & CAPD:** 6 mg per kg q48h (during or after q48h dialysis if possible). If next planned dialysis is 72 hrs away, give 9 mg/kg (AAC 57:864, 2013; JAC 69:200,2014).	
Linezolid	5-6/6-8	600 mg po/IV q12h	None	600 mg q12h	600 mg q12h **Same dose for CRRT**	600 mg q12h AD	**HEMO & CAPD:** As for CrCl <10. CAPD & CRRT: No dose adjustment	Accumulation of 2 metabolites—risk unknown (JAC 56:172, 2005)
Metronidazole	6-14/7-21	7.5 mg per kg q6h	D	100%	100% **Same dose for CRRT**	50%	HEMO: Dose as for CrCl <10 AD. CAPD: Dose for CrCl <10	
Nitrofurantoin	0.5/1	50-100 mg	D	100%	Avoid	Avoid	Not applicable	
Sulfamethoxazole (SMX)	10/20-50	1 gm q8h	I	q12h	q18h Same dose for CAVH	q24h	HEMO: Extra 1 gm AD. CAPD: 1 gm q24h	
Teicoplanin^NUS	45/62-230	6 mg per kg per day	I	q24h	q48h **Same dose for CRRT**	q72h	HEMO: Dose for CrCl <10. CAPD: Dose for CrCl <10	
Telithromycin	10/15	800 mg q24h	D	800 mg q24h	600 mg q24h	600 mg q24h (<30 mL per min.)	HEMO: 600 mg AD. CAPD: No data	
Telavancin	7-8/17.9	10 mg/kg q24h	D&I	10 mg/kg q24h	30-50: 7.5 mg/kg q24h <30: 10 mg/kg q48h	<30: 10 mg/kg q48h	No data	If CrCl <30, reduce dose to 600 mg once daily. If both liver and renal failure, dose is 400 mg once daily
Temocillin		1-2 gm q12h	I	1-2 gm q12h	1-2 gm q24h	1 gm q48h	HEMO: 1 gm q48h AD. CAPD: 1 gm q8h	No data

Abbreviation Key: Adjustment Method: **D** = dose adjustment; **I** = interval adjustment; **CAPD** = continuous ambulatory peritoneal dialysis; **CRRT** = continuous renal replacement therapy; **HEMO** = hemodialysis; **AD** = after dialysis; "**Supplement**" or "**Extra**" is to replace drug lost during dialysis – additional drug beyond continuation of regimen for CrCl < 10 mL/min.

TABLE 17A (5)

ANTIMICROBIAL	HALF-LIFE (NORMAL/ ESRD) hr	DOSE FOR NORMAL RENAL FUNCTION	METHOD (see footer)	ADJUSTMENT FOR RENAL FAILURE Estimated creatinine clearance (CrCl), mL/min			HEMODIALYSIS, CAPD	COMMENTS & DOSAGE FOR CRRT
				>50-90	10-50	<10		
ANTIBACTERIAL ANTIBIOTICS *(continued)*								
Trimethoprim (TMP)	11/20-49	100-200 mg q12h	I	q12h	**>30:** q12h; **10-30:** q18h; **Same dose for CRRT**	q24h	HEMO: Dose AD CAPD: q24h	CRRT dose: q18h
Trimethoprim-sulfamethoxazole-DS (Doses based on TMP component)								
Treatment (based on TMP component)	As for TMP	5-20 mg/kg/day divided q6-12h	I	No dose adjustment	**30-50:** No dose adjustment **10-29:** Reduce dose by 50%	Not recom- mended; but if used: 5-10 mg/kg q24h	Not recommended; but if used: 5-10 mg/kg q24h AD CRRT: 5-7.5 mg/kg q8h	
TMP-SMX Prophylaxis	As for TMP	1 tab po q24h or 3 times per week	No change	100%	100%	100%		
Vancomycin[1]	6/200-250	1 gm q12h	D&I	15-30 mg/kg q12h	15 mg/kg q24-96h	7.5 mg/kg q2-3 days	HEMO: For trough conc of 15-20 μg/mL, give 15 mg/kg if next dialysis in 1 day; give 25 mg/kg if next dialysis in 2 days; give 35 mg/kg if next dialysis in 3 days (CID 53:124, 2011)	CAVH/CVVH: 500 mg q24-48h. New hemodialysis membranes ↑ clear. of vanco; **check levels**
Penicillins								
Amoxicillin Ampicillin	1/5-20 1/7-20	250-500 mg q8h 250 mg-2 gm q6h	I I	q8h q6h	q8-12h q6-12h	q12-24h q12-24h	HEMO: Dose AD CAPD: 250 mg q12h	
Amoxicillin/ Clavulanate[2]	1.3 AM/1 5-20/4	500/125 mg q8h (see Comments)	D&I	500/125 mg q8h	250-500 mg AM component q12h	250-500 mg AM component q24h	HEMO: As for CrCl <10; extra dose after dialysis	**If CrCl <30 per mL, do not use 875/125 or 1000/62.5 AM/CL**
Amoxicillin ext. rel. tabs	1.5/?	775 mg once daily		Once daily	CrCl <30, no data, avoid usage			
Ampicillin (AM)/ Sulbactam(SB)	1 (AM)/1 (SB) 9 (AM)/10 (SB)	2 gm AM + 1 gm SB q6h	I	q6h	q8-12h	q24h	HEMO: Dose AD CAPD: 2 gm AM/1 gm SB q24h	CRRT dose: 1.5 AM/0.75 SB q12h
Aztreonam	2/6-8	2 gm q8h	D	100%	50-75%	25%	HEMO: Extra 0.5 gm AD CAPD: Dose for CrCl <10	Technically is a β-lactam antibiotic.
Penicillin G	0.5/6-20	0.5-4 million U q4h	D	0.5-4 million U q4h	0.5-4 million U q6h	0.5-4 million U q12h	HEMO: Dose AD CAPD: Dose for CrCl <10	1.7 mEq potassium per million units. ↑s potential of seizure. 10 million units per day max. dose in ESRD
Piperacillin	1/3.3-5.1	3-4 gm q4-6h	I	q4-6h	q6-8h; **Same dose for CRRT**	q8h	HEMO: 2 gm q8h plus 1 gm extra AD CAPD: Dose for CrCl <10	1.9 mEq sodium per gm

[1] If renal failure, use EMIT assay to measure levels; levels overestimated by RIA or fluorescent immunoassay.

[2] Clavulanate cleared by liver, not kidney. Hence as dose of combination decreased, a deficiency of clavulanate may occur (*JAMA 285:386, 2001*).

Abbreviation Key: Adjustment Method: **D** = dose adjustment; **I** = interval adjustment; "**Supplement**" or "**Extra**" is to replace drug lost during dialysis – additional drug beyond continuation of regimen for CrCl < 10 mL/min.
HEMO = hemodialysis; **AD** = after dialysis; **CAPD** = continuous ambulatory peritoneal dialysis; **CRRT** = continuous renal replacement therapy;

TABLE 17A (6)

ANTIMICROBIAL	HALF-LIFE (NORMAL/ESRD) hr	DOSE FOR NORMAL RENAL FUNCTION	METHOD (see footer)	ADJUSTMENT FOR RENAL FAILURE — Estimated creatinine clearance (CrCl), mL/min >50-90	10-50	<10	HEMODIALYSIS, CAPD	COMMENTS & DOSAGE FOR CRRT
ANTIBACTERIAL ANTIBIOTICS *(continued)*								
Pip (P)/Tazo(T)	0.71-1.2 (both)/2-6	3.375 – 4.5 gm q6-8h	D&I	100%	2.25 gm q6h <20: 2.25 gm q8h Same dose for CRRT	2.25 gm q8h	HEMO: Dose for CrCl <10 + extra 0.75 gm AD CAPD: 4.5 gm q12h; CRRT: 2.25 gm q8h	
Ticarcillin	1.2/13	3 gm q4h	D&I	1-2 gm q4h	1-2 gm q8h Same dose for CRRT	1-2 gm q12h	HEMO: Extra 3.0 gm AD CAPD: Dose for CrCl <10	5.2 mEq sodium per gm
Ticarcillin/ Clavulanate[2]	1.2/11-16	3.1 gm q4h	D&I	3.1 gm q4h	3.1 gm q8-12h Same dose for CRRT	2 gm q12h	HEMO: Extra 3.1 gm AD CAPD: 3.1 gm q12h	See footnote[a]
Tetracycline Antibiotics								
Tetracycline	6-10/57-108	250-500 mg qid	I	q8-12h	q12-24h Same dose for CRRT	q24h	HEMO/CAPD/CAVH: None	Avoid in ESRD
ANTIFUNGAL ANTIBIOTICS								
Amphotericin B & Lipid-based ampho B	24h-15 days/unchanged	Non-lipid: 0.4-1 mg/kg/day ABLC: 5 mg/kg/day LAB: 3-5 mg/kg/day	I	q24h	q24h Same dose for CRRT	q24h	HEMO/CAPD/CRRT: No dose adjustment	For ampho B, toxicity lessened by saline loading; risk amplified by concomitant cyclosporine A, aminoglycosides, or pentamidine
Fluconazole	37/100	100-400 mg q24h	D	100%	50%	50%	HEMO: 100% of recommended dose AD CAPD: Dose for CrCl <10	CRRT: 200-400 mg q24h
Flucytosine	3-6/75-200	37.5 mg per kg q6h	I	q6h	q12h Same dose for CRRT	q24h	HEMO: Dose AD CAPD: 0.5-1 gm q24h	Goal is peak serum level >25 mcg per mL and <100 mcg per mL
Itraconazole, po soln	21/25	100-200 mg q12h	D	100%	100% Same dose for CRRT	50%	HEMO/CAPD oral solution: 100 mg q12-24h	HEMO/CAPD (cyclodextrin). Switch to po or DC
Itraconazole, IV	21/25	200 mg IV q12h		200 mg IV bid	Do not use IV titra if CrCl <30 due to accumulation of carrier: cyclodextrin			
Posaconazole, IV	20-66/ND	300 mg IV q24h		300 mg IV q24h	Not recommended due to accumulation of IV vehicle (SBECD); consider switch to po rx			
Terbinafine	36-200?	250 mg po per day		Use has not been studied. Recommend avoidance of drug.				
Voriconazole, IV	Non-linear kinetics	6 mg per kg IV q12h times then 4 mg per kg q12h	I	No change	If CrCl <50 mL per min. accum. of IV vehicle (cyclodextrin). Switch to po or DC For CRRT: 4 mg/kg po q12h			
ANTIPARASITIC ANTIBIOTICS								
Pentamidine	3-12/73-18	4 mg per kg per day	I	q24h	q24h Same dose for CRRT	q24-36h	HEMO: 4 mg/kg q48h AD CAPD: Dose for CrCl <10	
Quinine	5-16/5-16	650 mg q8h	I	650 mg q8h	650 mg q8-12h Same dose for CRRT	650 mg q24h	HEMO: Dose AD CAPD: Dose for CrCl <10	Marked tissue accumulation

TABLE 17A (7)

ANTIMICROBIAL	HALF-LIFE (NORMAL/ESRD) hr	DOSE FOR NORMAL RENAL FUNCTION	METHOD (see footer)	ADJUSTMENT FOR RENAL FAILURE Estimated creatinine clearance (CrCl), mL/min			HEMODIALYSIS, CAPD	COMMENTS & DOSAGE FOR CRRT
				>50-90	10-50	<10		
ANTITUBERCULOUS ANTIBIOTICS *(See http://11ntcc.ucsd.edu/TB)*								
Amikacin/ Streptomycin (see page 205)								
Bedaquiline	24-30	400 mg po qd x 2 wks, then 200 mg tiw x 22 wks		No adjustment for mild-moderate renal impairment; **use with caution if severe renal impairment or ESRD**				
Capreomycin		15 mg/kg q24h	I	15 mg/kg q24h	15 mg/kg q24h CRRT: 25 mg/kg q24h (max 2.5 gm q24h)	15 mg/kg AD 3x/wk	HEMO: 15 mg/kg AD 3x/wk	
Cycloserine		10-15 mg/kg/day in 2 div doses	I	10-15 mg/kg/day in 2 div doses	CrCl 10-20: 10-15 mg/kg q12-24h	10-15 mg/kg q24h	HEMO: 10-15 mg/kg AD 3x/wk	
Ethambutol	4/7-15	15-25 mg per kg q24h	I	15-25 mg/kg q24h	**CrCl 30-50:** 15 mg/kg q24-36h **For CrCl 10-20:** 15-25 mg/kg q24-48h	15-25 mg/kg q48h	HEMO: 20 mg/kg 3x/wk AD CAPD: 25 mg/kg q48h	If possible, do serum levels on dialysis pts
Ethionamide	2/9	250-500 mg q12h	D	500 mg bid	500 mg bid	250 mg bid	HEMO/CAPD/CRRT: No dosage adjustment	
Isoniazid	0.7-4/8-17	5 mg per kg per day (max. 300 mg)	D	100%	100%	100%	HEMO: Dose AD CAPD: Dose for CrCl <10	
Pyrazinamide	9/26	25 mg per kg q24h (max. dose 2.5 gm q24h)	D	25 mg/kg q24h	**CrCl 21-90:** 25 mg/kg q24h **Same dose for CRRT** **For CrCl 10-20:** 25 mg/kg q48h **Same dose for CRRT**	12-25 mg per kg 3x/wk	HEMO: 25 mg/kg 3x/wk AD CAPD: No reduction	
Rifampin	1.5-5/1.8-11	600 mg per day	D	600 mg q24h	300-600 mg q24h	300-600 mg q24h	HEMO: No adjustment CAPD: Dose for CrCl <10	Biologically active metabolite
ANTIVIRAL/ANTIRETROVIRAL AGENTS								
Acyclovir, IV	2-4/20	5-12.4 mg per kg q8h	D&I	100% q8h	100% q12-24h	50% q24h	HEMO: Dose AD CAPD: Dose for CrCl <10	Rapid IV infusion can cause ↑ Cr. CRRT dose: 5-10 mg/kg q24h
Adefovir	7.5/15	10 mg po q24h	I	10 mg q24h	10 mg q48-72h[3]	10 mg q72h[3]	HEMO: 10 mg q week AD	CAPD: No data; CRRT: Dose?
Amantadine	12/500	100 mg po bid	I	q12h	q24-48h	q 7 days	HEMO/CAPD: Dose for CrCl <10/	CRRT: Dose for CrCl 10-50
Atripla	See each drug	200 mg emtricitabine + 300 mg tenofovir + 600 mg efavirenz	I	Do not use if CrCl <50				

Cidofovir: **Complicated dosing**—see package insert

[3] Ref: *Transplantation* 80:1086, 2005

Abbreviation Key: Adjustment Method: **D** = dose adjustment; **I** = interval adjustment; **D** = dose adjustment; **AD** = after dialysis; **"Supplement"** or **"Extra"** is to replace drug lost during dialysis – additional drug beyond continuation of dialysis
HEMO = hemodialysis; **CAPD** = continuous ambulatory peritoneal dialysis; **CRRT** = continuous renal replacement therapy; continuation of regimen for CrCl < 10 mL/min.

TABLE 17A (8)

ANTIMICROBIAL	HALF-LIFE (NORMAL/ ESRD) hr	DOSE FOR NORMAL RENAL FUNCTION	METHOD (see footer)	ADJUSTMENT FOR RENAL FAILURE Estimated creatinine clearance (CrCl), mL/min			HEMODIALYSIS, CAPD	COMMENTS & DOSAGE FOR CRRT
				>50-90	10-50	<10		
ANTIVIRAL/ANTIRETROVIRAL AGENTS *(continued)*								
Induction	2.5/unknown	5 mg per kg once per wk for 2 wks	–	Contraindicated in pts with CrCl < 55 mL/min.				Major toxicity is renal. No efficacy, safety, or pharmacokinetic data in pts with moderate/severe renal disease.
Maintenance	2.5/unknown	5 mg per kg q2wks	–	Contraindicated in pts with CrCl < 55 mL/min.				
Didanosine tablets[a]	0.6–1.6/4.5	125–200 mg q12h buffered tabs	D	200 mg q12h	200 mg q24h	<60 kg: 150 mg q24h; >60 kg 100 mg q24h	HEMO/CAPD/CRRT: Dose for CrCl <10	Based on incomplete data. Data are estimates.
		400 mg q24h enteric-coated tabs	D	400 mg q24h	125–200 mg q24h	**Do not use EC tabs**	HEMO/CAPD: Dose for CrCl <10	**If <60 kg & CrCl <10 mL per min, do not use EC tabs**
Emtricitabine (CAPS)	10/>10	200 mg q24h	I	200 mg q24h	200 mg q48h	200 mg q96h	HEMO: Dose for CrCl <10	*See package insert for oral solution.*
Emtricitabine + Tenofovir	See each drug	No change		No change	**30–49:** 200 mg q48h; **10–29:** 200 mg q72h	**CrCl <30:** Do not use	HEMO/CAPD: 0.05 mg q24h	Give after dialysis on dialysis days
Entecavir	128–149/?	0.5 mg q24h	D	0.5 mg q24h	**30–50:** 1 tab q48h; **10–30:** 0.15–0.25 mg q24h	0.05 mg q24h	HEMO/CAPD: 0.05 mg q24h	
Famciclovir	2.3–3/10–22	500 mg q8h	D&I	500 mg q8h	500 mg q12–24h	250 mg q24h	HEMO: Dose AD; CAPD: No data	CRRT: Not applicable
Foscarnet (CMV dosage). Dosage adjustment based on est. CrCl divided by wt (Kg)	Normal half-life (T½) 3 hrs with terminal T½ of 18-88 hrs. T½ very long with ESRD							*See package insert for further details.*

CrCl (mL/min per kg body weight—only for Foscarnet)

	METHOD	>1.4	>1-1.4	>0.8-1	>0.6-0.8	>0.5-0.6	>0.4-0.5	<0.4
Induction: 60 mg/kg IV q8h x 2-3 wks	D&I	60 q8h	45 q8h	50 q12h	40 q12h	60 q24h	50 q24h	Do not use
Maintenance: 90-120 mg/day IV	D&I	120 q24h	90 q24h	65 q24h	105 q48h	80 q48h	65 q48h	Do not use

ANTIMICROBIAL	HALF-LIFE (NORMAL/ ESRD) hr	DOSE FOR NORMAL RENAL FUNCTION	METHOD	>50-90	10-50	<10	HEMODIALYSIS, CAPD	COMMENTS & DOSAGE FOR CRRT
Ganciclovir IV:	3.6/30	Induction 5 mg per kg q12h IV	D&I	**70-90:** 5 mg per kg q12h; **50-60:** 2.5 mg per kg q12h	**25-49:** 2.5 mg per kg q24h; **10-24:** 1.25 mg/kg q24h	1.25 mg per kg 3 times per wk	HEMO: Dose AD; CAPD: Dose for CrCl <10	Continuous venovenous hemodiafiltration: 2.5 mg/kg IV once daily (AAC 58:94, 2014)
		Maintenance 5 mg per kg q24h IV	D&I	2.5–5.0 mg per kg q24h	0.6-1.25 mg per kg q24h	0.625 mg per kg 3 times per week	HEMO: 0.6 mg per kg AD; CAPD: Dose for CrCl <10	
po:		1 gm tid po	D&I	0.5-1 gm tid	0.5-1 gm q24h	0.5 gm 3 times per week	HEMO: 0.5 gm AD	
Maraviroc	14-18/No data	300 mg bid	D&I	300 mg bid		300 mg q24h	HEMO: 300 mg q24h	Risk of side effects increased if concomitant CYP3A inhibitor
Lamivudine	5-7/15-35	300 mg po q24h	D&I	300 mg po q24h	50-150 mg q24h	25-50 mg q24h	HEMO q24h; CAPD: Dose for CrCl<10	CRRT: 100 mg 1st day, then 50 mg/day

[a] Ref. for NRTIs and NNRTIs: *Kidney International 60:821, 2001*

Abbreviation Key: Adjustment Method: **D** = dose adjustment; **I** = interval adjustment; **D&I** = dose and interval adjustment. "**Supplement**" or "**Extra**" is to replace drug lost during dialysis – additional drug beyond continuation of regimen for CrCl < 10 mL/min.
HEMO = hemodialysis; **AD** = after dialysis; **CAPD** = continuous ambulatory peritoneal dialysis; **CRRT** = continuous renal replacement therapy;

TABLE 17A (9)

ANTIMICROBIAL	HALF-LIFE (NORMAL/ ESRD) hr	DOSE FOR NORMAL RENAL FUNCTION	METHOD (see footer)	ADJUSTMENT FOR RENAL FAILURE Estimated creatinine clearance (CrCl), mL/min			HEMODIALYSIS, CAPD	COMMENTS & DOSAGE FOR CRRT
				>50-90	10-50	<10		
ANTIVIRAL/ANTIRETROVIRAL AGENTS (continued)								
Oseltamivir, therapy	6-10/>20	75 mg po bid – treatment	I	75 mg q12h	**30-50:** 75 mg bid **<30:** 75 mg once daily	No data	HEMO: 30 mg qd non-dialysis days[5]; CAPD: 30 mg once per week	Dose for prophylaxis if CrCl <30: 75 mg once daily CRRT: 75 mg po bid
Peramivir		600 mg once daily	P&I	600 mg q24h	**31-49:** 200 mg q24h **10-30:** 100 mg q24h	100 mg (single dose) then 15 mg q24h	HEMO: 100 mg (single dose) then 100 mg 2 hrs AD (dialysis days only)	CRRT: http://www.cdc.gov/h1n1flu/eva/peramivir.htm
Ribavirin	Use with caution in patients with creatinine clearance <50 mL per min.							
Rimantadine, po	13-65/Prolonged	100 mg bid po	I	100 mg bid	100 mg q24h-bid	100 mg q24h	HEMO/CAPD: No data	Use with caution, little data
Stavudine, po	1-1.4/5.5-8	30-40 mg q12h	D&I	100%	50% q12-24h	≥60 kg: 20 mg per day <60 kg: 15 mg per day	HEMO: Dose as for CrCl <10 AD CAPD: No data CRRT: Full dose	
Stribild		1 tab daily	I	If CrCl <70: contraindicated	If CrCl < 50: discontinue			
Telbivudine	40-49/No data	600 mg po daily	I	600 mg q24h	**30-49:** 600 mg q48H **<30:** 600 mg q72h	600 mg q96h	HEMO: As for CrCl <10 AD	
Tenofovir, po	17/?	300 mg q24h	I	300 mg q24h	**30-49:** 300 mg q48h **10-29:** 300 mg q72-96h	No data	HEMO: 300 mg q7d or after 12 hrs of HEMO.[5]	
Valacyclovir	2.5-3.3/14	1 gm q8h	D&I	1 gm q8h	1 gm q12-24h	0.5 gm q24h	HEMO: Dose AD CAPD: Dose for CrCl <10	CAVH dose: As for CrCl 10-50
Valganciclovir	4/67	900 mg po bid	D&I	900 mg q24h	450 mg q24h to 450 mg every other day	DO NOT USE	See package insert	
Zalcitabine	2/>8	0.75 mg bid	D&I	0.75 mg q8h	0.75 mg q12h **Same dose for CRRT**	0.75 mg q24h	HEMO: Dose AD CAPD: No data	CRRT dose: As for CrCl 10-50
Zidovudine	1.1-1.4/1.4-3	300 mg q12h	D&I	300 mg q12h	300 mg q12h **Same dose for CRRT**	100 mg q8h	HEMO: Dose for CrCl <10 AD CAPD: Dose for CrCl <10	

[5] HEMO wt-based dose adjustments for children age >1 yr (dose after each HEMO): ≤15 kg: 7.5 mg; 16-23 kg: 10 mg; 24-40 kg: 15 mg; > 40 kg: 30 mg (CID 50:127, 2010).
[6] Acute renal failure and Fanconi syndrome reported.

Abbreviation Key. Adjustment Method: **D** = dose adjustment; **I** = interval adjustment; **D&I** = dose adjustment; **"Supplement"** or **"Extra"** is to replace drug lost during dialysis – additional drug beyond continuation of regimen for CrCl < 10 mL/min.
CAPD = continuous ambulatory peritoneal dialysis; **CRRT** = continuous renal replacement therapy;
HEMO = hemodialysis; **AD** = after dialysis.

TABLE 17B – NO DOSAGE ADJUSTMENT WITH RENAL INSUFFICIENCY BY CATEGORY

Antibacterials		Antifungals	Anti-TBc	Antivirals	
Azithromycin	Minocycline	Anidulafungin	Bedaquiline	Abacavir	
Ceftriaxone	Moxifloxacin	Caspofungin	Ethionamide	Atazanavir	Nelfinavir
Chloramphenicol	Nafcillin	Itraconazole oral solution	Isoniazid	Darunavir	Nevirapine
Ciprofloxacin XL	Oritavancin	Ketoconazole	Rifampin	Delavirdine	Raltegravir
Clindamycin	Polymyxin B	Micafungin	Rifabutin	Efavirenz	Ribavirin
Doxycycline	Pyrimethamine	Posaconazole, **po only**	Rifapentine	Enfuvirtide[1]	Saquinavir
Linezolid	Rifaximin	Voriconazole, **po only**		Fosamprenavir	Simeprevir[2]
	Tedizolid			Indinavir	Sofosbuvir[2]
	Tigecycline			Lopinavir	Tipranavir

[1] Enfuvirtide: Not studied in patients with CrCl <35 mL/min. DO NOT USE
[2] No data for CrCl <30 mL/min

TABLE 17C – ANTIMICROBIAL DOSING IN OBESITY

The number of obese patients is increasing. Intuitively, the standard doses of some drugs may not achieve effective serum concentrations. Pertinent data on anti-infective dosing in the obese patient is gradually emerging. Though some of the data needs further clarification, the following table reflects what is currently known. **Obesity is defined as ≥ 20% over Ideal Body Weight (Ideal BW) or Body Mass Index (BMI) > 30. Dose =** suggested body weight (BW) for dose calculation in obese patient, or specific dose if applicable. In general, the absence of a drug in the table indicates a lack of pertinent information in the published literature.

Drug	Dose	Comments
Acyclovir	Use **Ideal BW** Example: for HSV encephalitis, give 10 mg/kg of Ideal BW q8h	Unpublished data from 7 obese volunteers (*Davis, et al., ICAAC abstract, 1991*).
Aminoglycosides	Use **Adjusted BW** Example: Critically ill patient, Gentamicin or Tobramycin (not Amikacin) 7 mg/kg of Adjusted BW IV q24h (See Comment)	Adjusted BW = Ideal BW + 0.4(Actual BW – Ideal BW). Ref: *Pharmacother 27:1081, 2007.* Follow levels so as to lower dose once hemodynamics stabilize.
Cefazolin (surgical prophylaxis)	No dose adjustment needed: 2 gm x 1 dose (repeat in 3 hours?)	Conflicting data; unclear whether dose should be repeated, or if an even higher dose is required. Patients with BMI 40-80 studied. Refs: *Surg 136:738, 2004; Eur J Clin Pharmacol 67:985, 2011; Surg Infect 13:33, 2012.*
Cefepime	Modest dose increase: 2 gm IV q8h instead of the usual q12h	Data from 10 patients (mean BMI 48) undergoing bariatric surgery; regimen yields free T > MIC of 60% for MIC of 8 μg/mL. Ref: *Obes Surg 22:465, 2012.*
Daptomycin	Use **Actual BW** Example: 4-12 mg/kg of Actual BW IV q24h	Data from a single-dose PK study in 7 obese volunteers. Ref: *Antimicrob Ag Chemother 51:2741, 2007.*
Flucytosine	Use **Ideal BW** Example: Crypto meningitis, give 25 mg/kg of Ideal BW po q6h	Date from one obese patient with cryptococcal disease. Ref: *Pharmacother 15:251, 1995.*
Levofloxacin	**No dose adjustment** required Example: 750 mg po/IV q24h	Data from 13 obese patients; variability in study findings renders conclusion uncertain. Refs: *Antimicrob Ag Chemother 55:3240, 2011; J Antimicrob Chemother 66:1653, 2011.*
Linezolid	**No dose adjustment required** Example: 600 mg po/IV q12h	Data from 20 obese volunteers up to 150 kg body weight suggest standard doses provide AUC values similar to nonobese subjects. In a recent case report, standard dosing in a 265 kg male with MRSA pneumonia seemed to have reduced clinical effectiveness. Refs: *Antimicrob Ag Chemother 57:1144, 2013; Ann Pharmacother 47: e25, 2013.*
Moxifloxacin	**No dose adjustment** required Example: 400 mg po/IV q24h	Data from 12 obese patients undergoing gastric bypass. Ref: *J Antimicrob Chemother 66:2330, 2011.*
Oseltamivir	**No dose adjustment** required Example: 75 mg po q12h	Data from 10 obese volunteers, unclear if applicable to patients >250 kg (OK to give 150 mg po q12h). Ref: *J Antimicrob Chemother 66:2083, 2011.*
Piperacillin-tazobactam	6.75 gm IV over 4 hours and dosed every 8 hours. No data for pt with impaired renal function	Data need confirmation. Based on 14 obese patients with actual BW >130 kg and BMI >40 kg/m². Ref: *Int J Antimicrob Ag 41:52, 2013.* High dose to optimize dose for pathogens with MIC ≤16 mcg/mL. May enhance bleeding propensity in uremic patients.

[1] Ref. for NRTIs and NNRTIs: *Kidney International 60:821, 2001*

See page 2 for other abbreviations

TABLE 17C (2)

Drug	Dose	Comments
Vancomycin	Use **Actual BW** Example: in critically ill patient give 25-30 mg/kg of Actual BW IV load, then 15-20 mg/kg of Actual BW IV q8h-12h (infuse over 1.5-2 hr). No single dose over 2 gm. Check trough levels.	Data from 24 obese patients; Vancomycin half-life appears to decrease with little change in Vd. Ref: *Eur J Clin Pharmacol* 54:621, 1998.
Voriconazole po	**No dose adjustment** required Example: 400 mg po q12h x2 doses then 200 mg po q12h. Check trough concentrations (underdosing common with Voriconazole).	Data from a 2-way crossover study of oral voriconazole in 8 volunteers suggest no adjustment required, but data from one patient suggest use of adjusted BW. Recommended IV voriconazole dose based on actual BW (no supporting data). Refs: *Antimicrob Ag Chemother* 55:2601, 2011; *Clin Infect Dis* 53:745, 2011.

TABLE 18 – ANTIMICROBIALS AND HEPATIC DISEASE: DOSAGE ADJUSTMENT*

The following alphabetical list indicates antibacterials excreted/metabolized by the liver **wherein a dosage adjustment may be indicated** in the presence of hepatic disease. Space precludes details; consult the PDR or package inserts for details. List is **not** all-inclusive:

Antibacterials		Antifungals	Antivirals[§]	
Ceftriaxone	Nafcillin	Caspofungin	Abacavir	Indinavir
Chloramphenicol	Rifabutin	Itraconazole	Atazanavir	Lopinavir/ritonavir
Clindamycin	Rifampin	Voriconazole	Darunavir	Nelfinavir
Fusidic acid	Synercid**		Delavirdine	Nevirapine
Isoniazid	Telithromycin[++]		Efavirenz	Rimantadine
Metronidazole	Tigecycline		Enfuvirtide	Ritonavir
	Tinidazole		Fosamprenavir	Stribild

[§] Ref. on antiretrovirals: *CID* 40:174, 2005   ** Quinupristin/dalfopristin   [++] Telitho: reduce dose in renal & hepatic failure

TABLE 19 – TREATMENT OF CAPD PERITONITIS IN ADULTS*
(Periton Dial Intl 30:393, 2010)[1]

EMPIRIC Intraperitoneal Therapy: Culture Results Pending *(For MRSA see footnote[2])*

Drug		Residual Urine Output	
		<100 mL per day	>100 mL per day
(Cefazolin or Vanco) +	Can mix in same bag	1 gm per bag, q24h	20 mg per kg BW per bag, q24h
Ceftazidime		3 gm LD, then 1-2 gm IP q24h *(AAC 58:19, 2014)*	20 mg per kg BW per bag, q24h

Drug Doses for SPECIFIC Intraperitoneal Therapy—Culture Results Known. NOTE: Few po drugs indicated

Drug	Intermittent Dosing (once per day)		Continuous Dosing (per liter exchange)	
	Anuric	Non-Anuric	Anuric	Non-Anuric
Amphotericin B	NA	NA	MD 1.5 mg	NA
Ampicillin	250–500 mg po bid	ND	No LD, MD 125 mg	ND
Amp-sulbactam	2 gm q12h	ND	LD 1 gm, MD 100 mg	LD 1 gm, MD ↑ 25%
Cefazolin	15 mg per kg	20 mg per kg	LD 500 mg, MD 125 mg	LD 500 mg, ↑ MD 25%
Cefepime	1 gm in one exchange/day	1.25 gm	LD 500 mg, MD 125 mg	LD 500 mg, ↑ MD 25%
Ceftazidime	1000–2000 mg	ND	LD 500 mg, MD 125 mg	LD 500 mg; ↑ MD 25%
Ciprofloxacin	500 mg po bid	ND	LD 50 mg, MD 25 mg	ND
Daptomycin			LD 100 mg, MD 20 mg	LD 500 mg, ↑ MD 25%
Fluconazole	200 mg q24h	ND	200 mg q24h	ND
Gentamicin	0.6 mg per kg	↑ dose 25%	Not recommended	Not recommended
Imipenem	1 gm in one exchange q12h		LD 250 mg, MD 50 mg	LD 250 mg, ↑ MD 25%
Itraconazole	100 mg q12h	100 mg q12h	100 mg q12h	100 mg q12h
Metronidazole	250 mg po bid	ND	250 mg po bid	ND
TMP-SMX	160/800 mg po bid	ND	LD 320/1600 mg po, MD 80/400 mg po q24h	ND
Vancomycin	15–30 mg per kg q3–7 days	↑ dose 25%	LD 1 gm; MD 25 mg	LD 1 gm, ↑ MD 25%

CAPD = continuous ambulatory peritoneal dialysis
Indications for catheter removal: 1) Relapse with same organism within 1 mo; 2) Failure to respond clinically within 5 days:
3) Exit site and tunnel infection; 4) Fungal peritonitis; 5) Fecal flora peritonitis (suggests bowel perforation).

[1] **All doses IP unless indicated otherwise.**
 LD = loading dose, **MD** = maintenance dose, **ND** = no data; **NA** = not applicable—dose as normal renal function.
 Anuric = <100 mL per day, **non-anuric** = >100 mL per day
[2] **Does not provide treatment for MRSA.** If gram-pos cocci on gram stain, include vanco.
See page 2 for other abbreviations

TABLE 20A – ANTI-TETANUS PROPHYLAXIS, WOUND CLASSIFICATION, IMMUNIZATION

WOUND CLASSIFICATION

Clinical Features	Tetanus Prone	Non-Tetanus Prone
Age of wound	> 6 hours	≤ 6 hours
Configuration	Stellate, avulsion	Linear
Depth	> 1 cm	≤ 1 cm
Mechanism of injury	Missile, crush, burn, frostbite	Sharp surface (glass, knife)
Devitalized tissue	Present	Absent
Contaminants (dirt, saliva, etc.)	Present	Absent

IMMUNIZATION SCHEDULE

History of Tetanus Immunization	Dirty, Tetanus-Prone Wound		Clean, non-Tetanus-Prone Wound	
	Td[1,2]	Tetanus Immune Globulin	Td[1,2]	Tetanus Immune Globulin
Unknown or < 3 doses[3]	Yes	Yes	Yes	No
3 or more doses	No[4]	No	No[5]	No

Ref: *MMWR 60:13, 2011; MMWR 61:468, 2012; MMWR 62:131, 2013 (pregnancy)*

[1] Td = Tetanus & diphtheria toxoids, adsorbed (adult). For adult who has not received Tdap previously, substitute one dose of Tdap for Td when immunization is indicated *(MMWR 61::468, 2012).*

[2] For children < 7 years, use DTaP unless contraindicated; for persons ≥ 7 years, Td is preferred to tetanus toxoid alone, but single dose of Tdap can be used if required for catch-up series.

[3] Individuals who have not completed vaccine series should do so.

[4] Yes, if >5 years since last booster.

[5] Yes, if >10 years since last booster.

TABLE 20B – RABIES POSTEXPOSURE PROPHYLAXIS

All wounds should be cleaned immediately & thoroughly with soap & water. This has been shown to protect 90% of experimental animals![1]

Animal Type	Evaluation & Disposition of Animal	Recommendations for Prophylaxis
Dogs, cats, ferrets	Healthy & available for 10-day observation	Don't start unless animal develops sx, then immediately begin HRIG + vaccine
	Rabid or suspected rabid	Immediate HRIG + vaccine
	Unknown (escaped)	Consult public health officials
Skunks, raccoons, bats,* foxes, coyotes, most carnivores	Regard as rabid	Immediate vaccination
Livestock, horses, rodents, rabbits; includes hares, squirrels, hamsters, guinea pigs, gerbils, chipmunks, rats, mice, woodchucks	Consider case-by-case	Consult public health officials. Bites of squirrels, hamsters, guinea pigs, gerbils, chipmunks, rats, mice, other small rodents, rabbits, and hares **almost never** require rabies post-exposure prophylaxis.

* Most recent cases of human rabies in U.S. due to contact (not bites) with silver-haired bats or rarely big brown bats but risk of acquiring rabies from non-contact bat exposure is exceedingly low (*CID 48:1493, 2009*). For more detail, see *CID 30:4, 2000; JAVMA 219:1687, 2001; CID 37:96, 2003 (travel medicine advisory); Ln 363:959, 2004; EID 11:1921, 2005; MMWR 55 (RR-5), 2006.*

Postexposure Rabies Immunization Schedule

IF NOT PREVIOUSLY VACCINATED

Treatment	Regimen[2]
Local wound cleaning	**All postexposure treatment should begin with immediate, thorough cleaning of all wounds with soap & water.**
Human rabies immune globulin (HRIG)	20 units per kg body weight given once on day 0. If anatomically feasible, the full dose should be infiltrated around the wound(s), the rest should be administered IM in the gluteal area. If the calculated dose of HRIG is insufficient to inject all the wounds, it should be diluted with normal saline to allow infiltration around additional wound areas. HRIG should **not** be administered in the **same syringe**, or into the **same anatomical site** as vaccine, or more than 7 days after the initiation of vaccine. Because HRIG may partially suppress active production of antibody, no more than the recommended dose should be given.[3]
Vaccine	Human diploid cell vaccine (HDCV), rabies vaccine adsorbed (RVA), or purified chick embryo cell vaccine (PCECV) 1 mL **IM (deltoid area[4])**, one each days 0, 3, 7, 14[5].

IF PREVIOUSLY VACCINATED[6]

Treatment	Regimen[2]
Local wound cleaning	All postexposure treatment should begin with immediate, thorough cleaning of all wounds with soap **& water.**
HRIG	HRIG should **not** be administered
Vaccine	HDCV or PCEC, 1 mL **IM (deltoid area[4])**, one each on days 0 & 3

CORRECT VACCINE ADMINISTRATION SITES

Age Group	Administration Site
Children & adults	**DELTOID[4]** only (**NEVER** in gluteus)
Infants & young children	Outer aspect of thigh (anterolateral thigh) may be used (**NEVER** in gluteus)

1. From *MMWR 48:RR-1, 1999; CID 30:4, 2000;* B. T. Matyas, Mass. Dept. of Public Health. *MMWR 57:1, 2008*
2. These regimens are applicable for all age groups, including children.
3. In most reported post-exposure treatment failures, only identified deficiency was failure to infiltrate wound(s) with HRIG (*CID 22:228, 1996*). However, several failures reported from SE Asia in patients in whom WHO protocol followed (*CID 28:143, 1999*).
4. The **deltoid** area is the **only** acceptable site of vaccination for adults & older children. For infants & young children, outer aspect of the thigh (anterolateral thigh) may be used. Vaccine should **NEVER** be administered in gluteal area.
5. Note that this is a change from previous recommendation of 5 doses (days 0, 3, 7, 14 & 28) based on new data & recommendations from ACIP. Note that the number of doses for persons with altered immunocompetence remains unchanged (5 doses on days 0, 3, 7, 14 & 28) and recommendations for pre-exposure prophylaxis remain 3 doses administered on days 0, 7 and 21 or 28 (*MMWR 59 (RR-2), 2010*).
6. Any person with a history of pre-exposure vaccination with HDCV, RVA, PCECV; prior post-exposure prophylaxis with HDCV, PCEC or rabies vaccine adsorbed (RVA); or previous vaccination with any other type of rabies vaccine & a documented history of antibody response to the prior vaccination.

TABLE 21 SELECTED DIRECTORY OF RESOURCES

ORGANIZATION	PHONE/FAX	WEBSITE(S)
ANTIPARASITIC DRUGS & PARASITOLOGY INFORMATION		
CDC Drug Line	Weekdays: 404-639-3670	http://www.cdc.gov/ncidod/srp/drugs/drug-service.html
	Evenings, weekends, holidays: 404-639-2888	
DPDx: Lab ID of parasites		www.dpd.cdc.gov/dpdx/default.htm
Gorgas Course Tropical Medicine		http://info.dom.uab.edu/gorgas
Malaria	daytime: 770-488-7788	www.cdc.gov/malaria
	other: 770-488-7100	
	US toll free: 855-856-4713	
Expert Compound. Pharm.	800-247-9767/818-787-7256	www.uniquerx.com
World Health Organization (WHO)		www.who.int
Parasites & Health		www.dpd.cdc.gov/dpdx/HTML/Para_Health.htm
BIOTERRORISM		
Centers for Disease Control & Prevention	770-488-7100	www.bt.cdc.gov
Infectious Diseases Society of America	703-299-0200	www.idsociety.org
Johns Hopkins Center Civilian Biodefense		www.jhsph.edu
Center for Biosecurity of the Univ. of Pittsburgh Med. Center		www.upmc-biosecurity.org
US Army Medical Research Institute of Inf. Dis.		www.usamriid.army.mil
HEPATITIS B		
Hepatitis B Foundation		www.hepb.org, www.natap.org
HEPATITIS C		
CDC		www.cdc.gov/ncidod/diseases/hepatitis/C
Individual		http://hepatitis-central.com
		www.natap.org
HCV Guidelines		www.hcvguidelines.org
HIV		
General		
HIV InSite		http://hivinsite.ucsf.edu
Johns Hopkins AIDS Service		www.hopkins-aids.edu
		www.natap.org
Drug Interactions		
Johns Hopkins AIDS Service		www.hopkins-aids.edu
Liverpool HIV Pharm. Group		www.hiv-druginteractions.org
Other		http://AIDS.medscape.com
Prophylaxis/Treatment of Opportunistic Infections; HIV Treatment		www.aidsinfo.nih.gov
IMMUNIZATIONS		
CDC, Natl. Immunization Program	404-639-8200	www.cdc.gov/vaccines/
FDA, Vaccine Adverse Events	800-822-7967	www.fda.gov/cber/vaers/vaers.htm
National Network Immunization Info.	877-341-6644	www.immunizationinfo.org
Influenza vaccine, CDC	404-639-8200	www.cdc.gov/vaccines/
Institute for Vaccine Safety		www.vaccinesafety.edu
OCCUPATIONAL EXPOSURE, BLOOD-BORNE PATHOGENS (HIV, HEPATITIS B & C)		
National Clinicians' Post-Exposure Hotline	888-448-4911	www.ucsf.edu/hivcntr
Q-T$_c$ INTERVAL PROLONGATION BY DRUGS		www.qtdrugs.org; www.crediblemeds.org
SEXUALLY TRANSMITTED DISEASES		www.cdc.gov/std/treatment/TOC2002TG.htm
		Slides: http://www.phac-aspc.gc.ca/slm-maa/slides/index.html
TRAVELERS' INFO: Immunizations, Malaria Prophylaxis, More		
Amer. Soc. Trop. Med. & Hyg.		www.astmh.org
CDC, general	877-394-8747/888-232-3299	http://www.cdc.gov/travel/default.asp
CDC, Malaria:		www.cdc.gov/malaria
Prophylaxis		http://wwwn.cdc.gov/travel/default.asp
Treatment	770-488-7788	www.who.int/health_topics/malaria
MD Travel Health		www.mdtravelhealth.com
Pan American Health Organization		www.paho.org
World Health Organization (WHO)		www.who.int/home-page
VACCINE & IMMUNIZATION RESOURCES		
American Academy of Pediatrics		www.cispimmunize.org
CDC, National Immunization Program		www.cdc.gov/vaccines/
National Network for Immunization Information		www.immunizationinfo.org

TABLE 22A – ANTI-INFECTIVE DRUG-DRUG INTERACTIONS

Importance: ± = theory/anecdotal; + = of probable importance; ++ = of definite importance
To check for interactions between more than 2 drugs, see: http://www.drugs.com/drug_interactions.html
and http://www.healthline.com/druginteractions

ANTI-INFECTIVE AGENT (A)	OTHER DRUG (B)	EFFECT	IMPORT
Abacavir	Methadone	↓ levels of B	++
Amantadine (Symmetrel)	Alcohol	↑ CNS effects	+
	Anticholinergic and anti-Parkinson agents (ex. Artane, scopolamine)	↑ effect of B: dry mouth, ataxia, blurred vision, slurred speech, toxic psychosis	+
	Trimethoprim	↑ levels of A & B	+
	Digoxin	↑ levels of B	±
Aminoglycosides— parenteral (amikacin, gentamicin, kanamycin, netilmicin, sisomicin, streptomycin, tobramycin)	Amphotericin B	↑ nephrotoxicity	++
	Cis platinum (Platinol)	↑ nephro & ototoxicity	+
	Cyclosporine	↑ nephrotoxicity	+
	Neuromuscular blocking agents	↑ apnea or respiratory paralysis	+
	Loop diuretics (e.g., furosemide)	↑ ototoxicity	++
	NSAIDs	↑ nephrotoxicity	+
	Non-polarizing muscle relaxants	↑ apnea	+
	Radiographic contrast	↑ nephrotoxicity	+
	Vancomycin	↑ nephrotoxicity	+
Aminoglycosides— oral (kanamycin, neomycin)	**Warfarin**	↑ prothrombin time	+
Amphotericin B and ampho B lipid formulations	Antineoplastic drugs	↑ nephrotoxicity risk	+
	Digitalis	↑ toxicity of B if K⁺ ↓	+
	Nephrotoxic drugs: aminoglycosides, cidofovir, cyclosporine, foscarnet, pentamidine	↑ nephrotoxicity of A	++
Ampicillin, amoxicillin	Allopurinol	↑ frequency of rash	++
Artemether-lumefantrine	CYP3A inhibitors: amiodarone, atazanavir, itraconazole, ritonavir, voriconazole	↑ levels of A; ↑ QTc interval	++
	CYP2D6 substrates: flecainide, imipramine, amitriptyline	↑ levels of B; ↑ QTc interval	++
Atazanavir	See protease inhibitors and Table 22B		
Atovaquone	Rifampin (perhaps rifabutin)	↓ serum levels of A; ↑ levels of B	+
	Metoclopramide	↓ levels of A	+
	Tetracycline	↓ levels of A	++

Azole Antifungal Agents [Flu = fluconazole; Itr = itraconazole; **Ket** = ketoconazole; **Posa** = posaconazole
Vor = voriconazole; + = occurs; **blank space** = either studied & no interaction OR
no data found (may be in pharm. co. databases)]

Flu	Itr	Ket	Posa	Vor			
+	+			+	Amitriptyline	↑ levels of B	+
+	+	+		+	Calcium channel blockers	↑ levels of B	++
	+			+	Carbamazepine (vori contraindicated)	↓ levels of A	++
+	+	+	+	+	Cyclosporine	↑ levels of B, ↑ risk of nephrotoxicity	+
	+	+			Didanosine	↓ absorption of A	+
	+	+	+	+	Efavirenz	↓ levels of A, ↑ levels of B	++ (avoid)
	+	+	+		H₂ blockers, antacids, sucralfate	↓ absorption of A	+
+	+	+	+	+	Hydantoins (phenytoin, Dilantin)	↑ levels of B, ↓ levels of A	++
	+	+			Isoniazid	↓ levels of A	+
	+	+	+	+	Lovastatin/simvastatin	Rhabdomyolysis reported; ↑ levels of B	++
				+	Methadone	↑ levels of B	+
+	+	+	+	+	Midazolam/triazolam, po	↑ levels of B	++
+	+			+	Warfarin	↑ effect of B	++
+	+			+	Oral hypoglycemics	↑ levels of B	++
			+	+	Pimozide	↑ levels of B — **avoid**	++
	+	+			Protease inhibitors	↑ levels of B	++
	+	+	+	+	Proton pump inhibitors	↓ levels of A, ↑ levels of B	++
+	+	+	+	+	Rifampin/rifabutin (vori contraindicated)	↑ levels of B, ↓ serum levels of A	++
	+				Rituximab	inhibits action of B	++
			+	+	Sirolimus (vori and posa contraindicated)	↑ levels of B	++
+		+	+	+	Tacrolimus	↑ levels of B with toxicity	++
+		+			Theophyllines	↑ levels of B	+
		+			Trazodone	↑ levels of B	++
+					Zidovudine	↑ levels of B	+

TABLE 22A (2)

ANTI-INFECTIVE AGENT (A)	OTHER DRUG (B)	EFFECT	IMPORT
Bedaquiline	Rifampin	↓ levels of A	+ +
	Ketoconazole	↑ levels of A	+ +
Caspofungin	Cyclosporine	↑ levels of A	+ +
	Tacrolimus	↓ levels of B	+ +
	Carbamazepine, dexamethasone, efavirenz, nevirapine, phenytoin, rifampin	↓ levels of A; ↑ dose of caspofungin to 70 mg/d	+ +
Chloramphenicol	Hydantoins	↑ toxicity of B, nystagmus, ataxia	+ +
	Iron salts, Vitamin B12	↓ response to B	+ +
	Protease inhibitors—HIV	↑ levels of A & B	+ +
Clindamycin (Cleocin)	Kaolin	↓ absorption of A	+ +
	Muscle relaxants, e.g., atracurium, baclofen, diazepam	↑ frequency/duration of respiratory paralysis	+ +
	St John's wort	↓ levels of A	+ +
Cobicistat	*See Integrase Strand Transfer Inhibitors*		
Cycloserine	Ethanol	↑ frequency of seizures	+
	INH, ethionamide	↑ frequency of drowsiness/dizziness	+
Dapsone	Atazanavir	↓ levels of A - Avoid	+ +
	Didanosine	↓ absorption of A	+
	Oral contraceptives	↓ effectiveness of B	+
	Pyrimethamine	↑ in marrow toxicity	+
	Rifampin/Rifabutin	↓ serum levels of A	+
	Trimethoprim	↑ levels of A & B (methemoglobinemia)	+
	Zidovudine	May ↑ marrow toxicity	+
Daptomycin	HMG-CoA inhibitors (statins)	Consider DC statin while on dapto	+ +
Delavirdine (Rescriptor)	*See Non-nucleoside reverse transcriptase inhibitors (NNRTIs) and Table 22B*		
Didanosine (ddl) (Videx)	Allopurinol	↑ levels of A—**AVOID**	+ +
	Cisplatin, dapsone, INH, metronidazole, nitrofurantoin, stavudine, vincristine, zalcitabine	↑ risk of peripheral neuropathy	+
	Ethanol, lamivudine, pentamidine	↑ risk of pancreatitis	+
	Fluoroquinolones	↓ absorption 2° to chelation	+
	Drugs that need low pH for absorption: dapsone, indinavir, itra/ ketoconazole, pyrimethamine, rifampin, trimethoprim	↓ absorption	
	Methadone	↓ levels of A	+ +
	Ribavirin	↑ levels ddl metabolite—**avoid**	+ +
	Tenofovir	↑ levels of A (**reduce dose of A**)	+ +
Dolutegravir	*See Integrase Strand Transfer Inhibitors*		
Doripenem	Probenecid	↑ levels of A	+ +
	Valproic acid	↓ levels of B	+ +
Doxycycline	Aluminum, bismuth, iron, Mg++	↓ absorption of A	+
	Barbiturates, hydantoins	↓ serum t/2 of A	+
	Carbamazepine (Tegretol)	↓ serum t/2 of A	+
	Digoxin	↑ serum levels of B	+
	Warfarin	↑ activity of B	+ +
Efavirenz (Sustiva)	*See non-nucleoside reverse transcriptase inhibitors (NNRTIs) and Table 22B*		
Elvitegravir	*See Integrase Strand Transfer Inhibitors*		
Ertapenem (Invanz)	Probenecid	↑ levels of A	+ +
	Valproic acid	↓ levels of B	+ +
Ethambutol (Myambutol)	Aluminum salts (includes didanosine buffer)	↓ absorption of A & B	+
Etravirine	*See non-nucleoside reverse transcriptase inhibitors (NNRTIs) and Table 22B*		

Fluoroquinolones (**Cipro** = ciprofloxacin; **Gati** = gatifloxacin; **Gemi** = gemifloxacin; **Levo** = levofloxacin; **Moxi** = moxifloxacin; **Oflox** = ofloxacin)

Cipro	Gati	Gemi	Levo	Moxi	Oflox	NOTE: Blank space = *either studied and no interaction OR no data found*		
+			+	+	+	**Antiarrhythmics (procainamide, amiodarone)**	↑ Q-T interval (torsade)	+ +
+	+		+	+	+	Insulin, oral hypoglycemics	↑ & ↓ blood sugar	+ +
+						Caffeine	↑ levels of B	+
+					+	Cimetidine	↑ levels of A	+
+					+	Cyclosporine	↑ levels of B	±
+	+		+	+	+	Didanosine	↓ absorption of A	+ +
+	+	+	+	+	+	**Cations: Al+++, Ca++, Fe++, Mg++, Zn++ (antacids, vitamins, dairy products), citrate/citric acid**	↓ absorption of A (some variability between drugs)	+ +
+						Methadone	↑ levels of B	+ +
+			+		+	NSAIDs	↑ risk CNS stimulation/seizures	+ +
+						Phenytoin	↑ or ↓ levels of B	+

Cipro	Gati	Gemi	Levo	Moxi	Oflox	OTHER DRUG (B)	EFFECT	IMPORT
ANTI-INFECTIVE AGENT (A)						**OTHER DRUG (B)**	**EFFECT**	**IMPORT**
Fluoroquinolones *(continued)*								
						NOTE: Blank space = either studied and no interaction OR no data found		
+	+	+			+	Probenecid	↓ renal clearance of A	+
+						Rasagiline	↑ levels of B	+ +
				+		Rifampin	↑ levels of A *(CID 45;1001, 2007)*	+ +
+	+	+	+		+	**Sucralfate**	**↓ absorption of A**	**+ +**
+						Theophylline	↓ levels of B	+ +
+						Thyroid hormone	↓ levels of B	+ +
+						Tizanidine	↑ levels of B	+ +
+			+	+	+	Warfarin	↑ prothrombin time	+
Ganciclovir (Cytovene) & **Valganciclovir** (Valcyte)						Imipenem	↑ risk of seizures reported	+
						Probenecid	↑ levels of A	+
						Zidovudine	↓ levels of A, ↑ levels of B	+
Gentamicin						*See Aminoglycosides—parenteral*		
Imipenem & Meropenem						BCG	↓ effectiveness of B–avoid combination	+ +
						Divalproex	↓ levels of B	+ +
						Ganciclovir	↑ seizure risk	+ +
						Probenecid	↑ levels of A	+ +
						Valproic acid	↓ levels of B	+ +
Indinavir						*See protease inhibitors and Table 22B*		

Integrase Strand Transfer Inhibitors (INSTI): Dolutegravir (**DTG**), Raltegravir (**RAL**), Elvitegravir (**ELV**)
NOTE: interactions involving Stribild (elvitegravir + cobicistat + emtricitabine + tenofovir) reflect one or more of its components (the specifics may not be known).

DTG	RAL	Stribild (ELV)	OTHER DRUG (B)	EFFECT	IMPORT
ANTI-INFECTIVE AGENT (A)			**OTHER DRUG (B)**	**EFFECT**	**IMPORT**
x	x	x	Antacids (polyvalent cations)	↓ levels of A—space dosing	+ +
		x	Antiarrhythmics, digoxin	↑ levels of A—monitor	+
	x		Atazanavir/RTV	↑ levels of A—monitor	±
		x	Atorvastatin	↑ levels of B—monitor	+
		x	Benzodiazepines	↑ levels of B—monitor	+
		x	Beta-blockers	↑ levels of B—monitor	+
		x	Bosentan	**↓ levels of B— adjust dose or avoid**	+ +
		x	Buprenorphine	↑ levels of B—monitor	+
		x	Buspirone	↑ levels of B—monitor	+
		x	Calcium channel blockers	↑ levels of B—monitor	+
x			Carbamazepine	**↓ levels of A—avoid**	+ +
		x		**↓ levels of A, ↑ levels of B—avoid**	+ +
		x	Clarithromycin	↑ levels of A and B—monitor	+
		x	Clonazepam	↑ levels of B—monitor	+
		x	Colchicine	↑ levels of B—adjust dose	+
		x	Cyclosporine	↑ levels of B—monitor	+
		x	Dexamethasone	**↓ levels of A—avoid**	+ +
x			Doletilide	**↓ levels of B—avoid**	+ +
x			Efavirenz	↓ levels of A—adjust dose	+ +
	x			↓ levels of A—monitor	+
		x	Ethosuximide	↑ levels of B—monitor	+
x			Etravirine	**↓ levels of A—avoid**	+ +
	x			↓ levels of A—monitor	+
		x	Fluticasone	**↑ levels of B—avoid**	+ +
x			Fosamprenavir/RTV	**↓ levels of A—adjust dose or avoid**	+ +
x		x	Fosphenytoin/phenytoin	**↓ levels of A—avoid**	+ +
		x	Fluconazole	**↑ levels of A—avoid**	+ +
		x	Itraconazole	**↑ levels of A and B—adjust dose or avoid**	+ +
		x	Ketoconazole	**↑ levels of A and B—adjust dose or avoid**	+ +
x			Metformin	↑ levels of B—monitor	+ +
x			Nevirapine	**↓ levels of A—avoid**	+ +
	x		Omeprazole	↑ levels of A—monitor	±
		x	Oral contraceptives	↑ or ↓ levels of B—avoid	+ +
x		x	Oxcarbazepine	**↓ levels of A—avoid**	+ +

TABLE 22A (4)

Integrase Strand Transfer Inhibitors (INSTI) *(continued)*

DTG	RAL	Strbid (ELV)	OTHER DRUG (B)	EFFECT	IMPORT
			ANTI-INFECTIVE AGENT (A)		
x		x	Phenobarbital	**↓ levels of A—avoid**	+ +
		x	Phenothiazines	↑ levels of B—monitor	+ +
		x	Phosphodiesterase-5 inhibitors	**↑ levels of B—adjust dose or avoid**	+ +
x			Primidone	**↓ levels of A—avoid**	+ +
x	x	x	Rifampin, rifabutin, rifapentine	**↓ levels of A—adjust dose or avoid**	+ +
		x	Risperidone	↑ levels of B—monitor	+
		x	Salmeterol	**↑ levels of B—avoid**	+ +
		x	Sirolimus	↑ levels of B—monitor	+
x		x	St. John's wort	**↓ levels of A—avoid**	+ +
		x	SSRIs	↑ levels of B—monitor	+
x	x	x	Sucralfate	**↓ levels of A—space dosing**	+ +
		x	Tacrolimus	↑ levels of B—monitor	+ +
x			Tipranavir/RTV	**↓ levels of A—adjust dose or avoid**	+ +
	x			↓ levels of A—monitor	±
		x	Trazodone	↑ levels of B—monitor	+
		x	Tricyclic antidepressants	↑ levels of B—monitor	+
		x	Voriconazole	**↑ levels of A and B—adjust dose or avoid**	+ +
		x	Warfarin	↑ or ↓ levels of B—monitor	+
		x	Zolpidem ("Z" drugs)	↑ levels of B—monitor	+

ANTI-INFECTIVE AGENT (A)	OTHER DRUG (B)	EFFECT	IMPORT
Isoniazid	Alcohol, rifampin	**↑ risk of hepatic injury**	+ +
	Aluminum salts	↓ absorption (take fasting)	+ +
	Carbamazepine, phenytoin	↑ levels of B with nausea, vomiting, nystagmus, ataxia	+ +
	Itraconazole, ketoconazole	↓ levels of B	+
	Oral hypoglycemics	↓ effects of B	+
Lamivudine	Zalcitabine	**Mutual interference—do not combine**	+ +
Linezolid (Zyvox)	Adrenergic agents	Risk of hypertension	+ +
	Aged, fermented, pickled or smoked foods —↑ tyramine	Risk of hypertension	+
	Clarithromycin	↑ levels of A	+ +
	Meperidine	Risk of serotonin syndrome	+ +
	Rasagiline (MAO inhibitor)	Risk of serotonin syndrome	+
	Rifampin	↓ levels of A	+ +
	Serotonergic drugs (SSRIs)	Risk of serotonin syndrome	+ +
Lopinavir	*See protease inhibitors*		

Macrolides [Ery = erythromycin; Azl = azithromycin; Clr = clarithromycin; + = occurs; blank space = either studied and no interaction OR no data]

Ery	Azi	Clr	OTHER DRUG (B)	EFFECT	IMPORT
			Calcium channel blockers	↑ serum levels of B	+ +
+		+	Carbamazepine	↑ levels of B, nystagmus, nausea, vomiting, ataxia	+ + (avoid w/ erythro)
+		+	Cimetidine, **ritonavir**	↑ levels of B	+
+			Clozapine	↑ serum levels of B, CNS toxicity	+
		+	**Colchicine**	**↑ levels of B (potent, fatal)**	+ + (avoid)
+			Corticosteroids	↑ effects of B	+
+	+	+	Cyclosporine	↑ serum levels of B with toxicity	+
+	+	+	Digoxin, digitoxin	↑ serum levels of B (10% of cases)	+
		+	Efavirenz	↓ levels of A	+ +
+		+	Ergot alkaloids	↑ levels of B	+ +
+		+	Linezolid	↑ levels of B	+ +
+		+	Lovastatin/simvastatin	↑ levels of B; rhabdomyolysis	+ +
+		+	Midazolam, triazolam	↑ levels of B, ↑ sedative effects	+
+		+	Phenytoin	↑ levels of B	+
+	+	+	Pimozide	**Q-T interval**	+ +
+		+	Rifampin, rifabutin	↑ levels of B	+
+		+	Tacrolimus	↑ levels of B	+ +
+		+	Theophylline	↑ serum levels of B with nausea, vomiting, seizures, apnea	+ +
+		+	Valproic acid	↑ levels of B	+
+		+	Warfarin	May ↑ prothrombin time	+
		+	Zidovudine	↓ levels of B	+

TABLE 22A (5)

ANTI-INFECTIVE AGENT (A)	OTHER DRUG (B)	EFFECT	IMPORT
Maraviroc	Clarithromycin	↑ serum levels of A	++
	Delavirdine	↑ levels of A	++
	Itraconazole/ketoconazole	↑ levels of A	++
	Nefazodone	↑ levels of A	++
	Protease Inhibitors (not tipranavir/ritonavir)	↑ levels of A	++
	Anticonvulsants: carbamazepine, phenobarbital, phenytoin	↓ levels of A	++
	Efavirenz	↓ levels of A	++
	Rifampin	↓ levels of A	++
Mefloquine	ß-adrenergic blockers, calcium channel blockers, quinidine, quinine	↑ arrhythmias	+
	Divalproex, valproic acid	↓ level of B with seizures	++
	Halofantrine	Q-T prolongation	++ (avoid)
	Calcineurin inhibitors	Q-T prolongation (avoid)	++
Meropenem	*See Imipenem*		
Methenamine mandelate or hippurate	Acetazolamide, sodium bicarbonate, thiazide diuretics	↓ antibacterial effect 2° to ↑ urine pH	++
Metronidazole /Tinidazole	Alcohol	Disulfiram-like reaction	+
	Cyclosporin	↑ levels of B	++
	Disulfiram (Antabuse)	Acute toxic psychosis	+
	Lithium	↑ levels of B	++
	Warfarin	↑ anticoagulant effect	++
	Phenobarbital, hydantoins	↑ levels of B	++
Micafungin	Nifedipine	↑ levels of B	+
	Sirolimus	↑ levels of B	+
Nafcillin	Warfarin	↓ Warfarin effect	++
Nelfinavir	*See protease inhibitors and Table 22B*		
Nevirapine (Viramune)	*See non-nucleoside reverse transcriptase inhibitors (NNRTIs) and Table 22B*		
Nitrofurantoin	Antacids	↓ absorption of A	+

Non-nucleoside reverse transcriptase inhibitors (NNRTIs): For interactions with protease inhibitors, *see Table 22B.*
Del = delavirdine; **Efa** = efavirenz; **Etr** = etravirine; **Nev** = nevirapine

Del	Efa	Etr	Nev	Co-administration contraindicated *(See package insert):*	IMPORT
+		+		Anticonvulsants: carbamazepine, phenobarbital, phenytoin	++
+		+		Antimycobacterials: rifabutin, rifampin	++
+				Antipsychotics: pimozide	++
+	+	+		Benzodiazepines: alprazolam, midazolam, triazolam	++
+	+			Ergotamine	++
+	+	+		HMG-CoA inhibitors (statins): lovastatin, simvastatin, atorvastatin, pravastatin	++
+		+		St. John's wort	++
				Dose change needed:	
+				Amphetamines	↑ levels of B—**caution**	++
+		+	+	Antiarrhythmics: amiodarone, lidocaine, others	↓ or ↑ levels of B—**caution**	++
+	+	+	+	Anticonvulsants: carbamazepine, phenobarbital, phenytoin	↓ levels of A and/or B	++
+	+	+	+	Antifungals: itraconazole, ketoconazole, voriconazole, posaconazole	Potential ↓ levels of B, ↑ levels of A	++ (avoid)
+			+	Antirejection drugs: cyclosporine, rapamycin, sirolimus, tacrolimus	↑ levels of B	++
+			+	Calcium channel blockers	↑ levels of B	++
+		+	+	Clarithromycin	↑ levels of B metabolite, ↑ levels of A	++
+	+	+	+	Cyclosporine	↑ levels of B	++
+		+		Dexamethasone	↓ levels of B	++
+	+	+	+	Sildenafil, vardenafil, tadalafil	↑ levels of B	++
+		+		Fentanyl, methadone	↓ levels of B	++
+				Gastric acid suppression: antacids, H-2 blockers, proton pump inhibitors	↓ levels of B	++
	+		+	Mefloquine	↓ levels of B	++
	+	+	+	Methadone, fentanyl	↓ levels of B	++
	+		+	Oral contraceptives	↑ or ↓ levels of B	++
+	+	+	+	Protease inhibitors—*see Table 22B*		
+	+	+	+	**Rifabutin, rifampin**	↑ or ↓ levels of rifabutin; ↓ levels of A—**caution**	++
+	+	+	+	St. John's wort	↓ levels of B	
+		+	+	Warfarin	↑ levels of B	++

ANTI-INFECTIVE AGENT (A)	OTHER DRUG (B)	EFFECT	IMPORT
Oritavancin	Warfarin	↑ levels of B	++
Pentamidine, IV	Amphotericin B	↑ risk of nephrotoxicity	+
	Pancreatitis-assoc drugs, eg, alcohol, valproic acid	↑ risk of pancreatitis	+
Piperacillin	Cefoxitin	Antagonism vs pseudomonas	++
Pip-tazo	Methotrexate	↑ levels of B	++
Polymyxin B	Curare paralytics	Avoid: neuromuscular blockade	++

TABLE 22A (6)

223

ANTI-INFECTIVE AGENT (A)	OTHER DRUG (B)	EFFECT	IMPORT
Polymyxin E (Colistin)	Curare paralytics	Avoid: neuromuscular blockade	++
	Aminoglycosides, Ampho B, Vanco	↑ nephrotoxicity risk	++
Primaquine	Chloroquine, dapsone, INH, probenecid, quinine, sulfonamides, TMP/SMX, others	↑ risk of hemolysis in G6PD-deficient patients	++

Protease Inhibitors—Anti-HIV Drugs. (**Atazan** = atazanavir; **Darun** = darunavir; **Fosampren** = fosamprenavir; **Indin** = indinavir; **Lopin** = lopinavir; **Nelfin** = nelfinavir; **Saquin** = saquinavir; **Tipran** = tipranavir). For interactions with antiretrovirals, see Table 22B Only a partial list—check package insert

Also see http://aidsinfo.nih.gov
To check for interactions between more than 2 drugs, see: http://www.drugs.com/drug_interactions.html and http://www.healthline.com/druginteractions

Atazan	Darun	Fosampren	Indin	Lopin	Nelfin	Saquin	Tipran			
							+	**Analgesics:** 1. Alfentanil, fentanyl, hydrocodone, tramadol	↑ levels of B	+
	+			+		+	+	2. Codeine, hydromorphone, morphine, methadone	↓ levels of B (JAIDS 41:563, 2006)	+
+	+	+	+	+	+		+	**Anti-arrhythmics: amiodarone, lidocaine, mexiletine, flecainide**	↑ levels of B; **do not co-administer or use caution** (See package insert)	++
	+		+	+	+	+		**Anticonvulsants: carbamazepine, clonazepam, phenobarbital**	↓ levels of A, ↑ levels of B	++
+		+		+			+	Antidepressants, all tricyclic	↑ levels of B	+
+	+			+			+	Antidepressants, all other	↑ levels of B; do not use pimozide	++
	+						+	Antidepressants: SSRIs	↓ levels of B - avoid	++
								Antihistamines	Do not use	++
+	+	+	+	+	+		+	**Benzodiazepines, e.g., diazepam, midazolam, triazolam**	↑ levels of B—do not use	++
+			+	+				Boceprevir	↓ levels of A & B	++
+	+	+	+	+		+	+	Calcium channel blockers (all)	↑ levels of B	++
+				+	+	+	+	Clarithro, erythro	↑ levels of B if renal impairment	+
+	+			+			+	Contraceptives, oral	↓ levels of A & B	++
	+	+	+			+		Corticosteroids: prednisone, dexamethasone	↓ levels of A, ↑ levels of B	+
+	+	+	+	+	+	+	+	Cyclosporine	↑ levels of B, monitor levels	+
						+		Digoxin	↑ levels of B	++
+		+	+	+	+	+	+	Ergot derivatives	**levels of B—do not use**	++
		+	+			+	+	Erythromycin, clarithromycin	↑ levels of A & B	+
			+		+	+		Grapefruit juice (>200 mL/day)	↓ indinavir & ↑ saquinavir levels	++
+	+	+	+	+	+	+		H2 receptor antagonists	↓ levels of A	++
+	+	+	+	+	+	+	+	**HMG-CoA reductase inhibitors (statins): lovastatin, simvastatin**	↑ levels of B—do not use	++
+								Irinotecan	**levels of B—do not use**	++
	+		+	+	+	+	+	Ketoconazole, itraconazole, ? vori.	↑ levels of A, ↑ levels of B	++
+	+	+	+	+	+	+	+	Posaconazole	↑ levels of A, no effect on B	++
			+					Metronidazole	Poss. disulfiram reaction, alcohol	+
			+					Phenytoin (JAIDS 36:1034, 2004)	↓ levels of A & B	++
+	+	+	+	+	+	+	+	Pimozide	**levels of B—do not use**	++
+	+			+	+	+	+	Proton pump inhibitors	↓ levels of A	++
+	+	+	+	+	+	+	+	Rifampin, rifabutin	↓ levels of A, ↑ levels of B **(avoid)**	++
+	+	+	+	+	+	+	+	Sildenafil (Viagra), tadalafil, vardenafil	Varies, some ↑ & some ↓ levels of B	++
+	+	+	+	+	+	+	+	**St. John's wort**	↓ levels of A—do not use	++
+	+	+	+	+	+	+	+	**Sirolimus, tracrolimus**	↑ levels of B	++
+								Tenofovir	↓ levels of A—add ritonavir	++
	+		+	+				Theophylline	↓ levels of B	+
+		+		+				Warfarin	↑ levels of B	+
Pyrazinamide								INH, rifampin	May ↑ risk of hepatotoxicity	±
Pyrimethamine								Lorazepam	↑ risk of hepatotoxicity	+
								Sulfonamides, TMP/SMX	↑ risk of marrow suppression	+
								Zidovudine	↑ risk of marrow suppression	+
Quinine								Digoxin	↑ digoxin levels; ↑ toxicity	++
								Mefloquine	↑ arrhythmias	+
								Warfarin	↑ prothrombin time	++
Quinupristin- dalfopristin (Synercid)								Anti-HIV drugs: NNRTIs & PIs	↑ levels of B	++
								Antineoplastic: vincristine, docetaxel, paclitaxel	↑ levels of B	++
								Calcium channel blockers	↑ levels of B	++
								Carbamazepine	↑ levels of B	++
								Cyclosporine, tacrolimus	↑ levels of B	++

TABLE 22A (7)

ANTI-INFECTIVE AGENT (A)	OTHER DRUG (B)	EFFECT	IMPORT
Quinupristin-dalfopristin (Synercid) *(continued)*	Lidocaine	↑ levels of B	++
	Methylprednisolone	↑ levels of B	++
	Midazolam, diazepam	↑ levels of B	++
	Statins	↑ levels of B	++
Raltegravir	*See Integrase Strand Transfer Inhibitors*		
Ribavirin	Didanosine	↑ levels of B → toxicity—**avoid**	++
	Stavudine	↓ levels of B	++
	Zidovudine	↓ levels of B	++
Rifamycins (rifampin, rifabutin) Ref.: *ArIM 162:985, 2002* The following is a partial list of drugs with rifampin-induced ↑ metabolism and hence lower than anticipated serum levels: ACE inhibitors, dapsone, diazepam, digoxin, diltiazem, doxycycline, fluconazole, fluvastatin, haloperidol, moxifloxacin, nifedipine, progestins, triazolam, tricyclics, voriconazole, zidovudine *(Clin Pharmacokinetic 42:819, 2003).*	Al OH, ketoconazole, PZA	↓ levels of A	+
	Atovaquone	↑ levels of A, ↓ levels of B	+
	Beta adrenergic blockers (metoprolol, propranolol)	↓ effect of B	+
	Caspofungin	↓ levels of B—increase dose	++
	Clarithromycin	↑ levels of A, ↓ levels of B	++
	Corticosteroids	replacement requirement of B	++
	Cyclosporine	↓ effect of B	++
	Delavirdine	**levels of A, ↓ levels of B—avoid**	++
	Digoxin	↓ levels of B	++
	Disopyramide	↓ levels of B	++
	Fluconazole	↑ levels of A	+
	Amprenavir, indinavir, nelfinavir, ritonavir	↑ levels of A (↓ dose of A), ↓ levels of B	++
	INH	Converts INH to toxic hydrazine	++
	Itraconazole, ketoconazole	↓ levels of B, ↑ levels of A	++
	Linezolid	↓ levels of B	++
	Methadone	↓ serum levels (withdrawal)	+
	Nevirapine	↓ levels of B—avoid	++
	Warfarin	Suboptimal anticoagulation	++
	Oral contraceptives	↓ effectiveness; spotting, pregnancy	+
	Phenytoin	↓ levels of B	+
	Protease inhibitors	↓ levels of A, ↑ levels of B—CAUTION	++
	Quinidine	↓ effect of B	+
	Raltegravir	↓ levels of B	++
	Sulfonylureas	↓ hypoglycemic effect	+
	Tacrolimus	↓ levels of B	++
	Theophylline	↑ levels of B	+
	TMP/SMX	↓ levels of A	+
	Tocainide	↓ effect of B	+
Rimantadine	*See Amantadine*		
Ritonavir	*See protease inhibitors and Table 22B*		
Saquinavir	*See protease inhibitors and Table 22B*		
Stavudine	Ribavirin	↓ levels of A—**AVOID**	++
	Zidovudine	Mutual interference—do not combine	++
Strand Transfer Integrase Inhibitors (STIIs)	*See Integrase Strand Transfer Inhibitors*		
Sulfonamides	Beta blockers	↑ levels of B	++
	Cyclosporine	↓ cyclosporine levels	+
	Methotrexate	↑ antifolate activity	+
	Warfarin	↑ prothrombin time; bleeding	+
	Phenobarbital, rifampin	↓ levels of A	+
	Phenytoin	↑ levels of B; nystagmus, ataxia	+
	Sulfonylureas	↑ hypoglycemic effect	+
Telithromycin (Ketek)	Carbamazine	↓ levels of A	++
	Digoxin	↑ levels of B—do digoxin levels	++
	Ergot alkaloids	↑ levels of B—avoid	++
	Itraconazole; ketoconazole	↑ levels of A; no dose change	+
	Metoprolol	↑ levels of B	++
	Midazolam	↑ levels of B	++
	Warfarin	↑ prothrombin time	+
	Phenobarbital, phenytoin	↓ levels of B	++
	Pimozide	**↑ levels of B; QT prolongation—AVOID**	++
	Rifampin	↓ levels of A—avoid	++
	Simvastatin & other "statins"	↑ levels of B (↑ risk of myopathy)	++
	Sotalol	↓ levels of B	++
	Theophylline	↑ levels of B	++

TABLE 22A (8)

ANTI-INFECTIVE AGENT (A)	OTHER DRUG (B)	EFFECT	IMPORT
Tenofovir	Atazanavir	↓ levels of B—add ritonavir	++
	Didanosine (ddI)	↑ levels of B (reduce dose)	++
Terbinafine	Cimetidine	↑ levels of A	+
	Phenobarbital, rifampin	↓ levels of A	+
Tetracyclines	*See Doxycycline, plus:*		
	Atovaquone	↓ levels of B	+
	Digoxin	↑ toxicity of B (may persist several months—up to 10% pts)	++
	Methoxyflurane	↑ toxicity; polyuria, renal failure	+
	Sucralfate	↓ absorption of A (separate by ≥2 hrs)	+
Thiabendazole	Theophyllines	↑ serum theophylline, nausea	+
Tigecycline	Oral contraceptives	↓ levels of B	++
Tinidazole (Tindamax)	*See Metronidazole—similar entity, expect similar interactions*		
Tobramycin	*See Aminoglycosides*		
Trimethoprim	Amantadine, dapsone, digoxin, methotrexate, procainamide, zidovudine	↑ serum levels of B	++
	Potassium-sparing diuretics	↑ serum K⁺	++
	Repaglinide	↑ levels of B (hypoglycemia)	++
	Thiazide diuretics	↓ serum Na⁺	+
Trimethoprim-Sulfamethoxazole	Ace inhibitors	↑ serum K+	++
	Amantadine	↑ levels of B (toxicity)	++
	Azathioprine	Reports of leukopenia	+
	Cyclosporine	↓ levels of B, ↑ serum creatinine	+
	Loperamide	↑ levels of B	+
	Methotrexate	Enhanced marrow suppression	++
	Oral contraceptives, pimozide, and 6-mercaptopurine	↓ effect of B	+
	Phenytoin	↑ levels of B	+
	Rifampin	↑ levels of B	+
	Warfarin	↑ activity of B	+
Valganciclovir (Valcyte)	*See Ganciclovir*		
Vancomycin	Aminoglycosides	↑ frequency of nephrotoxicity	++
Zalcitabine (ddC) (HIVID)	Valproic acid, pentamidine (IV), alcohol, lamivudine	↑ pancreatitis risk	+
	Cisplatin, INH, metronidazole, vincristine, nitrofurantoin, d4T, dapsone	↑ risk of peripheral neuropathy	+
Zidovudine (ZDV) (Retrovir)	Atovaquone, fluconazole, methadone	↑ levels of A	+
	Clarithromycin	↓ levels of A	±
	Indomethacin	↑ levels of ZDV toxic metabolite	+
	Nelfinavir	↓ levels of A	++
	Probenecid, TMP/SMX	↑ levels of A	+
	Rifampin/rifabutin	↓ levels of A	++
	Stavudine	**Interference—DO NOT COMBINE!**	++
	Valproic Acid	↑ levels of A	++

TABLE 22B – DRUG-DRUG INTERACTIONS BETWEEN NON-NUCLEOSIDE REVERSE TRANSCRIPTASE INHIBITORS (NNRTIS) AND PROTEASE INHIBITORS
(Adapted from Guidelines for the Use of Antiretroviral Agents in HIV-Infected Adults & Adolescents; see www.aidsinfo.nih.gov)

NAME (Abbreviation, Trade Name)	Atazanavir (ATV, Reyataz)	DARUNAVIR (DRV, Prezista)	Fosamprenavir (FOS-APV, Lexiva)	Indinavir (IDV, Crixivan)	Lopinavir/Ritonavir (LP/R, Kaletra)	Nelfinavir (NFV, Viracept)	Saquinavir (SQV, Invirase)	Tipranavir (TPV)
Delavirdine (DLV, Rescriptor)	No data	No data	Co-administration not recommended	IDV levels ↑ 40%. Dose: IDV 600 mg q8h. DLV standard	Expect LP levels to ↑. No dose data	NFV levels ↑ 2X, DLV levels ↓ 50%. Dose: No data	SQV levels ↑ 5X. Dose: SQV 800 mg q8h. DLV standard	No data
Efavirenz (EFZ, Sustiva)	ATV AUC ↓ 74%. Dose: EFZ standard; ATA/RTV 300/100 mg q24h with food	Standard doses of both drugs	FOS-APV levels ↓. Dose: EFZ standard; FOS-APV 1400 mg + RTV 300 mg q24h or 700 mg FOS-APV + 100 mg RTV q12h	Levels: IDV ↓ 31%. Dose: IDV 1000 mg q8h. EFZ standard	Level of LP ↓ 40%. Dose: LP/R 533/133 mg q12h, EFZ standard	Standard doses	Level: SQV ↓ 62%. Dose: SQV 400 mg + RTV 400 mg q12h	No dose change necessary
Etravirine (ETR, Intelence)	↑ ATV & ↑ ETR levels.	Standard doses of both drugs	↑ levels of FOS-APV.	↓ level of IDV.	↑ levels of ETR, ↓ levels of LP/R.	↑ levels of NFV.	↓ ETR levels 33%; SQV/R no change. Standard doses of both drugs	↓ levels of ETR, ↑ levels of TPV & RTV. **Avoid combination.**
Nevirapine (NVP, Viramune)	Avoid combination. ATZ increases NVP concentrations > 25%; NVP decreases ATZ AUC by 42%	Standard doses of both drugs	Use with caution. NVP AUC increased 14% (700/100 Fos/rit); NVP AUC inc. 29% (Fos 1400 mg bid)	IDV levels ↓ 28%. Dose: IDV 1000 mg q8h or combine with RTV. NVP standard	LP levels ↓ 53%. Dose: LP/R 533/133 mg q12h; NVP standard	Standard doses	Dose: SQV + RTV 400/400 mg, both q12h	Standard doses

TABLE 23 – LIST OF GENERIC AND COMMON TRADE NAMES

GENERIC NAME: TRADE NAMES	GENERIC NAME: TRADE NAMES	GENERIC NAME: TRADE NAMES
Abacavir: Ziagen	Doxycycline: Vibramycin	Nitrofurantoin: Macrobid, Macrodantin
Abacavir + Lamivudine: Epzicom	Efavirenz: Sustiva	Nystatin: Mycostatin
Abacavir + Lamivudine + Dolutegravir: Triumeq	Efavirenz/Emtricitabine/Tenofovir: Atripla	Ofloxacin: Floxin
Abacavir + Lamivudine + Zidovudine: Trizivir	Elvitegravir: Vitekta	Olysio: Simeprevir
	Elvitegravir + Cobicistat + Emtricitabine + Tenofovir: Stribild	Oritavancin: Orbactiv
Acyclovir: Zovirax		Oseltamivir: Tamiflu
Adefovir: Hepsera	Emtricitabine: Emtriva	Oxacillin: Prostaphlin
Albendazole: Albenza	Emtricitabine + tenofovir: Truvada	Palivizumab: Synagis
Amantadine: Symmetrel	Emtricitabine + tenofovir + rilpivirine: Complera	Paromomycin: Humatin
Amikacin: Amikin		Pentamidine: NebuPent, Pentam 300
Amoxicillin: Amoxil, Polymox	Enfuvirtide (T-20): Fuzeon	Peramivir:Rapivab
Amoxicillin extended release: Moxatag	Entecavir: Baraclude	Piperacillin: Pipracil
Amox./clav.: Augmentin, Augmentin ES-600; Augmentin XR	Ertapenem: Invanz	Piperacillin/tazobactam: Zosyn, Tazocin
	Etravirine: Intelence	Piperazine: Antepar
Amphotericin B: Fungizone	Erythromycin(s): Ilotycin	Podophyllotoxin: Condylox
Ampho B-liposomal: AmBisome	*Ethyl succinate:* Pediamycin	Polymyxin B: Poly-Rx
Ampho B-lipid complex: Abelcet	*Glucoheptonate:* Erythrocin	Posaconazole: Noxafil
Ampicillin: Omnipen, Polycillin	*Estolate:* Ilosone	Praziquantel: Biltricide
Ampicillin/sulbactam: Unasyn	Erythro/sulfisoxazole: Pediazole	Primaquine: Primachine
Artemether-Lumefantrine: Coartem	Ethambutol: Myambutol	Proguanil: Paludrine
Atazanavir: Reyataz	Ethionamide: Trecator	Pyrantel pamoate: Antiminth
Atovaquone: Mepron	Famciclovir: Famvir	Pyrimethamine: Daraprim
Atovaquone + proguanil: Malarone	Fidaxomicin: Dificid	Pyrimethamine/sulfadoxine: Fansidar
Azithromycin: Zithromax	Fluconazole: Diflucan	Quinupristin/dalfopristin: Synercid
Azithromycin ER: Zmax	Flucytosine: Ancobon	Raltegravir: Isentress
Aztreonam: Azactam, Cayston	Fosamprenavir: Lexiva	Retapamulin: Altabax
Bedaquiline: Sirturo	Foscarnet: Foscavir	Ribavirin: Virazole, Rebetol
Boceprevir: Victrelis	Fosfomycin: Monurol	Rifabutin: Mycobutin
Caspofungin: Cancidas	Fusidic acid: Taksta	Rifampin: Rifadin, Rimactane
Cefaclor: Ceclor, Ceclor CD	Ganciclovir: Cytovene	Rifapentine: Priftin
Cefadroxil: Duricef	Gatifloxacin: Tequin	Rifaximin: Xifaxan
Cefazolin: Ancef, Kefzol	Gemifloxacin: Factive	Rilpivirine: Edurant
Cefdinir: Omnicef	Gentamicin: Garamycin	Rimantadine: Flumadine
Cefditoren pivoxil: Spectracef	Griseofulvin: Fulvicin	Ritonavir: Norvir
Cefepime: Maxipime	Halofantrine: Halfan	Saquinavir: Invirase
Cefixime^NUS: Suprax	Idoxuridine: Dendrid, Stoxil	Spectinomycin: Trobicin
Cefoperazone-sulbactam: Sulperazon^NUS	INH + RIF: Rifamate	Stavudine: Zerit
	INH + RIF + PZA: Rifater	Stibogluconate: Pentostam
Cefotaxime: Claforan	Interferon alfa: Intron A	Silver sulfadiazine: Silvadene
Cefotetan: Cefotan	Interferon, pegylated: PEG-Intron, Pegasys	Sulfamethoxazole: Gantanol
Cefoxitin: Mefoxin		Sulfasalazine: Azulfidine
Cefpodoxime proxetil: Vantin	Interferon + ribavirin: Rebetron	Sulfisoxazole: Gantrisin
Cefprozil: Cefzil	Imipenem + cilastatin: Primaxin, Tienam	Tedizolid: Sivextro
Ceftaroline: Teflaro	Imiquimod: Aldara	Telaprevir: Incivek
Ceftazidime: Fortaz, Tazicef, Tazidime	Indinavir: Crixivan	Telavancin: Vibativ
Ceftibuten: Cedax	Itraconazole: Sporanox	Telbivudine: Tyzeka
Ceftizoxime: Cefizox	Iodoquinol: Yodoxin	Telithromycin: Ketek
Ceftobiprole: Zeftera	Ivermectin: Stromectol, Sklice	Temocillin: Negaban, Temopen
Ceftolozane-tazobactam:Zerbaxa	Kanamycin: Kantrex	Tenofovir: Viread
Ceftriaxone: Rocephin	Ketoconazole: Nizoral	Terbinafine: Lamisil
Cefuroxime: Zinacef, Ceftin	Lamivudine: Epivir, Epivir-HBV	Thalidomide: Thalomid Thiabendazole: Mintezol
Cephalexin: Keflex	Lamivudine + abacavir: Epzicom	
Cephradine: Anspor, Velosef	Levofloxacin: Levaquin	Ticarcillin: Ticar
Chloroquine: Aralen	Linezolid: Zyvox	Tigecycline: Tygacil
Cidofovir: Vistide	Lomefloxacin: Maxaquin	Tinidazole: Tindamax
Ciprofloxacin: Cipro, Cipro XR	Lopinavir/ritonavir: Kaletra	Tipranavir: Aptivus
Clarithromycin: Biaxin, Biaxin XL	Loracarbef: Lorabid	Tobramycin: Nebcin
Clindamycin: Cleocin	Mafenide: Sulfamylon	Tretinoin: Retin A
Clofazimine: Lamprene	Maraviroc: Selzentry	Trifluridine: Viroptic
Clotrimazole: Lotrimin, Mycelex	Mebendazole: Vermox	Trimethoprim: Primsol
Cloxacillin: Tegopen	Mefloquine: Lariam	Trimethoprim/sulfamethoxazole: Bactrim, Septra
Colistimethate: Coly-Mycin M	Meropenem: Merrem	
Cycloserine: Seromycin	Mesalamine: Asacol, Pentasa	Valacyclovir: Valtrex
Daptomycin: Cubicin	Methenamine: Hiprex, Mandelamine	Valganciclovir: Valcyte
Dalbavancin: Dalvance	Metronidazole: Flagyl	Vancomycin: Vancocin
Darunavir: Prezista	Micafungin: Mycamine	Voriconazole: Vfend
Delavirdine: Rescriptor	Minocycline: Minocin	Zalcitabine: HIVID
Dicloxacillin: Dynapen	Moxifloxacin: Avelox	Zanamivir: Relenza
Didanosine: Videx	Mupirocin: Bactroban	Zidovudine (ZDV): Retrovir
Diethylcarbamazine: Hetrazan	Nafcillin: Unipen	Zidovudine + 3TC: Combivir
Diloxanide furoate: Furamide	Nelfinavir: Viracept	Zidovudine + 3TC + abacavir: Trizivir
Dolutegravir: Tivicay	Nevirapine: Viramune	
Doripenem: Doribax	Nitazoxanide: Alinia	

TABLE 23 (2)
LIST OF COMMON TRADE AND GENERIC NAMES

TRADE NAME: GENERIC NAME	TRADE NAME: GENERIC NAME	TRADE NAME: GENERIC NAME
Abelcet: Ampho B-lipid complex	Herplex: Idoxuridine	Rimactane: Rifampin
Albenza: Albendazole	Hiprex: Methenamine hippurate	Rocephin: Ceftriaxone
Aldara: Imiquimod	HIVID: Zalcitabine	Selzentry: Maraviroc
Alinia: Nitazoxanide	Humatin: Paromomycin	Septra: Trimethoprim/sulfa
Altabax: Retapamulin	Ilosone: Erythromycin estolate	Seromycin: Cycloserine
AmBisome: Ampho B-liposomal	Ilotycin: Erythromycin	Silvadene: Silver sulfadiazine
Amikin: Amikacin	Incivek: Telaprevir	Sirturo: Bedaquiline
Amoxil: Amoxicillin	Intelence: Etravirine	Sivextro: Tedizolid
Ancef: Cefazolin	Intron A: Interferon alfa	Sklice: Ivermectin lotion
Ancobon: Flucytosine	Invanz: Ertapenem	Spectracef: Cefditoren pivoxil
Anspor: Cephradine	Invirase: Saquinavir	Sporanox: Itraconazole
Antepar: Piperazine	Isentress: Raltegravir	Stoxil: Idoxuridine
Antiminth: Pyrantel pamoate	Kantrex: Kanamycin	Stribild: Elvitegravir + Cobicistat +
Aptivus: Tipranavir	Kaletra: Lopinavir/ritonavir	Emtricitabine + Tenofovir
Aralen: Chloroquine	Keflex: Cephalexin	Stromectol: Ivermectin
Asacol: Mesalamine	Ketek: Telithromycin	Sulfamylon: Mafenide
Atripla: Efavirenz/emtricitabine/tenofovir	Lamisil: Terbinafine	Sulperazon^{NUS}: Cefoperazone-sulbactam
Augmentin, Augmentin ES-600	Lamprene: Clofazimine	Suprax: Cefixime^{NUS}
Augmentin XR: Amox./clav.	Lariam: Mefloquine	Sustiva: Efavirenz
Avelox: Moxifloxacin	Levaquin: Levofloxacin	Symmetrel: Amantadine
Azactam: Aztreonam	Lexiva: Fosamprenavir	Synagis: Palivizumab
Azulfidine: Sulfasalazine	Lorabid: Loracarbef	Synercid: Quinupristin/dalfopristin
Bactroban: Mupirocin	Macrodantin, Macrobid: Nitrofurantoin	Taksta: Fusidic acid
Bactrim: Trimethoprim/	Malarone: Atovaquone + proguanil	Tamiflu: Oseltamivir
sulfamethoxazole	Mandelamine: Methenamine mandel	Tazicef: Ceftazidime
Baraclude: Entecavir	Maxaquin: Lomefloxacin	Teflaro: Ceftaroline
Biaxin, Biaxin XL: Clarithromycin	Maxipime: Cefepime	Tegopen: Cloxacillin
Biltricide: Praziquantel	Mefoxin: Cefoxitin	Tequin: Gatifloxacin
Cancidas: Caspofungin	Mepron: Atovaquone	Thalomid: Thalidomide
Cayston: Aztreonam (inhaled)	Merrem: Meropenem	Ticar: Ticarcillin
Ceclor, Ceclor CD: Cefaclor	Minocin: Minocycline	Tienam: Imipenem
Cedax: Ceftibuten	Mintezol: Thiabendazole	Timentin: Ticarcillin-clavulanic acid
Cefizox: Ceftizoxime	Monocid: Cefonicid	Tinactin: Tolnaftate
Cefotan: Cefotetan	Monurol: Fosfomycin	Tindamax: Tinidazole
Ceftin: Cefuroxime axetil	Moxatag: Amoxicillin extended release:	Tivicay: Dolutegravir
Cefzil: Cefprozil	Myambutol: Ethambutol	Trecator SC: Ethionamide
Cipro, Cipro XR: Ciprofloxacin	Mycamine: Micafungin	Triumeq: Abacavir + Lamivudine +
& extended release	Mycobutin: Rifabutin	Dolutegravir
Claforan: Cefotaxime	Mycostatin: Nystatin	Trizivir: Abacavir + ZDV + 3TC
Coartem: Artemether-Lumefantrine	Nafcil: Nafcillin	Trobicin: Spectinomycin
Coly-Mycin M: Colistimethate	Nebcin: Tobramycin	Truvada: Emtricitabine + tenofovir
Combivir: ZDV + 3TC	NebuPent: Pentamidine	Tygacil: Tigecycline
Complera: Emtricitabine + tenofovir +	Nizoral: Ketoconazole	Tyzeka: Telbivudine
rilpivirine	Norvir: Ritonavir	Unasyn: Ampicillin/sulbactam
Crixivan: Indinavir	Noxafil: Posaconazole	Unipen: Nafcillin
Cubicin: Daptomycin	Olysio: Simeprevir	Valcyte: Valganciclovir
Cytovene: Ganciclovir	Omnicef: Cefdinir	Valtrex: Valacyclovir
Dalvance: Dalbavancin	Omnipen: Ampicillin	Vancocin: Vancomycin
Daraprim: Pyrimethamine	Orbactiv: Oritavancin	Vantin: Cefpodoxime proxetil
Dificid: Fidaxomicin	Pediamycin: Erythro. ethyl succinate	Velosef: Cephradine
Diflucan: Fluconazole	Pediazole: Erythro. ethyl succinate +	Vermox: Mebendazole
Doribax: Doripenem	sulfisoxazole	Vfend: Voriconazole
Duricef: Cefadroxil	Pegasys, PEG-Intron: Interferon,	Vibativ: Telavancin
Dynapen: Dicloxacillin	pegylated	Vibramycin: Doxycycline
Edurant: Rilpivirine	Pentam 300: Pentamidine	Victrelis: Boceprevir
Emtriva: Emtricitabine	Pentasa: Mesalamine	Videx: Didanosine
Epivir, Epivir-HBV: Lamivudine	Pipracil: Piperacillin	Viracept: Nelfinavir
Epzicom: Lamivudine + abacavir	Polycillin: Ampicillin	Viramune: Nevirapine
Factive: Gemifloxacin	Polymox: Amoxicillin	Virazole: Ribavirin
Famvir: Famciclovir	Poly-Rx: Polymyxin B	Viread: Tenofovir
Fansidar: Pyrimethamine + sulfadoxine	Prezista: Darunavir	Vistide: Cidofovir
Flagyl: Metronidazole	Priftin: Rifapentine	Vitekta: Elvitegravir
Floxin: Ofloxacin	Primaxin: Imipenem + cilastatin	Xifaxan: Rifaximin
Flumadine: Rimantadine	Primsol: Trimethoprim	Yodoxin: Iodoquinol
Foscavir: Foscarnet	Prostaphlin: Oxacillin	Zerit: Stavudine
Fortaz: Ceftazidime	Rapivab: Peramivir	Zeftera: Ceftobiprole
Fulvicin: Griseofulvin	Rebetol: Ribavirin	Zerbaxa: Ceftolozane-tazobactam
Fungizone: Amphotericin B	Rebetron: Interferon + ribavirin	Ziagen: Abacavir
Furadantin: Nitrofurantoin	Relenza: Zanamivir	Zinacef: Cefuroxime
Fuzeon: Enfuvirtide (T-20)	Rescriptor: Delavirdine	Zithromax: Azithromycin
Gantanol: Sulfamethoxazole	Retin A: Tretinoin Retrovir: Zidovudine (ZDV)	Zmax: Azithromycin ER
Gantrisin: Sulfisoxazole	Reyataz: Atazanavir	Zovirax: Acyclovir
Garamycin: Gentamicin	Rifadin: Rifampin	Zosyn: Piperacillin/tazobactam
Halfan: Halofantrine	Rifamate: INH + RIF	Zyvox: Linezolid
Hepsera: Adefovir	Rifater: INH + RIF + PZA	

INDEX OF MAJOR ENTITIES

PAGES (page numbers bold if major focus)   PAGES (page numbers bold if major focus)

Bold numbers indicate major considerations. Antibiotic selection often depends on modifying circumstances and alternative agents.